OUTCOME PREDICTION IN CANCER

OUTCOME PREDICTION IN CANCER

Editors

AZZAM F.G. TAKTAK

and

ANTHONY C. FISHER

Department of Clinical Engineering
Royal Liverpool University Hospital
United Kingdom

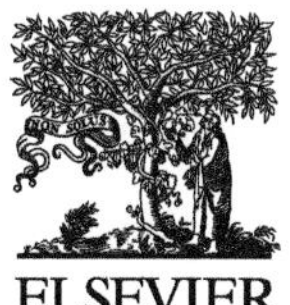

ELSEVIER

Amsterdam • Boston • Heidelberg • London • New York • Oxford
Paris • San Diego • San Francisco • Singapore • Sydney • Tokyo

ELSEVIER
Radarweg 29, PO Box 211, 1000 AE Amsterdam, The Netherlands
The Boulevard, Langford Lane, Kidlington, Oxford OX5 1GB, UK

First edition 2007

Copyright © 2007 Elsevier B.V. All rights reserved

No part of this publication may be reproduced, stored in a retrieval system
or transmitted in any form or by any means electronic, mechanical, photocopying,
recording or otherwise without the prior written permission of the publisher

Permissions may be sought directly from Elsevier's Science & Technology Rights
Department in Oxford, UK: phone (+44) (0) 1865 843830; fax (+44) (0) 1865 853333;
Email: permissions@elsevier.com. Alternatively you can submit your request online by
visiting the Elsevier web site at http://elsevier.com/locate/permissions, and selecting:
Obtaining permission to use Elsevier material

Notice
No responsibility is assumed by the publisher for any injury and/or damage to persons
or property as a matter of products liability, negligence or otherwise, or from any use
or operation of any methods, products, instructions or ideas contained in the material
herein. Because of rapid advances in the medical sciences, in particular, independent
verification of diagnoses and drug dosages should be made

ISBN-13: 978-0-444-52855-1
ISBN-10: 0-444-52855-5

For information on all Elsevier publications
visit our website at books.elsevier.com

Printed and bound by CPI Antony Rowe, Eastbourne

Working together to grow
libraries in developing countries

www.elsevier.com | www.bookaid.org | www.sabre.org

ELSEVIER BOOK AID International Sabre Foundation

To my wife
Diane

for all the help and support in preparing this book

A. Taktak

Foreword

We live in an era of contrasts, when rapidly developing science and technology from genetic research to availability of astounding computing power, still fall short of addressing societal expectations of individualized patient care. This is especially relevant in the clinical management of cancer, where prediction of the likely outcome from standard or alternative treatments is criticial.

This book reviews recent advances across a range of disciplines, including integrated decision support systems comprising molecular markers, from histopathology to clinical signs, which combine with sophisticated non-linear mathematical and statistical methods to accurately predict outcome from standard treatment. These developments make way for personalized inferences using as much as possible of the individual's bioprofile, in order to explore the covariate dependence of outcomes of interest—typically, diagnosis of malignancy, tumour grading, or time-to-event statistics for mortality and recurrence.

Current improvements in generic non-linear algorithms enable explicit modelling of complex decision boundaries and survival curves, without resorting to limiting assumptions regarding parameter linearity or hazard proportionality. Nevertheless, it is advisable to adopt a realistic approach to complex non-linear modelling, with a clear understanding of the biological significance of the candidate biomarkers for predictive inference, since the availability of vast numbers of genetic indicators, for example, runs the risk of identifying spurious correlations that would not stand up in the analysis of unseen data. Recommendations for robust non-linear processing, illustrated by real-world case studies, have been made in several chapters of this book. Several analyses of censored time-to-event data, so crucial to modelling cancer outcomes, are benchmarked against proven statistical methods. This demonstrates the robustness, flexibility and predictive accuracy achieved by powerful new analytical frameworks. Difficult issues essential for obtaining reliable predictions are addressed, including model selection and efficient regularization.

Practical decision support systems also require an infrastructure supporting standardized data acquisition from remote centres and for remote access. These issues are equally as critical as the use of advanced analysis methods, since reliance on data-based models depends on the completeness, integrity and consistency of the underlying data. An important message of the book is that the added value from data analysis now justifies an investment on standardized protocols for data acquisition and monitoring. This enables multicentre modelling and evaluation studies to take place on a large scale, beyond what is possible solely on the basis of existing historical patient records.

In conclusion, this book is an up-to-date review of the state-of-the-art in several key elements for practical outcome prediction, which is of special importance for the management of cancer. It makes the case for collaborative efforts between technical and scientific disciplines, such as cytogenetics, healthcare informatics and machine learning, and, beyond them, into the clinical arena.

Strictly standardized practices in data acquisition, laboratory measurements, clinical protocols and data recording will magnify the value already abstracted through the use of sophisticated numerical methods. They will bridge the gap between "dead data", representing clinical audit trails, and prospective data, from which solid insights are gained into the phenomenology of cancer. They also serve as practical clinical instruments for predictive inference evidence on the basis of previous patient histories. My hope is that this book will, in some way, inspire the beginning of this momentous transformation.

Paulo J.G. Lisboa, BSc, PhD, CEng, FIEE, FIMA
School of Computing and
Mathematical Sciences
Liverpool John Moores University
United Kingdom

Contents

Contributors

Corneliu T.C. Arsene, PhD, School of Computing and Mathematical Sciences, Liverpool John Moores University, Byrom Street, Liverpool L3 3AF, UK

Flavio Baronti, MSc, Dipartimento di Informatica, University of Pisa, Largo Bruno Pontecorvo, 3, 56127 Pisa, Italy

Pedro Barroso, BSc, UNINOVA, Campus da FCT/UNL, Monte de Caparica, 2829-516 Caparica, Portugal

Elia Biganzoli, PhD, Unità di Statistica Medica e Biometria, Istituto Nazionale per lo Studio e la Cura dei Tumori, Via Venezian 1, 20133 Milano, Italy

Patrizia Boracchi, PhD, Istituto di Statistica Medica e Biometria, Università degli Studi di Milano, Milano, Italy

Lutgarde M.C. Buydens, MSc, PhD, Laboratory for Analytical Chemistry, Radboud University Nijmegen, PO Box 9010, 6500 GL Nijmegen, The Netherlands

Adrian Cassidy, BSc, MSc, Roy Castle Lung Cancer Research Programme, The University of Liverpool Cancer Research Centre, The University of Liverpool, 200 London Road, Liverpool L3 9TA, UK

Bertil E. Damato, MD, PhD, FRCOphth., Ocular Oncology Service, Royal Liverpool University Hospital, Liverpool L7 8XP, UK

Andy Devos, MSc, PhD, SCD-SISTA, Department of Electrical Engineering, Katholieke Universiteit Leuven, Kasteelpark Arenberg 10, 3001 Heverlee (Leuven), Belgium

Tadeusz A. Dyba, Sc.D., Finnish Cancer Registry, Liisankatu 21 B, FIN-00170, Helsinki, Finland

Antonio Eleuteri, PhD, Dipartimento di Scienze Fisiche, Università degli Studi di Napoli "Federico II", Italy

John K. Field, MA, PhD, BDS, FRCPath, Roy Castle Lung Cancer Research Programme, The University of Liverpool Cancer Research Centre, The University of Liverpool, 200 London Road, Liverpool L3 9TA, UK

José Manuel Fonseca, PhD, UNINOVA, Campus da FCT/UNL, Monte de Caparica, 2829-516 Caparica, Portugal

Mithat Gönen, PhD, Department of Biostatistics and Epidemiology, Memorial Sloan-Kettering Cancer Center, New York, NY, USA

Marinette van der Graaf, MSc, PhD, Department of Radiology, Radboud University Nijmegen Medical Centre, PO Box 9101, 6500 HB Nijmegen, The Netherlands

Roger Green, PhD, Faculty of Medicine, Memorial University of Newfoundland, St. John's, Newfoundland, Canada

Timo R. Hakulinen, Sc.D., Finnish Cancer Registry, Liisankatu 21 B, FIN-00170, Helsinki, Finland

Arend Heerschap, MSc, PhD, Department of Radiology, Radboud University Nijmegen Medical Centre, PO Box 9101, 6500 HB Nijmegen, The Netherlands

Peter Jančovič, PhD, Electronic, Electrical & Computer Engineering, University of Birmingham, Birmingham, UK

Andrew S. Jones, MD, FRCS, Section of Head and Neck Surgery, Faculty of Medicine, University of Liverpool, Clinical Sciences Centre, University Hospital Aintree, Longmoor Lane, Liverpool L9 7AL, UK

Michael W. Kattan, PhD, Department of Quantitative Health Sciences, The Cleveland Clinic Foundation, 9500 Euclid Avenue / Wb-4, Cleveland, Ohio 44195, USA

Münevver Köküer, PhD, Biomedical Computing Research Group (BIOCORE), School of Mathematical and Information Sciences, Coventry University, Priory Street, Coventry CV1 5FB, UK

Xenofon Kotsiakis, MD, Department of Neurosurgery, General Hospital of Chania, Chania, Crete, Greece

Michail G. Kounelakis, M.A.Sc, PhD, Department of Electronic and Computer Engineering, Technical University of Crete, Kounoupidiana, Chania, Crete, Greece – PC 73100

Michele de Laurentiis, MD, Dipartimento di Endocrinologia ed Oncologia Molecolare e Clinica, Università degli Studi di Napoli "Federico II", Italy

Paulo J.G. Lisboa, BSc, PhD, CEng, FIEE, FIMA, School of Computing and Mathematical Sciences, Liverpool John Moores University, Byrom Street, Liverpool L3 3AF, UK

Alberto Mario Marchevsky, MD, Department of Pathology, Cedars-Sinai Medical Center, 8700 Beverly Blvd, Los Angeles CA 90048, USA

Alessio Micheli, PhD, Dipartimento di Informatica, University of Pisa, Largo Bruno Pontecorvo, 3, 56127 Pisa, Italy

Leopoldo Milano, PhD, Dipartimento di Scienze Fisiche, Università degli Studi di Napoli "Federico II" Napoli, Italy

André Damas Mora, MSc, UNINOVA, Campus da FCT/UNL, Monte de Caparica, 2829-516 Caparica, Portugal

Raouf N.G. Naguib, PhD, DIC, CEng, CSci, Biomedical Computing Research Group (BIOCORE), School of Mathematical and Information Sciences, Coventry University, Priory Street, Coventry CV1 5FB, UK

Alessandro Passaro, MSc, Dipartimento di Informatica, University of Pisa, Largo Bruno Pontecorvo, 3, 56127 Pisa, Italy

Peter T. Scardino, MD, Department of Urology, Memorial Sloan-Kettering Cancer Center, New York, NY, USA

Christian Setzkorn, MSc, PhD, Department of Clinical Engineering, Royal Liverpool University Hospital, 1st Floor, Duncan Building, Daulby Street, Liverpool L7 8XP, UK

Arjan W. Simonetti, MSc, PhD, SCD-SISTA, Department of Electrical Engineering, Katholieke Universiteit Leuven, Kasteelpark Arenberg 10, 3001 Heverlee (Leuven), Belgium

Antonina Starita, PhD, Dipartimento di Informatica, University of Pisa, Largo Bruno Pontecorvo, 3, 56127 Pisa, Italy

Roberto Tagliaferri, PhD, DMI, Università degli Studi di Salerno, Napoli, Italy

Azzam F.G. Taktak, BEng, PhD, CEng, CSci, Department of Clinical Engineering, Royal Liverpool University Hospital, 1st Floor, Duncan Building, Daulby Street, Liverpool L7 8XP, UK

Sabine van Huffel, MEng, PhD, SCD-SISTA, Department of Electrical Engineering, Katholieke Universiteit Leuven, Kasteelpark Arenberg 10, 3001 Heverlee (Leuven), Belgium

Julia A. Woolgar, PhD, FRCPath, FDS RCS Eng., Oral Pathology, Liverpool University Dental Hospital, Pembroke Place, Liverpool L3 5PS, UK

H. Banfield Younghusband, PhD, Faculty of Medicine, Memorial University of Newfoundland, St. John's, Newfoundland, Canada

Michalis Zervakis, PhD, Department of Electronic and Computer Engineering, Technical University of Crete, Kounoupidiana, Chania, Crete, Greece – PC 73100

Introduction

Outcome prediction in cancer has been the subject of interest to clinicians, healthcare workers and patients for many decades. Survival is the most important outcome to patients since it helps them plan their lives and provide care to their family members. However, there are other outcomes of equal importance such as loss of functionality, disfigurement and quality of life.

Traditional methods of outcome prediction in cancer include the Kaplan–Meier non-parametric model and the Cox regression semi-parametric model. There has also been considerable interest in the use of artificial neural networks (ANNs) in outcome prediction due to the number of theoretical advantages they offer. ANNs can provide much wider (but not infinite) flexibility in fitting models to data where patterns are not so obvious (Ripley, 1996). The main advantages of using ANNs in modelling are: first, they allow arbitrary non-linear relationships between independent and dependent variables, second, they allow all possible interactions between dependent variables and third, ANNs do not require explicit distributional assumption.

Many clinicians have realised the potential of ANNs as an aid tool in the analysis. The main concern over the "black box" issue has been addressed by a number of researchers who have provided a statistical framework for ANNs (Biganzoli et al., 1998; Ripley and Ripley, 2001; Lisboa et al., 2003; Bishop, 2004).

A useful measure for the success of new technologies in integrating into clinical practice is the number of clinical trials in the literature. Despite a large number of publications describing the use of ANNs in medicine, the number of clinical trials in this area remains small (Gant et al., 2001; Lisboa, 2002; Lisboa and Taktak, 2006). The reluctance of clinicians to readily embrace these powerful tools in everyday practice can be attributed to many factors. In the past, a number of researchers have experimented with these techniques taking advantage of their "black-box" nature. Whilst the benefit of such feature does have its appeal, it can also be the curse on these powerful tools. Lack of understanding of the underpinning mathematical science often leads to inappropriate use of the technique which ultimately leads to wrong conclusions. A common mistake, for example, is the use of far too few samples with a limited number of events in the test set (Bottaci et al., 1997; Das et al., 2003). In such cases, quoting the accuracy alone of the test set as a measure of performance is not very useful since this figure would be high even if the networks did not detect the event at all (Ripley and Ripley, 2001; Kaiserman et al., 2005).

The majority of clinical trial studies compared the performance of ANNs with other methods such as clinical indicators (Stephan et al., 2003) and statistical analysis (Remzi et al., 2003). In cervical cancer, there are many examples on the use of the widely known PAPNET system, one of very few ANN systems to gain FDA approval for clinical use. The system uses ANNs to extract abnormal cell appearance from vaginal smear slides and describe them in histological terms (Boon and Kok, 2001). The alternative more conventional way is to re-screen the slides under the microscope. Mango and Valente (1998) have shown that the PAPNET system has uncovered a higher proportion of false negatives than conventional microscopic re-screening as confirmed by cytologists. Sherman et al. (1997) looked at the results of PAPNET in 200 specific cases where initial screening was inconclusive and compared them with conventional microscopy, DNA analysis and biopsy. The study showed that for these cases, PAPNET would have reduced unnecessary biopsies but at the expense of increasing false positives. Parekattil et al. (2003) showed in a clinical trial on bladder cancer that their ANN model was more accurate in identifying patients who required cystoscopy thereby providing possible savings.

This book provides an insight into survival analysis from different perspectives. It is aimed at bringing together specialists from different disciplines who deal with the problem from an entirely different angle but share a common goal. The book is organised into the following five main sections:

The clinical problem

The first section of this book contains chapters highlighting the traditional methods for providing prognosis. Such methods involve the widely used TNM staging system based on the extent of tumour involvement at the primary site (T), lymph node involvement (N) and metastasis (M). The system provides a number which reflects the stage of the tumour which influences the prognosis and choice of treatment. A number of studies in the literature have looked into the true value of this system for different types of cancer. In Chapter 1, Woolgar provides an overall review of the prognostic value of traditional and contemporary pathological features in oral cancer and suggests practical tips to aid reporting pathologists in producing their assessment. In Chapter 2, Damato and Taktak highlight some of the limitations of traditional methods including inappropriate categorisation of baseline variables, competing outcome, bias resulting in under- or over-reporting of outcomes and speculative interpretation of outcome data. Competing risks becomes obvious when using age, for example, as one of the input variables in tumour-specific survival. As older patients withdraw from the study at a higher rate than younger ones, this introduces a bias in the model. In Chapter 3, Hakulinen and Dyba explain how to deal with the issue of competing risks.

Biological and genetic factors

In Chapter 4, Cassidy and Field outline various risk factors and the interactions between them in studying lung cancer. The chapter looks at developing an individual molecular genetic and epidemiological risk assessment model to identify high-risk individuals who may subsequently be recruited into an appropriate intervention programme. In the next chapter in this section, Jones proposes a model for cellular pathways illustrating the chaotic nature of cancerous cells and explains how a "top-down" system from gene to phenotype (such as biochemistry models), each employing rigid pathways is far too inferior against a system which allows for fluid interconnections such as a neural network. A pilot study in this chapter involving 1000 patients with laryngeal carcinoma is also described.

Mathematical background of prognostic models

In this section, the mathematical background of prognostic models and ANNs in particular are described in detail. In Chapter 6, Biganzoli and Boracchi explain the mathematical background of non-linear interactions of the explanatory variables in survival models. This aspect is of great importance in applying these models to genetic and proteomic data with very high throughput of data. In Chapter 7, Eleuteri et al. observe the fact that the use of conventional models may involve making too strict assumptions and they describe how feature selections can be carried out mathematically in ANN models. In Chapter 8, Arsene and Lisboa provide an in-depth analysis into the role of neural networks within the context of statistical methods and parametric techniques and apply the model developed in node-negative breast cancer patients.

Application of machine learning methods

A number of applications using various types of machine learning algorithms are included in this section. In Chapter 9, Marchevsky provides a useful overview on the practical aspects of applying ANN models and discusses some of the difficulties in validating the accuracies of these models. In Chapter 10, Baronti et al. describe the application of machine learning methods in head and neck squamous cell carcinoma and how the individual risk is modified by genetic factors, such as polymorphisms of enzymes involved in the metabolism of tobacco carcinogens and in the DNA repair mechanisms. Devos et al. discuss the use of magnetic resonance spectroscopic imaging (MRSI) and the combination with conventional magnetic resonance imaging (MRI) for the automated characterisation of brain tumours in Chapter 11. The importance of a medical decision support system for clinical purposes fusing data from several MR and non-MR techniques is also discussed. In Chapter 12, Kokuer et al. propose various statistical and artificial intelligence models in studying hereditary non-polyposis colorectal cancer with the view of screening those at higher risk more regularly. In the final chapter of this section, Kounelakis et al. review several genomic-based methods for brain cancer analysis with the emphasis on DNA microarrays technology.

Dissemination of information

A very important aspect which is often overlooked is disseminating the information and sharing the knowledge. This is crucial in order to achieve effective communication between clinicians, healthcare workers and patients. The make-or-break of the most sophisticated systems is sometimes dependent on the manner in which information is translated into clinical practice such as building user-friendly interface tools. The internet provides the ideal medium for ease of dissemination making information readily available to clinicians, literally at their fingertips. In Chapter 14, Fonseca et al. review the state-of-the-art intelligent medical information systems, the main problems associated with their development and the currently adopted solutions. The final two chapters provide examples of current systems. Setzkorn et al. describe the development of a web-based system for standardising and sharing information which is essential in multi-centre collaboration in Chapter 15, whilst Kattan et al. focus on simple and effective communication tool called the nomogram; in Chapter 16. A nomogram is a graphical depiction of a multivariable model which has been used for a long time, but (sadly) not as widely as one might expect given its advantages.

Azzam F.G. Taktak
Department of Clinical Engineering
Royal Liverpool University Hospital, UK

References

Biganzoli, E., P. Boracchi, L. Mariani and E. Marubini, 1998, Feed forward neural networks for the analysis of censored survival data: a partial logistic regression approach. Stat. Med., 17(10), 1169–1186.

Bishop, C.M., 2004, Error functions. In: Neural networks for pattern recognition. Oxford University Press, Oxford, pp. 230–236.

Boon, M.E. and L.P. Kok, 2001, Using artificial neural networks to screen cervical smears: how new technology enhances health care. In: G.V. Dybowski R. (Ed.), Clinical Applications of Artificial Neural Networks. Cambridge University Press, Cambridge pp. 81–89.

Bottaci, L., P.J. Drew, J.E. Hartley, M.B. Hadfield, R. Farouk, P.W. Lee, I.M. Macintyre, G.S. Duthie, and J.R. Monson, 1997, Artificial neural networks applied to outcome prediction for colorectal cancer patients in separate institutions. Lancet, 350(9076), 469–472.

Das, A., T. Ben Menachem, G.S. Cooper, A. Chak, M.V. Sivak, J.A. Gonet Jr. and R.C. Wong, 2003, Prediction of outcome in acute lower-gastrointestinal haemorrhage based on an artificial neural network: internal and external validation of a predictive model. Lancet, 362(9392), 1261–1266.

Gant, V., S. Rodway and J. Wyatt, 2001, Artificial neural networks: practical considerations for clinical applications. In: G.V. Dybowski R. (Ed.), Clinical Applications of Artificial Neural Networks. Cambridge University Press, Cambridge pp. 329–356.

Kaiserman, I., M. Rosner and J. Pe'er, 2005, Forecasting the prognosis of choroidal melanoma with an artificial neural network. Ophthalmology, 112(9), 1608.

Lisboa, P.J., 2002, A review of evidence of health benefit from artificial neural networks in medical intervention. Neural Netw., 15(1), 11–39.

Lisbosa, P.J., H. Wong, P. Harris and R. Swindell, 2003, A Bayesian neural network approach for modelling censored data with an application to prognosis after surgery for breast cancer. Artif. Intell. Med., 28(1), 1–25.

Lisboa, P.J. and A.F.G. Taktak, 2006, The use of artificial neural networks in decision support in cancer: A Systematic Review. Neural Netw., 19, 408–415.

Mango, L.J. and P.T. Valente, 1998, Neural-network-assisted analysis and microscopic rescreening in presumed negative cervical cytologic smears. A comparison. Acta Cytol., 42(1), 227–232.

Parekattil, S.J., H.A. Fisher and B.A. Kogan, 2003, Neural network using combined urine nuclear matrix protein-22, monocyte chemoattractant protein-1 and urinary intercellular adhesion molecule-1 to detect bladder cancer. J. Urol., 169(3), 917–920.

Remzi, M., T. Anagnostou, V. Ravery, A. Zlotta, C. Stephan, M. Marberger and B. Djavan 2003, An artificial neural network to predict the outcome of repeat prostate biopsies. Urology, 62(3), 456–460.

Ripley, B.D., 1996, Pattern Recognition and Neural Networks. Cambridge University Press, Cambridge.

Ripley, B.D. and R.M. Ripley, 2001, Neural networks as statistical methods in survival analysis. In: G.V. Dybowski R. (Ed.), Clinical Applications of Artificial Neural Networks. Cambridge University Press, Cambridge, pp. 237–255.

Sherman, M.E., M.H. Schiffman, L.J. Mango, D. Kelly, D. Acosta, Z. Cason, P. Elgert, S. Zaleski, D.R Scott, R.J Kurman, M. Stoler and A.T. Lorincz, 1997, Evaluation of PAPNET testing as an ancillary tool to clarify the status of the "atypical" cervical smear. Mod. Pathol., 10(6), 564–571.

Stephan, C., B. Vogel, H. Cammann, M. Lein, V. Klevecka, P. Sinha, G. Kristiansen, D. Schnorr, K. Jung and S.A. Loening, 2003, An artificial neural network as a tool in risk evaluation of prostate cancer. Indication for biopsy with the PSA range of 2–20 mg/l. Urologe A, 42(9), 1221–1229.

Section 1

The Clinical Problem

Chapter 1

The Predictive Value of Detailed Histological Staging of Surgical Resection Specimens in Oral Cancer

Julia A. Woolgar

Clinical Dental Sciences, University of Liverpool, Liverpool, UK
Email: jaw@liverpool.ac.uk

Abstract

It is well known that the outcome of squamous cell carcinoma of the oral cavity and oropharynx is related to the stage (i.e. extent) of the tumour, and detailed histopathological assessment of the surgical resection specimen provides information that is central to determining the post-operative treatment needs and prognosis for an individual patient. This chapter reviews in detail the prognostic value of traditional and contemporary pathological features of the primary tumour and the cervical lymph node metastases; and outlines general patient factors such as age, gender and co-morbidity, and considers their relative importance. Practical tips to aid the reporting pathologist in producing a standardized pathological staging assessment are included. The value of the current pathological TNM staging classification is considered and possible amendments and alternatives are explored. The chapter ends with "the way ahead"? – a brief review of molecular and biological markers in oral and oropharyngeal squamous cell carcinoma.

Contents

Outcome Prediction in Cancer
Edited by A.F.G. Taktak and A.C. Fisher
© 2007 Elsevier B.V. All rights reserved

1. INTRODUCTION

Oral cancer – squamous cell carcinoma arising from the surface epithelium lining the mouth and oropharynx (OSCC) – is an important and serious disease. It ranks among the ten most common cancers in the world, accounting for 3–5% of all malignancies (Silverman, 2001). In Europe, the incidence has risen sharply in recent years, particularly in females and younger age groups, apparently due to changing patterns of exposure to tobacco and alcohol, the main aetiological factors which act on a genetically susceptible individual (Bettendorf et al., 2004). Survival has remained at a disappointingly stable level despite significant development in multimodality treatment (Silverman, 2001; Bettendorf et al., 2004), and in the United Kingdom, the death: registration ratio is 0.6 (1400 deaths and 2500 new cases per year) (Hindle et al., 1996). In addition to the high mortality, the disease causes great morbidity, with patients having to cope with both the aesthetic and functional changes resulting from the disease and its treatment.

The extent of the disease at presentation has a major influence on outcome and survival. The disease begins within the surface epithelium and invades the surrounding tissues. In addition to the local spread, metastatic deposits develop in the regional (cervical) lymph nodes in the neck in at least 50% of cases. Blood-borne systemic metastases, mainly to the lungs, liver and bone, are common in the later stages of the disease but death usually occurs as a result of uncontrolled locoregional disease and malignant cachexia (Woolgar et al., 1999; Funk et al., 2002). Outcome is usually measured by actuarial (life tables) survival analysis but consideration of only disease-specific deaths probably underestimates the true impact of the disease due to the frequency of deaths due to cardiovascular and respiratory diseases in the post-operative period, and also deaths indirectly related to the disease, such as suicide (Woolgar et al., 1999).

OSCC can be treated by surgery, radiotherapy or chemotherapy, either alone or in combination, depending on the site and stage of the disease and general factors such as co-morbidity. Clinical staging of the extent of disease at both the primary site and in the neck is notoriously inaccurate, and the value of CT, MRI and SPECT imaging remains uncertain (Woolgar et al., 1995a; Woolgar, 1999a; Chong et al., 2004). The importance of pathological staging of resection specimens, both in selecting patients for adjuvant therapies and in predicting survival, has been increasingly recognized in recent years. Although the TNM staging classification (UICC, 2002) is widely used throughout the world, it is too crude to offer an accurate prediction in an individual patient, since it considers only the surface diameter of the primary tumour (T); the number, laterality and size of positive lymph nodes (N); and the presence or absence of systemic metastases (M). In recent years, interest has been focused on the histological features of the deep invasive tumour front, and molecular and genetic markers (Bryne et al., 1992, 1995; Martinez-Gimenco et al., 1995; Po Wing Yuen et al., 2002; Sawair et al., 2003).

The main objective of this chapter is to discuss the predictive value of detailed histological assessment of routine surgical specimens from patients with OSCC and to highlight practical considerations including the development of minimum datasets. In addition, it will provide a brief overview of molecular and biological markers, and look at current predictive models and consider future possibilities.

2. PREDICTIVE FEATURES RELATED TO THE PRIMARY TUMOUR

2.1. Surface greatest dimension (tumour diameter)

Surface greatest dimension – "tumour diameter" – is the feature used to indicate tumour size in both the clinical (cTNM) and pathological (pTNM) arms of TNM staging classification system (UICC, 2002). The prognosis of oral cancer worsens as the size at presentation increases and several independent reports in the 1980s showed that large size at presentation is predictive of poor survival (Platz et al., 1983; Crissman et al., 1984; Maddox, 1984).

The diameter (and T stage) of the primary tumour affects both the choice and outcome of treatment. The size of the primary tumour is an important factor in determining the surgeon's ability to obtain tumour-free margins (Scholl et al., 1986; Sutton et al., 2003), and a higher rate of local recurrence is associated with tumours of increasing diameter and T stage (Scholl et al., 1986; Woolgar et al., 1999; Sutton et al., 2003). In patients treated by radiotherapy, tumour size is an important determinant of the dose necessary to effect a cure (Bentzen et al., 1991).

Tumour size is an important predictor of cervical metastasis, and this is a major factor in the correlation between diameter and outcome (Maddox, 1984; Woolgar et al., 1999). Hibbert et al. (1983) attempted to study the prognostic effect of diameter alone, and their results showed that in patients without cervical metastasis, diameter was not significantly related to the 5-year survival. This finding may reflect the poor correlation between tumour diameter and tumour thickness seen in patients without metastasis (Woolgar and Scott, 1995), since tumour thickness rather than diameter appears to be the more important size criterion in relation to both metastasis and survival (see below).

Diameter has the advantage that its clinical assessment is relatively simple compared to the clinical assessment of tumour thickness, and this explains its pivotal role in the TNM staging system. In the routine pathological staging assessment, no account is made for tissue shrinkage during fixation and processing – around 15% of the fresh tissue volume (Batsakis, 1999) – and the maximum diameter of invasive (not merely intraepithelial) carcinoma is measured to the nearest millimetre using an optical micrometer to supplement the macroscopic inspection of the resection specimen (Woolgar and Scott, 1995; Helliwell and Woolgar, 1998, in press). In addition to tissue shrinkage, discrepancies between the clinical and pathological assessment of tumour diameter may occur due to the inability to distinguish between premalignant lesions and invasive carcinoma without microscopy, and the presence of a poorly cohesive invasive tumour front with extensive undermining of intact mucosa and satellite islands ahead of the main tumour mass, again features that are only detectable on microscopy.

2.2. Tumour thickness

Tumour thickness measurement as a prognostic indicator was first introduced by Breslow (1970) in relation to cutaneous malignant melanomas and the measurement proved to be more objective and reproducible than an assessment of the Clarke level of invasion (Clark et al., 1969) in which histological depth is expressed by reference to the anatomical deep structures reached by the advancing edge of the tumour. The technique was soon applied to squamous cell carcinomas of the skin (Friedman et al., 1985), lip and intra-oral mucosa (Frierson and Cooper, 1986; Mohit-Tabatabai et al., 1986; Shingaki et al., 1988), and the superiority of thickness over diameter was soon recognized. Several independent studies (Shingaki et al., 1988; Nathanson and Agren, 1989; Po Wing Yuen et al., 2002), have shown that tumour thickness is the only size criterion to have independent predictive value on multivariate analysis, particularly when the tumours are from a single intra-oral site or restricted to TNM T1 and T2 categories (diameter less than 40 mm), and it is now widely accepted that thickness is a more accurate predictor of sub-clinical nodal metastasis, local recurrence and survival than diameter (Po Wing Yuen et al., 2002). Nevertheless, the critical thickness differs widely in different reports and it is highly site dependent. For example, the critical thickness in relation to metastasis in floor-of-mouth tumours was only 1.5 mm in the study by Mohit-Tabatabai et al. (1986) compared to 6 mm for tumours of the buccal mucosa (Urist et al., 1987). In tumours of the oral tongue, the critical thickness is less for tumours of the ventral aspect than the lateral border, possibly due to differences in the depth, calibre and richness of the lymphatic vessels at the two sites (Woolgar and Scott, 1995). The reconstructed thickness – which compensates for both nodular and ulcerative growth by measuring to an imaginary reconstructed mucosal surface (Moore et al., 1986; Woolgar and Scott, 1995; Helliwell and Woolgar, 1998, in press) – is recommended as a more accurate and robust predictor than actual tumour thickness (Woolgar and Scott, 1995; Woolgar et al., 1999; Po Wing Yuen et al., 2002). In the study of Woolgar et al. (1999), the tumours were from diverse sites within the mouth and oropharynx, yet the mean thickness in patients dying of/with OSCC was twice that of survivors/patients dying free of OSCC.

Accurate pathological assessment of the thickness measurement (and other measurements such as diameter and excision margins) relies on thorough sampling of the surgical specimen by slicing the complete resection specimen into thin (3–4 mm) slices to ensure that any streaks and satellites, for example, due to vascular or neural invasion, are not overlooked. The micrometer measurement must include all tumour islands, including those well ahead of the main advancing tumour front. Immunohistochemical staining for pan-cytokeratins is useful for highlighting stray islands and individual tumour cells in difficult cases.

Systems for T-staging based on tumour thickness rather than diameter have been proposed (Martinez-Gimenco et al., 1995; Howaldt et al., 1999; Po Wing Yuen et al., 2002) but not yet adopted by the TNM system (UICC, 2002), partly because the critical site at the different oral sub-sites is still uncertain and also because of the desire to maintain uniformity of staging criteria and categories in both the clinical and pathological systems. Initial studies using intra-oral ultrasonography to measure tumour thickness appear promising (Helbig et al., 2001) and clinical staging based on tumour thickness may become routine in the future.

2.3. Other indicators of tumour size

Other histological indicators of the size of the primary tumour include pathological cross-sectional area, exophytic: endophytic ratio, shape and form (ulcerative, nodular papillary, etc.) (Po Wing Yuen et al., 2002), but these seem to offer no advantages over a simple measurement of tumour thickness.

Tumour thickness and diameter are used as surrogates for tumour volume which is a significant factor during radiotherapy of malignant tumours (Bentzen et al., 1991). The prognostic significance of tumour volume in terms of survival in oral cancer is unknown but recent advances in imaging techniques (Chong et al., 2004) should facilitate its evaluation in the future.

2.4. Histological grade of conventional OSCC

It has been customary to grade OSCC according to the method originally described by Broders (1920), which takes into account a subjective assessment of the degree of keratinization, cellular and nuclear pleomorphism, and mitotic activity. Three categories are described by the WHO (1997): grade 1 (well differentiated); grade 2 (moderately differentiated) and grade 3 (poorly differentiated), with optional grouping of well and moderately differentiated as low grade, and poorly differentiated and undifferentiated as high grade. In a tumour showing different grades, the higher grade determines the final categorization. Similar terminology is recommended by the UICC pTNM system (2002). Although several large studies in the 1970s (Shear et al., 1976; Langdon et al., 1977) reported a correlation between histological grade and survival, most authorities now recognize that Broders' grade alone shows poor correlation with outcome and response to treatment in an individual patient (WHO, 1997; Po Wing Yuen et al., 2002). The subjective nature of the assessment; small biopsies from tumours showing histological heterogeneity and inadequate sampling; poor tissue preservation; reliance on structural characteristics of the tumour cells rather than functional ones; and evaluation of tumour cells in isolation from the supporting stroma and host tissues have all been cited as possible explanations for the disappointing findings (WHO, 1997). In general terms, most OSCC are well or moderately well differentiated lesions and in recent years, there appears to have been little interest in evaluating the prognostic role of the WHO tumour grade and its association with other features such as tumour site and size, and nodal metastasis.

2.5. Multifactorial and invasive front histological malignancy grading

In an attempt to overcome some of the problems associated with the Broders' grading system, Jakobbson et al. (1973) introduced the multifactorial histological malignancy grading system in which multiple features of both the tumour cells and the interface between the tumour cells and the host tissues are assigned points according to strictly defined criteria. Several modifications followed (Anneroth and Hansen, 1984; Anneroth et al., 1987, Shinghaki et al., 1988; Martinez-Gimenco et al., 1995), the most successful being consideration of solely the most dysplastic areas at the deep advancing edge of the tumour (invasive front grading) (Bryne et al., 1992; Woolgar and Scott, 1995). Woolgar and Scott (1995) found a significant association between five of the six assessed features (degree of keratinization, number of mitoses, pattern of invasion, stage of invasion and density of the lymphoplasmacytic infiltrate – but not the degree of nuclear pleomorphism) and the presence of histological nodal metastasis. There was a significant positive correlation between the total score and both tumour diameter and tumour thickness, vascular invasion, and perineural invasion, and a logistic regression model based on total score and vascular invasion correctly classified 39 out of the 45 tongue tumours under study. Other workers have also found invasive front grading useful in predicting nodal metastasis, local recurrence and survival (Bryne et al., 1995; Martinez-Gimenco et al., 1995; Sawair et al., 2003). For example, in a study of 102 tumours from different intra-oral sites, Sawair et al. (2003) found that the total score was associated with overall survival on multivariate analysis and pattern of invasion was the most useful feature in predicting nodal metastasis. Pattern of invasion correlates with several in vitro markers of malignancy such as loss of contact inhibition, tumour cell mobility and secretion of proteolytic enzymes (Crissman, 1986), and its observation in routine histological preparations provides a simple measure of tumour behaviour.

Improved reproducibility was one of the aims of multifactorial histological malignancy grading and several workers have reported good levels of intra-observer agreement but inter-observer agreement is less satisfactory (Bryne et al., 1995; Sawair et al., 2003). Suggestions to improve reproducibility include simplification of the categories, clarification of definitions, and omission of less reproducible features such as nuclear pleomorphism (Sawair et al., 2003) particularly since the value of the latter feature seems doubtful (Woolgar and Scott, 1995; Woolgar, 1999b). In addition to tumour factors such as histological heterogeneity, differences in experiences of the assessors, varying interpretation of the category definitions, subconscious baseline shift and fatigue which can all affect the quality of the assessment (Sawair et al., 2003) are difficult to eliminate and hence limit the validity and predictive value of invasive front grading in the clinical setting.

2.6. Histological subtypes of OSCC

In addition to conventional OSCC, the WHO recognizes several histological subtypes (WHO, 1997). Correct recognition and documentation are necessary for full assessment of their prognostic significance. However, it is uncertain what proportion of the tumour should show the specific features to qualify for sub-categorization and several subtypes can co-exist in a single tumour.

2.6.1. Verrucous carcinoma

This variant is characterised by a predominantly exophytic growth of well-differentiated keratinizing epithelium and a locally destructive pushing margin at its interface with the underlying connective tissue. It is often preceded by verrucous hyperplasia or proliferative verrucous leukoplakia (WHO, 1997). The prognosis is generally excellent since nodal metastases do not occur. However, verrucous carcinoma may co-exist with conventional OSCC in 20% of cases, with a consequent reduced prognosis. Correct diagnosis requires thorough sampling, particularly since the histological differential diagnosis of verrucous carcinoma is wide and the initial biopsy specimen may be too superficial to include the deep advancing front.

2.6.2. Carcinoma cuniculatum

In the mouth, this lesion arises on mucoperiosteum as multiple deeply penetrating burrows and cysts lined by well-differentiated orthokeratotic epithelium (Kao et al., 1982), and it is characterised by extensive local spread (to bone and overlying skin) and absence of metastases. Occurrence in the mouth is not well documented in the British literature and some cases are probably misdiagnosed as conventional SCC or pseudocarcinomatous hyperplasia.

2.6.3. Papillary squamous cell carcinoma

This tumour is characterised by an exophytic growth of folded non-keratinizing fronds of dysplastic epithelium which may co-exist with (or precede to) conventional OSCC. The prognosis of this controversial lesion is uncertain (Batsakis and Suarez, 2000).

2.6.4. Adenoid (acantholytic) squamous cell carcinoma

This variant has pseudoglandular spaces produced by degeneration within islands of SCC, and, hence probably not a distinct clinicopathological entity (WHO, 1997). The prognostic importance of acantholysis is uncertain.

2.6.5. Adenosquamous carcinoma

In contrast to adenoid SCC, the adenosquamous carcinoma has features of both adenocarcinoma and SCC, and hence contains glandular structures and mucin-secreting cells (WHO, 1997). The prognosis is said to be poor due to early, multiple nodal metastases, but this may be due, at least in part, to confusion with the high-grade mucoepidermoid carcinoma and further evaluation is necessary.

2.6.6. Basaloid squamous cell carcinoma

Basaloid SCC has a mixed composition of basaloid and squamous cells, often arranged as lobules with peripheral pallisading and central focal squamous differentiation or cystic change (WHO, 1997). The co-existence of focal conventional SCC or dysplasia of the overlying mucosa is helpful in differentiation from ameloblastoma and adenoid cystic carcinoma. Prognosis appears poor due to extensive local spread, and regional and distant metastases.

2.6.7. Spindle cell carcinoma

In a true spindle cell carcinoma, the malignant spindle cells should be demonstrably of epithelial origin and therefore, distinguishable from an SCC with a fibroblastic stromal proliferation, a carcinosarcoma in which an SCC is accompanied by a sarcoma, other types of sarcomas and malignant melanoma (WHO, 1997). Polypoid spindle cell lesions appear less invasive and less likely to metastasize than conventional SCC, while flat and ulcerative forms behave as conventional SCC (WHO, 1997).

2.6.8. Giant cell (pleomorphic) carcinoma

As in the lung lesion, malignant multinucleate giant cells of osteoclast-like size lie amidst sheets of pleomorphic mononuclear or spindle cells (Ferlito et al., 1985). Too few cases have been reported in the mouth to allow comment on prognosis.

2.6.9. Undifferentiated carcinoma

Some tumours consist of a syncytial mass of undifferentiated epithelial cells with vesicular nuclei and prominent nucleoli but their prognosis is uncertain (WHO, 1997).

2.7. Vascular invasion

Assessment of the presence and extent of vascular invasion was part of the multifactorial grading system proposed by Jakobbson et al. (1973). Later systems (Anneroth and Hansen, 1984; Bryne et al., 1992) omitted this characteristic since they considered it was difficult to define and recognize with certainty. Nevertheless, an assessment of vascular invasion is still thought valuable since its detection in random tissue sections statistically implies a considerable number of tumour cells are entering the vascular compartment, thus increasing the likelihood of successful metastatic growth (Close et al., 1987; Helliwell and Woolgar, 1998, in press). Our own studies – in which vascular invasion was defined as the presence of aggregates of tumour cells within endothelial-lined channels or invasion of the media of a vessel with ulceration of the intima – have shown a significant association with tumour site, diameter and thickness; perineural invasion; invasive front multifactorial histological malignancy score and pattern of invasion; nodal metastasis; status of resection margins; local recurrence; and survival (Woolgar and Scott, 1995; Woolgar et al., 1999; Sutton et al., 2003).

2.8. Perineural invasion

Our studies (Woolgar and Scott, 1995; Woolgar et al., 1999; Sutton et al., 2003) show that infiltration of the perineural space of nerves at the advancing front of the tumour (taking care to exclude mere juxtaposition) is related to the site, the diameter and thickness of the tumour, pattern of invasion at the advancing tumour front, presence of nodal metastasis; close/involved resection margins and survival. Rahima et al. (2004) also showed a significant association with tumour differentiation; depth of invasion; nodal metastasis;

local and regional recurrence, distant metastasis, and survival; and the association with both regional recurrence and distant metastasis was maintained on multivariate analysis. Similar findings have been reported by Fagan et al. (1998). The failure to demonstrate the prognostic value of perineural invasion in earlier studies such as that of Carter et al. (1982) is likely due to their inclusion of salvage post-radiotherapy cases where extensive perineural invasion is almost ubiquitous.

2.9. Bone involvement

In the TNM staging classification (UICC, 2002), involvement of bone with penetration of the mandibular or maxillary cortical plate to involve cancellous bone qualifies for T4, stage IVA status, with its implied poor prognosis. Bone involvement influences the type and extent of treatment, but it is uncertain whether the stage IVA status is justified (Ash et al., 2000). Tumours of the gingiva and alveolar ridge are most likely to involve bone, but the risk of nodal metastases in these sites is low (Woolgar, 1997; Woolgar et al., 1999), leading to the anticipation that T4N0 tumours involving bone have a better prognosis than the other stage IVA categories. In our studies of mandibular resections from previously untreated patients (Brown et al., 2002a,b; Shaw et al., 2004), an infiltrative, but not an erosive, pattern of invasion (Slootweg and Muller, 1989) was predictive for local recurrence and survival even after taking into account the prevailing soft tissue prognosticators (Shaw et al., 2004). These findings may explain the previous uncertainties on the prognostic significance of bone involvement and Shaw et al. (2004) advocate a change in the pTNM staging classification so that the infiltrative pattern is a prerequisite for pT4 status.

2.10. Sialoadenotropism and ductal invasion

The influence of sialoadenotropism and ductal invasion on survival is uncertain but both features are associated with increased local recurrence and second primary tumours.

2.11. Skin involvement

Direct spread to the skin in conventional OSCC is indicative of a poor prognosis – Cole and McGuirt (1995) reported a median survival of seven months. Lymphatic spread to the skin was an even more ominous sign with a median survival of only three months.

2.12. Velocity of tumour growth

Evans et al. (1982) reported that velocity of growth (estimated by dividing the surface area of the tumour at presentation by the time elapsed since initial symptoms) had significant prognostic value, with slow growing tumours having a better prognosis. The method relies on the patient's memory and the prognostic significance of velocity of growth derived in this way has not been confirmed by other authorities.

2.13. Tumour site

The gradual decrease in the 5-year survival for more posteriorly located tumours has been recognized for many years (Farr et al., 1980), and the association between tumour site and survival is largely explained by tumour site's influence on nodal metastasis, and to a lesser extent, site's influence on stage at presentation; degree of differentiation; features of the advancing tumour front including the pattern of invasion and perineural invasion; vascular invasion; the surgeon's ability to achieve clear resection margins, and the occurrence of second primary tumours (Woolgar et al., 1995b, 1999; Sutton et al., 2003). Nodal metastases were diagnosed histologically in 59–64% of tumours of the tongue, retromolar area and oropharynx compared to 22% of buccal tumours and less than 7% of gingival/alveolar tumours in the study reported by Woolgar et al. (1999). Between 38 and 41% of patients with retromolar, oropharyngeal and lateral tongue tumours had died of/with OSCC compared to only 10–17% of patients with floor-of-mouth and buccal tumours.

2.14. Status of the resection margins

The resection margins include both the surface mucosa at the edge of the tumour and the submucosal and deeper connective tissues all around the defect, yet few authorities state which aspect is unsatisfactory. The distinction is important. Unsatisfactory mucosal margins are more amenable to surgical revision and recurrences due to re-growth of the OSCC at the superficial margin are usually evident on clinical inspection and can often be successfully treated (Woolgar et al., 1999; Sutton et al., 2003). In contrast, recurrences due to re-growth of tumour cells left behind at the deep margin may grow undetected under the skin-flap or reconstruction and thus, they tend to be large at diagnosis, and their size and position makes them less amenable to salvage surgery. Studies on the prognostic importance of the surgical resection margin have been further hampered by the lack of agreement on what constitutes a satisfactory margin (Batsakis, 1999). In routine assessment (Helliwell and Woolgar, 1998, in press), no account is made for tissue shrinkage which can result in a reduction of 30–47% in the margin width when the clinical pre-incision ("in situ") width is compared with the margin seen in the microscope slide (Johnson et al., 1997). The UK Royal College of Pathologists designates margins of 5 mm or more as clear, 1–5 mm as close and less than 1 mm as involved, and records the status of both the mucosal and deep margins (Helliwell and Woolgar, 1998, in press), and we follow these guidelines. Other authorities apply less stringent criteria and classify close margins as 2 mm (Sawair et al., 2003) or even 1 mm (Sheahan et al., 2003), and involved margins as only those with tumour cut-through (Sawair et al., 2003). Even 5 mm may not be "clear" when the tumour has a highly unfavourable pattern of invasion with widely spaced, tiny groups of poorly cohesive cells at the invasive front. Our own studies show that mucosal margins are rarely involved and an unsatisfactory mucosal margin is more often due to an unexpected synchronous primary tumour, or a multifocal superficial tumour, than failure to clear the index tumour (Woolgar et al., 1999; Sutton et al., 2003). Our studies found that the status of the resection margin is related to tumour diameter and thickness; tumour site; and features of the invasive front such as the pattern of invasion, perineural and vascular invasion; local and regional recurrence; and survival. The association with survival was maintained on multivariate analysis (Woolgar et al., 1995b, 1999, 2003; Woolgar, 1999b; Sutton et al., 2003; Shaw et al., 2004). At five years, only 11% of patients with an involved margin were disease free (that is, alive and well or dead, free of disease), compared with 47% of those with close margins and 78% with clear margins. The relative risk of death associated with even a close margin was similar to that associated with nodal metastasis (Sutton et al., 2003). Adjuvant post-operative radiotherapy does not appear to decrease the risk of local recurrence in patients with involved/close margins to a level similar to patients with clear margins (Loree and Strong, 1990; Sutton et al., 2003). Even a positive margin on evaluation of the initial intra-operative frozen section increases the risk of local recurrence, despite a negative result being achieved on frozen-section evaluation of the revised margin (Scholl et al., 1986).

2.15. Peripheral epithelial dysplasia, multifocal carcinoma and second primary tumours

Both peripheral epithelial dysplasia and an index (first) tumour of multifocal origin are associated with an increased risk of second (and serial) primary tumours (Woolgar, 1999b; Woolgar et al., 1999). Second (and serial) primary SCCs have been reported in 7–33% of oral cancer patients (Berg et al., 1970). The wide range probably reflects factors as diverse as the criteria for diagnosis and division from recurrent/persistent disease; the duration of the study; the extent of the follow-up clinical assessment; and the implementation and success of anti-smoking/drinking campaigns. Second primary tumours are usually diagnosed at a routine follow-up examination and hence tend to be small and amenable to treatment (Woolgar et al., 1999). Nevertheless, second, and in particular, serial, primary tumours together with systemic metastases account for most of the disease-specific deaths occurring after 24 months (Jones et al., 1995; Woolgar et al., 1999).

2.16. Local relapse

Local relapse – the re-appearance of SCC within the oral cavity/oropharynx – can be classified as a true recurrence developing from foci of tumour cells left in the operative site (persistent disease); or a new primary (metachronous) SCC developing from the mucosa adjacent to the operative site (often at the edge of the skin-flap used to reconstruct the surgical defect); or elsewhere within the mouth/oropharynx well away from the site of the first (index) tumour (Woolgar et al., 1999). True recurrences develop much earlier than metachronous tumours and carry the worst prognosis. In our study on 200 patients (Woolgar et al., 1999), 20 patients developed a true recurrence (median time to diagnosis, 8 months) and

18 had died of their disease (median survival, 14 months). In contrast, the median time to diagnosis of metachronous SCC was 18 months and only four of the 15 patients had died of disease.

2.17. Incisional surgical biopsy specimens

Although many of the features discussed in this section can only be adequately assessed in surgical resection specimens, a good incisional biopsy specimen – one that includes part of the invasive tumour front – can prompt useful comment or provisional information on the tumour type and subtype; the tumour grade; features of the invasive front including pattern of invasion and perineural invasion; vascular invasion; tumour thickness, and the presence of epithelial dysplasia at the periphery of the tumour and sialoadenotropism.

3. PREDICTIVE FEATURES RELATED TO THE REGIONAL LYMPH NODES

The prognostic importance of the presence and extent of lymph node metastasis has been recognized for many decades. Different studies have reported an association between outcome (in terms of regional recurrence and/or survival) and:

- metastatic status – nodal metastasis present versus absent (Maddox, 1984; Callery et al., 1984);
- laterality of positive nodes (Spiro et al., 1974; Grandi et al., 1985; Kowalski et al., 2000);
- number of positive nodes (Snow et al., 1982; Greenberg et al., 2003; Sawair et al., 2003);
- size of metastatic deposit (Spiro et al., 1974; Snow et al., 1982; Richard et al., 1987);
- anatomical level of involvement (Grandi et al., 1985; Carter et al., 1987; Kowalski et al., 2000);
- extracapsular spread (ECS) (extracapsular rupture) (Myers et al., 2001; Greenberg et al., 2003; Shingaki et al., 2003; Woolgar et al., 2003);
- embolization/permeation of perinodal lymphatics (Richard et al., 1987); and
- pathological N (pN) stage (Calhoun et al., 1994).

Some of the studies present conflicting data and there is no general agreement on which features are the best prognosticators. The lack of agreement may be due to factors influencing the stringency of the pathological assessment (including multiple pathologists with differing experience and expertise; lack of standard protocols; subjective interpretation of protocols and definitions; and sampling errors in harvesting lymph nodes and sectioning tissue blocks, etc.), and factors related to the cohort under study. The latter category includes factors such as the criteria for entry into the study (some studies have included irradiated cases, for example); differing proportions of therapeutic (clinically positive) and elective (clinically negative) neck dissections; and different protocols for post-operative radiotherapy.

In our studies, all the pathological assessments were made by a single pathologist (the author) following guidelines recommended by the UK Royal College of Pathologists (Helliwell and Woolgar, 1998, in press). The neck dissections are orientated and the anatomical levels are marked by the surgeon prior to immersion of the complete specimen in a formaldehyde-based solution for 24–48 h fixation. Lymph nodes are identified by inspection and palpation, dissected out and bisected or sliced. If the node appears negative, all slices are processed. "Size of metastasis" refers to the total profile diameter of the metastatic deposit not the size of the lymph node. When some positive nodes are matted, the "number of positive nodes" includes an estimate of the number of nodes contributing to the matted mass. Isolated tumour nodules in the region of the lymphatic drainage are regarded as a nodal metastasis and only nodules within 10 mm of the primary carcinoma, without any evidence of residual nodal tissues, are designated as a discontinuous extension of the primary tumour. The detection of minor degrees of ECS is aided by harvesting lymph nodes with their immediate pericapsular adipose tissue in position. The extent of ECS is recorded as involving

- the surrounding anatomical structures such as the internal jugular vein or sternocleidomastoid muscle;
- the perinodal adipose tissue; and
- the immediate pericapsular fibrous tissue.

Equivocal examples of ECS are upstaged. Around 50% of the neck dissections in our studies are elective procedures and previously irradiated cases are excluded. Post-operative radiotherapy is prescribed for cases with multiple positive nodes or ECS or close/involved margins around the primary tumour.

Only a few studies have used multiple regression analysis to assess the most predictive features of OSCC mortality. In our study of 173 positive neck dissections (Woolgar et al., 2003), ECS was the most important feature in the stepwise regression model of Cox. It was even more important than involved margins at the primary site. The Kaplan–Meier survival curves showed patients with macroscopic ECS tended to die within the first 15 months, while patients with microscopic ECS tended to die during the second year so that the survival probability was similar – 33 and 36%, respectively – by three years. In contrast, the three-year survival probability for patients with metastases confined to lymph nodes was 72% – approaching the 81% survival probability seen in patients without metastasis in our previous article on survival (Woolgar et al., 1999). Hence, our findings challenge the traditional view that the presence of lymph node metastasis reduces the survival by 50%. It has been suggested that the prognostic significance of ECS is obliterated by post-operative radiotherapy (Pinsolle et al., 1997). This is not our experience. Many of our cases with ECS relapse initially in the mouth rather than in the neck. ECS shows a significant correlation with unfavourable histological features at the primary tumour site such as a non-cohesive pattern of invasion, vascular and perineural invasion, and close/involved resection margins. Hence, we believe ECS is a simple, readily detectable indicator of tumour aggression. Furthermore, it is applicable even in cases with small volume metastatic disease since it occurs in a substantial number of patients with a single positive node (36%) or metastatic deposits of 10 mm or less (34%). The prognostic importance of ECS has also been emphasized by Myers et al. (2001). In their study, it was the best predictor of both regional recurrence and development of distant metastases and consequent decreased survival. Shingaki et al. (2003) also found a correlation between ECS and distant metastases. Greenberg et al. (2003) found there was no difference in survival of patients with ECS of less than, or more than, 2 mm. Despite the convincing evidence in these independent reports, the prognostic significance of ECS has been disputed by other recent studies (Pinsolle et al., 1997; Howaldt et al., 1999). However, Howaldt et al. (1999) postulated that their failure to demonstrate a significant association was probably due to the lack of standardization of the pathological observation and definition of ECS, and they considered the same explanation could be applied to the study reported by Pinsolle et al. (1997).

Sawair et al. (2003) found that the number of positive nodes was the most useful factor in predicting regional recurrence and survival. In our study (Woolgar et al., 2003), there were no significant differences in cases with two or more positive nodes. Only patients with a single positive node had a better prognosis. In our study, classification by maximum node size gave good separation of the survival curves when the categories were <10, 11–30 and ≥ 31 mm (Woolgar et al., 2003). Only 10% of patients had a nodal metastasis of ≥ 31 mm and only 3% had a metastasis of ≥ 60 mm. Nevertheless, the number of positive nodes and size of the metastatic deposit (with its seldom used pN3 category of more than 60 mm) remain pivotal in the TNM staging system (UICC, 2002), and ECS is not mentioned. In our study (Woolgar et al., 2003), ECS showed a significant correlation with the number of positive nodes, largest metastatic deposit, highest anatomical level and pN stage. All five features reflect the tumour volume but only ECS reflects tumour behaviour and it is unfortunate that this simple assessment is not part of pTNM staging.

The prognostic significance of micrometastases (profile diameter of ≤ 2 mm) and isolated tumour cells (profile diameter of ≤ 0.2 mm), features that are included in the pTNM classification (UICC, 2002), is yet to be determined. Also, the prognostic importance of other features of nodal metastasis such as necrosis and cystic change, and features of negative lymph nodes such as the different types of reaction, remain uncertain.

Relapse in the neck is a significant cause of death in OSCC (Woolgar et al., 1995b, 1999, 2003; Slootweg et al., 1996). It may result from growth of occult metastases when initial treatment has been confined to the primary site, or it may reflect metastasis to nodes outside the original field of treatment, or recurrence (persistence) in the operated or irradiated field. In addition, there may be relapse in the contralateral neck. In the study reported by Cunningham et al. (1986), 42% of patients with T1/T2 tumours of the oral tongue treated by local therapy alone later developed clinically overt disease. The reported frequency of recurrent disease in the operated neck ranges from 15 to 50% of cases (Farr et al., 1980; Byers et al., 1988). Factors influencing the rate of recurrence include the pathological extent of metastatic disease at the time of initial surgery; the type of surgical neck dissection procedure; and the use of adjuvant therapy (Kowalski et al., 2000; Myers et al., 2001; Greenberg et al., 2003; Shingaki et al., 2003). The cure rates for salvage procedures in patients with recurrent regional disease are poor (Slootweg et al., 1996; Myers et al., 2001). In our study (Woolgar et al., 1999), the median time to diagnosis of recurrence in the operated positive field was five months (range 1–11 months) and the median survival time was seven months (range 2–15 months). Furthermore, no patients survived recurrence in the operated positive field.

4. DISTANT (SYSTEMIC) METASTASES

Between 5 and 25% of OSCC patients have clinical evidence of distant metastases within 2 years of initial diagnosis (Calhoun et al., 1994). Traditionally, cases initially staged N2 or N3, and those with uncontrolled locoregional disease were thought to be most at risk (Calhoun et al., 1994), but more recent reports have shown ECS is the single best predictor (Myers et al., 2001; Shingaki et al., 2003). The mean survival following diagnosis of distant metastases is less than 6 months and 90% of cases are dead within 2 years (Calhoun et al., 1994).

5. GENERAL PATIENT FEATURES

The prognostic importance of general patient features is weak compared to the pathological extent and characteristics of the tumour but survival is reportedly associated with

- trismus, reduced tongue mobility or referred otalgia at presentation (Ho et al., 2004);
- geographical location (Carvalho et al., 2004);
- race (Funk et al., 2002);
- gender (Platz et al., 1983; Funk et al., 2002);
- age (Platz et al., 1983; Callery et al., 1984; Funk et al., 2002);
- co-morbid conditions secondary to tobacco and alcohol abuse (Platz et al., 1983; Funk et al., 2002);
- immune status (Reichert et al., 2001);
- absence of usual risk factors (Koch et al., 1999); and
- the development of second (and serial) primary tumours (Jones et al., 1995).

The evidence tends to be inconsistent and at times contradictory possibly due, at least in part, to the use of different statistical methods, and complex inter-relationships with the possibility of one feature acting as surrogate for one or more other features.

6. MOLECULAR AND BIOLOGICAL MARKERS

Evaluation of the predictive role of molecular and biological markers has been hampered by conflicting data from molecular and genetic studies; technical variability; and the expense (and consequent tendency for small patient numbers). Currently, there is no clear indication of the prognostic value of molecular markers, despite the escalating number of markers and reports, and they are still regarded as research, rather than routine, tools (Helliwell and Woolgar, 1998, in press; Bettendorf et al., 2004). Recently, attention has been started to focus on tumour–host interactions at the invasive front and the tumour's ability to circumvent the immune response (Schliephake, 2003).

6.1. Angiogenic factors

The correlation between tumour angiogenesis and tumour growth, metastasis, recurrence and prognosis is well established in several types of solid neoplasms (Craft and Harris, 1994) and there is mounting evidence that it is a useful prognosticator in OSCC (Williams et al., 1994; Schliephake, 2003). Histological assessment of tumour angiogenesis involves quantifying the vessel concentration following immunostaining of endothelial cell markers such as vascular endothelial growth factor/receptor (VEGF/VEGF-R), platelet-derived endothelial cell growth factor (PD-ECGF); endoglin, factor VIII-related antigen, ABH blood groups antigens, CD31, CD34, CD36, and the lectin, UEA-1. The results are not clear-cut since some markers are only expressed transiently and factors determining the overall balance of angiogenesis are poorly understood. The enzyme nitric oxide synthase type II (NOS2) (Brennan et al., 2001) and the lymphatic endothelial marker, PA2.26, (Munoz-Guerra et al., 2004) may also prove useful. Serum, urine and cerebrospinal fluid levels of vascular markers, and visualization of the microvasculature by colour Doppler, magnetic resonance imaging and positron emission spectroscopy are other possibilities.

6.2. Adhesion molecules

Adhesion molecules – such as integrins, cadherins, catenins, desmoplakin and plakoglobin – together with matrix degradation factors are involved in tumour invasion and metastasis (Lo Muzio et al., 1999). Loss of expression of desmoplakin/plakoglobin and CD44 reportedly correlate with distant metastases and poor survival in OSCC (Gonzales-Moles et al., 2003) but further studies are needed to define the precise role of adhesion molecules and their predictive value.

6.3. Matrix degradation factors

These include the matrix metalloproteinases (MMPs), cathepsines and hyaluronan but their value as prognosticators in oral cancer has not been adequately evaluated (Kosunen et al., 2004).

6.4. Cell cycle markers

These include the cyclins and the cyclin-dependent kinases (CDKs), proliferating cell nuclear antigen (PCNA), p120, Ki67, MIB1, nucleolar organiser regions (AgNORs), S-phase kinase-interacting protein 2 (Skp2), bcl2 and BAG1 (which also control apoptosis), and telomerase. Immunohistochemical studies have tended to concentrate on the predictive value of PCNA, Ki67/MIB and AgNORs but the results have been disappointingly inconsistent (Schliephake, 2003).

6.5. Growth factors and growth factor receptors

Oral cancer studies have tended to concentrate on epidermal growth factor (EGF) and its receptor (EGF-R, c-erbl-4, Her-2/neu), and hepatocyte growth factor (HGF) and its receptor (c-met protein) but their prognostic value remains uncertain (Xia et al., 1999; Ulanovski et al., 2004).

6.6. Immune response and apoptosis

Most markers of tumour suppression and anti-tumour defence show complex interactions and often trigger key events (or contribute to cascades) in the cell cycle or apoptosis. Early attention was focussed on retinoblastoma protein (pRb), a key factor in the G1 checkpoint of the cell cycle; and p53, which controls the cell cycle by either arresting cells in the G1 phase or by triggering apoptosis (Schoelch et al., 1999). More promising components of the immune response/apoptosis in terms of predicting survival could be:

- cyclin-dependent kinase inhibitors (CDKIs) of the p53-regulated p21 family and the p53-independent INK4 family (Schoelch et al., 1999);
- Bax which induces apoptosis (Schoelch et al., 1999; Folkman, 2003);
- Fas and its ligand FasL, mediators of apoptosis (Folkman, 2003);
- dendritic cells, which trigger the T-cell anti-tumour immune response (Reichert et al., 2001); and
- zeta chains, T-cell receptors (Reichert et al., 2001).

6.7. Oncogenes

The role of oncogenes – genes whose products are associated with neoplastic transformation – in the development of OSCC is well recognized (Bettendorf et al., 2004). Xia et al. (1999) reported that overexpression of the proto-oncogene epidermal growth factor receptor (*EGFR/c-erbB 1*) is associated with advanced T stage, unfavourable pattern of invasion, high incidence of nodal metastasis and shortened survival. Little is known about the predictive value of the *Ras* oncogene family, *c-Myc*, and *Cyclin D1* and their interactions with other oncogenes and tumour suppressor genes.

6.8. Tumour suppression genes

The importance of the major tumour suppression genes, *p53*, *retinoblastoma* (*Rb*) gene and *p16/p21/p27*, in cancer development is well documented but their prognostic significance in terms of survival is still largely uncertain (Gleich and Salamone, 2002). The *p16*, *p21* and *p27* suppressor genes that act as modulators of the cell cycle appear to be the most promising.

6.9. DNA content

The prognostic impact of DNA patterns in neoplastic OSCC cells measured by static and flow cytometry was reviewed by Stell (1991) using meta-analysis. He concluded that survival was better for patients with DNA diploid tumours than those with non-diploid tumours.

The degree of aneuploidy appears to correlate with the response to induction/adjuvant chemotherapy with a higher response in non-diploid groups (Tennvall et al., 1993).

6.10. Cytogenetic changes

There are numerous reports of specific genetic alterations, such as chromosome deletions, in OSCC and premalignant lesions, and recent evidence (Field et al., 1995; Yamamoto et al., 2003) suggests that allelic imbalance (loss of heterozygosity) at key chromosomal loci is predictive of reduced survival.

7. THE WAY AHEAD?

In summary, it is clear that the identification of accurate predictive models in oral and oropharyngeal cancer has been hampered by the relatively small number of cases of the disease, especially in any one treatment centre; the heterogeneity of clinical features such as the extent of the disease at presentation; and, in particular, by the lack of standard clinical, management and laboratory protocols combined with inconsistent recording and reporting of data. The dearth of translational research on biological and molecular markers, despite the huge volume of "academic" reports, exemplifies the tendency to focus on single markers, rather than their clinical effects and position in the multi-step processes of tumour development, growth and dissemination.

Even two of the well-established histological predictive factors – tumour thickness and extracapsular spread of nodal metastases – have not become part of the routine TNM pathological staging classification. The introduction of guidelines and minimum datasets into routine diagnostic pathology should minimize inconsistencies and produce reliable, standardized data with the potential for realistic multi-centre research, pooling of data, etc. An "evidence-based" minimum dataset – together with regular audit – prevents, or at least minimizes, issues associated with compliance; calibration, consistency, clarity and completeness of data; and time and cost efficiency. The dataset introduced by the UK Royal College of Pathologists (Helliwell and Woolgar, 1998, in press) is one such example (Fig. 1).

Other pathways leading to more efficient research and development could include:

- The wider use of standardized computerised databases with improved retrieval and exchange of information.
- Reduced reliance on subjective interpretation and wider use of automated techniques and quantitative data.
- The replacement of tumour diameter and thickness measurements by a total tumour load (volume) measurement.
- The use of biological markers to assess the velocity of tumour growth.
- The development of accurate predictive models, applicable to individual patients, and with the opportunity to incorporate multiple independent variables, and eventually, the development of models using neural networks and artificial intelligence.
- The development of survival data that takes account of deaths indirectly due to the disease in addition to disease-specific deaths.

HEAD AND NECK CARCINOMA MINIMUM DATASET

Surname:.................. Forenames:...................... Date of Birth:...............Sex:.....
Hospital:......................... Hospital No...................... NHS No.....................
Date of receipt................ Date of report................... Report No..................
Pathologist..................... Surgeon........................
Clinical TNM stage.............................. Previous radiotherapy Yes ® No ® Unknown ®
T...... N...... M...... Previous chemotherapy Yes ® No ® Unknown ®

Primary Tumour
Site...
Subsite(s)..............................
Right ® Left ® Midline ®
Type of Resection...................................
Histological type: squamous carcinoma ®
Other/subtype................

Differentiation well ® moderate ® poor ®
Invasive front cohesive ® non-cohesive ®

Maximum diameter ....(mm)
Maximum depth of invasion ....(mm)
Distance from invasive tumour to
mucosal margin ....(mm)
deep margin ....(mm)

	Yes	No
Vascular invasion	®	®
Nerve invasion	®	®
Bone/cartilage invasion	®	®
Severe dysplasia present	®	®
Severe dysplasia at margin	®	®

Right Neck Dissection Yes ® No ®
Comprehensive Selective ®
Node levels present 1 2 3 4 5 6 other
Total number of nodes.................
Number positive nodes..................
Levels with metastases 1 2 3 4 5 6 other
Largest metastasis ....(mm)
Extracapsular spread Yes ® No ®
Levels with ECS...........................

Left Neck Dissection Yes ® No ®
Comprehensive ® Selective ®
Node levels present 1 2 3 4 5 6 other
Total number of nodes..................
Number positive nodes..................
Levels with metastases 1 2 3 4 5 6 other
Largest metastasis ....(mm)
Extracapsular spread Yes ® No ®
Levels with ECS...........................

COMMENTS/ADDITIONAL INFORMATION

SUMMARY OF PATHOLOGICAL DATA

TUMOUR SITE.......................................
New primary ® Recurrence ® Not known ®
TUMOUR TYPE...................................

pTNM STAGE pT...... pN....... pM........
SNOMED CODES
T.................. M...................
T.................. M...................

RESECTION OF PRIMARY TUMOUR CLEAR ® CLOSE ® INVOLVED ®

Signed:

Reproduced from *"Minimum Datasets for Histopathology Reports on Head and Neck Carcinomas and Salivary Neoplasms"* with permission of The Royal College of Pathologists, London, UK.

Fig. 1. UK Royal College of Pathologists' dataset.

Models based on multiple independent variables that predict outcome in terms of lymph node metastasis already exist (Williams et al., 1994; Martinez-Gimenco et al., 1995; Woolgar and Scott, 1995), and seem to be more accurate than prediction based on single variables. For example, the system proposed by Martinez-Gimenco et al. (1995) which uses seven variables and a simple weighted scoring system, correctly classified 80% of cases into low-risk and high-risk groups. The system proposed by Williams et al. (1994) combined tumour thickness and immunohistochemical markers of angiogenesis and correctly predicted nodal metastasis and local recurrence in 90 and 98% of cases, respectively.

Prediction of outcome in terms of survival is less accurate, probably due to the greater influence of general patient and management factors. Studies by the DOSAK co-operative group (Platz et al., 1983, 1986; Howaldt et al., 1993, 1994, 1999) are impressive in terms of patient numbers and well-established tumour registry but the results have been disappointing probably due, at least in part, to over reliance on subjectively defined factors and, by their own admission, failure to achieve the required standardization among the pathologists at the 23 participating centres (Howaldt et al., 1999). The authors highlighted the lack of standardization with reference to the failure to define, or agree on, extranodal spread (ECS).

The recent shift in attention to the invasive tumour front and the prospect of studies combining traditional histological and molecular/genetic markers is welcome and provides hope that research in the present decade will shift from the "superficial exposition" of molecular and biological markers to real understanding of biological processes and the identification of key stages. Finally, it is essential that a universally accepted staging classification, such as the TNM system, can make opportune changes in response to new evidence.

REFERENCES

Anneroth, G. and L.S. Hansen, 1984, A methodologic study of histologic classification and grading of malignancy in oral squamous cell carcinoma. Scand. J. Dent. Res., 92, 448–468.

Anneroth, G., J. Batsakis and M. Luna, 1987, Review of the literature and a recommended system of malignancy grading in oral squamous cell carcinomas. Scand. J. Dent. Res., 95, 229–249.

Ash, C.S., R.W. Nason, A.A. Abdoh and M.A. Cohen, 2000, Prognostic implications of mandibular invasion in oral cancer. Head Neck, 22, 794–798.

Batsakis, J.G., 1999, Surgical excision margins: a pathologist's perspective. Adv. Anat. Pathol., 6, 140–148.

Batsakis, J.G. and P. Suarez, 2000, Papillary squamous cell carcinoma: will the real one please stand up? Adv. Anat. Pathol., 7, 2–8.

Bentzen, S.M., L.V. Johansen and J. Overgaard, 1991, Clinical radiobiology of squamous carcinoma of the oropharynx. Int. J. Radiat. Oncol. Biol. Phys., 20, 1197–1206.

Berg, J.W., D. Schottenfeld and F. Ritier, 1970, Incidence of multiple primary cancer, 3: Cancers of the respiratory and upper digestive system as multiple primary cancers. J. Natl. Cancer Inst., 44, 263–274.

Bettendorf, O., J. Piffko and A. Bankfalvi, 2004, Prognostic and predictive factors in oral squamous cell cancer: important tools for planning individual therapy? Oral Oncol., 40, 110–119.

Brennan, P.A., M. Palacios-Callender, G.A. Zaki, A.V. Spedding and J.D. Langdon, 2001, Type II nitric oxide synthase (NOS2) expression correlates with lymph node status in oral squamous cell carcinoma. J. Oral Pathol. Med., 30, 129–134.

Breslow, A., 1970, Thickness, cross-sectional areas and depth of invasion in the prognosis of cutaneous melanoma. Ann. Surg., 172, 902–908.

Broders, A.C., 1920, Squamous cell epithelioma of the lip; a study of five hundred and thirty seven cases. JAMA, 74, 656–664.

Brown, J.S., N. Kalavrezos, J. D'Souca, P. Magennis and J.A.Woolgar, 2002a, Factors that influence the method of mandibular resection in the management of oral squamous cell carcinoma. Br. J. Oral Maxillofac. Surg., 40, 275–284.

Brown, J.S., D. Lowe, N. Kalavrezos, J. D'Souca, P. Maggenis and J. Woolgar, 2002b, Patterns of invasion and routes of tumor entry into the mandible by oral squamous cell carcinoma. Head Neck, 24, 370–383.

Bryne, M., H. Koppang, R. Lilleng and A. Kjaerheim, 1992. Malignancy grading of the deep invasive margins of oral squamous cell carcinomas has high prognostic value. J. Pathol., 166, 375–381.

Bryne, M., N. Jenssen and M. Boysen, 1995, Histologic grading in the deep invasive front of T1 and T2 glottic squamous cell carcinomas has high prognostic value. Virch. Archiv., 427, 277–281.

Byers, R.M., P.F. Wolf and A.J. Ballantyne, 1988, Rationale for elective modified neck dissection. Head Neck Surg., 10, 160–167.

Calhoun, K.H., P. Fulmer and R. Weiss, 1994, Distant metastases from head and neck squamous cell carcinomas. Laryngoscope, 104, 1199–1205.

Callery, C.D., R.H. Spiro and E.W. Strong, 1984, Changing trends in the management of squamous carcinoma of the tongue. Am. J. Surg., 148, 449–454.

Carter, R.L., M.R. Pittam, N.S.B. Tanner, 1982, Pain and dysphagia in patients with squamous carcinomas of the head and neck: The role of perineural spread. J. R. Soc. Med., 75, 598–606.

Carter, R.L., J.M. Bliss, K.C. Soo and C.J. O'Brien, 1987, Radical neck dissections for squamous carcinomas: pathological findings and their clinical implications with particular reference to transcapsular spread. Int. J. Radiat. Oncol. Biolo. Phys., 13, 828–832.

Carvalho, A.L., B. Singh, R.H. Spiro, L.P. Kowalski and J.P. Shah, 2004, Cancer of the oral cavity: a comparison between institutions in a developing and a developed nation. Head Neck, 26, 31–38.

Chong, V.F., J.Y. Zhou, J.B. Khoo, J. Huang and T.K. Lim, 2004, Tongue carcinoma: tumor volume measurement. Int. J. Radiat. Oncol. Biol. Phys., 59, 59–66.

Clark, W.H., L. From, E. Bernardino and M. Mihm, 1969, Histogenesis and biologic behaviour of primary human malignant melanoma of the skin. Cancer Res., 29, 705– 727.

Close, L.G., D.K. Burns and J. Reisch, 1987, Microvascular invasion in cancer of the oral cavity and oropharynx. Arch. Otolaryngol. Head Neck Surg., 113, 1191–1195.

Cole, R.D. and W.F. McGuirt, 1995, Prognostic significance of skin involvement for mucosal tumors of the head and neck. Arch. Otolaryngol. Head Neck Surg., 121, 1246–1248.

Craft, P.S. and A.L. Harris, 1994, Clinical prognostic significance of tumour angiogenesis. Annals Oncol., 5, 301–311.

Crissman, J.D., W.Y. Liu, J.L. Gluckman and G. Cummings, 1984, Prognostic value of histopathologic parameters in squamous cell carcinoma of the oropharynx. Cancer, 54, 2995–3001.

Crissman, J.D., 1986, Tumor-host interactions as prognostic factors in the histologic assessment of carcinomas. Pathol. Annu., 21, 29–52.

Cunningham, M.J., J.T. Johnson, E.N. Myers, V.L. Schramm and P.B. Thearle, 1986, Cervical lymph node metastasis after local excision of early squamous cell carcinoma of the oral cavity. Am. J. Surg., 152, 361–365.

Evans, S.J.W., J.D. Langdon, A.D. Rapidis and N.W. Johnson, 1982, Prognostic significance of STNMP and velocity of tumour growth in oral cancer. Cancer, 49, 773–776.

Fagan, J.J., B. Collins, L. Barnes, F. D'Amico, E.N. Myers and J.T. Johnson, 1998, Perineural invasion in squamous cell carcinoma of the head and neck. Arch. Otolaryngol. Head Neck Surg., 124, 637–640.

Farr, H.W., P.M. Goldfarb and C.M. Farr, 1980, Epidermoid carcinoma of the mouth and pharynx at the Sloan Kettering Cancer Center. Am. J. Surg., 140, 563–567.

Ferlito, A., J. Friedmann and G. Recher, 1985, Primary giant cell carcinoma of the larynx. A clinicopathological study of four cases. J. Otorhinolaryngol., 47, 105–112.

Field, J.K., H. Kiaris, J.M. Risk, C. Tsiriyotis, R. Adamson, V. Zoumpourlis, H. Rowley, K. Taylor, J. Whittaker, P. Howard, J.C. Beirne, J.R. Gosney, J. Woolgar, E.D. Vaughan, D.A. Spandidos and A.S. Jones, 1995, Allelotype of squamous cell carcinoma of the head and neck: fractional allele loss correlates with survival. Br. J. Cancer, 72, 1180–1188.

Folkman, J., 2003, Angiogenesis and apoptosis. Semin. Cancer Biol., 13(2), 159–167.

Friedman, H.I., P.H. Cooper and H.J. Wanebo, 1985, Prognostic and therapeutic use of microstaging of cutaneous squamous cell carcinoma of the trunk and extremities. Cancer, 56, 1099–1105.

Frierson, H.F. and P.H. Cooper, 1986, Prognostic factors in squamous cell carcinoma of the lower lip. Hum. Pathol., 17, 346–354.
Funk, G.F., L.H. Karnell and R.A. Robinson, 2002, Presentation, treatment, and outcome of oral cavity cancer: a National Cancer Database report. Head Neck, 24, 165–180.
Gleich, L.L. and F.N. Salamone, 2002, Molecular genetics of head and neck cancer. Cancer Control, 9, 369–378.
Gonzales-Moles, M.A., M. Bravo, I. Ruiz-Avila, F. Esteban, A. Rodriguez-Archilla, S. Gonzalez-Moles and B. Arias, 2003, Adhesion molecule CD44 as a prognostic factor in tongue cancer. Anticancer Res., 23, 5197–5202.
Grandi, C., M. Alloisio, D. Moglia, S. Podrecca, L. Sala, P. Salvatori and R. Molinari, 1985, Prognostic significance of lymphatic spread in head and neck carcinomas: therapeutic implications. Head Neck Surg., 8, 67–73.
Greenberg, J.S., R. Fowler, J. Gomez, V. Mo, D. Roberts, A.K. El Naggar and J.N. Myers, 2003, Extent of extracapsular spread. A critical prognosticator in oral tongue cancer. Cancer, 97, 1464–1470.
Helbig, M., C. Flechtenmacher, J. Hansmann, A. Dietz and A.J. Tasman, 2001, Intraoperative B-mode endosonography of tongue carcinoma. Head Neck, 23, 233–237.
Helliwell, T. and J.A. Woolgar, 1998, Standards and Minimum Datasets for Reporting Common Cancers. Minimum Dataset for Head and Neck Carcinoma Histopathology Reports, The Royal College of Pathologists, London.
Helliwell, T. and J.A. Woolgar, 2006, Minimum Dataset for Histopathology Reports on Head and Neck Carcinomas and Salivary Neoplasms, The Royal College of Pathologists, London.
Hibbert, J., N.J. Marks, P.J. Winter and O.H. Shaheen, 1983, Prognostic factors in oral squamous cell carcinoma and their relation to clinical staging. Clin. Otolaryngol., 8, 197–203.
Hindle, I., M.C. Downer and P.M. Speight, 1996, The epidemiology of oral cancer. Br. J. Oral Maxillofac. Surg., 34, 471–476.
Ho, T., M. Zahurak and W.M. Koch, 2004, Prognostic significance of presentation-to-diagnosis interval in patients with oropharyngeal carcinoma. Arch. Otolaryngol. Head Neck Surg., 130, 45–51.
Howaldt, H.P., M. Frenz and H. Pitz, 1993, Proposal for a modified T classification. J. Craniomaxillofac. Surg., 21, 96–101.
Howaldt, H.P., M. Frenz and H. Pitz, 1994, Results of the DOSAK observational studies. Recent results. Cancer Res., 134, 173–182.
Howaldt, H.P., M. Kainz, B. Euler and H. Vorast, 1999, Proposal for modification of the TNM staging classification of cancer of the oral cavity. J. Craniomaxillofac. Surg., 27, 275–288.
Jakobbson, P.A., C.M. Eneroth, D. Killander, G. Moberger and B. Martensson, 1973, Histologic classification and grading of malignancy in carcinoma of the larynx. Acta Radiol., 12, 1–8.
Johnson, R.E., J.D. Sigman and G.F. Funk, 1997, Quantification of surgical margin shrinkage in the oral cavity. Head Neck, 19, 281–286.
Jones, A.S., P. Morar and D.E. Phillips, 1995, Second primary tumours in patients with head and neck squamous cell carcinoma. Cancer, 75, 1343–1352.
Kao, G.F., J.H. Graham and E.B. Helwig, 1982, Carcinoma cuniculatum (verrucous carcinoma of the skin): a clinicopathologic study of 46 cases with ultrastructural observations. Cancer, 49, 2395–2403.
Koch, W.M., M. Largo and D. Sewell, 1999, Head and neck cancer in non-smokers: a distinct clinical and molecular entity. Laryngoscope, 109, 1544–1551.
Kosunen, A., K. Ropponen, J. Kellokoski, M. Pukkila, J. Virtaniemi and H. Valtonen, 2004, Reduced expression of hyaluronan is a strong indicator of poor survival in oral squamous cell carcinoma. Oral Oncol., 40, 257–263.
Kowalski, L.P., R. Bagietto, J.R. Lara, R.L. Santos, J.F. Silva and M. Magrin, 2000, Prognostic significance of the distribution of neck node metastasis from oral carcinoma. Head Neck, 22, 207–214.
Langdon, J.D., P.W. Harvey, A.D. Rapidis, M.F. Patel and N.W. Johnson, 1977, Oral cancer: the behaviour and response to treatment of 194 cases. J. Maxillofac. Surg., 5, 221–237.
Loree, T.R. and E.W. Strong, 1990, Significance of positive margins in oral cavity squamous carcinoma. Am. J. Surg., 160, 410–414.
Lo Muzio, L., S. Staibano, G. Pannone, M. Grieco, M.D. Mignogna, A. Cerrato, N.F. Testa and G. De Rosa, 1999, Beta- and gamma-catenin expression in oral squamous cell carcinomas. Anticancer Res., 19, 3817–3826.
Maddox, W.A., 1984, Vicissitudes of head and neck cancer. Am. J. Surg., 148, 428–432.
Martinez-Gimenco, C., E.M. Rodriguez, C.N. Vila and C.L. Varela, 1995, Squamous cell carcinoma of the oral cavity: a clinicopathologic scoring system for evaluating risk of cervical lymph node metastasis. Laryngoscope, 105, 728–33.

Mohit-Tabatabai, M.A., H.J. Sobel, B.F. Rush and A. Mashberg, 1986, Relation of thickness of floor of mouth stage I and II cancers to regional metastasis. Am. J. Surg., 152, 351–353.

Moore, C., J.G. Kuhns and R.A. Grennberg, 1986, Thickness as prognostic aid in upper aerodigestive tract cancer. Arch. Surg., 121, 1410–1414.

Munoz-Guerra, M.F., E.G. Marazuela, E. Martin-Villar, M. Quintanilla and C. Gamallo, 2004, Prognostic significance of intratumoral lymphangiogenesis in squamous cell carcinoma of the oral cavity. Cancer, 100, 553–560.

Myers, J.N., J.S. Greenberg, V. Mo and D. Roberts, 2001, Extracapsular spread. A significant predictor of treatment failure in patients with squamous carcinoma of the tongue. Cancer, 92, 3030–3036.

Nathanson, A. and K. Agren, 1989, Evaluation of some prognostic factors in small squamous cell carcinoma of the mobile tongue: a multicenter study in Sweden. Head Neck, 11, 387–392.

Pinsolle, J., V. Pinsolle, C. Majoufre, S. Duroux and H. Demeaux, 1997, Prognostic value of histologic findings in neck dissections for squamous cell carcinoma. Arch. Otolargol. Head Neck Surg., 123, 145–148.

Platz, H., R. Fries, M. Hudec, A.M. Tjoa and R.R. Wagner, 1983, The prognostic relevance of various factors at the time of first admission of the patient. J. Maxillofac. Surg., 11, 3–12.

Platz, H., R. Fries and M. Hudec, 1986, Prognosis of Oral Cavity Carcinomas. Results of a Multicentric Retrospective Observational Study. Hanser, Munich.

Po Wing Yuen, A., K.Y. Lam, L.K. Lam, C.M., A. Wong, T.L. Chow, W.F. Yuen and W.I. Wei, 2002, Prognostic factors of clinically stage I and II oral tongue carcinoma – a comparative study of stage, thickness, shape, growth pattern, invasive front malignancy grading, Martinez-Gimenco score, and pathologic features. Head Neck, 24, 513–520.

Rahima, B., S. Shingaki, M. Nagata and C. Saito, 2004, Prognostic significance of perineural invasion in oral and oropharyngeal carcinoma. Oral Surg. Oral Med. Oral Pathol. Oral Radiol. Endod., 97, 423–431.

Reichert, T.E., C. Scheuer, R. Day, W. Wagner and T.L. Whiteside, 2001, The number of intratumoral dendritic cells and zeta-chain expression in T-cells as prognostic and survival biomarkers in patients with oral carcinoma. Cancer, 91, 2136–2147.

Richard, J.M., H. Sancho-Garnier, C. Micheau, D. Saravane and Y. Cachin, 1987, Prognostic factors in cervical lymph node metastasis in upper respiratory and digestive tract carcinomas: study of 1,713 cases during a 15-year period. Laryngoscope, 97, 97–101.

Sawair, F.A., C.R. Irwin, D.J. Gordon, A.G. Leonard, M. Stephenson and S.S. Napier, 2003, Invasive front grading: reliability and usefulness in the management of oral squamous cell carcinoma. J. Oral Pathol. Med., 32, 1–9.

Schliephake, H., 2003, Prognostic relevance of molecular markers of oral cancer – a review. Int. J. Oral Maxillofac. Surg., 32, 233–245.

Schoelch, M.L., Q.T. Le, S. Silverman, A. McMillan, N.P. Dekker, K.K. Fu, B.L. Ziober and J.A. Regezi, 1999, Apoptosis-related proteins and the development of oral squamous cell carcinoma. Oral Oncol., 35, 77–85.

Scholl, P., R.M. Byers, J.G. Batsakis, P. Wolf and H. Santini, 1986, Microscopic cut-through of cancer in the surgical treatment of carcinoma of the tongue. Prognostic and therapeutic implications. Am. J. Surg., 152, 354–360.

Shaw, R.J., J.S. Brown, J.A. Woolgar, D. Lowe, S.N. Rogers and E.D. Vaughan, 2004, The influence of the pattern of mandibular invasion on recurrence and survival in oral squamous cell carcinoma. Head Neck, 26, 861–869.

Sheahan, P., C. O'Keane, J.N. Sheahan and T.P. O'Dwyer, 2003, Effect of tumour thickness and other factors on the risk of regional disease and treatment of the N0 neck in early oral squamous carcinoma. Clin. Otolaryngol., 28, 461–471.

Shear, M., D.M. Hawkins and H.W. Farr, 1976, The prediction of lymph node metastases from oral squamous carcinoma. Cancer, 37, 1901–1907.

Shingaki, S., I. Suzuki and T. Wakajima, 1988, Evaluation of histopathologic parameters in predicting cervical lymph node metastasis of oral and oropharyngeal carcinomas. Oral Surg. Oral Med. Oral Pathol., 66, 683–688.

Shingaki, S., M. Takada, K. Sasai, R. Bibi, T. Kobayashi and T. Nomura, 2003, Impact of lymph node metastasis on the pattern of failure and survival in oral carcinomas. Am. J. Surg., 185, 278–284.

Silverman, S., 2001, Demographics and occurrence of oral and pharyngeal cancer. The outcomes, the trends, the challenge. J. Am. Dent. Assoc., 132, 7S–11S.

Slootweg, P.J. and H. Muller, 1989, Mandibular invasion by oral squamous cell carcinoma. J. Craniomaxillofac. Surg., 17, 69–74.

Slootweg, P.J., G.J. Hordijk and R. Koole, 1996, Autopsy findings in patients with head and neck squamous cell cancer and their therapeutic relevance. Oral Oncol. Eur. J. Cancer, 32B, 413–415.

Snow, G.B., A.A. Annyas, E.A. van Slooten, H. Bartelink, A.A.M. Hart, 1982, Prognostic factors of neck node metastasis. Clin. Otolaryngol., 7, 185–192.

Spiro, R.H., A.E. Alfonso, H.W. Farr and E.W. Strong, 1974, Cervical node metastasis from epidermoid carcinoma of the oral cavity and oropharynx. A critical assessment of current staging. Am. J. Surg., 128, 562–567.

Stell, P.M., 1991, Ploidy in head and neck cancer: a review and meta-analysis. Clin. Otolaryngol., 16, 510–516.

Sutton, D.N., J.S. Brown, S.N. Rogers, E.D. Vaughan and J.A. Woolgar, 2003, The prognostic implications of the surgical margin in oral squamous cell carcinoma. Int. J. Oral Maxillofac. Surg., 32, 30–34.

Tennvall, J., J. Wennerberg and H. Anderson, 1993, DNA analysis as a predictor of the outcome of induction chemotherapy in advanced head and neck carcinomas. Arch. Otolaryngol. Head Neck Surg., 119, 867–880.

UICC, 2002, In: L.H. Sobin and C. Wittekind. (Eds.), International Union Against Cancer, TNM Classification of Malignant Tumours, 6th ed, Wiley-Liss, New York.

Ulanovski, D., Y. Stern, P. Roizman, T. Shpitzer and A. Popovtzer, 2004, Expression of EGFR and Cerb-B2 as prognostic factors in cancer of the tongue. Oral Oncol., 40, 532–537.

Urist, M.M., C.J. O'Brien, S.J. Soong, D.W. Visscher, W.A. Maddox, 1987, Squamous cell carcinoma of the buccal mucosa: analysis of prognostic factors. Am. J. Surg., 154, 411–414.

Williams, J.K., G.W. Carlson and C. Cohen, 1994, Tumor angiogenesis as a prognostic factor in oral cavity tumors. Am. J. Surg., 168, 373–380.

Woolgar, J.A. and J. Scott, 1995, Prediction of cervical lymph node metastasis in squamous cell carcinoma of the tongue/floor of mouth. Head Neck, 17, 463–472.

Woolgar, J.A., J.C. Beirne, H.G. Vaughan, J. Lewis-Jones, J. Scott and J.S. Brown, 1995a, Correlation of histopathologic findings with clinical and radiologic assessments of cervical lymph-node metastases in oral cancer. Int. J. Oral Maxillofac. Surg., 24, 30–37.

Woolgar, J.A., J. Scott, E.D. Vaughan, J.S. Brown, C.R. West and S. Rogers, 1995b, Survival, metastasis and recurrence of oral cancer in relation to pathological features. Ann. R. Coll. Surg. Engl., 77, 325–331.

Woolgar, J.A., 1997, Detailed topography of cervical lymph-node metastases from oral squamous cell carcinoma. Int. J. Oral Maxillofac. Surg., 26, 3–9.

Woolgar, J.A., 1999a, Pathology of the N0 neck. Br. J. Oral Maxillofac. Surg., 37, 205–209.

Woolgar, J.A., 1999b, T2 carcinoma of the tongue: the histopathologist's perspective. Br. J. Oral Maxillofac. Surg., 37, 187–193.

Woolgar, J.A., S. Rogers, C.R. West, R.D. Errington, J.S. Brown, and E.D. Vaughan, 1999, Survival and patterns of recurrence in 200 oral cancer patients treated by radical surgery and neck dissection. Oral Oncol., 35, 257–265.

Woolgar, J.A., S.N. Rogers, D. Lowe, J.S. Brown and E.D. Vaughan, 2003, Cervical lymph node metastasis in oral cancer: the importance of even microscopic extracapsular spread. Oral Oncol., 39, 130–137.

Woolgar, J.A. and A. Triantafyllou, A histopathological appraisal of surgical resection margins in oral and oropharyngeal cancer resection specimens. Oral Oncol. In press.

World Health Organisation Histological Typing of Cancer and Precancer of the Oral Mucosa, 1997, In: J.J. Pindborg, P.A. Reichart, C.J. Smith, I. van der Waal, (Eds), 2nd ed, Springer, New York.

Xia, W., Y.-K. Lau, H.-Z. Zhang, F.-Y. Xiao, D.A. Johnston and A.R. Liu, 1999, Combination of EGFR, HER-2/neu, and HER-3 is a stronger predictor for the outcome of oral squamous cell carcinoma than any individual family members. Clin. Cancer Res., 5, 4164–4174.

Yamamoto N., J. Mizoe, H. Mumasawa, H. Tsujii and T. Shibhara, 2003, Allelic loss on chromosomes 2q, 3p, and 21q: possibly a poor prognostic factor in oral squamous cell carcinoma. Oral Oncol., 39, 796–805.

Chapter 2

Survival after Treatment of Intraocular Melanoma

Bertil Damato[1] and Azzam Taktak[2]

[1]*Ocular Oncology Service, Royal Liverpool University Hospital, Prescot St, Liverpool L7 8XP, UK*
[2]*Department of Clinical Engineering, Duncan Building, Royal Liverpool University Hospital, Prescot St, Liverpool L7 8XP, UK*

Abstract

Intraocular melanomas tend to occur in Caucasians, with an incidence of approximately six per million per year. Untreated, these tumours tend to make the eye blind and painful. Despite successful treatment of the ocular tumour, about 50% of patients develop metastatic disease, which usually involves the liver and which is usually fatal within a year of the onset of symptoms. Recent cytogenetic studies have identified two types of melanoma: tumours of low grade malignancy, which rarely or never spread outside the eye, and which are characterized by two copies of chromosome 3; and high-grade melanomas, characterized by loss of chromosome 3 (i.e monosomy 3), which seem to be fatal in all patients. Most studies have used Kaplan-Meier survival curves to report mortality and to demonstrate the predictive value of factors such as age, gender, tumour diameter and tumour cell type. These estimates have been subject to errors caused by incorrect diagnosis of cause of death, biased censoring, loss to follow-up, and competing risks. Survival analyses are also subject to limitations of Cox analysis and Log rank analysis, which make a number of assumptions about correlations. Attempts have been made to overcome some of these problems with neural networks, reporting overall mortality in patients in comparison with survival in the matched general population. The entire approach to patient care depends greatly on whether survival curves are believed to reflect the influence of treatment or the prevalence of high-grade melanoma, a debate which is still unresolved.

Acknowledgements

The project is partially funded by the BIOPATTERN EU Network of Excellence (Grant number: EU 508803). The Liverpool Ocular Oncology Centre is funded by the National Specialist Commissioning Advisory Group (NSCAG) of the Department of Health of England.

Contents

© 2007 Elsevier B.V. All rights reserved

1. INTRODUCTION

Randomised, prospective studies for evaluating new treatments are especially difficult when a disease is rare, even if there is an efficient infrastructure for multicentre collaboration. Therefore, there is scope for reducing the sample size needed by refining outcomes analysis. This requires enhanced statistical power, which in turn depends on good disease categorisation, precise measurement of baseline variables, accurate recording of all relevant outcomes, and avoidance of bias.

In this chapter, we discuss our approach to survival analysis after treatment of rare cancers, using intraocular melanoma as our model. Our aims are to highlight the limitations and pitfalls of conventional outcomes analysis, and to propose possible solutions.

2. INTRAOCULAR MELANOMA

Intraocular melanomas are malignant neoplasms arising from melanocytes in the uvea, which is a pigmented tissue comprising the iris, the ciliary body and the choroid (Damato, 2000).

2.1. Epidemiology

Uveal melanomas are the most common primary ocular malignant tumours in adults, with an incidence of approximately 5 per million per year in Caucasians (Singh et al., 2005). They are about two or three times more common in blue and grey eyes than in brown eyes and are extremely rare in individuals with dark skin. They occur as commonly in males as in females.

About 90% of all uveal melanomas arise in the choroid, which is a cup-shaped tissue lying between retina and the sclera. Approximately 5–7% occur in ciliary body, a ring of muscular tissue covered by secretory epithelium, which focuses the lens and produces aqueous humor. About 3–5% of melanomas arise in the iris, the pigmented, muscular tissue regulating the size of the pupil.

2.2. Presentation

Patients with choroidal melanoma present mostly because of blurred or distorted vision, visual field loss, or photopsia (i.e. seeing flashing lights) (Damato, 2001). Ciliary body melanomas tend to press on the lens, causing cataract and astigmatism. Iris melanomas present as a cosmetic blemish or with raised intraocular pressure. In the UK, about 40% of patients are asymptomatic, being detected on routine examination by an optometrist or ophthalmologist.

2.3. Clinical features

Choroidal melanomas first appear as a dome-shaped, pigmented, choroidal mass, often with specks of orange pigment, and usually with exudative retinal detachment. These tumours often break through Bruch's membrane and retinal pigment epithelium to develop a mushroom shape, eventually perforating the retina. Ciliary body tumours damage the lens, as mentioned above, and can spread posteriorly into the choroid and anteriorly into the iris. Iris melanomas form a discrete or diffuse tumour and, in addition, tend to grow circumferentially along the angle of the anterior chamber, obstructing the trabecular meshwork which drains aqueous humor from the eye, thereby causing a raised intraocular pressure, glaucomatous optic nerve damage, and loss of vision. Advanced uveal melanomas result in a blind, painful eye and can spread extraocularly into the orbit and conjunctiva.

2.4. Diagnosis

Uveal melanomas can usually be diagnosed by inspection, using a slit-lamp or ophthalmoscope. Ultrasonography measures tumour dimensions, particularly the longest basal dimension and height, and demonstrates tumour shape, extent, and internal acoustic reflectivity. If after these investigations the diagnosis is still uncertain, biopsy may be required. The differential diagnosis is extensive and includes conditions such as choroidal naevus, haemangioma, and metastasis.

2.5. Treatment of the ocular tumour

Previously, the standard treatment was enucleation (i.e. amputation of the eye), but this has largely been superseded by a variety of therapies aimed at conserving the eye with as much useful vision as possible (Damato, 2004). Such "conservative" forms of treatment include plaque radiotherapy, proton beam radiotherapy, stereotactic radiotherapy, trans-scleral local resection, trans-retinal local resection, transpupillary thermotherapy, and photodynamic therapy (Damato, 2004). Facilities for these treatments are usually available only at specialist ocular oncology centres. When conservation of the eye is attempted, the eye is preserved in about 90% of patients, with vision depending greatly on the size of the tumour and its distance from the optic nerve and fovea (Damato and Lecuona, 2004).

2.6. Presentation of metastatic disease

Approximately 50% of all patients ultimately develop metastatic disease, which occurs by haematogenous spread (i.e. through the blood circulation) (Diener West et al., 1992). Such disease nearly always involves the liver, less common sites being lung, skin, bone, and brain. Metastatic disease is only rarely evident at the time of diagnosis and treatment of the primary intraocular tumour, usually developing from the second post-treatment year onwards. Metastatic disease usually presents with abdominal pain, weakness, and weight loss, eventually causing liver failure, jaundice, confusion, cachexia, and death. Increasingly, metastatic disease is detected before the development of symptoms, by performing ultrasonography and liver function tests. Depending on where the patient is treated, these investigations are undertaken either once or twice a year, either in all patients or only those considered to be at high risk of developing metastatic disease (Eskelin et al., 1999). Diagnosis is based either on clinical examination or liver biopsy. The rate of post-mortem examination varies greatly from one country to another.

2.7. Treatment of metastatic disease

Systemic chemotherapy is the most common form of treatment, but this only rarely produces prolonged remissions, although newer agents seem more effective. Intra-hepatic chemotherapy is more effective at treating liver metastases, but patients who respond to this treatment tend to develop disease in other parts of the body. Rarely, hepatic metastases are amenable to surgical resection, which can prolong life by several years. Immunotherapy can also induce long remission, although this is rare.

Death usually occurs within a year of diagnosis of metastatic disease, with survival time depending on size of the largest metastasis, biochemical liver function test results, and state of health at diagnosis (Eskelin et al., 2003).

2.8. Prediction of metastatic disease

Clinical features associated with poor survival probability include:

- large basal tumour dimension;
- ciliary body involvement; and
- extraocular spread (Kujala and Kivelä, 2005).

There are conflicting reports regarding the prognostic significance of older age at diagnosis and male gender. Histopathological features indicating poor prognosis include:

- presence of epithelioid cells (as opposed to spindle-shaped cells) (McLean et al., 1978);
- increased microvascular density (Mäkitie et al., 1999); and
- certain extravascular matrix patterns, particularly closed, laminin loops (Chen et al., 2003).

Uveal melanomas tend to develop characteristic cytogenetic abnormalities, which include:

- partial or complete loss of chromosome 3;
- gains in the long arm of chromosome 8; and
- abnormalities in the short arm of chromosome 6 (Horsman et al., 1990; Parrella et al., 1999).

The chromosome 3 and 8 abnormalities, which often occur together, are associated with a poor prognosis whereas the chromosome 6 abnormalities correlate with good survival (Prescher et al., 1996; Parrella et al., 1999; Scholes et al., 2003). There is currently some debate as to whether the different cytogenetic types represent different classes of uveal melanoma, which are distinct from the very outset, or different grades, with the high-grade, monosomy-3 tumours being more life-threatening than the disomy-3 variants.

3. STATISTICAL METHODS FOR PREDICTING METASTATIC DISEASE

3.1. Proportion surviving at 5 years and other time periods

When there is complete long-term follow-up for all cases, the simplest way to summarise the data is by measuring the proportion surviving at the selected time point (e.g. five years); and these proportions can be compared across subgroups by relatively simple statistical methods such as a Chi squared test, with confidence intervals. However, this type of analysis lacks power because it cannot take into account cases with a shorter time since treatment or those lost to follow-up, or those who have died of unrelated causes. Also, the choice of time period at which to carry out the analysis is arbitrary and can introduce subjective bias.

3.2. Kaplan–Meier analysis

The Kaplan–Meier method is a more sophisticated method of summarising survival data, which uses all the cases in a series, not just those followed up until the selected cut-off. The technique is to divide the follow-up period into a number of small time intervals, determining for each interval the number of cases followed up over that interval and the number of events of interest (e.g. deaths) during each period.

When the surviving proportion is multiplied by the surviving proportions for each of the preceding time periods, a probability of surviving to the end of that time period is obtained. This survival probability is then plotted against time. With modern software, the time interval used is just one day. A stepped "curve" is obtained, with each step representing an event. Any case whose follow-up is curtailed because of incomplete follow-up or because of loss to follow-up is censored and represented as a tag, which is placed on the survival curve at a point corresponding to the relevant follow-up time. With increasing follow-up time, the curve is based on fewer and fewer cases, therefore becoming progressively less reliable; hence it is conventional to truncate the survival curve when fewer than five cases remain.

The Kaplan–Meier method gives an unbiased estimate of survival only if censored cases are typical of the whole series. If patients are lost to follow-up for reasons related to the event being studied, e.g. because they appear to be cured and so are discharged from the clinic, or conversely because they are too ill to attend the clinic, then the Kaplan–Meier method will underestimate or overestimate the true survival. Consequently, Kaplan–Meier methods should be used only when follow-up is reasonably complete and when losses to follow-up are clearly due to unrelated events.

3.3. Logrank test

The logrank test is similar to the Kaplan–Meier analysis in that all cases are used to compare two or more groups e.g. treated versus control group in a randomised trial. Again, the follow-up is divided into small time periods (e.g. days), and the number of actual events occurring in each time period are compared.

This test is most powerful in detecting a higher cured proportion in one group than the other group. It is much less effective at detecting a difference when survival is merely prolonged in one group as compared with the other, the proportion of those surviving being unchanged (i.e. when the two Kaplan–Meier curves first separate and then come together again).

As with the Kaplan–Meier method, the logrank test should be used only when follow-up is reasonably up to date, and when losses to follow-up are clearly caused by unrelated events. A limitation of the logrank test is that it only assesses the effect of one variable at a time on prognosis. To assess multiple variables, a more complex method such as the Cox model is needed.

3.4. Cox proportional hazards model

When several clinical and pathological variables are analysed by a logrank test, it is common to find that most or all correlate with prognosis in some way, and these variables are often associated with each other. For example, an analysis looking at several baseline factors in a univariate fashion may find that prognosis is worse in elderly patients, in those with a large tumour, and in patients whose tumour is poorly differentiated, respectively. If in the same sample, elderly patients tend to have larger and more undifferentiated tumours, the question arises as to whether old age itself increases the risk of metastatic death or whether elderly patients have a worse prognosis because they have larger and less well-differentiated tumours. Multivariate analysis can help answer this question, and in survival studies the standard method of analysis is using Cox's proportional hazard model.

Like other multivariate techniques, the Cox model can be used to derive a prognostic index, where the coefficients from the model are rounded to integers to give a simple scoring system that will predict a patient's overall risk of an event (e.g. death) from the patient's individual risk factors.

The Cox model has several limitations. First, it assumes that the effect of prognostic variables is constant over time. Therefore, if, for example, large tumours are twice as likely as small tumours to cause death during the first year after treatment, then the same will be true in those patients without death at the start of year two, and similarly for year three and so on; that is, the hazard (of death) remains in the same proportion – hence the name "proportional hazards model". Second, it assumes that when multiple risk factors are present, the risk of death is calculated by multiplying rather than adding the risks associated with each adverse factor. For example, if a large tumour size trebles the risk of death and if poor tumour differentiation also trebles the risk of death, then the effect of both factors together is estimated to be a ninefold increase and not a sixfold increase. Third, it relies on the baseline population to calculate the h_0 parameter, which is a nonsense parameter. Fourth, it does not allow non-linear interactions between the input variables (such as the product of two variables) unless this is entered manually, and this requires prior knowledge. Finally, in common with all regression models, the fitness increases with increased number of variables without any warning when over-fitting might occur.

4. PREDICTING METASTATIC DEATH WITH NEURAL NETWORKS

Artificial Neural Networks (ANNs) have been used in conjunction with statistical methods to model survival in cancer. As with statistical methods, ANNs allow the combination of categorical and continuous variables. ANNs may offer advantages over linear statistical models. They allow:

- arbitrary non-linear relationships between independent and dependent variables; and
- all possible interactions between dependent variables.

Moreover, ANNs do not require explicit distributional assumption. Their main disadvantage is their "black box" nature, which makes it difficult to get an insight into the problem. A study comparing ANNs with statistical regression analysis has found that for small sample sizes (i.e. $n < 2000$) the ANNs tended to outperform regression; however, this investigation could not rule out the possibility of publication bias.

The application of ANNs to censored data provides potential advantages over traditional linear models that assume proportional hazards. ANNs deal with the censorship issue by including time as one of the covariates. By including patients only for the time intervals when outcomes are observed and omitting them when they are unknown, the network weights are optimised to a partial log-likelihood. This is described in the literature as a Partial Logistic Artificial Neural Network (PLANN) model (Ravdin and Clark, 1992; Biganzoli et al., 2002; Lisboa et al., 2003; Bishop, 2004). The combination of ANNs with probabilistic algorithms has proved to be a powerful technique in survival prediction studies.

Another approach is to combine ANNs with Bayes' theorem in order to transform the binary outcome of the network into a probability figure (Taktak et al., 2004). First, the ANN classifies the input into two classes, high risk (e.g. of death) and low risk. Next, the actual mortality is determined by dividing the number of observed deaths by the total study sample. Then, the neural network estimates the probability of death given the class. Then, the sensitivity of the neural network is calculated by dividing the estimated probability of death by the actual mortality. Finally, the probability of death estimated by the neural network is corrected for the networks sensitivity.

5. MISCELLANEOUS ERRORS

5.1. Mistaken cause of death

The diagnosed cause of death might be incorrect if it relies on clinical examination, without biopsy or post-mortem examination. For example, a patient dying of hepatic cancer after treatment of uveal melanoma might be assumed to have liver metastases from the eye whereas these may have originated from an unrecognised tumour in another part of the body. Conversely, cardiac arrest might be attributed to ischaemic heart disease when in fact it has been caused by a metastasis to the heart (Makitie and Kivelä, 2001).

It is possible to estimate the disease-related mortality in patients with uveal melanoma by subtracting the all-cause mortality in these patients from the all-cause mortality in the age-matched and gender-matched population, using census data. This is possible because uveal melanomas are so rare.

5.2. Biased censoring

Most patients with uveal melanoma are eventually discharged from the ocular oncology centre where they were treated, particularly if they live far from this centre. Many are also discharged from the local eye department, especially if their eye has been removed. Such loss to follow-up may result in complications being under-reported.

Outcomes analysis can be distorted by biased uncensoring. For example, after being discharged, and hence censored, patients developing metastatic disease tend to get in touch with the oncology centre to ask whether any further help can be provided. This results in their being "uncensored". Those who remain well and who do not contact the oncology centre remain censored at an earlier date. Such a bias has the effect of exaggerating the proportion of patients reported to develop metastatic disease.

Both these forms of bias can be avoided by ensuring that all patients are followed up even after being discharged from the oncology centre. We have done this by sending all our patients a questionnaire on the anniversary of their treatment. This problem is also avoided by using data from a national cancer registry. With this system, patients are assumed to be alive at the close of the study, unless of course the study centre has been informed of the patient's death by the cancer registry.

5.3. Competing risks

Some patients with occult metastatic spread will inevitably die of other causes before the metastases have had time to cause fatal disease. The risk of non-metastatic death therefore competes with the risk of metastatic death. If patients dying of non-metastatic causes are merely censored, this will have the effect of exaggerating reported rates of metastatic death. Statistical programs have therefore been developed to cope with such competing risks when analysing outcomes.

5.4. Categorisation

There is a tendency to divide continuous variables, such as largest basal tumour diameter, into categories when drawing Kaplan–Meier survival curves. For example, uveal melanomas are categorised as "small", "medium", and "large", according to whether the basal tumour diameter is less than 10, 10–15 mm, and more than 15 mm respectively (Kujala and Kivelä, 2005). By reducing the number of survival curves in the graph to only three, such categorisation makes the diagram easier to view. However, the precision of any prognostication is diminished; for example, the estimated survival prognosis with a 15-mm diameter melanoma will be the same as that of a 10 mm tumour but much better than that of a 16-mm diameter lesion. The situation would be improved by reducing the range of each category to only 1–2 mm or removing categorisation altogether, for example, if an electronic medium is used instead of a paper chart.

6. A NEURAL NETWORK FOR PREDICTING SURVIVAL IN UVEAL MELANOMA PATIENTS

6.1. Description of ANN for uveal melanoma

To overcome the limitations mentioned above, we have developed two types of ANN, a Bayesian and a partial logistic ANN. These ANNs predict all-cause mortality according to age, gender, largest basal tumour diameter, and ciliary body involvement. The output also displays the all-cause mortality in the age- and gender-matched general population so that disease-specific mortality can be estimated. Largest basal tumour diameter is categorised in 2 mm intervals, improving precision. Our neural network displays survival both in the form of conventional curves (Figs. 1 and 2) and also in a pictogram (Fig. 3), which is more easily understood by patients. Furthermore, our program also takes account

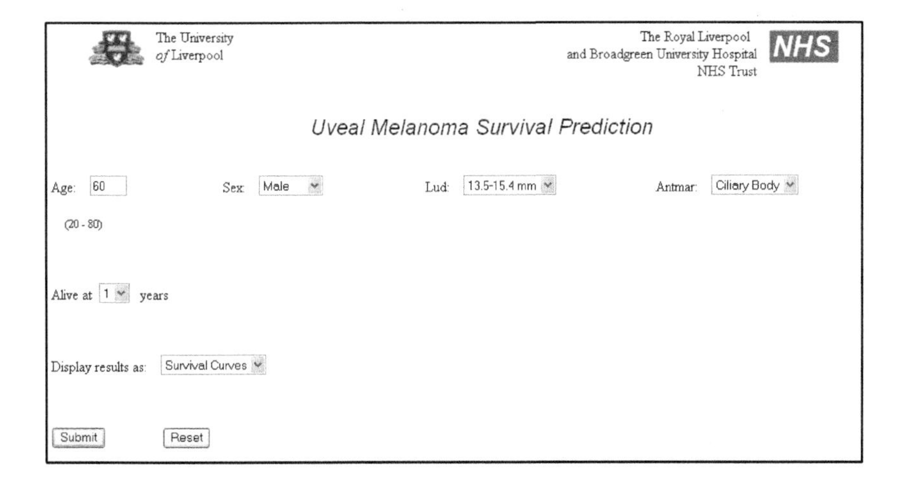

Fig. 1. User interface for a uveal melanoma survival prediction software using ANNs.

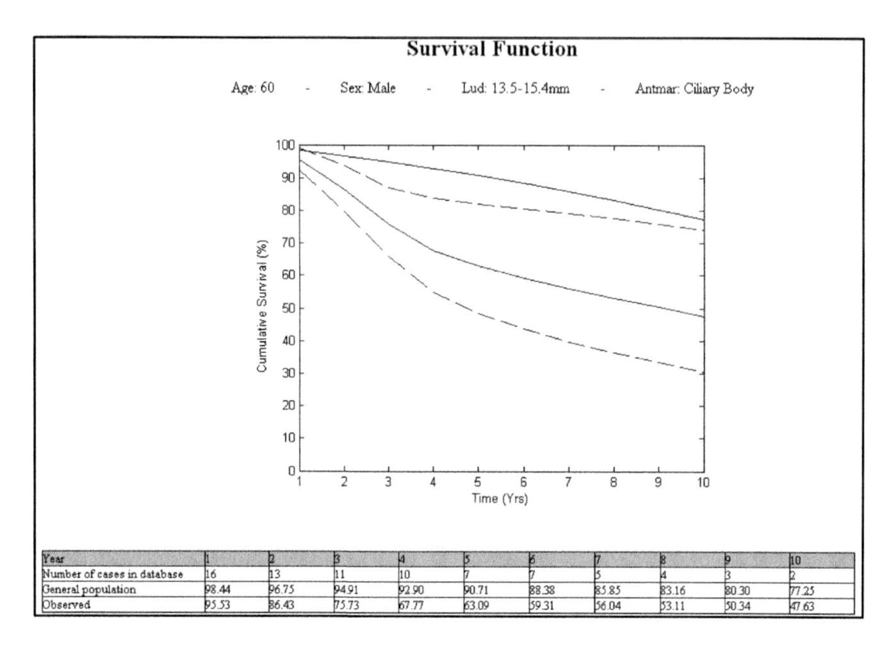

Year	1	2	3	4	5	6	7	8	9	10
Number of cases in database	16	13	11	10	7	7	5	4	3	2
General population	98.44	96.75	94.91	92.90	90.71	88.38	85.85	83.16	80.30	77.25
Observed	95.53	86.43	75.73	67.77	63.09	59.31	56.04	53.11	50.34	47.63

Fig. 2. Survival prediction curve for a 60-year-old male with a 13–15 mm tumour involving the ciliary body compared with a 60-year-old male from the general population.

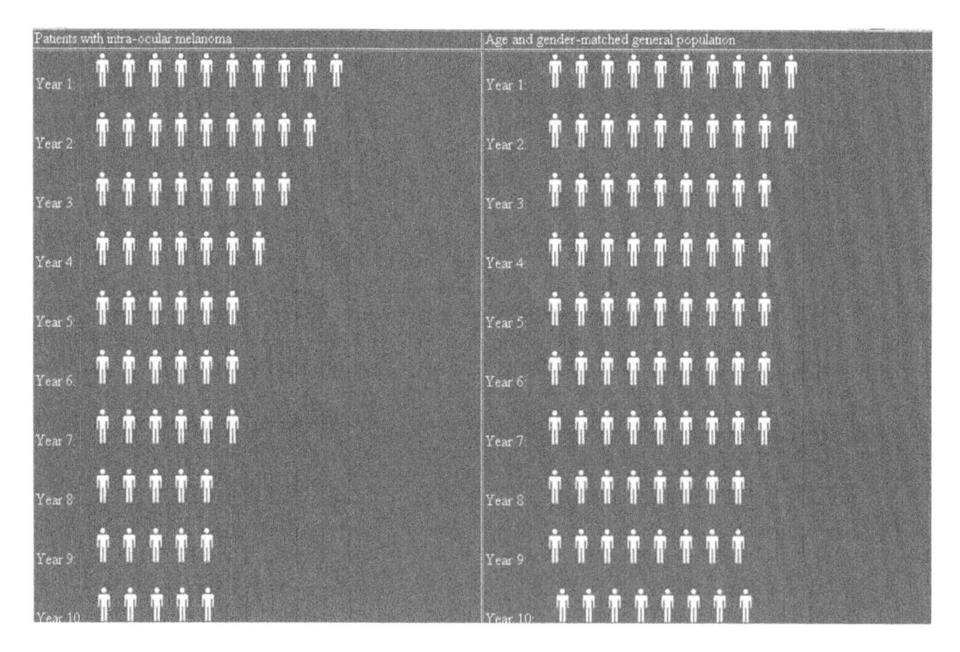

Fig. 3. A pictogram for the same patient compared with age-and gender-matched group from the general population.

of the improvement in survival probability with time after treatment. For example, after treatment of uveal melanoma, most metastatic deaths occur in the first five years after treatment (Fig. 4). Therefore, a patient given a 47% chance of surviving ten years who is still alive in the fifth post-operative year has a much better chance of surviving another five years than he or she did originally (Fig. 5). Such an improvement in the survival probability can be very reassuring for patients especially if it can be demonstrated to them, as with our program.

6.2. Limitations of ANN for uveal melanoma

Our neural network for predicting survival in patients with uveal melanoma has several limitations. First, although our program matches our patients with the general population having the same age and gender, it takes no account of the date of birth, so that, for example, an individual born in 1920 is treated similarly to a person born in 1970, who would have a longer life-expectancy. Second, our neural network does not adjust for concurrent diseases, such as diabetes mellitus and ischaemic heart disease, which reduce survival probability. Third, no use is made of histological and cytogenetic data, which would greatly enhance prognostication. We hope to address these shortcomings in future models.

7. CAVEATS REGARDING INTERPRETATION OF SURVIVAL STATISTICS

Problems can arise even with an accurate prognostic model for predicting survival after treatment of uveal melanoma, if the data are not interpreted correctly.

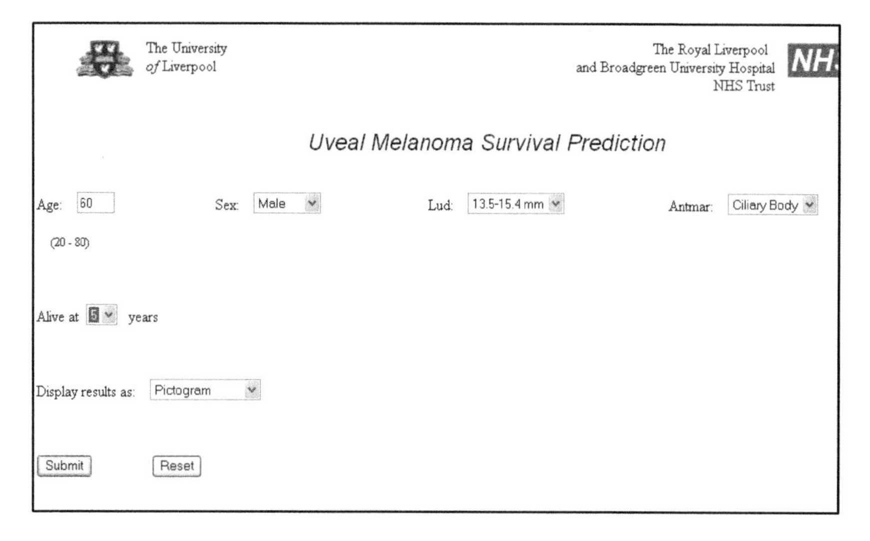

Fig. 4. Entering the original information for the same patient having survived 5 years after treatment.

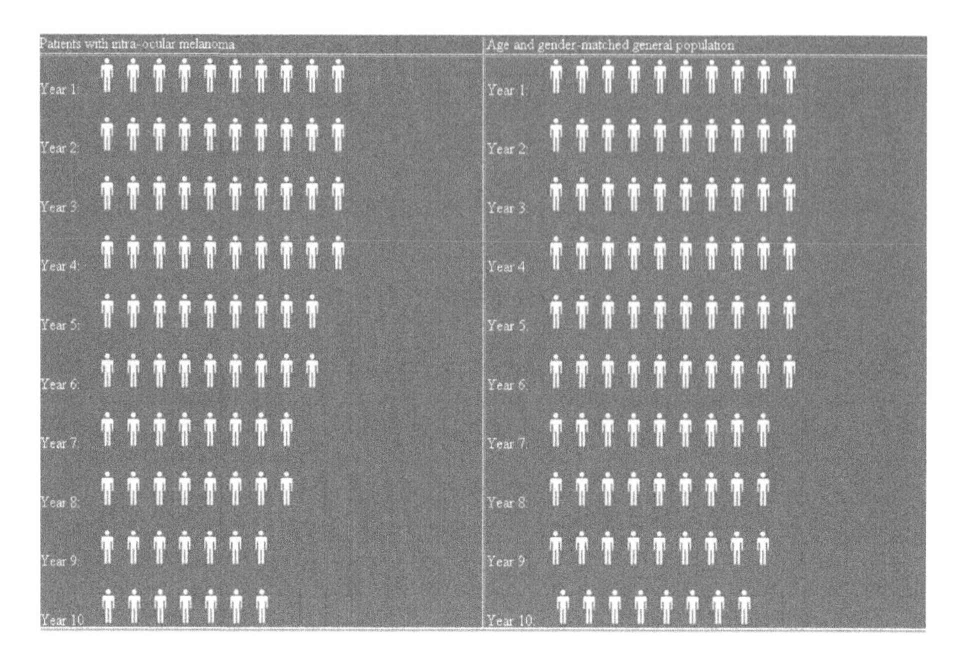

Fig. 5. A pictogram for the same patient having survived 5 years after treatment.

7.1. Lead-time bias

A strong correlation between tumour size and metastatic death rate might merely be the result of lead-time bias, both the primary tumour and the metastases having been present for a longer period. Other time-dependent variables, such as extraocular tumour extension, have the same limitation. The TNM Classification of uveal melanomas, developed by the World Health Organization, groups these tumours according to largest basal diameter and extraocular extension. The term "classification" and the survival variation between categories might be interpreted to mean that there are different "classes" of uveal melanoma whereas only progressive "stages" of the same disease are being differentiated.

7.2. Grades versus classes

Uveal melanomas without abnormalities in chromosomes 3 and 8 are associated with a 90% five-year survival whereas those with abnormalities in both these chromosomes indicate only a 45% five-year survival probability. It has been suggested that these two types of melanoma are entirely distinct "classes", that is, totally different from their very inception and incapable of transforming from one class to another. Another possibility is that the two varieties are different grades of the same disease, with the "high-grade" melanomas evolving from the "low-grade" tumours over time. A small melanoma without chromosome 3 and 8 abnormalities might be left untreated by those who consider it to belong to a non-lethal class of tumour, which can never develop any metastatic potential. The same tumour would be treated urgently and aggressively by those who regard it as a low-grade variant, which can de-differentiate into a more malignant grade at any time.

7.3. Causality

If after taking lead-time bias into account, there is indeed a statistical correlation between large tumour size and metastatic death, this can be explained in two ways.

The prevailing hypothesis is that uveal melanomas metastasise after they grow large, perhaps because large tumour size:

- enhances any opportunities for the tumour to develop more aggressive features, increasing its capacity to metastasise; or because
- the greater volume allows more intense seeding of tumour cells into the general circulation.

This view has led to large melanomas being considered more dangerous than small tumours. Large tumours therefore tend to be treated more urgently and aggressively than small melanomas. In fact, it is accepted practice to delay treatment of small uveal melanomas until growth has been documented. The concept of late metastatic spread has also encouraged beliefs that:

- Treatment of uveal melanomas is often life-saving, especially with small and medium-sized tumours;
- Local tumour recurrence causes metastatic disease, if conservative treatment fails; and
- Screening of the population for uveal melanoma should improve survival.

An alternative explanation is that metastases begin to develop before the tumour grows large. According to this hypothesis, large tumour size is considered only an indicator of increased tumour malignancy, assuming that there is indeed an inverse correlation between cell doubling time and metastatic potential. In other words, non-lethal tumours tend to grow slowly so that they are usually small when diagnosed whereas tumours that have metastasised usually grow quickly, so that they are usually large by the time of treatment. According to this hypothesis:

- Treatment of uveal melanomas is only palliative, perhaps preventing metastatic spread only with very small tumours;
- Small tumours should be treated urgently and aggressively, because it is with these tumours that opportunities for preventing metastatic spread are greatest;
- Local tumour recurrence is more likely to be an indicator of a tumour's metastatic potential than the cause of spread, except perhaps in very small tumours; and
- Screening is unlikely to improve survival, unless perhaps melanomas are treated at a very early stage, maybe when they are indistinguishable from naevi.

It is perhaps surprising that patient management is so profoundly influenced by intuitive beliefs as to whether metastasis occurs before or after the intraocular tumour grows large. This perplexing situation will continue as long as the natural history of uveal melanomas remains unknown. It is hoped that molecular biology will determine whether small melanomas are less malignant than large tumours or less likely to be malignant.

8. FURTHER STUDIES

With uveal melanoma, randomised, prospective studies are needed to determine how survival is influenced by:

- immediate versus delayed treatment of the primary tumour, in patients with asymptomatic or indeterminate lesions;
- curative versus palliative treatment of uveal melanoma, the two therapeutic approaches differing in the measures taken to prevent local tumour recurrence or visual loss; and
- adjuvant systemic therapy in patients with high-grade uveal melanoma.

These studies require:

- a meaningful classification for uveal melanoma;
- large numbers of patients to ensure that these studies have sufficient statistical power;
- multicentre collaboration for achieving adequate patient numbers;
- organisations and web-based environments for facilitating such collaboration; and
- efficient analytical methods for minimising the number of patients needing to be accrued to clinical trials, thereby enhancing the feasibility of these studies and shortening their duration.

9. CONCLUSIONS

Survival analyses demonstrate correlations between outcomes and baseline variables thereby enabling tumours to be described according to their class, grade, and stage of development. This information allows any planning of life-management and clinical care to be based on prognostication. It also enhances treatment comparisons in randomised prospective studies. The refinements to survival analysis discussed in this chapter should reduce the number of patients needed for such studies thereby enabling results to be obtained more quickly and making it easier to investigate rare diseases such as uveal melanoma.

REFERENCES

Biganzoli, E., P. Boracchi, and E. Marubini, 2002, A general framework for neural network models on censored survival data. Neural. Netw., 15(2), 209–218.

Bishop, C.M. 2004, Error functions. In: Neural Networks for Pattern Recognition, Oxford University Press, Oxford, pp. 194–252.

Chen, X., Z. Ai, M. Rasmussen, P. Bajcsy, L. Auvil, M. Welge, L. Leach, S. Vangveeravong, A.J. Maniotis and R. Folberg, 2003, Three-dimensional reconstruction of extravascular matrix patterns and blood vessels in human uveal melanoma tissue: techniques and preliminary findings. Invest. Ophthalmol. Vis. Sci., 44(7), 2834–2840.

Damato, B., 2000, Ocular Tumours: Diagnosis and Treatment. Butterworth Heinemann, Oxford.

Damato, B., 2001, Detection of uveal melanoma by optometrists in the United Kingdom. Ophthalmic. Physiol. Opt., 21, 268–271.

Damato, B., 2004, Developments in the management of uveal melanoma. Clin. Exp. Ophthalmol., 32(6), 639–647.

Damato, B. and K. Lecuona, 2004, Conservation of eyes with choroidal melanoma by a multimodality approach to treatment: an audit of 1632 patients. Ophthalmol. 111, 977–983.

Diener West, M., B.S. Hawkins, J.A. Markowitz and A.P. Schachat, 1992, A review of mortality from choroidal melanoma. II. A meta- analysis of 5-year mortality rates following enucleation, 1966 through 1988. Arch. Ophthalmol., 110, 245–250.

Eskelin, S., S. Pyrhonen, P. Summanen, J.U. Prause and T. Kivelä, 1999, Screening for metastatic malignant melanoma of the uvea revisited. Cancer, 85(5), 1151–1159.

Eskelin, S., S. Pyrhonen, M. Hahka-Kemppinen, S. Tuomaala and T. Kivelä, 2003, A prognostic model and staging for metastatic uveal melanoma. Cancer, 97(2), 465–475.

Horsman, D.E., H. Sroka, J. Rootman and V.A. White, 1990, Monosomy 3 and isochromosome 8q in a uveal melanoma. Cancer Genet. Cytogenet., 45(2), 249–253.

Kujala, E. and T. Kivelä, 2005, Tumor, node, metastasis classification of malignant ciliary body and choroidal melanoma evaluation of the 6th edition and future directions. Ophthalmol. 112(6), 1135–1144.

Lisboa, P.J., H. Wong, P. Harris and R. Swindell, 2003, A Bayesian neural network approach for modelling censored data with an application to prognosis after surgery for breast cancer. Artif. Intell. Med., 28(1), 1–25.

Mäkitie, T. and T. Kivelä, 2001, Cardiac metastasis from uveal melanoma. Arch. Ophthalmol., 119(1), 139–140.

Mäkitie, T., P. Summanen, A. Tarkkanen and T. Kivelä, 1999, Microvascular loops and networks as prognostic indicators in choroidal and ciliary body melanomas. J. Natl. Cancer Inst., 91(4), 359–367.

McLean, I.W., L.E. Zimmerman and R.M. Evans, 1978, Reappraisal of Callender's spindle a type of malignant melanoma of choroid and ciliary body. Am. J. Ophthalmol., 86, 557–564.

Parrella, P., D. Sidransky and S.L. Merbs, 1999, Allelotype of posterior uveal melanoma: implications for a bifurcated tumor progression pathway. Cancer Res., 59(13), 3032–3037.

Prescher, G., N. Bornfeld, H. Hirche, B. Horsthemke, K.H. Jockel and R. Becher, 1996, Prognostic implications of monosomy 3 in uveal melanoma. Lancet, 347(9010), 1222–1225.

Ravdin, P.M. and G.M. Clark, 1992, A practical application of neural network analysis for predicting outcome of individual breast cancer patients. Breast Cancer Res. Treat., 22(3), 285–293.

Scholes, A.G., B.E. Damato, J. Nunn, P. Hiscott, I. Grierson and J.K. Field, 2003, Monosomy 3 in uveal melanoma: correlation with clinical and histologic predictors of survival. Invest. Ophthalmol. Vis. Sci., 44(3), 1008–1011.

Singh, A.D., L. Bergman and S. Seregard, 2005, Uveal melanoma: epidemiologic aspects. Ophthalmol. Clin. North Am., 18(1), 75–84, viii.

Taktak, A.F., A.C. Fisher and B.E. Damato, 2004, Modelling survival after treatment of intraocular melanoma using artificial neural networks and Bayes theorem. Phys. Med. Biol., 49(1), 87–98.

Chapter 3

Recent Developments in Relative Survival Analysis

Timo R. Hakulinen and Tadeusz A. Dyba

Finnish Cancer Registry, Liisankatu 21 B, FIN-00170 Helsinki, Finland
Email: timo.hakulinen@cancer.fi, tadek.dyba@cancer.fi

Abstract

Relative survival is used to summarize the excess mortality the cancer patients have in comparison with a corresponding general population group. It is often interpreted as the patients' survival if the mortality from other competing causes of death than the cancer of the patients were eliminated.

An analysis of the total patient mortality does not differentiate whether variables such as age and sex are related to the disease-specific mortality, the "natural" mortality in the source population or to both of them. However, information on causes of death may be unavailable or non-reliable preventing the cause-specific survival analysis. Relative survival thus provides an "objective" way to account for mortality due to competing risks or for natural mortality, and as such is commonly used by population-based cancer registries.

Relative survival is based on an additive hazards model where the total hazard of dying is regarded as a sum of a known baseline hazard (of a comparable general population group) and an excess hazard associated with the diagnosis of cancer. The excess hazard is assumed to depend on prognostic factors, and non-proportional effects can also be accommodated in the calculations. In fact, non-proportional excess hazards are rather a rule than an exception.

There are at least five methods to perform the analyses. The regression analyses of relative survival can be conducted easily using mainstream statistical software packages (e.g. SAS and STATA), thereby removing the reliance on special-purpose software. The relative survival methodology has been recently generalized also to analyses of cancer-specific relative survival of patients with multiple tumours.

The main alternative to relative survival analysis is cause-specific survival analysis, where it assumes patient-specific knowledge of the causes of death. Additionally, multiplicative hazards models may be considered as alternatives.

Acknowledgment

The work was supported by a grant from the Academy of Finland.

Keywords: Relative survival, excess mortality, actuarial method, cause-specific survival, regression analysis.

Contents

© 2007 Elsevier B.V. All rights reserved

1. INTRODUCTION

Survival is regarded as the most important outcome for cancer treatment (Peto et al., 1976, 1977). It is also used more generally as a quality indicator for cancer service provision (Ries et al., 2002; Berrino et al., 2003). In a population-based cancer registration system, the cancer registry collects information on all patients diagnosed with cancer in a certain time period and follows-up these patients with respect to death or emigration. The resulting survival figures give an unbiased representation of cancer patient survival, as opposed to figures coming from clinical trials or hospitals based on selected patient materials which are not likely to be generalizable in the same way.

2. CAUSE-SPECIFIC SURVIVAL

Survival as such is not necessarily the best indicator to reflect what happens to patients as far as their cancer is concerned. Patients do die also from other diseases during their follow-up time. Thus, estimated proportions of survivors, commonly referred to as observed survival rates (contrary to accurate terminology, see Elandt-Johnson, 1975), give an unduly pessimistic picture on cancer patient survival with respect to the risk of death the patients have because of their cancer. Moreover, as older patients tend to die more than the younger ones from other causes, observed survival rates are not strictly comparable between patient groups with different age structures. For example, Fig. 1 shows the observed survival rates by age and follow-up time for female patients diagnosed with localized stomach cancer in Finland during 1985–2002. These rates are the lowest for the oldest age groups, but it is uncertain whether or to which extent this depends on deaths due to other causes which are more frequent in older patients.

This can, of course, be checked by using the information on patients' causes of death. If it can be assumed that within the age groups dying from other causes and dying from cancer are independent processes, deaths due to other causes may be treated as events censoring the follow-up time. This assumption has been made in Fig. 2. The resulting cause-specific (stomach-cancer specific) survival rates for the stomach-cancer patients are still the lowest for the oldest patients but a large part of the differences has disappeared and can thus be accounted for by deaths due to other causes. For example, the five-year observed survival rates were 81 and 30% for patients aged 0–44 and 75 years or more at diagnosis, respectively. The corresponding cause-specific survival rates were 83 and 45% indicating that one quarter of the difference between the age groups can be accounted for by deaths due to other causes, remaining three quarters attributable to stomach cancer.

Fortunately, it is possible for the Finnish Cancer Registry to obtain the causes of death of the individual patients from the Central Statistical Office. As the Registry receives several notifications per case, there is also the possibility of correcting the information in the official cause-of-death records (Hakulinen and Teppo, 1977). Particularly, with respect

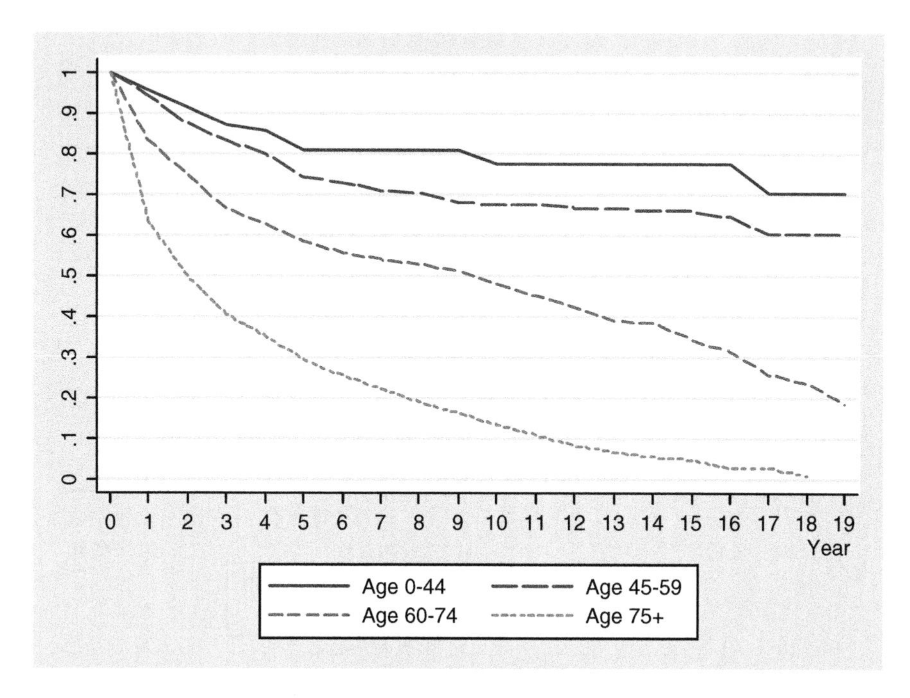

Fig. 1. The observed survival rates of female stomach-cancer patients diagnosed in Finland during 1985–2002 with a localized tumour, by age at diagnosis and follow-up time.

to causes of death due to cancer, the Registry is often better aware of the original location of the tumour than the person signing the death certificate. In many other cancer registries, however, it is not possible for the registry to obtain any information on patients' causes of death, due to a strict legislation on confidentiality. Even when the registry is able to receive information on the cause of death, it does not often make any correction for it due to the "official" nature of the cause of death. Thus, in general, the use of cause-specific survival rates is often complicated by the non-availability or inferior quality of the cause-of-death records.

3. INDEPENDENCE ASSUMPTION

Another problem for cause-specific survival analysis is the assumption of independence made between the disease of the patients and the other causes of death, within the age groups applied. If no stratification by age is made, it is clear that such an assumption is not necessarily valid. For example, for the stomach-cancer patients the cause-specific survival is lower for the older than for the younger patients. Thus, the deaths due to stomach cancer are more frequent in the older age groups, precisely where the deaths due to other causes are also more frequent. Clearly, without stratification for age, there would be dependence between these two causes of death.

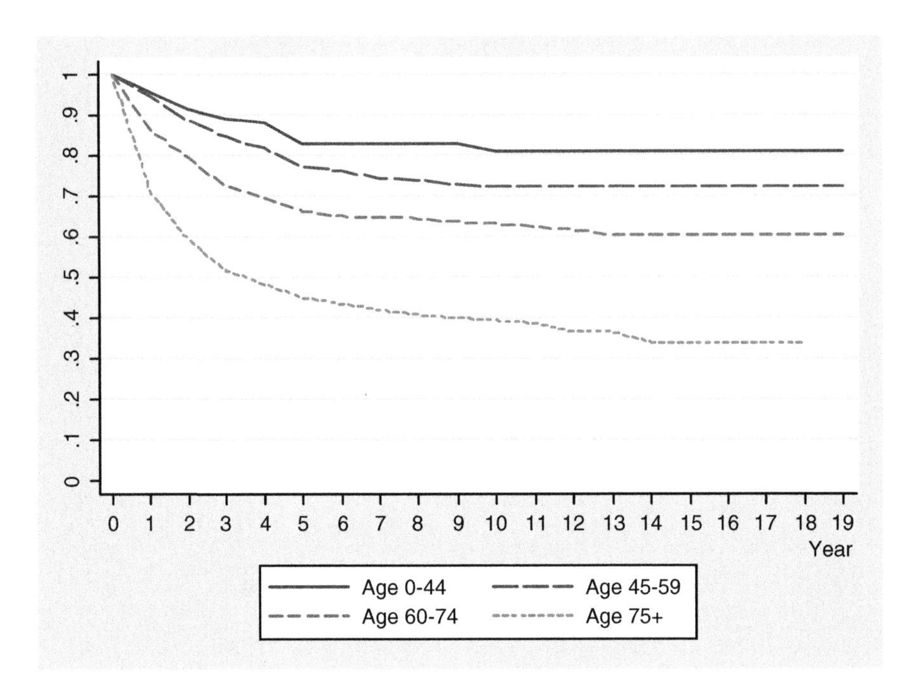

Fig. 2. The cause-specific survival rates of female stomach-cancer patients diagnosed in Finland during 1985–2002 with a localized tumour, by age at diagnosis and follow-up time.

Normally in survival analysis, it is assumed that the risks of dying and censoring are independent, and that the survival for the censored patients would, on average, be the same as for patients that can be followed beyond the time point of censoring. Often, this is likely to be true as the risk of being censored does not depend on the factors that determine the risk of dying.

The normal independence assumption in survival analysis means, for cause-specific survival analysis, that the cause-specific (e.g. stomach-cancer specific) survival for patients dying from other causes would, on average, be the same as for patients that can be followed beyond the time point of death due to other causes. This is not likely to be true, at least, for the stomach-cancer patients. Old patients will be censored relatively early due to their higher mortality due to other causes. Had this censoring not taken place, it would nevertheless been likely that their survival prospects with respect to stomach cancer had been worse than average as stomach-cancer mortality is higher for the older patients.

A control for age by stratification certainly decreases the problem but does not eliminate it completely. With overall dependencies on age it is likely that dependencies, although to a smaller extent, remain within age groups. The problem is similar to residual confounding in epidemiology (Greenland, 1999). Moreover, there may be variables other than age that cause similar complications. Some of them like sex or place of residence may be recorded and thus taken into account, but others like smoking habits or social class may well be unavailable and thus, no direct correction for differences in them can be made.

Let us consider the amount of bias due to dependence between the causes of death that would be introduced by not making the stratification by age. The overall cause-specific survival rates without bias (by assuming independence of the causes of death within the age groups) are obtainable as weighted averages of the age-specific cause-specific survival rates, weights being proportional to the number of patients by age group at the beginning of the follow-up. A comparison between this weighted analysis and a non-weighted analysis, where all age groups have been analysed together, shows that there is a bias towards more favourable survival (Fig. 3). The 15-year unweighted and weighted cause-specific survival rates are 54.5 and 52.1%, respectively, with an upward bias of 54.5 – 52.1 = 2.4% units. As usually both the deaths due to the cancer of the patients and due to other causes are more common in older age groups, the bias resulting from pooling over the age group will be towards more optimistic cause-specific survival rates.

4. EXPECTED SURVIVAL

When the causes of death of individual patients are not available or unreliable, the cause-specific survival analysis introduced above can be substituted with the analysis of relative

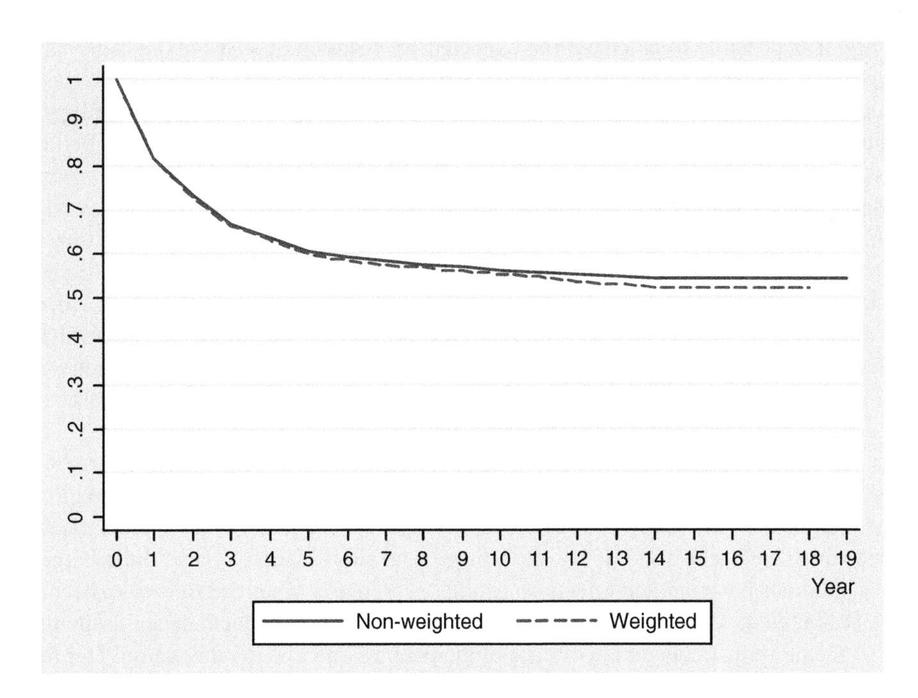

Fig. 3. Weighted averages of the cause-specific survival rates by age and the unweighted cause-specific survival rates of female stomach-cancer patients diagnosed in Finland during 1985–2002 with a localized tumour, by follow-up time.

survival rates. This analysis has been the standard practice at population-based cancer registries for decades (Cutler, 1964; Ries et al., 2002; Berrino et al., 2003).

In relative survival analysis, the mortality due to diseases other than cancer is obtained from the mortality observed in a comparable group of persons in the general population in the geographical area where the cancer registration is in operation. In principle, the mortality due to the patients' disease should be subtracted from the general population mortality, but in practice this subtraction has such a small effect that it may be neglected (Ederer et al., 1961). This analysis does not require cause-specific mortality rates for the general population, which is a clear practical advantage. However, there is also the theoretical advantage that the mortality in a comparable general population group will be independent of the disease of the patients. Clearly, this was a particular advantage in terms of data processing before the advent of readily available modern computing. Further, there is the advantage for interpretation, when relative survival cannot be interpreted as a probability estimate, see Section 5 for relative survival curve.

The life tables (mortality tables) of the general population in the geographical area of cancer registration (or as close to it as possible) are thus used to estimate the mortality due to other causes. It is customary to call this estimate the patients' expected mortality, in the sense that this would be the mortality expected for the patients if they were a sample of the general population, given their age, sex and calendar time of observation. Also other variables, such as place of residence or social class, can be involved when general population life tables are available for these variables (Coleman et al., 1999). Based on the expected mortality, it is possible to calculate the expected proportions of survivors, usually called the expected survival rates, and to create the expected survival curves for the patient groups. These curves show the expected survival rates by follow-up time for the patient groups, by assuming that the patients were subject to general population mortality only. Figure 4 shows the expected survival curves for the stomach-cancer patient groups considered previously. For the youngest patient group, 0–44 years, the rates are closer to 100% whereas for patients aged 75 years or more at diagnosis they fall markedly with follow-up time.

It is of interest to compare the expected survival rates by follow-up time with cause-specific survival rates calculated for other causes of death for the patients, by considering death due to cancer as a censoring event to the follow-up. The comparison shows that in ages below 60 years, up to ten years of follow-up, these rates are not far from each other, but in higher ages, the long-term expected survival rates tend to be somewhat lower than the cause-specific survival rates due to other causes (Table 1).

The expected survival rates may be calculated in a number of ways. The three most common ways in the literature are called the Ederer I, Ederer II and the "Hakulinen" (1982) methods. If the analysis is stratified by age group, it does not matter much in practice which method is used. If however, there is no stratification by age, the differences between methods have marked effects on results, particularly when the follow-up becomes longer (Hakulinen, 1982). The reason is the violation of the independence assumption between the mortalities due to the disease of the patients and due to other causes (for independence assumption, see Section 3) which is equally important for relative survival as it is for cause-specific survival. This is discussed in Section 5 for relative survival.

Here, initially, it may be useful to characterize the differences between the three methods. The Ederer I method calculates the expected survival rate from diagnosis up to a certain length of follow-up as the average of the patient-specific expected survival

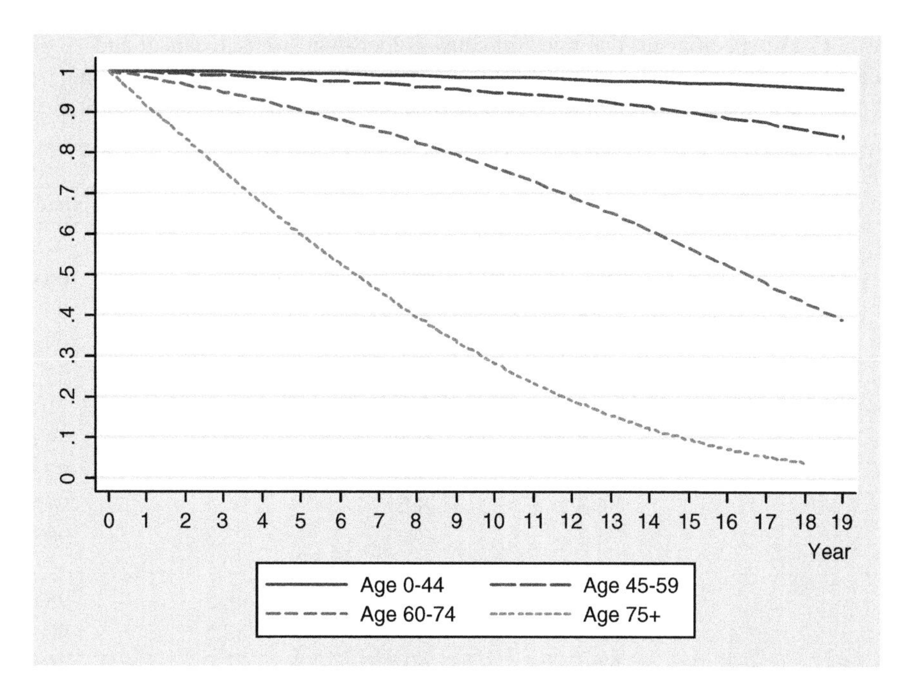

Fig. 4. The expected survival rates of female stomach-cancer patients diagnosed in Finland during 1985–2002 with a localized tumour, by age at diagnosis and follow-up time. The "Hakulinen" method has been used.

probabilities, under the assumption that each patient would be a member of the general population. This method has a conceptual problem for recently diagnosed patients for whom it is not possible to calculate expected 10- or 15-year survival probabilities, as these would be dependent on the mortality experience of the general population in the future. To overcome this problem, it is customary to assume that the general population will have in the future the same mortality as it has had in the most recent period of observation. However, it is probably unwise to compare observed survival of patients with survival that would be expected for some of the patients in the future years yet to come.

The "Hakulinen" method takes the potential follow-up times of the patients into account and produces the expected survival rates from an expected life table where the follow-up times have been censored when the patients cannot be followed any longer. Thus, no general population life tables for future years are needed.

The Ederer II method calculates at each point of follow-up an expected mortality rate for patients under observation. However, which patients are under observation depends also on the mortality due to the disease of the patients before that observation point. Thus, the Ederer II method introduces a dependence between the cause-specific and the expected mortalities which is at variance with the independence assumption between the two causes of death introduced in Section 5 for relative survival.

Table 2 shows the expected survival rates calculated by the three methods for all patients combined. When the follow-up time is prolonged, differences between the methods start

Table 1. Cause-specific survival rates for causes other than stomach cancer and expected survival rates (%) of stomach-cancer patients diagnosed in Finland during 1985–2002 with a localized tumour, by sex and age at diagnosis and follow-up time

Age and follow-up time (years)	Males		Females	
	Other causes	Expected	Other causes	Expected
0–44				
1	100	99.7	100	99.9
5	96.9	98.3	97.5	99.4
10	94.2	96.0	95.4	98.5
15	84.5	92.9	95.4	97.1
45–59				
1	97.8	99.0	99.7	99.6
5	92.7	94.5	96.8	97.9
10	84.3	87.1	95.5	94.9
15	74.2	76.6	93.3	90.0
60–74				
1	93.3	96.5	96.2	98.4
5	82.6	81.6	88.5	90.4
10	63.7	60.8	77.7	76.3
15	42.2	39.4	59.8	56.8
75+				
1	87.6	89.1	90.0	91.6
5	63.4	52.3	68.2	59.9
10	28.1	21.8	37.3	28.4
15	11.3	6.4	15.9	9.5

Table 2. Expected survival rates (%) of stomach-cancer patients diagnosed in Finland during 1985–2002 with a localized tumour, by sex and method of calculation, all ages combined (Hak – "Hakulinen" method, EI – Ederer I method and EII – Ederer II method)

Follow-up time (years)	Males			Females		
	Hak	EI	EII	Hak	EI	EII
1	94.8	94.8	94.8	95.8	95.8	95.8
5	75.9	75.6	78.9	79.1	79.1	82.2
10	56.0	55.1	61.5	60.0	60.1	65.7
15	40.0	38.6	46.1	43.9	44.0	51.0

to emerge. In particular, when the follow-up time is more than ten years, the Ederer II method gives much higher expected survival rates than the two other methods. However, age-specifically, the results given by the different methods do not practically differ from each other (results not shown).

The different methods of calculation of the expected survival rates are not introduced in detail here. There are specialized software for the methods (Hakulinen and Abeywickrama, 1985) but the calculation can also be achieved with general-purpose applications in SAS and STATA (Dickman et al., 2004).

5. RELATIVE SURVIVAL

The relative survival rate is calculated as the ratio between the observed and expected survival rates. The basis for interpreting relative survival as a survival rate, or probability depending on the disease of the patients only, is the independence assumption between the mortality due to the disease of the patients and that due to other causes. Thus, analogously with the cause-specific survival, control for age and other variables is needed and often attempted through stratification of the analysis. The problem of "residual confounding" introduced above for independence assumption remains with relative survival. A particular problem with relative survival that does not have to exist for the cause-specific analysis is that the patients are not necessarily a sample from the general population, not even given age, sex and calendar period. Often the disease risks differ by social class and a number of background variables: consequently, it is impossible to take all this into account in making up a comparable general population group. The study by Dickman et al. (1998) estimated that for Finland the bias by omitting social class is small, but this result may not necessarily hold in many other countries or for other omitted background variables. In Britain, degree of deprivation, corresponding to social class, was taken into account in calculating comparable expected survival rates (Coleman et al., 1999).

Under the independence assumption, the relative survival can be interpreted as the probability of survival given that the disease of the patients was the only cause of death. If this assumption is not valid, a more general interpretation which is still useful may be applied: the relative survival is the ratio between the observed and expected survival rates. In a way, the latter interpretation tells which proportion of the theoretically "maximal" survival rate the patients have had. It is advantageous in that the "maximum" does not depend on the disease see Section 4 for expected survival.

Actually, it is possible that the expected survival rate in the comparable general population group is not a theoretical maximum, as the mortality in the patient group may also be smaller than in the comparable general population group. It may be so due to chance, to the possibility that the patients are under thorough surveillance, or, for example, to the fact that the patients come more from upper than lower social groups or from areas with better than average health services.

Figure 5 shows the relative survival rates by age and follow-up time for the stomach-cancer patients. Although they resemble the cause-specific survival rates in Fig. 2, there is one minor difference, though, between the curves: the relative survival rates may experience counter-intuitive upward turns in some parts of the follow-up. This happens

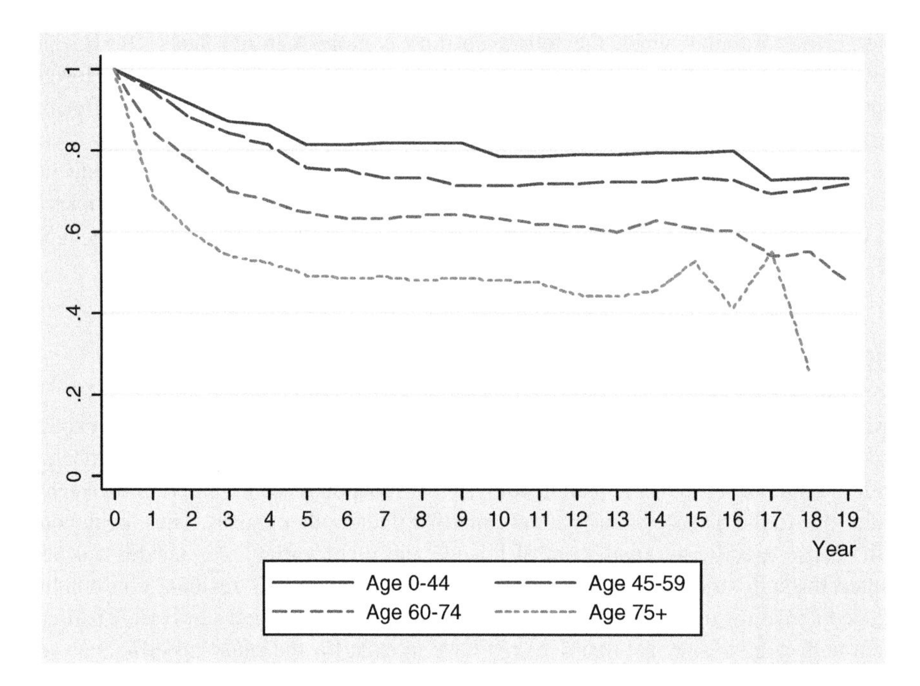

Fig. 5. The relative survival rates of female stomach-cancer patients diagnosed in Finland during 1985–2002 with a localized tumour, by age at diagnosis and follow-up time. The "Hakulinen" method has been used for the expected survival rates.

as there are occasionally periods with no deaths in the patient group even though a very small number of deaths was expected in the comparable general population group, for example, in the age group 0–44 years. In practice, relative survival analysis has to be always conducted using some small, e.g. annual, subintervals of follow-up. In small intervals it is not rare to observe no deaths in a group of patients.

For the stomach-cancer patients the relative and cause-specific survival rates are in a fair agreement, except for longer follow-up times for the older patients where the relative survival rates are clearly higher (Table 3). This is in keeping with the corresponding comparison between the expected and cause-specific survival rates for other causes (Table 1).

If the age groups are combined in a single analysis of observed survival, and the expected survival calculated with the three alternative methods, large differences are found when the follow-up time is longer than ten years (Table 4). It is particularly noteworthy, that the Ederer II method gives a more pessimistic long-term survival prospect than would be expected on the basis of the age-specific relative survival rates (Table 3).

It would, in principle, be best to do the relative survival analyses age-specifically and to calculate the overall relative survival rates by follow-up time as weighted averages of the age-specific relative survival rates, with weights proportional to the number of patients at the beginning of follow-up by age group (method WRR in Fig. 3 in Hakulinen, 1977, p. 437).

Table 3. Observed, cause-specific and relative survival rates (%) of stomach-cancer patients diagnosed in Finland during 1985–2002 with a localized tumour, by sex and age at diagnosis and follow-up time

	Males			Females		
Age and follow-up time (years)	Observed	Cause-specific	Relative	Observed	Cause-specific	Relative
0–44						
1	94.9	95.7	95.2	95.7	95.7	95.8
5	79.4	82.6	80.8	80.8	82.9	81.3
10	74.2	79.5	77.3	77.3	81.1	78.6
15	64.0	76.3	68.9	77.3	81.1	79.6
45–59						
1	89.8	92.1	90.7	94.2	94.5	94.6
5	66.3	72.1	70.1	74.2	77.3	75.8
10	55.8	68.1	64.1	67.6	72.3	71.2
15	47.8	66.4	62.4	66.0	72.3	73.3
60–74						
1	78.0	84.2	80.8	83.1	86.4	84.5
5	49.6	62.0	60.8	58.5	66.3	64.7
10	32.6	56.5	53.7	48.2	63.1	63.2
15	20.3	53.0	51.4	34.5	60.5	60.9
75+						
1	57.7	67.0	64.8	63.2	71.2	69.0
5	24.4	41.3	46.7	29.5	45.0	49.3
10	9.3	36.9	42.5	13.6	39.4	48.1
15	3.4	34.0	53.2	5.0	34.1	52.6

Table 4. Relative survival rates (%) of stomach-cancer patients diagnosed in Finland during 1985–2002 with a localized tumour, by sex and method of expected rate calculation, all ages combined (Hak – "Hakulinen" method, EI – Ederer I method and EII – Ederer II method)

	Males			Females		
Follow-up time (years)	Hak	EI	EII	Hak	EI	EII
1	78.8	78.8	78.8	80.4	80.4	80.4
5	61.4	61.6	59.0	62.9	62.8	60.4
10	58.0	59.0	52.8	63.4	63.3	57.9
15	58.1	60.2	50.3	67.1	67.0	57.8

The problem with this approach is that for the oldest age group it will be difficult to obtain long-term relative survival rates. For example, for the oldest age group of the stomach-cancer patients, 75 years or more at diagnosis, a 15-year follow-up means that the patients have to age up to 90 years or more. The expected survival rate is low, and the relative survival rate is based on very few observed patients and thus very unstable. On the other hand, this unstable rate has a large weight because of the high proportion of old patients at the beginning of the follow-up, and thus the overall weighted relative survival rate is unstable, too. The relative survival rate might well also be unavailable as none of the surviving patients would have had a sufficiently long follow-up. This is the situation after 18 years of follow-up for the oldest age group in the figures.

For these reasons, arguments have been given for unstratified analysis (Brenner and Hakulinen, 2004a), where relative survival simply has the interpretation of a ratio between the observed and expected survival rates. The unstratified analysis is biased by the dependence between the disease-specific and the expected mortality. When the dependence has not been adjusted for, counter-intuitive results by long-term relative survival rates increasing with follow-up time are occasionally observed (Hakulinen, 1977). Most problematic is, however, that biases will be hidden in long-term survival rates even when they do not look counter-intuitive.

Figure 6 shows the results of weighted (stratified) and non-weighted relative survival analyses of the stomach-cancer patients. The non-weighted results (RSR) tend to be higher than in the long-term follow-up more unstable weighted results (WRR), which do possess the desired interpretation of survival rate estimates for the patients when their cancer only is considered as a possible cause of death. This interpretation, however desirable, is nevertheless theoretical in nature. The non-stratified result has the more general rather simple interpretation of a ratio between the observed and expected survival rates: this ratio does not have an interpretation as a probability estimate and therefore a cumulative relative survival curve (RSR) does not look anything like a real survival curve. This issue has been, unfortunately, mostly neglected in the relative survival analysis literature. Moreover, this ratio is dependent on the patterns of censoring by age which may vary between populations (Hakulinen, 1982).

One could imagine that the bias in long-term relative survival rates from the probability interpretation viewpoint could be avoided by calculating a ratio between the appropriately weighted observed survival rates and the similarly weighted expected survival rates (i.e. in the extreme, each patient making a separate age stratum, the Ederer I method for expected survival rates). This does not, however, remove the inherent dependence between the disease-specific mortality and the mortality due to other causes (see the WOR method in Hakulinen (1977), and the corresponding curve in Fig. 6). This method only controls for differences in the age-specific patterns of censoring.

Most relative survival analyses are conducted for survival times up to five years. The age-specific analyses usually do not create any problems whichever method is used to calculate expected survival, and the biases introduced by not stratifying for age are unlikely to be overly large. It is, nevertheless, good to be aware of them so that they can be quantified and corrected whenever needed by more appropriate analytical approaches.

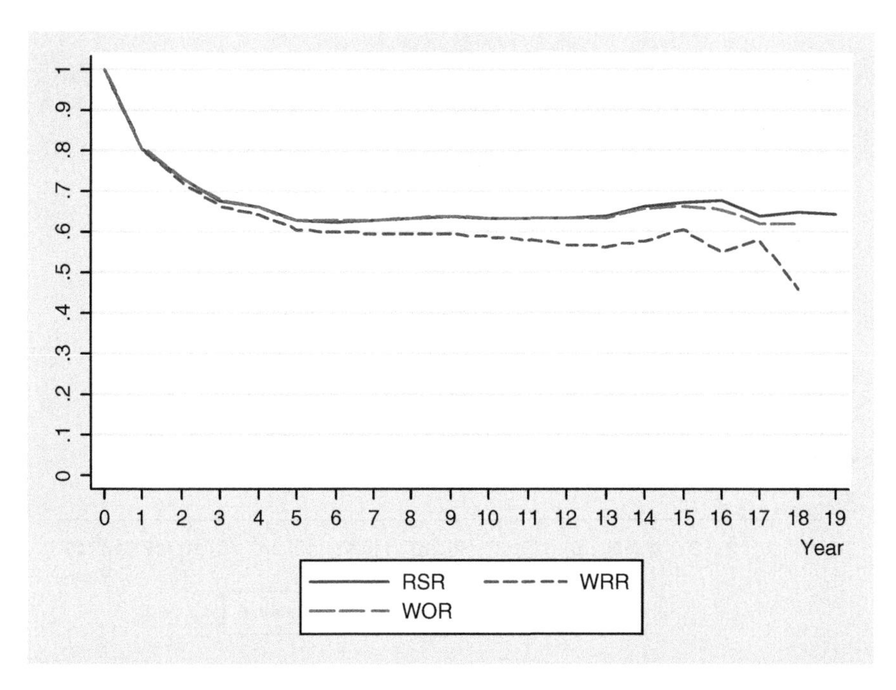

Fig. 6. Weighted averages of the age-specific relative survival rates (WRR), the unweighted relative survival rates (RSR) and ratios between the weighted averages of the age-specific observed and expected survival rates (WOR) of female stomach-cancer patients diagnosed in Finland during 1985–2002 with a localized tumour, by follow-up time.

6. POINT OF CURE

Often it is of interest to know when the patients under follow-up are cured. For cause-specific survival analysis that point of follow-up time is the earliest after which the patients no longer die from their disease. For the relative survival analysis that point is the earliest time after which the patients have the same mortality as the comparable general population group. As introduced in Section 4 for expected survival, the Ederer II method is the one that produces expected mortality for patients under follow-up at a particular time of follow-up. It is thus possible using this method to compare, e.g. the observed one-year survival rates of the patients under observation at the beginning of each follow-up year with those expected for a comparable general population group.

Figure 7 shows the results of such a comparison for the stomach-cancer patients. The ratio between the annual observed and expected survival rates is approximately 100% after six years of follow-up. The annual cause-specific survival rates calculated for comparison agree with this estimate: there are virtually no deaths due to stomach cancer after six years of follow-up.

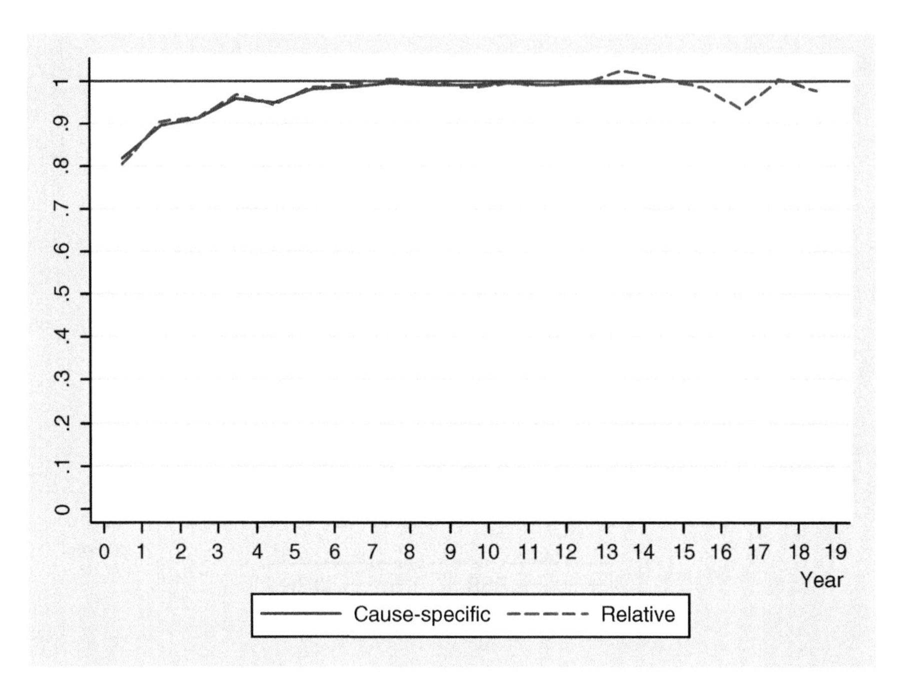

Fig. 7. Annual cause-specific and relative survival rates of female stomach-cancer patients diagnosed in Finland during 1985–2002 with a localized tumour.

The appropriately estimated cause-specific and relative survival rates for patients at the beginning of follow-up up to the point of cure give the estimates for the proportion of patients cured. The six-year cause-specific and relative survival rates for that purpose from the weighted analyses are 58.5 and 59.9%, respectively. The non-weighted analyses give 59.1 and 62.5% for these two rates, respectively. Between the relative survival rates there is thus a 2.6% unit (62.5 – 59.9%) difference which may be considered as a bias for the probability interpretation.

7. REGRESSION ANALYSIS

There are several factors related to the patient and tumour that affect the cause-specific and relative survival. The cause-specific analyses can be conducted analogously to overall survival analyses by using death due to patients' cancer as the "death" and death due to other causes as an event censoring the follow-up time. The independence assumption remains, but conditionally on the factors included in the model of analysis. The most usual model for these analyses is the Cox proportional hazards (mortalities) model with its time-dependent extensions. These extensions are often needed with materials from the population-based cancer registries, as the cause-specific hazards (mortalities) tend to be non-proportional with follow-up time, particularly with respect to variables such as age and stage at diagnosis. For example for stage, the effect on the cause-specific hazard is marked during the early years of follow-up but disappears later on in the longer term follow-up. The analysis by the Cox model and its extensions is taught in many textbooks of survival analysis and can be conducted using major statistical software packages.

There are also analogous regression models for relative survival. Basically, all the five models cited in the literature are equivalent although they differ from each other with respect to assumptions about the data aggregation level and error structures (Dickman et al., 2004). In relative survival regression, the cause-specific hazard is substituted with excess hazard (mortality). The excess hazard or excess mortality of the patients is defined as the difference between the total mortality of the patients and the mortality expected in the comparable general population group.

Taking the male and female stomach-cancer patients as an example, the five-year relative survival rates of the patients depend strongly on tumour stage but much less on age or sex (Table 5). The regression model for the first five years of follow-up confirms this fact but also shows strong non-proportionality for the stage- and age-specific excess hazards. In Cox regression the effects are measured with hazard ratios. In relative survival analysis the corresponding quantities are the excess hazard ratios (EHRs), also called as relative excess risks. For example, when the tumour is localized the females have a significant advantage over the males (EHR = 1.18) that can be assumed to hold for the five years of follow-up (Table 6). The EHR decreases significantly by 21% between each consecutive six-year period of diagnosis. Due to non-proportionality of the excess hazards by age, the EHR for patients with a localized tumour does not remain constant over the five-year follow-up. In the first year of follow-up, the EHR in the oldest age group is more than nine times that in the youngest age group, whereas this difference disappears by the fifth year of follow-up (Table 6).

Table 5. Five-year observed and relative survival rates (%) of stomach-cancer patients diagnosed in Finland during 1985–2002 by sex, age and stage at diagnosis

	Males		Females	
Stage and age (years)	Observed	Relative	Observed	Relative
Localized				
0–44	79.4	80.8	80.8	81.3
45–59	66.2	70.1	74.2	75.8
60–74	49.6	60.8	58.5	64.7
75+	24.4	46.7	29.5	49.3
Non-localized				
0–44	7.1	7.3	13.4	13.5
45–59	9.5	10.1	9.2	9.4
60–74	5.6	6.9	8.6	9.6
75+	3.7	7.0	3.8	6.2

Table 6. The model-based excess hazard ratios (EHRs), with 95% confidence intervals, for stomach-cancer patients diagnosed in Finland during 1985–2002 with a localized tumour

Variable	EHR	95% CI
Sex		
Males	1.18	1.05–1.32
Females	1.00	Reference
Six-year period of diagnosis	0.79	0.74–0.86
Follow-up year and age		
1		
0–44	1.09	0.34–3.53
45–64	1.88	0.68–5.17
65–74	4.67	1.75–12.5
75+	9.91	3.72–26.4
2		
0–44	1.15	0.36–3.72
45–64	2.04	0.74–5.62
65–74	2.02	0.75–5.49
75+	3.64	1.34–9.90
3		
0–44	0.97	0.27–3.30
45–64	1.41	0.50–3.99
65–74	2.41	0.89–6.53
75+	2.99	1.08–8.32
4		
0–44	0.74	0.20–2.76
45–64	0.70	0.23–2.16
65–74	1.24	0.44–3.51
75+	1.78	0.59–5.38
5		
0–44	0.97	0.28–3.41
45–64	1.58	0.56–4.49
65–74	1.06	0.37–3.08
75+	1.00	Reference

The biases between the different methods of calculation of the expected survival rates do not enter the regression analyses of relative survival rates when the relevant variables, particularly age, have been accounted for by a proper model in the analyses. In practice, patients' mortality is compared with expected mortality in each subinterval of follow-up. Thus, for the regression analyses, the Ederer II method is used to derive the expected mortality.

Relatively little work has so far been devoted to summarize the model-based excess hazard ratios by using model-based relative survival rates (Esteve et al., 1990), particularly with non-proportional excess hazards (Giorgi et al., 2003). Dyba and Hakulinen (1994)

using GLIM (Generalized Linear Interactive Modelling, see The GLIM System, 1993) have produced model-based confidence intervals for them. The model-based relative survival rates are free from biases cited above for the various approaches in simple relative survival analysis. Thus, the analyses should become more model-based in practice. It is important that the model used fits the empirical data appropriately.

When the model does fit, the model-based estimates have a smaller standard error than the empirical estimates (Table 7). The empirical and model-based estimates differ as the entire data set has been used in the modelling instead of a particular subset. From the modelling point of view, the difference may be accounted for by the removal of unnecessary randomness in the estimates.

8. PERIOD ANALYSIS

Traditionally, the problem with all longer term survival analyses has been that their results are too out of date to be generalized to currently diagnosed patients. Brenner and Gefeller (1996) suggested that the practice from demography for the estimation of the expectation of life should be followed in order to achieve survival rates that are more up-to-date. In demography, the population is, in principle, followed up from birth to death but the last deaths will occur more than 100 years after the birth. The expectation of life is calculated using observed survival rates by one-year age groups in the population. Instead of waiting for more than 100 years, demographers have decided to use always most up-to-date observed one-year survival rates, i.e. from the most recent calendar year: thus, the resulting expectation of life is more up-to-date for the persons currently under observation. On the other hand, it is interpreted as a theoretical expectation of life for a person who would have the one-year observed probabilities of survival equal to those prevailing in the most recent calendar year.

This approach, called period analysis by Brenner and Gefeller, works also for observed and relative survival analysis although, in order to achieve statistical precision in the estimates, the annual follow-up year-specific observed or relative survival rates may have to be adopted from patients under observation during a few recent calendar years instead

Table 7. The model-based and the empirical five-year relative survival rates (RSR, %) for female stomach-cancer patients diagnosed in Finland during 1985–1990 with a localized tumour, with standard errors, by age. The model in Table 6 has been applied

	Model-based		Empirical	
Age (years)	RSR	SE	RSR	SE
0–44	80.0	3.1	69.5	7.2
45–64	70.8	2.2	69.1	4.3
65–74	59.7	2.0	59.1	3.3
75+	41.7	2.5	39.5	3.9

of one calendar year (Brenner and Hakulinen, 2002). There is statistical software to take care of the analysis (Brenner et al., 2004b; Dickman et al., 2004).

For example, the five-year relative survival rates for male and female stomach-cancer patients diagnosed during 1985–2002 with a localized tumour and followed up until the end of 2003 were 61 and 63%, respectively. If the follow-up of patients is restricted to the period 1998–2003 both of these rates are much higher, 69 and 73%, respectively. These may be regarded as predictions for recently diagnosed patients.

9. AGE STANDARDIZATION

It is clear that the comparison between relative survival rates in different patient groups could be based on regression models. However, there is also a need for tools to make simple descriptive comparisons. The relative survival rates depend on age, and comparisons between them have been made using the direct method of age standardization: the age-specific relative survival rates have been weighted with a constant set of weights, typically proportional to a real or hypothetical distribution of patients at diagnosis (Cutler, 1964; Black and Bashir, 1998; Corazziari et al., 2004). These weights work well and for shorter term follow-up give estimates for relative survival rates that can be interpreted as survival rates of patients if the disease was the only cause of death and if the age distribution of the patients were the same as that in the standard population from which the weights have been derived.

Brenner and Hakulinen (2003, 2004a) have pointed out that often the traditionally standardized rates appear rather low, particularly compared to the non-standardized rates. They have suggested two new methods of age standardization of which one does not even require a relative survival analysis by age groups. These methods give results that are consistent with the non-standardized relative survival rates when the relative survival rates are standardized by using the patient material itself as the standard. This is, of course, a useful feature, but makes the standardized rates subject to the biases introduced earlier as a result of the dependence between the cause-specific and expected mortalities.

Thus, the rates standardized in these new methods cannot be interpreted as survival probabilities when the disease of the patients is the only cause of death. They can be interpreted as ratios between the observed and expected survival rates if the patients have the same age distribution at the beginning of the follow-up as the reference population and, in one of the methods (Brenner and Hakulinen, 2003), also the same age-specific expected survival rates as the reference population. Using the other method (Brenner and Hakulinen, 2004a), also differences in the age-specific patterns of censoring affect the standardized rates.

The traditional method of age standardization does not have these problems. Thus, the choice of method of age standardization depends on which interpretation is desired for the standardized rates and on how much precision is desirable in the comparison.

10. PARAMETRIC METHODS

It is possible to combine the regression analyses of relative survival and of proportion cured. The idea is that the patients can be partitioned to a proportion cured, subject to the mortality in the comparable general population group only, and to a proportion bound to die from the disease of the patients, subject additionally to excess mortality (Verdecchia et al., 1998; de Angelis et al., 1999; Sposto, 2002). Both components may depend on factors related to the patient or tumour.

In order to achieve efficiency in the analysis, parametric models are called for. The proportion cured is modelled as a logistic function of the factors, whereas Weibull models have had success when fitted to the excess hazard.

The results of these analyses are particularly useful when interpreting changes over time or differentials between patient groups. For example, it may be possible to distinguish whether an improvement in relative survival over time may be attributable to an increased proportion cured, or to an increased length of life of those bound to die from the disease, or to both of these possibilities. These may thus help in interpreting whether the increase in relative survival is a genuine improvement in patient survival or merely the result of an earlier diagnosis with no real effect on survival.

11. MULTIPLE TUMOURS

The cause-specific and relative survival rate analyses can be generalized for analyses of multiple tumours. These generalizations may also involve parametric methods and proportions of cure (Heinävaara and Hakulinen, 2002a).

The cause-specific analyses, even with various factors affecting cause-specific mortality, can be generalized in a rather straightforward way when the cause of death information can be used, provided that the different (usually two) tumours of the patient are not located in the same organ. When they are, the cancer registry may have additional information as to which one of the tumours was the cause of death (Heinävaara et al., 2002).

The relative survival analyses are based on the assumption that each new tumour brings an additional component of excess hazard with relevant factors affecting it (Heinävaara and Hakulinen, 2002b). The additional components can be estimated by, for example, comparing the survival in the patient group with two tumours with that in a group with one tumour only. Although the principles of these analyses are clear, their implementation may be rather technically challenging.

The interesting question in these analyses is whether a certain cancer as a subsequent tumour is more severe to the patient than as the first tumour, given the relevant factors affecting the survival. The results so far indicate that this is not necessarily the case always (Heinävaara, 2003).

12. CONCLUSION

Relative survival analysis is a useful technique, particularly for the analysis of population-based cancer survival rates but may also be useful for other diseases (Heinämäki et al., 1986). There is still some progress to be made in improving its user-friendliness, particularly in converting the results on the excess hazard ratios of the regression analyses to relative survival rates with interpretation. The simple analysis results are subject to biases that may not be marked with short follow-up times but may be quite severe with longer periods of follow-up.

Relative survival analysis and its extensions have been used successfully in estimating cancer incidence on the basis of cancer mortality (Verdecchia et al., 1989) and in predicting cancer mortality and prevalence on the basis of cancer incidence (Hakulinen et al., 1989; Verdecchia et al., 2002). They can be used in estimating the expectations of life for cancer patients (Hakama and Hakulinen, 1977). Simple generalizations of the log-rank tests have been made for the relative survival rates (Hakulinen et al., 1987) but they can also be easily implemented as special cases in regression modelling. Multiplicative hazards, with a possibility of individual follow-up time scale transformations based on expected hazard may provide interesting alternative insights into the data (Stare et al., 2005).

The relative survival analyses make the cause-specific analysis of cancer patient survival independent of whether the causes of death of the patients are available or not. In so doing, any difference between the mortality of the patients and the expected mortality in a comparable general population group will be attributed to the patients' cancer. For example, lung-cancer patients have an increased mortality also due to the other causes of death, attributable to the main cause of lung cancer, smoking. This additional mortality will in relative survival analyses be included in the excess hazard of lung-cancer patients. This excess hazard is of interest by itself but caution must be exercised when attributing that excess hazard to lung cancer.

Relative survival analysis is a useful but challenging method. With a good knowledge on problems related to it and a careful application, it may be used and developed to solve many important problems in cancer care in the population.

REFERENCES

Berrino, F., R. Capocaccia, M.P. Coleman, J. Esteve, G. Gatta, T. Hakulinen, A. Micheli, M. Sant and A. Verdecchia (Eds.), 2003, Survival of cancer patients in Europe: the Eurocare-3 study. Ann. Oncol. 14 (Suppl. 5): V1–V155.

Black, R.J. and S.A Bashir, 1998, World standard cancer patient populations: a resource for comparative analysis of survival data. In: R. Sankaranarayanan, R.J. Black and D.M. Parkin (Eds.), Cancer Survival in Developing Countries. IARC Scientific Publications, No. 145, Lyon, pp. 9–11.

Brenner, H. and O. Gefeller, 1996, An alternative approach to monitoring cancer patient survival. Cancer, 78, 2004–2010.

Brenner, H. and T. Hakulinen, 2002, Up-to-date long-term survival curves of patients with cancer by period analysis. J. Clin. Oncol., 20, 826–832.

Brenner, H. and T. Hakulinen, 2003, On crude and age-adjusted relative survival rates. J. Clin. Epidemiol., 56, 1185–1191.

Brenner, H., V. Arndt, O. Gefeller and T. Hakulinen, 2004a, An alternative approach to age adjustment of cancer survival rates. Eur. J. Cancer, 40, 2317–2322.

Brenner, H., O. Gefeller and T. Hakulinen, 2004b, Period analysis for "up-to-date" cancer survival data: theory, empirical evaluation, computational realisation and applications. Eur. J. Cancer, 40, 326–335.

Coleman, M.P., P. Babb, P. Damiecki, P. Grosclaude, S. Honjo, J. Jones, G. Knerer, A. Pitard, M. Quinn, A. Sloggett and B. de Stavola, 1999, Cancer Survival Trends in England and Wales, 1971–1995: Deprivation and NHS Region. Studies in Medical and Population Subjects No. 61. The Stationery Office, London.

Corazziari, I., M. Quinn and R. Capocaccia, 2004, Standard cancer patient populations for age standardising survival ratios. Eur. J. Cancer, 40, 2307–2316.

Cutler, S.J. (Ed.), 1964, International Symposium on End Results of Cancer Therapy. National Cancer Institute Monograph 15, Washington.

de Angelis, R., R. Capocaccia, T. Hakulinen, B. Söderman and A. Verdecchia, 1999, Mixture models of cancer survival analysis: application to population-based data with covariates. Stat. Med., 18, 441–454.

Dickman, P., A. Auvinen, E.T. Voutilainen and T. Hakulinen, 1998, Measuring social class differences in cancer patient survival: is it necessary to control for social class differences in general population mortality? A Finnish population-based study. J. Epidemiol. Comm. Health, 52, 1–8.

Dickman, P., A. Sloggett, M. Hills and T. Hakulinen, 2004, Regression models for relative survival. Stat. Med., 23, 51–64.

Dyba, T. and T. Hakulinen, 1994, Confidence intervals for model-based cumulative relative survival rates using GLIM. GLIM Newsl., 23, 29–35.

Ederer, F., L.M. Axtell and S.J Cutler, 1961, The relative survival rate: a statistical methodology. Natl. Cancer Inst. Monogr., 6, 101–121.

Elandt-Johnson, R., 1975, Definition of rates: some remarks on their use and misuse. Amer. J. Epidemiol., 102, 267–271.

Esteve, J., E. Benhamou, M. Croasdale and L. Raymond, 1990, Relative survival and the estimation of net survival: elements for further discussion. Stat. Med., 9, 529–538.

Giorgi, R., M. Abrahamowicz, C. Quantin, P. Bolard, J. Esteve, J. Gouvernet and J. Faivre, 2003, A relative survival regression model using B-spline functions to model non-proportional hazards. Stat. Med., 22, 2767–2784.

Greenland, S., 1999, Confounding. In: P. Armitage and T. Colton (Eds.), Encyclopedia of Biostatistics, Vol. 1, Wiley, Chichester, pp. 900–907.

Hakama, M. and T. Hakulinen, 1977, Estimating the expectation of life in cancer survival studies with incomplete follow-up information. J. Chron. Dis., 30, 585–597.

Hakulinen, T., 1977, On long-term relative survival rates. J. Chron. Dis., 30, 431–443.

Hakulinen, T., 1982, Cancer survival corrected for heterogeneity in patient withdrawal. Biometrics, 38, 933–942.

Hakulinen, T. and K.H. Abeywickrama, 1985, A computer program package for relative survival analysis. Comp. Progr. Biomed., 19, 197–207.

Hakulinen, T. and L. Teppo, 1977, Causes of death among female patients with cancer of the breast and intestines. Ann. Clin. Res., 9, 15–24.

Hakulinen, T., L. Tenkanen, K. Abeywickrama and L. Päivärinta, 1987, Testing equality of relative survival patterns based on aggregated data. Biometrics, 43, 313–325.

Hakulinen, T., M. Kenward, T. Luostarinen, H. Oksanen, E. Pukkala, B. Söderman and L. Teppo, 1989, Cancer in Finland in 1954–2008. Incidence, Mortality and Prevalence by Region. Cancer Society of Finland Publ. No. 42, Helsinki.

Heinämäki, P., M. Haavisto, T. Hakulinen, K. Mattila and S. Rajala, 1986, Mortality in relation of urinary characteristics in the very aged. Gerontology, 32, 167–171.

Heinävaara, S., 2003, Modelling Survival of Patients with Multiple Cancers. Statistical Research Reports 18, The Finnish Statistical Society, Helsinki.

Heinävaara, S. and T. Hakulinen, 2002a, Parametric mixture model for analysing relative survival of patients with multiple cancers. J. Cancer Epidemiol. Prev., 7, 147–153.

Heinävaara, S. and T. Hakulinen, 2002b, Relative survival of patients with subsequent cancer. J. Cancer Epidemiol. Prev., 7, 173–179.

Heinävaara, S., L.Teppo and T. Hakulinen, 2002, Cancer-specific survival of patients with multiple cancers: an application to patients with multiple breast cancers. Stat. Med., 21, 3183–3195.

Peto, R., M.C. Pike, P. Armitage, N.E. Breslow, D.R. Cox, S.V. Howard, N. Mantel, K. McPherson, J.Peto and P.G. Smith, 1976, Design and analysis of randomized clinical trials requiring prolonged observation of each patient. I. Introduction and design. Br. J. Cancer, 34, 585–612.

Peto, R., M.C. Pike, P. Armitage, N.E. Breslow, D.R. Cox, S.V. Howard, N. Mantel, K. McPherson, J.Peto and P.G. Smith, 1977, Design and analysis of randomized clinical trials requiring prolonged observation of each patient. II. Analysis and examples. Br. J. Cancer, 35, 1–39.

Ries, L.A.G., M.P. Eisner, C.L. Kosary, B.F. Hankey, B.A. Miller, L. Clegg and B.K. Edwards (Eds.), 2002, SEER Cancer Statistics Review, 1973–1999. National Cancer Institute, Bethesda.

Sposto, R., 2002, Cure model analysis in cancer: an application to data from the Children's Cancer Group. Stat. Med., 21, 293–312.

Stare, J., R. Henderson and M. Pohar, 2005, An individual measure of relative survival, Appl. Stat., 54, 115–126.
The GLIM System, 1993, Release 4 Manual, Clarendon Press, Oxford.
Verdecchia, A., R. Capocaccia, V. Egidi and A. Golini, 1989, A method for the estimation of chronic disease morbidity and trends from mortality data. Stat. Med., 8, 201–216.
Verdecchia, A., R. de Angelis, R. Capocaccia, M. Sant, A. Micheli, G. Gatta and F. Berrino, 1998, The cure for colon cancer: results from the EUROCARE study. Int. J. Cancer, 77, 322–329
Verdecchia, A., G. de Angelis and R. Capocaccia, 2002, Estimation and projections of cancer prevalence from cancer registry data. Stat. Med., 21, 3511–3526.

Section 2

Biological and Genetic Factors

Chapter 4

Environmental and Genetic Risk Factors of Lung Cancer

Adrian Cassidy and John K. Field

Roy Castle Lung Cancer Research Programme, The University of Liverpool Cancer Research Centre, The University of Liverpool, 200 London Road, Liverpool L3 9TA, UK
Email: cassidya@livac.uk and J.K.Field@liv.ac.uk

Abstract

Lung cancer accounts for more than one million deaths per year worldwide. Disease survival is poor with a 5-year mortality of approximately 90% and the only option for control is through avoidance of exposure to lung carcinogens. Although the molecular changes that characterise lung cancer are complex, tobacco smoking is well established as the major aetiological risk factor for lung cancer. Risk factors that have been shown to increase the risk of lung cancer can be grouped into genetic and environmental, with both positive and negative associated risks. Environmental risk factors can be further subdivided into those encountered through smoking, occupation, domestic and outdoor environment, and diet. This chapter examines the major known lung cancer risk factors and endeavours to place each in perspective.

The way forward for improved management and prognosis for individuals who are at risk of developing lung cancer lies with early detection of disease prior to clinical symptoms. Ultimately our understanding of the genetic and environmental basis of lung cancers will enable us to identify high-risk populations and to develop effective prevention, early detection and chemoprevention strategies.

Keywords: Lung cancer, incidence, mortality, smoking, occupation, air pollution, diet, genetic susceptibility, socioeconomic status, gender, prior lung disease, familial, polymorphism, gene, prevention, early detection.

Contents

Outcome Prediction in Cancer
Edited by A.F.G. Taktak and A.C. Fisher
© 2007 Elsevier B.V. All rights reserved

1. INTRODUCTION

Lung cancer is the result of molecular changes that occur in the cell, resulting in the deregulation of pathways, which control normal cellular growth, differentiation and apoptosis (Ross and Rosen, 2002). It is the most common cancer in the world, both in terms of incidence (1.35 million new cases, representing 12.4% of all new cancers) and mortality (1.18 million deaths, or 17.6% of the world total) (Parkin et al., 2005). Lung cancer is clinically divided into two categories: non-small cell lung cancer (NSCLC), including squamous cell carcinoma, adenocarcinoma and large cell carcinoma, representing approximately 80% of all lung cancers and small cell lung cancer (SCLC). These two major types of lung cancers are in essence two completely different diseases, each of which has its own recommended therapies. NSCLCs (squamous cell, adenocarcinoma and large cell carcinoma) are potentially curable with surgery, but largely unresponsive to chemotherapy. Patients with distant metastases from NSCLC can be treated palliatively with radiation. Conversely SCLCs do respond to chemotherapy and radiation, but are usually too far advanced at diagnosis for a surgical cure.

Despite advances in the treatment of lung cancer, survival rates have changed little in the last decade, and long-term survival remains poor. The 5-year survival of all patients with lung cancer is only 6% in the UK (Coleman et al., 2004). The major reason for these dismal statistics is that lung cancer is typically diagnosed at an advanced stage and hence, is unresectable for cure. In contrast, the 5-year survival of stage 1 lung cancer is approximately 70%, thereby suggesting that if the diagnosis were to be made at an earlier stage, the outcome in these individuals could be vastly improved (Ganti and Mulshine, 2005).

Although the molecular changes that characterise lung cancer are complex, tobacco smoking is well established as the major aetiological risk factor for lung cancer. Risk factors that have been shown to increase the risk of lung cancer can be grouped into genetic and environmental (with both positive and negative associated risks) (Beckett, 1993). Environmental risk factors can be further subdivided into those encountered through smoking, occupation, domestic and outdoor environment, and diet. The discussion that follows examines the major known lung cancer risk factors and attempts to place each in perspective.

2. LUNG CANCER INCIDENCE AND MORTALITY

Lung cancer incidence varies markedly throughout the world (Parkin et al., 2005). In men, the incidence rate, including all histologic types, varies up to 35-fold between high and low-risk areas. The highest rates are recorded among African Americans in the United States and in Lower Silesia, Poland, while the lowest rates are recorded in Africa. Males consistently show higher lung cancer incidence than females in all populations, with male: female ratios varying approximately from 1.5 to 20 (Parkin et al., 2003). At present, more men than women die each year from lung cancer, but in recent years a rapid increase in lung cancer mortality has been observed among women in developed countries, contrasting with a levelling off or decrease among men (Bray et al., 2004; Tyczynski et al., 2004; Parkin et al., 2005).

The estimated number of lung cancer cases worldwide has increased by 51% since 1985 (+44% in men and +76% in women) (Parkin et al., 2005). This overall upward trend disguises substantial differences between countries. In men, several populations have now passed the peak of the tobacco-related epidemic, and incidence and mortality rates are now declining, such as in the United States (Jemal et al., 2001) and the countries of northern and western Europe (Bray et al., 2004). In contrast, incidence and mortality are increasing rapidly in Southern and Eastern European countries (Tyczynski et al., 2004). In women, the epidemic is less advanced; a rising trend in incidence and morality is observed in most Western countries, although in the United Kingdom, it seems that the peak may now have been reached (Jemal et al., 2004). The observed patterns in lung cancer rates reflect the historical prevalences of smoking among men and women, variations in cigarette composition and more recent cessation rates (Forey et al., 2002; Bray et al., 2004). As the lung cancer epidemic begins to subside in the developed countries, it is on the rise in the developing world (Boffetta and Parkin, 1994).

2.1. Smoking and lung cancer

Smoking of tobacco products, and in particular of cigarettes, is responsible for most cases of lung cancer with an attributable proportion estimated to be in the order of 90% in men and 80% in women (Peto et al., 1992; Mannino et al., 2001; Simonato et al., 2001; Jemal et al., 2003; Crispo et al., 2004). Among the 4000 identified chemicals in cigarette smoke, more than 60 are established carcinogens (IARC, 2004). In relation to human lung cancer, arguably the most important carcinogens are polycyclic aromatic hydrocarbons (PAHs) such as benzo[*a*]pyrene and the tobacco-specific nitrosamine 4-(methylnitrosamino)-1-(3-pyridyl)-1-butanone (also known as nicotine-derived nitrosaminoketone (NNK)) (Hecht, 1999).

Most tobacco carcinogens require metabolic activation to exert their carcinogenic effects; there are competing detoxification pathways and the balance between metabolic activation and detoxification differs among individuals and affects cancer risk (Fig. 1) (Wogan et al., 2004). Metabolic activation leads to the formation of DNA adducts, which are carcinogen metabolites bound covalently to DNA. DNA adducts are absolutely central to the carcinogenic process (Hecht, 1999; Tang et al., 2001). If their formation is inhibited or blocked, so is carcinogenesis (Hecht, 2003). If DNA adducts escape cellular

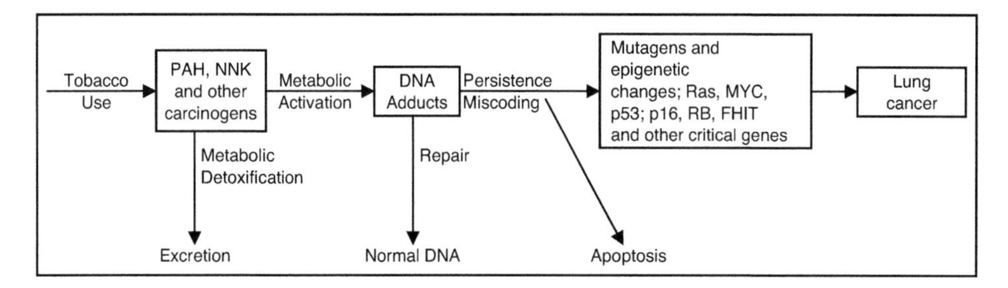

Fig. 1. Scheme linking lung cancer and tobacco smoke carcinogens and their induction of multiple mutations in critical genes.

repair mechanisms and persist, they may lead to miscoding, resulting in permanent mutations (Westra et al., 1993; Denissenko et al., 1996). Cells with DNA damage may be removed by apoptosis or programmed cell death. If a permanent mutation occurs in a critical region of an oncogene or tumour suppressor gene, it can lead to activation of the oncogene or deactivation of the tumour suppressor gene. Multiple events of this type lead to aberrant cells with loss of normal growth control and ultimately to cancer (Hecht, 2003; Wogan et al., 2004).

There is a clear dose–response relationship between lung cancer risk and the number of cigarettes smoked per day, the degree of inhalation and the age at initiation of smoking (Engeland et al., 1996; Agudo et al., 2000; Kreuzer et al., 2000). Peto et al. (2000) recently estimated that the cumulative risk of death from lung cancer by age 75 among current smokers was 16%, rising to 24% for current smokers of at least 25 cigarettes per day. Doll and Peto (1978) reported that a tripling of the number of cigarettes smoked per day was estimated to triple the risk, whereas a tripling of the duration of smoking was estimated to increase the lung cancer risk 100-fold. The type of cigarette smoked also influences the risk; those who smoke filtered cigarettes have a lower lifetime risk than those who smoke non-filtered cigarettes (Lubin et al., 1984). In general, someone who has smoked all their life has 20–40 times greater risk of developing lung cancer than a non-smoker (Peto et al., 2000; Simonato et al., 2001; Crispo et al., 2004). Cigar smoking is also an established cause of lung cancer. The lung cancer risks associated with cigar smoking are substantial, but are less than the risks observed for cigarette smoking due to differences in smoking frequency and depth of inhalation. The same pattern holds true for pipe smoking (Boffetta et al., 1999).

Smoking increases the risk of all histological types of lung cancer, although the relative risk is greater for squamous-cell and small-cell carcinomas than for adenocarcinomas (Jedrychowski et al., 1992; Dosemeci et al., 1997; Simonato et al., 2001). Adenocarcinoma has always been more common in women than in men, in both smokers and non-smokers. There is evidence of a temporal change in the distribution of histological types (Watkin, 1989). The most frequent histological type is squamous cell carcinoma; however, since the mid-1980s the rate for adenocarcinoma has increased significantly (Janssen-Heijnen et al., 1995; Travis et al., 1996; Charloux et al., 1997a,b). Changes in cigarette design and manufacturing technology in the latter half of the twentieth century may partly explain these changes because the composition and carcinogenicity of tobacco smoke has been altered (Tyczynski et al., 2003).

Many studies show a decreased risk of lung cancer in ex-smokers compared to current smokers (Chyou et al., 1992; Jedrychowski et al., 1992; Kabat, 1996; Peto et al., 2000; Simonato et al., 2001; Crispo et al., 2004). The decline in risk appears to be slower, the longer the smoking history (Lubin et al., 1984). However, it is clear that the risk of lung cancer may be substantially reduced, dependent on the duration of smoking and age at cessation. Peto et al. (2000) demonstrated the benefit of quitting smoking with cumulative risks of lung cancer of 10, 6, 3 and 2% for men who stopped smoking at ages 60, 50, 40 and 30, respectively. Therefore smokers who quit, even well into middle age, avoid a large proportion of their subsequent risk of lung cancer. However, it is also apparent that many ex-smokers remain at high risk because genetic damage to the smoking-exposed respiratory epithelium persists for decades after smoking cessation (Wistuba et al., 1997) and that these individuals never return to the baseline level of risk seen for non-smokers.

2.1.1. Involuntary smoking

Because smoking is an established cause of lung cancer in smokers, it follows that there must also be some risk of lung cancer to lifelong non-smokers exposed to environmental tobacco smoke (IARC, 1986). Involuntary smoking was first considered a possible risk factor for lung cancer in 1981 when two studies were published that described increased lung cancer risk among never-smoking women who were married to smokers (Hirayama, 1981; Trichopoulos et al., 1981). Studies have since been directed at the specific environments where non-smokers are exposed to tobacco smoke, including home, workplaces and public places. In general, these studies indicate an increased risk especially for persons with high exposure (Vineis et al., 2004a). A meta-analysis by Hackshaw et al. (1997) found an excess risk of 24% among lifelong non-smokers with partners who smoked (relative risk (RR) 1.24, 95% CI: 1.13–1.36). Furthermore, a significant dose–response relationship was identified. This excess risk could not be explained by confounding or misclassification. An updated meta-analysis of epidemiological studies of lung cancer and adult exposure to environmental tobacco smoke was recently conducted, resulting in RRs of 1.22 (95% CI: 1.12–1.32) in women and 1.36 (95% CI: 1.02–1.82) in men from spousal exposure, and of 1.15 (95% CI: 1.05–1.26) in women and 1.28 (95% CI: 0.88–1.84) in men from workplace exposure (IARC, 2004). Studies of involuntary smoking provide further evidence documenting the dose–response relationship between cigarette smoke and lung cancer. The doses extend to far lower levels than those of active smoking, and increased risk is observed, suggesting that there is no threshold for tobacco carcinogenesis (Alberg and Samet, 2003).

2.2. Occupational exposure and lung cancer

Apart from cigarette smoking, most other risk factors for lung cancer have been identified in occupational settings. Results on occupations known to entail exposure to lung carcinogens consistently indicate an association, but there is wide variation in the magnitude of the risk estimates, probably because of changes in industrial processes over time and between countries (Richiardi et al., 2004). Whilst it is clear that the contribution of occupational exposure to the lung cancer burden is small compared to that of cigarette smoking, it is large compared to the contributions of most other exposure classes (Alberg and Samet, 2003).

Twenty nine chemicals, groups of chemicals or mixtures which are used in industrial or agricultural settings have been classified in the IARC Monograph series as established human carcinogens (Group 1), of which 12 exert their influence on the lung (Siemiatycki et al., 2004). Occupational carcinogens may initiate and/or promote the development of cancer through many biochemical pathways and micromolecular alterations in the cellular constituents (Vallyathan et al., 1998). The most common defects observed in lung cancers associated with occupational exposure are loss of control of cellular differentiation and proliferation due to activation of oncogenes and/or mutations of tumour suppressor genes, such as *p53* (Harris and Hollstein, 1993; Taylor et al., 1994; Roth, 1995; Hussain and Harris, 1998). Current available data provides evidence for associations between specific genes and certain workplace aetiological agents (Table 1). However, further investigations in this field are required to elucidate the mechanisms involved in lung carcinogenesis.

Table 1. Main acquired genetic alterations in human lung cancer and their relationship with environmental exposures

Gene	Alteration	%SCC	%AC	%SqCC	%LCC	Exposure
p53	D, M(G:C->T:A), HM	70–90	30	50	?	Tobacco, radon, asbestos, PAH
K-ras	M (GGT->TGT)	<1	15–60	8–9	?	Tobacco, asbestos
FHIT	D, LOH	70		40-80		Tobacco, asbestos

Alteration: D, deletion; M, mutation; HM, hypermethylation; LOH, loss of heterozygosity;

Histological type: SCC, small cell carcinoma; AC, adenocarcinoma; SqCC, squamous cell carcinoma; LCC, large cell carcinoma.

Exposure: PAH, polycyclic aromatic hydrocarbons.

Asbestos is a well-established occupational carcinogen; the epidemiologic evidence dating to the 1950s (Doll, 1955). The risk of lung cancer has been noted to increase with increased exposure to asbestos (Newhouse and Berry, 1979) and to be associated with the principal commercial forms of asbestos (Lemen et al., 1980). Workplace exposure, particularly the widespread exposure to asbestos in the 1940s through the 1960s, has contributed to the current burden of lung cancer (Alberg et al., 2005). Investigations of occupational groups, who are often heavily exposed over many years to workplace agents, have provided a substantial understanding of the carcinogenicity of a number of chemical and physical agents. Many studies have shown that people in certain occupations are at increased risk of lung cancer. For example: asphalt workers and roofers (Partanen and Boffetta, 1994); printers (Lynge et al., 1995); rubber industry workers (Weiland et al., 1996); aluminium smelter workers (Selden et al., 1997); asbestos cement workers (Magnani and Leporati, 1998); iron and steel workers (Grimsrud et al., 1998); workers exposed to high levels of lead (Anttila et al., 1995).

Cigarette smoking potentiates the effect of many of the known occupational lung carcinogens (Saracci and Boffetta, 1994). Given the multifactorial aetiology of lung cancer, synergistic interactions among risk factors may have substantial consequences for lung cancer risk (Alberg and Samet, 2003). These interactions typically have been considered on an agent-by-agent basis, as for example the synergistic effect of cigarette smoking on the lung cancer risk from asbestos exposure (Vainio and Boffetta, 1994; Steenland and Stayer, 1997; Nelson and Kelsey, 2002). A review by Coultas and Samet (1992) reported an increased lung cancer risk in workers who smoked and were exposed to the following chemicals: arsenic; asbestos; chloromethyl ethers; chromium; nickel; PACs; radon; vinyl chloride. Vallyathan et al. (1998) suggest that cigarette smoking in synergy with occupational factors may account for as much as 40% of lung cancers. Given the multistage process underlying cell carcinogenesis, it is therefore important when assessing the relative contribution of any one exposure, to address whether it is influenced by other exposures.

Knowledge on the occupational causes of lung cancer is more advanced than in the case of other groups of carcinogens. Estimates of the global burden of occupational cancer show figures in the order of 2–4% (Doll and Peto, 1981; Peto, 2001). It should be stressed, however, that these cancers concentrate among exposed individuals (mainly blue-collar workers), among whom they may represent up to 20% of total cancers (Boffetta et al., 1995). Furthermore, unlike lifestyle factors such as cigarette smoking, exposure is involuntary and can be, to a large extent, avoided (Boffetta, 2004).

2.3. Air pollution and lung cancer

2.3.1. Outdoor air pollution

Outdoor air pollution has long been suspected of increasing the risk of lung cancer (Cohen, 2000). There is a biological rationale for carcinogenic potential of numerous components of air pollution, including benzo[*a*]pyrene, benzene, various heavy metals (arsenic, chromium, nickel, cadmium and beryllium), particles (especially fine particles) and possibly ozone (Boffetta and Nyberg, 2003).

Earlier analytical studies generally compared residence in urban areas, where the air is considered more polluted, to residence in rural areas (Vena, 1982; Pershagen and Simonato, 1990; Nyberg et al., 2000). The evidence suggests that urban air pollution may be a risk factor for lung cancer with estimated relative risks (RR) up to 1.5 in most situations. An obvious limitation of these comparisons is the difficulty of disentangling air pollution from other factors associated with urban life (Anto et al., 2001). An association between air pollution and lung cancer has also been reported in a number of case-control studies, which have incorporated data on smoking and occupational exposures (Barbone et al., 1995; Katsouyanni and Pershagen, 1997; Nyberg et al., 2000). However, a major drawback of previous studies has been the inadequate characterisation of air pollution exposure (Katsouyanni and Pershagen, 1997).

Several well-conducted cohort studies have shown a relation between several indicators of air pollution levels and lung cancer risk among residents (Dockery et al., 1993; Abbey et al., 1999; Hoek et al., 2002; Pope et al., 2002). The main advantage of the cohort studies is that exposure is ascertained independently of and prior to the onset of disease, reducing the likelihood of bias (Vineis et al., 2004b). Abbey et al. (1999) reported substantial increases in RRs of lung cancer mortality among men in relation to long-term ambient concentrations of PM10 (RR = 3.36, 95% CI: 1.57–7.19) and SO_2 (RR = 1.99, 95% CI: 1.24–3.20). Hoek et al. (2002) reported the risk of lung cancer to be slightly elevated for a 10 $\mu g/m^3$ increment in exposure to black smoke (RR = 1.06, 95% CI: 0.43–2.63) and for a 30 $\mu g/m^3$ increment in SO_2 (RR = 1.25, 95% CI: 0.42–3.72). However, results from both studies were based on relatively few lung cancer cases. Two of the largest cohort studies suggest an excess risk of lung cancer of approximately 19% per 10 $\mu g/m^3$ increment in long-term average PM2.5, after adjustment for confounding factors (Dockery et al., 1993; Pope et al., 2002). More recently, a cohort study conducted in Norway with a 27-year follow-up found that the adjusted RRs for developing lung cancer among men was 1.08 (95% CI: 1.02–1.15) for a 10 μg/m^3 increment in NO_2 (Nafstad et al., 2003).

Despite the small relative risks, the number of lung cancer cases that might be caused by air pollution (assuming a causal relationship), is relatively large due to the high prevalence of exposure (Boffetta and Nyberg, 2003). In a review of the causes of cancer, Doll and Peto (1981) estimated that perhaps 1–2% of lung cancer cases were related to air pollution. More recently, Boffetta and Nyberg (2003) estimated the proportion of lung cancers attributable to air pollution in the EU at approximately 3.6%, corresponding to some 7000 lung cancer cases per year. On the basis of the available evidence, there are reasonable grounds for concern that air pollution may increase lung cancer risk, especially in combination with other known risk factors, such as active and passive smoking and occupational exposures (Vineis et al., 2004b).

2.3.2. Indoor air pollution

Exposure to indoor air pollution from combustion sources used for heating and cooking, as well as high levels of cooking oil vapours resulting from some cooking methods, have been identified as risk factors for lung cancer. Recently, a large case-control study conducted in Central and Eastern European countries and the UK observed a modestly increased risk of lung cancer related to solid fuel use for cooking OR 1.22 (95% CI: 1.05–1.47) rather than heating OR 1.37 (95% CI: 0.90–2.09) (Lissowska et al., 2005). Given the long latency of lung cancer, cooking and heating methods may still play a role in the risk of lung cancer among middle-aged and older generations in Europe, although its importance should be diminishing (Boffetta and Nyberg, 2003).

The carcinogenicity of radon decay products has been widely studied in occupationally exposed populations, in particular underground miners (Lubin et al., 1995). Radon can leach into homes from the ground and levels are, therefore, high in granite-rich areas. Lung cancer due to domestic exposure to radon daughters is accepted to be a risk in such areas. A pooled RR of 1.06 (95% CI: 1.01–1.10) has recently been calculated for individuals exposed to residential radon at 100 Bq/m^3 compared to unexposed individuals (Darby et al., 2005). Darby and colleagues estimated that radon is responsible for 6.5% of all deaths from lung cancer in the UK, including 5.5% attributable to the joint effect of radon and smoking and 1% to residential radon alone.

2.4. Diet and lung cancer

Dietary factors may also play a role in the aetiology of lung cancer. Scores of epidemiologic studies have reported a lower risk of lung cancer among persons whose diet includes a relatively large amount of vegetables, fruits and other plant products (Kvåle et al., 1983; Jain et al., 1990; Ziegler et al., 1992; Dorgan et al., 1993; Steinmetz et al., 1993; Voorrips et al., 2000b). Evidence from cohort studies published since 2000 has tended to reinforce this pattern of associations (Feskanich et al., 2000; Holick et al., 2002; Neuhouser et al., 2003; Wright et al., 2003; Skuladottir et al., 2004). In the European Prospective Investigation into Cancer and Nutrition study (Miller et al., 2004), and in a pooled analysis of cohort studies (Mannisto et al., 2004), the protective association was stronger for fruit than for vegetable consumption. It is possible, however, that the decrease in risk is actually due to some other compound in foods containing these substances, or an aspect of lifestyle related to consumption of such foods. While it is generally accepted that a diet of large amounts of vegetables, fruits and other plant products lowers cancer incidence, there is still a need to identify the most effective constituents of the diet as well as to elucidate their mechanism of action (Walaszek et al., 2004).

Many studies have focused on identifying the specific components of foods that may be responsible for reducing the risk of lung cancer. As a result, a protective role has been suggested for micronutrients such as β-carotene, vitamin C, vitamin E and selenium (Koo, 1988; Voorrips et al., 2000a). β-carotene has been extensively studied because of its antioxidant properties and the importance of this pro-vitamin for epithelial growth and differentiation (van Zandwijk and Hirsch, 2003). Other micronutrients with antioxidant capacity, and therefore the potential to decrease lung cancer risk, include vitamin E, selenium, allyl sulphur compounds and tea polyphenols.

New lines of inquiry have also emerged, such as studies of phytochemicals such as flavonoids and isothiocyanates. Phytochemicals are low molecular weight molecules produced by plants. Of the many classes of phytochemicals, those studied in relation to lung cancer include phytoestrogens, flavonoids and glucosinoids (Alberg et al., 2005). Flavonoids exhibit potent antioxidant activity and flavonoid intake has been at least weakly associated with lung cancer in some of the preliminary studies of this topic (Knekt et al., 1997; Le Marchand et al., 2000a). Isothiocyanates are metabolites of the class of phytochemicals known as glucosinoids. Isothiocyanates could exert anticancer effects by blocking carcinogens via induction of phase II detoxification enzymes, such as glutathione *S*-transferase. Cruciferous vegetables contain high concentrations of glucosinolates, and hence consumption leads to higher endogenous isothiocyanate concentrations. As with cruciferous vegetables (Neuhouser et al., 2003; Brennan et al., 2005), lung cancer risk is consistently lower with higher intakes of isothiocyanates (London et al., 2000; Spitz et al., 2000; Zhao et al., 2001).

2.4.1. Diet, genetic susceptibility and lung cancer

Epidemiological evidence suggests that genes controlling the metabolism of carcinogens and antioxidant or nutritional status are associated with lung cancer risk, possibly through their ability to modulate DNA damage by carcinogens. Since many carcinogenic compounds require metabolic activation to enable them to react with cellular macromolecules, individual features of carcinogen metabolism may play an essential role in the development of environmental cancer (Hietanen et al., 1997). A sizeable number of studies have examined associations between genetic polymorphisms in the detoxification loci and the risk of lung cancer often reporting contradictory results (d'Errico et al., 1999; Bouchardy et al., 2001; Kiyohara et al., 2002). Fewer studies have examined associations among genetic polymorphisms, specific dietary components and lung cancer risk (Seow et al., 1998; London et al., 2000; Spitz et al., 2000).

The glutathione-*S*-transferase (GST) family is a group of multifunctional proteins. One of their major roles is to catalyse the conjugation of electrophilic compounds to glutathione (GSH). Approximately 40–50% of the population is deficient in the best characterised GST of the Mu subgroup, *GST1* or *GSTM1* (Brockmoller et al., 1994). Polymorphisms in inherited metabolic traits and intake of dietary antioxidants may be associated with higher risk of lung cancer in smokers. Plasma retinol, β-carotene, α-tocopherol and zeaxanthin are reported to be inversely correlated with DNA damage, especially in individuals with the *GSTM1* null genotype (Cheng et al., 1995; Mooney and Perera, 1996). Lower consumption of isothiocyanates has been associated with elevated lung cancer risk in current smokers with null genotypes at both *GSTT1* and *GSTM1* (London et al., 2000; Spitz et al., 2000). More recently, a large case-control study reported that weekly consumption of cruciferous vegetables protected against lung cancer in those who were *GSTM1* null (OR = 0.67, 95% CI: 0.49–0.91), *GSTT1* null (OR = 0.63, 95% CI: 0.37–1.07), or both (OR = 0.28, 95% CI: 0.11–0.67) (Brennan et al., 2005). In addition, it has been suggested that while male smokers with a *GSTM1* null genotype may have a greater risk of lung cancer than smokers with non-null genotypes, the risk can be attenuated by α-tocopherol supplementation (Woodson et al., 1999). These studies would suggest that, at the very least, it may be important to consider micronutrient intake when examining the relationship between polymorphisms in the phase I and II loci and lung cancer (Tsai et al., 2003).

2.5. Socioeconomic status and lung cancer

Socioeconomic variations in lung cancer incidence and mortality have been reported for a number of European countries (Vagero and Persson, 1986; Davey Smith et al., 1991; Beer et al., 1993; Faggiano et al., 1994; Regidor et al., 1995; van Loon et al., 1997; Levi et al., 1998; Fernandez and Borrell, 1999; Hart et al., 2001). Many studies have suggested that the risk of developing lung cancer is significantly higher in the more disadvantaged sections of society. A study examining the relationship between social deprivation and cancer in Scotland (Bain and McLaren, 1998) observed a threefold difference for lung cancer between the most and least deprived areas. Factors that could explain the association between lung cancer and lower socioeconomic status include smoking, diet, occupational exposures and exposure to environmental pollution in the area of residence. In two Scottish studies, smoking accounted for approximately 55% of the higher lung cancer mortality rate in manual compared with non-manual men (Hart et al., 2001) suggesting other risk factors play a more important role than was previously thought, particularly in the lower socioeconomic groups (Mackenbach et al., 2004). van Loon et al. (1995) observed a higher risk for lung cancer in blue-collar workers which could only be partially explained by smoking habits and diet, indicating occult links between lung cancer and socioeconomic status. Furthermore, Faggiano et al. (1997) using longitudinal data relating to England and Wales, observed a widening of social class differences in lung cancer in men over time. A recent study from Norway reported an increased risk of lung cancer-related mortality among men who were exposed to worse housing conditions during childhood, independent of adult socioeconomic circumstances (Naess et al., 2004). As lung cancer is a disease affecting many older people, an additional group who may be socially disadvantaged is the elderly, who have lower levels of diagnostic investigation and treatment than their younger counterparts.

Lower socioeconomic status has also been associated with later stage at diagnosis (Schwartz et al., 2003), which may partly explain why lung cancer survival among men is significantly lower for the poor than the rich (Coleman et al., 2004). Among adults living in the most deprived areas of England and Wales, who were diagnosed with cancer during 1981–1990, 5-year survival was significantly lower than for those in the most affluent areas for 44 out of 47 different cancers (Coleman et al., 1998). Five-year survival for lung cancer patients diagnosed in England and Wales during 1996–1999 was 6% in men and women, not significantly better than for patients diagnosed around a decade earlier (Coleman et al., 2004).

Further work is required to ascertain the robustness of the relationships between various measures of socioeconomic status and cancer (Krieger et al., 2003). There is also a need for further development and broader application of multilevel models to tease out the different roles of society, culture, behaviour, and the environment, and elucidate how they manifest themselves through individual behaviours and biologic pathways (Diez-Roux, 2000). Advancing our understanding of the complex linkages between components of socioeconomic status and lung cancer risk is essential to effectively address the social class disparities and reduce lung cancer rates in the poorest segments of society (Alberg et al., 2005).

2.6. Prior lung disease and lung cancer

A long-standing inflammatory reaction in the bronchi is accompanied by a continual cycle of injury and repair and could therefore play a key role in lung carcinogenesis (Ames et al., 1993; Pages and Fuchs, 2002). Indeed, several studies have suggested that prior lung diseases, such as asthma, chronic bronchitis, emphysema, pneumonia, tuberculosis, hay fever and impaired pulmonary function may modify lung cancer risk (Alavanja et al., 1992; Wu et al., 1995; Mayne et al., 1999; Osann et al., 2000; Brenner et al., 2001; Santillan et al., 2003; Talbot-Smith et al., 2003; Littman et al., 2004; Schabath et al., 2005). Brenner et al. (2001) reported significantly increased risk for individuals diagnosed with emphysema within 10 years of lung cancer onset. In the same study Brenner et al. found a six-fold increase in lung cancer in individuals diagnosed with pneumonia within 5 years of lung cancer onset, but no apparent risk for persons diagnosed 5 or more years prior to the diagnosis of cancer. One plausible explanation for this dichotomy is that the development of chronic respiratory disease may merely identify those persons who received higher doses of cigarette smoke at target sites in the respiratory tract (Samet et al., 1986). A recent prospective cohort study found evidence supporting the hypothesis that chronic bronchitis or emphysema increases lung cancer risk after controlling for cigarette smoking (Hazard Ratio (HR) = 1.29, 95% CI: 1.09–1.53). The association was particularly strong for squamous cell carcinoma and persons below the age of 65 years at diagnosis (Littman et al., 2004). Schabath et al. (2005) reported an increased risk of lung cancer among individuals with a prior diagnosis of emphysema (OR = 2.87, 95% CI: 2.20–3.76), while there was a protective effect for lung cancer among those with a prior diagnosis of hay fever (OR = 0.58, 95% CI: 0.48–0.70). However, the authors did not find any evidence for an aetiologic association between lung cancer and other respiratory diseases, including asthma, bronchitis and emphysema.

Previous studies have shown that polymorphisms in the *CYP1A1* (Cantlay et al., 1995), *GSTM1* (Cantlay et al., 1994; Harrison et al., 1997) and *mEPHX* (Smith and Harrison, 1997) are weakly associated with susceptibility to emphysema. In a recent case-control study (Schabath et al., 2005), the MMP-1 2G/2G genotype was associated with a 1.7-fold increase in lung cancer risk (95% CI: 1.35–2.19). The risk associated with the "adverse" 2G/2G genotype was substantially higher in the presence of emphysema (OR = 4.45, 95% CI: 2.34–8.47), and the risk was reduced for individuals with emphysema and the putatively "protective" 1G genotypes (OR = 2.58, 95% CI: 1.63–4.09). Interestingly, these protective 1G genotypes exhibited a greater protective effect in individuals with a history of hay fever.

Several prospective studies have also examined the association between lung function, based on spirometry, and future lung cancer risk (Skillrud et al., 1988; Islam and Schottenfeld, 1994; Eberly et al., 2003; Mannino et al., 2003). These studies found that individuals with evidence of obstructive lung disease at baseline, or a higher rate of decline in pulmonary function during follow-up, had an increased risk of developing lung cancer.

In some instances, the association between respiratory disease and lung cancer remains controversial. For instance, there are conflicting epidemiologic data and no proven hypothesis for the role of asthma and hay fever in lung carcinogenesis. Consequently, doubt remains on the causal nature of these associations and confirmation of findings in additional populations will lend strength to earlier observations.

2.7. Gender and lung cancer

In the past several decades the incidence of lung cancer has risen among women, especially in North America and Northern Europe (Blot and McLaughlin, 2004; Parkin et al., 2005). The increase in the incidence of lung cancer in women is primarily due to an increase in their tobacco use. Controversy exists as to whether women are more or less susceptible to the carcinogenic effects of cigarette smoke than men (Patel, 2005). Risch et al. (1993) report that women with a history of 40 pack years of smoking relative to non-smokers had an odds ratio of 27.9 (95% CI: 14.9–52.0) compared to that of men of 9.6 (95% CI: 5.6–16.3). Zang and Wynder (1996) estimated that female smokers had a 1.5-fold higher risk of developing lung cancer than male smokers. In a study of lung cancer patients, Mollerup et al. (1999) found that female smokers had a significantly higher level of PAH adducts in their lungs compared to male smokers, supporting the epidemiological data on lung cancer risk. More recently, Henschke and Miettinen (2004) evaluated the absolute risk for lung cancer in men and women smokers undergoing baseline computed tomography (CT) and concluded that for a given level of smoking, more women than men developed lung cancer.

Conversely, a number of well-conducted cohort studies have reported that women are not more susceptible to tobacco carcinogens than men (Patel, 2005). A recent analysis of over 60 000 women from the Nurses Health Study and over 25 000 men from the Health Professionals Follow-up Study showed no convincing evidence of increased lung cancer risk in women (Bain et al., 2004). The clear picture emerging from large cohort studies is that women do not have higher rates of smoking-induced lung cancer than men (Blot and McLaughlin, 2004).

Regardless of sex differences in the relative risk of lung cancer in smokers, lung cancer appears to be a biologically different disease in women (Patel, 2005). The histologic distribution of lung cancer among women is distinctly different than that among men (Osann et al., 1993; Travis et al., 1996: Radzikowska et al., 2002). Female smokers are more likely to develop adenocarcinoma of the lung than squamous cell carcinoma, which is more common in men (Ferguson et al., 1990; Thun et al., 1997). Never smokers with lung cancer almost uniformly have adenocarcinoma and are also approximately 2.5 times more likely to be female than male (Keohavong et al., 1996). Biologic rationales have emerged to attempt to explain why women might be more susceptible to tobacco or other lung carcinogens. The factors included were sex differences in the metabolism or detoxification of nicotine and other compounds in tobacco (Kure et al., 1996; Toyooka et al., 2003); hormonal interactions as suggested by the detection of oestrogen and progesterone receptors in human lung tumour tissue (Taioli and Wynder, 1994; Omoto et al., 2001; Stabile et al., 2002; Patrone et al., 2003; Spivack et al., 2003); and differential proliferative or growth stimulation effects indicated by gastrin-releasing peptide receptor expression markers more common among female non-smokers and smokers (Keohavong et al., 1996; Shriver et al., 2000).

The available evidence suggests that the development of lung cancer is different in women compared to men. Women smokers are more likely than men to develop adenocarcinoma of the lung. Women who have never smoked are more likely to develop lung cancer than their male counterparts. These differences are due to hormonal, genetic and metabolic differences between the sexes (Patel, 2005).

2.8. Familial risk of lung cancer

More than 40 years ago, Tokuhata and Lilienfeld (1963) provided epidemiologic evidence for familial aggregation of lung cancer after accounting for personal smoking, which suggested the possible interaction of genes, shared environment and common lifestyle factors in the aetiology of lung cancer. Familial aggregation and increased familial risk for lung cancer have since been reported in several studies, providing indirect evidence that genetic factors contribute to susceptibility to lung cancer (Amos et al., 1992; Yang et al., 1999; Etzel et al., 2003; Xu et al., 2005). Results from a recent meta-analysis of the published literature on familial aggregation of lung cancer are consistent with a twofold increase associated with family history, with evidence of risk being related to early age of diagnosis and number of relatives affected (Matakidou et al., 2005). In a recent study (Jonsson et al., 2004), a familial factor for lung cancer was shown to extend beyond the nuclear family, as relative risks for first-, second- and third-degree relatives of individuals with lung cancer were all significantly increased. This effect was the strongest for relatives of individuals with early-onset lung carcinoma.

Familial association is most readily detected in lung cancer occurring in non-smokers (Sellers et al., 1990). The majority of inherited lung cancer risk probably comes from small but significant effects arising from genetic polymorphisms that are frequent in the population (Amos et al., 1999). Several studies have suggested that a number of low-penetrance, high-frequency polymorphisms are likely to account for a proportion of lung cancer risk (Spitz et al., 1999). Polymorphisms in these genes could explain individual differences in susceptibility to tobacco carcinogens and are likely to include genes involved in decreasing or increasing the activity of carcinogens (e.g. *CYP1A*, *CYP2E* and *GSTM1*) and genes involved in monitoring and repairing tobacco carcinogen-induced DNA damage (e.g. *p53* and *ERCC1*) (Wei et al., 2000; Bosken et al., 2002; Wu et al., 2002). Recently a major lung cancer susceptibility locus was mapped to chromosome 6q23-35 through a genome-wide linkage analysis, further supporting the role of genetic factors in the susceptibility of lung cancer (Bailey-Wilson et al., 2004). Further, the authors found a genotype–smoking interaction with carriers having an increased risk with any amount of smoking, whereas non-carriers have an increasing risk with increasing smoking level. This finding could explain why people who never smoke can still develop lung cancer.

2.9. Genetic susceptibility

While 80–90% of lung cancers can be attributed to cigarette smoking, only 10–15% of all smokers develop lung cancer (Mattson et al., 1987). Investigators have long hypothesised that individuals differ in their susceptibility to environmental insults (Motulsky, 1957; Heath, 1958; Friberg, 1959) and that these differences may be the result of genetic predisposition (Schwartz, 2004). Analysis of the genetic variability that affects the capacity to metabolise carcinogens in humans has shown that a number of genes may play an important role in lung carcinogenesis (Table 2). The following section provides an overview of the most widely studied polymorphisms including P4501A1 (*CYP1A1*), glutathione-*S*-transferase M1 (*GSTM1*), myeloperoxidase (*MPO*), and NAD(P)H: quione oxidoreductase (*NQO1*). This subject is extraordinarily large and therefore we have not attempted to conduct a comprehensive review.

2.9.1. Cytochrome P450s (CYPs)

CYPs are a superfamily of oxidising enzymes, the majority of which are involved in the metabolism of xenobiotics (Gonzalez and Gelboin, 1993). Their principal function is to convert xenobiotics into derivatives that can be more easily excreted from the body. Based on sequence homology, the *CYP* superfamily is divided into 10 subfamilies, *CYP1–CYP10*. Subfamilies *CYP1*, *CYP2*, *CYP3* and *CYP4* are primarily involved in drug metabolism (Kamataki, 1993). The metabolic pathway includes an activation step at which point the metabolite is capable of reaction with macromolecules. These include DNA, which via the formation of adducts, may lead to mutation. At several points in this pathway there are opportunities for detoxification, where the modified xenobiotic is conjugated to water-soluble moieties, such as glutathione, glucuronide and sulphate, which facilitate excretion. The relationship between activation and detoxification may determine an individual's risk, with those with high levels of activation by CYPs and low levels of detoxification by, for example, *GSTM1*, at the highest risk of contracting lung cancer.

The *CYP1A1* gene is important for the metabolism of PACs (Omura et al., 1993). The gene product, aromatic hydrocarbon hydrolase catalyses the first step in the conversion of many environmental carcinogens, such as benzo[*a*]pyrene in cigarette smoke, to

Table 2. Categories of genes studied in relation to lung cancer susceptibility

Gene type	Examples	Studies
Phase 1	*CYP1A1*	Vineis et al. (2003)
	CYP1A2	Seow et al. (2001)
	CYP2C9	London et al. (1997c)
	CYP2D6	Rostami-Hodjegan et al. (1998)
Phase 2	*GSTM1*	Taioli et al. (2003)
	NQO1	Xu et al. (2001)
	MPO	Feyler et al. (2002)
	NAT2	Zhou et al. (2002)
	hGPX1	Ratnasinghe et al. (2000)
Cell cycle	*Cyclin D1*	Qiuling et al. (2003)
	p16	Gonzalez-Quevedo et al. (2002)
	p53	Saintigny et al. (1999)
	p21	Shoji et al. (2002)
	Rb	Geradts et al. (1999)
DNA repair	*ERCC*	Cheng et al. (2000)
	XRCC	Spitz et al. (2001)
	hOGG1	Park et al. (2004)
Apoptosis	*BCL2*	Bandala et al. (2001)
	p53	Robles et al. (2001)
	FAS	Zhang et al. (2005)
	Caspase 3	Takata et al. (2001)

their ultimate DNA-binding carcinogenic form. The *CYP1A1* gene has been located near the MPI locus at 15q22-24. A positive association between development of lung cancer and the mutant homozygous genotype of *CYP1A1 Msp I* or *CYP1A1* Ile-Val polymorphism has been reported in several Japanese populations (Kawajiri et al., 1990; Le Marchand et al., 2000b). The *CYP1A1 Msp* I polymorphism has a higher variant allele frequency than the *CYP1A1* Ile-Val polymorphism. Nakachi et al. (1993) found that individuals with either of these genotypes that were also deficient in *GST1* were at greater risk of lung cancer; with susceptible MspI or Ile-Val gene type. The impact of genetically determined predisposition was found to be more appreciable at low levels of cigarette consumption (Nakachi et al., 1991). A meta-analysis based on 15 studies reported a non-significant OR of 1.27 associated with the MspI polymorphism and a non-significant OR of 1.62 for the exon 7 polymorphism in *CYP1A1* (Houlston, 2000). Recent studies have reported that two polymorphisms in the *CYP1A1* gene, a T3801C substitution at the 3′ end of the gene and an A2455G substitution resulting in an *Ile*462*Val* exchange in the heme-binding region of exon 7, appear to increase lung cancer risk in Caucasians (Le Marchand et al., 2003; Taioli et al., 2003; Vineis et al., 2003). In a pooled analysis of 22 studies, Vineis et al. (2003) reported a significant 2.4-fold increase for the homozygote MspI variant, however, this finding was based on very small number of cases and controls carrying the risk genotype. The *CYP1A1 Ile462Val* polymorphism might also play a role in lung carcinogenesis among non-smokers (Hung et al., 2003).

CYP2D6 is associated with the oxidation of a wide range of therapeutic drugs. A polymorphism at the *CYP2D6* gene locus has been shown to have a significant effect on the rate of metabolism of many drugs. Poor metabolisers (PM) would activate less of the carcinogens they were exposed to and hence would be at a reduced risk of lung cancer, however if *CYP2D6* catalyses the detoxification of a particular carcinogen then PM individuals would be at increased risk and extensive and intermediate metabolisers (EM + IM) would have comparatively lower risks. Ayesh et al. (1990) showed a strong association between the *CYP2D6* (PM) polymorphism and reduced lung cancer susceptibility. This work has been supported by other studies, which were summarised by Wolf et al. (1994) who concluded that among lung cancer patients there is approximately a 4% prevalence of PM compared to 8% in the general population. Other meta-analyses subsequently confirmed the inheritance of the *CYP2D6* PM genotype as a risk factor (d'Errico et al., 1996; Christensen et al., 1997). Additionally, London et al. (1997b) co-analysed a number of variables, including smoking history and occupational exposure to environmental pollutants, also found the *CYP2D6* PM phenotype to be a significant risk factor. Bouchardy et al. (1996) collected detailed smoking history for their study and found a statistically significant association between the *CYP2D6* extensive metaboliser (EM) phenotype and susceptibility to lung cancer but the PM phenotype was only protective for heavy smokers. Higher carcinogen DNA levels have been associated with *CYP2D6* genotypes and *CYP2E1* minor alleles (Kato et al., 1995) suggesting that these polymorphisms can be predictive of an individual's lifetime response to carcinogen exposure. More recent studies that have assessed genotype have generated inconsistent results (Christensen et al., 1997) suggesting the possibility that the *CYP2D6* genotype may be weakly associated with increased risk of lung cancer (Rostami-Hodjegan et al., 1998).

2.9.2. Glutathione-S-transferases (GST)

The glutathione-*S*-transferase (GST) family is a group of multifunctional proteins. One of their major roles is to catalyse the conjugation of electrophilic compounds to glutathione (GSH). *GST* genes form a super family of at least 13 genes consisting of five distinct families, named alpha (*GSTA*), sigma (*GSTS*), mu (*GSTM*), pi (*GSTP*) and theta (*GSTT*). GST1 or *GSTM1*, the best characterised GST, belongs to the Mu subgroup. Approximately 40–50% of the population are deficient in this enzyme (Brockmoller et al., 1994), which is shown to be due to a homozygous nulled *GST1* gene by Seidegard et al. (1988). To be deficient in a major detoxification pathway is likely to increase the risk of carcinogenesis. Kihara et al. (1994) showed that lung cancer risk of those with a *GSTM1* null phenotype is dependent on the extent of tobacco exposure but that the proportion of patients with *GSTM1* null phenotype increases progressively in the squamous cell carcinoma group. London et al. (1997a) found no significant association between homozygous deletion of the *GSTM1* gene and the risk of lung cancer, however, they did find an elevated risk for lighter smokers with this genotype. Many studies have produced conflicting data but several meta-analyses indicate that the null genotype confers a small increased risk of lung cancer (McWilliams et al., 1995; d'Errico et al., 1996). More recently, a meta-analysis estimated an overall OR of 1.13 (95% CI: 1.04–1.25), suggesting a modest increased risk associated with the *GSTM1* null genotype (Houlston, 1999). An updated meta-analysis reported similar findings (OR, 1.17 (95% CI: 1.07–1.27) but did not indicate that this susceptibility was stronger among cigarette smokers than among non–smokers (Benhamou et al., 2002). A pooled analysis (Taioli et al., 2003) in whites <45 years of age also found an OR of 1.1 (95% CI: 0.9–1.3), while a study on an African-American population reported a twofold increased risk (95% CI: 1.07–4.11) among those persons with the null genotype (Ford et al., 2000).

2.9.3. Combined phase I and II polymorphisms

Since genetic polymorphisms have been found for both phase I and II enzymes, risk assessment could be increased sensitivity if polymorphisms in both phases of enzymes are taken into consideration as biomarkers for susceptibility to cancer. It is likely that an individual with the high-risk genotype (either a genotype coding for a more active phase I enzyme or a less efficient phase II enzyme, or both of those) might be at a higher risk of cancer than that with the opposite genotype (combination) (Kiyohara et al., 2002). Analyses of combined *CYP1A1* and *GSTM1* risk genotypes have generally showed risk increases of more than threefold, however, sample sizes have usually been small (Hayashi et al., 1992; Alexandrie et al., 1994; Quinones et al., 2001). The importance of interactions between genes is highlighted by the joint assessment of the *CYP1A1* and *GSTM1* null polymorphisms in non-smokers, which indicated that the combination of the two variant genotypes was associated with a more than fourfold increased likelihood of lung cancer compared with the combination of the two nonvariant genotypes (Hung et al., 2003). Combined *CYP1A1* and *GSTM1* genotype is thus a potential predictor of genetic susceptibility to lung cancer in populations where *CYP1A1* alleles are common (Kiyohara et al., 2002).

2.9.4. NAD(P)H quinone oxidoreductase (DT-diaphorase)

NAD(P)H quinone oxidoreductase 1 (NQO1), formerly referred to as DT-diaphorase, is a cytosolic enzyme catalysing the two-electron reduction of quinone substrates. NQO1 either metabolically activates or detoxifies carcinogens present in cigarette smoke. Benzo[*a*]pyrene (BP) is one of the most important carcinogens and the formation of BP quinone–DNA adduct is prevented by NQO1 (Joseph and Jaiswal, 1994). In contrast, carcinogenic heterocyclic amines present in smoke are metabolically activated by NQO1 (de Flora et al., 1994). Therefore, this enzyme is thought to be involved in both metabolic activation and detoxification of carcinogenic agents that could be involved in lung carcinogenesis.

Conflicting findings also have been reported in investigations of polymorphism in the *NQO1* gene, which can act in both carcinogen activation and detoxification. Because of its dual role in metabolism, there is little agreement in the literature about which genotype is the "risk genotype", making comparisons across studies difficult (Schwartz, 2004). Lewis et al. (2001) reported that the variant allele was associated with a non-significant increased risk of lung cancer and a significant increased risk (OR = 3.80, 95% CI: 1.19–12.1) of SCLC. Other studies that have reported significant associations between *NQO1* genotype and lung cancer risk have been based on fairly small sample sizes and/or subgroup analyses (Wiencke et al., 1997; Chen et al., 1999; Xu et al., 2001; Sunaga et al., 2002). In the largest study, risk was increased at lower levels of cigarette consumption and was decreased at higher levels of cigarette consumption (Xu et al., 2001). However, there was a gene–environment interaction between the genotype and smoking: current smokers with the T/T genotype had a smaller cancer risk that those with C/C genotype (OR = 0.38, 95% CI: 0.19–1.00).

2.9.5. Myeloperoxidase (MPO)

Neutrophil recruitment into lung tissue occurs after exposure to variety of insults known to increase lung cancer risk, including tobacco smoke particles, infection, asbestos and ozone (Hunninghake et al., 1979; Schmekel et al., 1990a,b). Following immunological and/or chemical insults, neutrophils release MPO and undergo a respiratory burst, which is characterised by a massive increase in oxygen consumption and a consequent NADPH-dependent production of superoxide and other free radicals (Hunninghake et al., 1979). MPO is present in the primary granules of neutrophils and catalyses the production of the potent bacteriotoxic oxidising agent hypochlorous acid (a one- and two-electron oxidant that can attack endogenous molecules including DNA) from hydroxyl radicals and chloride ions. A significant proportion (25–40%) of the hydrogen peroxide formed by activated neutrophils may be converted to hypochlorous acid (Foote et al., 1983; Prutz, 1998). MPO metabolically activates a wide range of tobacco smoke mutagens and environmental pollutants to DNA-damaging metabolites, including aromatic amines (Tsuruta et al., 1985), the promutagenic derivatives of PAHs (Trush et al., 1985; Mallet et al., 1991; Petruska et al., 1992) and heterocyclic amines (Williams et al., 1998). It is possible that possession of two copies of the A allele of the *MPO* gene reduces the risk of lung cancer. The wild-type G allele is present in 75% of Caucasians (London et al., 1997d; Cascorbi et al., 2000; Le Marchand et al., 2000b). Studies investigating the *MPO* gene have shown fairly consistent, although not always statistically significant, reductions in the risk of lung cancer to be associated with the variant allele (Le Marchand et al., 2000b; Feyler et al., 2002; Schabath et al., 2002) suggesting an important role for *MPO* in lung cancer aetiology, possibly through activation of carcinogens and/or production of free radicals in or near the target cells. In the largest study of *MPO* and lung cancer risk conducted to date, the adjusted odds ratios for the A/A and A/G genotypes were 1.15 (95% CI: 0.7–1.9, $p > 0.2$) and 1.03 (95% CI: 0.8–1.3, $p > 0.20$), respectively, compared with the wild-type G/G genotype. These findings are in contrast to the earlier studies suggesting a protective effect of carrying the variant A allele (Xu et al., 2002). For further information, see a recent review by Kiyohara et al. (2005).

3. CONCLUSION

Lung cancer has the highest worldwide rate of cancer mortality, exceeding the combined rate of the next three leading causes of death due to cancer: colon, breast and prostate (Hirsch and Lippman, 2005). Detection of lung cancer usually occurs late in the disease when it is beyond effective treatment. More than 40% of all lung cancer patients present with metastasised disease at diagnosis (Ginsberg et al., 2001). In these clinically advanced tumour stages, long-term survival is rarely achieved with conventional cytotoxic agents (Schiller et al., 2002). Consequently, there is a high mortality rate with 5-year survival ranging from 6% in the UK (Coleman et al., 2004) to 15% in the United States (Parkin et al., 2005).

Changes in modifiable risk factors, including occupational exposures, second-hand tobacco smoke and dietary factors may all have an effect on lung cancer incidence in the future. The dominant role of cigarette smoking in lung cancer causation, however, indicates that efforts to limit the use of tobacco are currently the most effective method to reduce the burden of lung cancer (Beckett, 1993). The best method of prevention is by persuading smokers to stop (using various smoking cessation strategies) and young people not to start smoking. In the UK, the prevalence of smoking among adults decreased from 44% in 1974 to 25% (26% of men and 24% of women) in 2002 (ONS, 2003). There has been a corresponding decrease in the male rate of death from lung cancer. Rates fell the fastest in the late 1970s and early 1980s since then decreases have been moderate. Despite major efforts to reduce smoking rates, lung cancer remains the largest cancer killer. Furthermore, the global burden of lung cancer will undergo drastic shifts from the developed to the developing world in the future (Alberg et al., 2005). China, the world's most populous country, has tripled cigarette consumption between 1978 and 1987 and as a result, mortality from lung cancer has risen sharply (Liu et al., 1998). Given the long latency period between exposure and peak incidence of cancer, coming of the potential epidemic stresses the urgent need to develop effective prevention strategies (Goodman, 2002). Realistically, in spite of knowing how to prevent lung cancer, the disease is likely to require treatment for many years to come.

Policies which encourage individuals to quit smoking must coincide with programmes to detect lung cancer before the onset of clinical symptoms. Even after stopping smoking, the long-term smokers remain at a high-risk of developing lung cancer and currently, there is no established cancer control policy for these individuals. Molecular studies show that genetic alterations persist many years after cessation of smoking in parallel to an increased lung cancer risk and most of the individuals who now develop lung cancer in the United States are ex-smokers (Strauss et al., 1995; Wistuba et al., 1997). Lung cancer is an ideal disease for a population-based screening programme because we can easily identify the at-risk group (Sethi, 2002). Advances in molecular and radiological approaches provide potential hope for early diagnosis and screening of high-risk individuals, which in turn may lead to identification of innovative treatments and improved survival (Huber and Stratakis, 2004).

Currently spiral computed tomographic (CT) imaging would appear to be the best clinical modality for identifying very early lung cancer (Mulshine and Sullivan, 2005). Two large studies have recently evaluated the efficacy of low-dose CT scanning as a screening tool for lung cancer (Henschke et al., 1999; Swenson et al., 2002). Although both studies found that screening detected most cancers at an earlier stage (majority stage 1A) than would be expected in an unscreened population, there was a high incidence of false-positive lung nodules. Although low-dose CT scanning is feasible, it is unclear at present whether mortality can be lowered. A large prospective randomised control trial is currently underway in the US to evaluate the cost effectiveness and mortality reduction of screening (Moore et al., 2005).

The way forward for improved management and prognosis for individuals who are at risk of developing lung cancer lies with early detection of disease prior to clinical symptoms. An increasing number of molecular and genetic lesions considered essential for the final malignant phenotype have been identified and some of these lesions are directly related to exposure to carcinogens from tobacco smoke (van Zandwijk et al., 2005). However, conclusions from genetic susceptibility studies of lung cancer have, in general, been limited by the low frequency of some polymorphisms in the population, the variability in allele frequencies by ethnicity, alternative definitions of risk genotype, the potential for heterogeneity by histologic type of lung cancer, and the variation in risk associated with the level of exposure to tobacco smoke (Schwartz, 2004). To overcome these potential limitations in the future, it will be essential to conduct well-designed, large studies that evaluate the risk along genetic pathways, since it is unlikely that one genotype has a strong effect on risk. The advances in genotyping platforms and throughput will facilitate the identification of new variants and also enable researchers to analyse multiple polymorphisms within genes and multiple genes within the same pathway (Goode et al., 2002). Indeed, it is likely that the defining feature of future studies will involve genome-wide SNP mapping of genes in much larger samples of cases and controls (Caporaso, 2002; Syvanen, 2005). Surrogate markers, found to be the most representative of molecular changes, will be used to develop quantitative risk assessment models and lead to a better understanding of the multistep carcinogenic process. Furthermore, these markers will have potential as an adjunct to new screening modalities, such as spiral CT (Spitz et al., 2005). To illuminate how the identification of susceptible individuals and early detection of lung cancer may work in practice, Field et al. (2006) have developed a "biomarker-based screening cascade" (Fig. 2). In the first instance, high-risk populations would be identified through epidemiological risk factors (e.g. smoking duration, respiratory

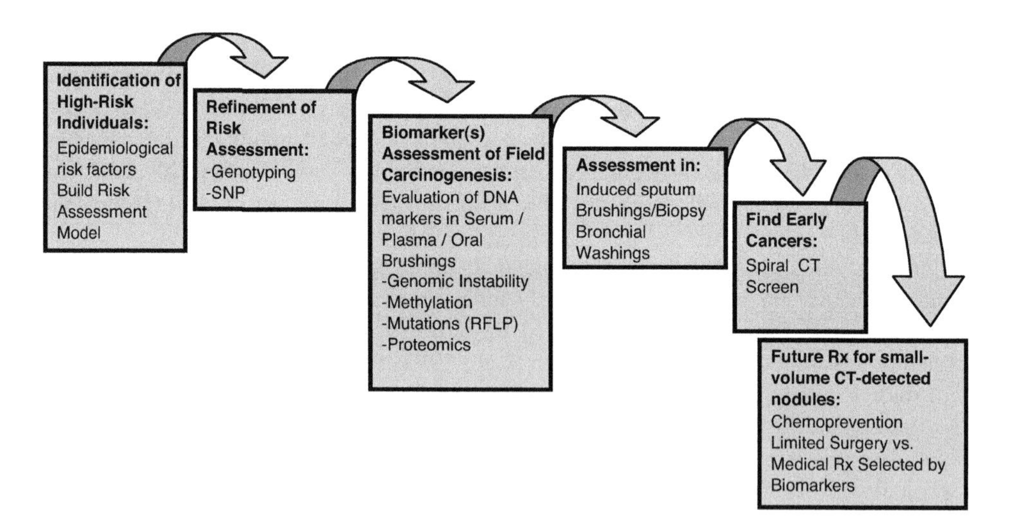

Fig. 2. Lung cancer screening cascade.

disease and occupational exposure) (Field et al., 2005; Cassidy et al., 2006). DNA-based susceptibility markers would be identified in high-risk individuals followed by detection of biomarkers in serum or plasma and bronchial lavage or induced sputum. The cumulative risk of developing lung cancer at this point would trigger clinical investigations through spiral CT imaging. The combined results of imaging and molecular–pathological investigations will determine the individual's future lung cancer treatment regime.

The death rate from lung cancer worldwide is unacceptably high, and this epidemic shows few signs of reversing in the foreseeable future. The eventual understanding of the genetic and environmental basis of lung cancers will enable us to identify high-risk populations and to develop effective prevention, early detection and chemoprevention strategies (Carbone, 2004). Prevention and early detection must be a healthcare priority for all nations if we are to have a major impact on this disease.

REFERENCES

Abbey, D.E., N. Nishino, W.F. McDonnell, R.J. Burchette, S.F. Knutsen, W. Lawrence Beeson and J.X. Yang, 1999, Long-term inhalable particles and other air pollutants related to mortality in nonsmokers. Am. J. Respir. Crit. Care Med., 159(2), 373–382.

Agudo, A., W. Ahrens, E. Benhamou, S. Benhamou, P. Boffetta, S.C. Darby, F. Forastiere, C. Fortes, V. Gaborieau, C.A. Gonzalez, K.H. Jockel, M. Kreuzer, F. Merletti, H. Pohlabeln, L. Richiardi, E. Whitley, H.E. Wichmann, P. Zambon and L. Simonato, 2000, Lung cancer and cigarette smoking in women: a multicenter case-control study in Europe. Int. J. Cancer, 88(5), 820–827.

Alavanja, M.C., R.C. Brownson, J.D. Boice Jr. and E. Hock, 1992, Preexisting lung disease and lung cancer among nonsmoking women. Am. J. Epidemiol., 136(6), 623–632.

Alberg, A.J. and J.M. Samet, 2003, Epidemiology of lung cancer, Chest, 123(1 Suppl), 21S–49S.

Alberg, A.J., M.V. Brock and J.M. Samet, 2005, Epidemiology of lung cancer: looking to the future. J. Clin. Oncol., 23(14), 3175–3185.

Alexandrie, A.K., M.I. Sundberg, J. Seidegard, G. Tornling and A. Rannug, 1994, Genetic susceptibility to lung cancer with special emphasis on CYP1A1 and GSTM1: a study on host factors in relation to age at onset, gender and histological cancer types. Carcinogenesis, 15(9), 1785–1790.

Ames, B.N., M.K. Shigenaga and L.S. Gold, 1993, DNA lesions, inducible DNA repair, and cell division: three key factors in mutagenesis and carcinogenesis. Environ. Health Perspect., 101(Suppl 5), 35–44.

Amos, C.I., N.E. Caporaso and A. Weston, 1992, Host factors in lung cancer risk: a review of interdisciplinary studies. Cancer Epidemiol. Biomarkers Prev., 1(6), 505–513.

Amos, C.I., W. Xu and M.R. Spitz, 1999, Is there a genetic basis for lung cancer susceptibility? Recent Results. Cancer Res., 151, 3–12.

Anto, J.M., P. Vermeire, J. Vestbo and J. Sunyer, 2001, Epidemiology of chronic obstructive pulmonary disease. Eur. Respir. J., 17(5), 982–994.

Anttila, A., P. Heikkila, E. Pukkala, E. Nykyri, T. Kauppinen, S. Hernberg and K. Hemminki, 1995, Excess lung cancer among workers exposed to lead. Scand. J. Work Environ. Health, 21(6), 460–469.

Ayesh, S.K., M. Ferne, B.M. Babior and Y. Matzner, 1990, Partial characterisation of a C5A-inhibitor in peritoneal fluid. J. Immunol., 144, 3066–3070.

Bailey-Wilson, J.E., C.I. Amos, S.M. Pinney, G.M. Petersen, M. de Andrade, J.S. Wiest, P. Fain, A.G. Schwartz, M. You, W. Franklin, C. Klein, A. Gazdar, H. Rothschild, D. Mandal, T. Coons, J. Slusser, J. Lee, C. Gaba, E. Kupert, A. Perez, X. Zhou, D. Zeng, Q. Liu, Q. Zhang, D. Seminara, J. Minna and M.W. Anderson, 2004, A major lung cancer susceptibility locus maps to chromosome 6q23-25. Am. J. Hum. Genet., 75(3), 460–474.

Bain, M. and G. McLaren, 1998, Deprivation and Health in Scotland: Insights from NHS Data. ISD Publications, Edinburgh.

Bain, C., D. Feskanich, F.E. Speizer, M. Thun, E. Hertzmark, B.A. Rosner and G.A. Colditz, 2004, Lung cancer rates in men and women with comparable histories of smoking. J. Natl. Cancer. Inst., 96(11), 826–834.

Bandala, E., M. Espinosa, V. Maldonado and J. Melendez-Zajgla, 2001, Inhibitor of apoptosis-1 (IAP-1) expression and apoptosis in non-small-cell lung cancer cells exposed to gemcitabine. Biochem. Pharmacol., 62(1), 13–19.

Barbone, F., M. Bovenzi, F. Cavallieri and G. Stanta, 1995, Air pollution and lung cancer in Trieste, Italy. Am. J. Epidemiol., 141(12), 1161–1169.

Beckett, W.S., 1993, Epidemiology and etiology of lung cancer. Clin. Chest Med., 14(1), 1–15.

Beer, V., B. Bisig and F. Gutzwiller, 1993, Social class gradients in years of potential life lost in Switzerland. Soc. Sci. Med., 37, 1011–1018.

Benhamou, S., W.J. Lee, A.K. Alexandrie, P. Boffetta, C. Bouchardy, D. Butkiewicz, J. Brockmoller, M.L. Clapper, A. Daly, V. Dolzan, J. Ford, L. Gaspari, A. Haugen, A. Hirvonen, K. Husgafvel-Pursiainen, M. Ingelman-Sundberg, I. Kalina, M. Kihara, P. Kremers, L. Le Marchand, S.J. London, V. Nazar-Stewart, M. Onon-Kihara, A. Rannug, M. Romkes, D. Ryberg, J. Seidegard, P. Shields, R.C. Strange, I. Stucker, J. To-Figueras, P. Brennan and E. Taioli, 2002, Meta- and pooled analyses of the effects of glutathione S-transferase M1 polymorphisms and smoking on lung cancer risk. Carcinogenesis, 23(8), 1343–1350.

Blot, W.J. and J.K. McLaughlin, 2004, Are women more susceptible to lung cancer? J. Natl. Cancer Inst., 96(11), 812–813.

Boffetta, P., 2004, Epidemiology of environmental and occupational cancer. Oncogene, 23(38), 6392–6403.

Boffetta, P. and F. Nyberg, 2003, Contribution of environmental factors to cancer risk. Br. Med. Bull., 68, 71–94.

Boffetta, P. and D.M. Parkin, 1994, Cancer in developing countries. CA Cancer J. Clin., 44(2), 81–90.

Boffetta, P., M. Kogevinas, L. Simonato, J. Wilbourn and R. Saracci, 1995, Current perspectives on occupational cancer risks. Int. J. Occup. Environ. Health, 1(4), 315–325.

Boffetta, P., G. Pershagen, K.H. Jockel, F. Forastiere, V. Gaborieau, J. Heinrich, I. Jahn, M. Kreuzer, F. Merletti, F. Nyberg, F. Rosch and L. Simonato, 1999, Cigar and pipe smoking and lung cancer risk: a multicenter study from Europe. J. Natl. Cancer Inst., 91(8), 697–701.

Bosken, C.H., Q. Wei, C.I. Amos and M.R. Spitz, 2002, An analysis of DNA repair as a determinant of survival in patients with non-small-cell lung cancer. J. Natl. Cancer Inst., 94(14), 1091–1099.

Bouchardy, C., S. Benhamou and P. Dayer, 1996, The effect of tobacco on lung cancer risk depends on CYP2D6 activity. Cancer Res., 56, 251–253.

Bouchardy, C., S. Benhamou, N. Jourenkova, P. Dayer and A. Hirvonen, 2001, Metabolic genetic polymorphisms and susceptibility to lung cancer. Lung Cancer, 32(2), 109–112.

Bray, F., J.E. Tyczynski and D.M. Parkin, 2004, Going up or coming down? The changing phases of the lung cancer epidemic from 1967 to 1999 in the 15 European Union countries. Eur. J. Cancer, 40(1), 96–125.

Brennan, P., C.C. Hsu, N. Moullan, N. Szeszenia-Dabrowska, J. Lissowska, D. Zaridze, P. Rudnai, E. Fabianova, D. Mates, V. Bencko, L. Foretova, V. Janout, F. Gemignani, A. Chabrier, J. Hall, R.J. Hung, P. Boffetta and F. Canzian, 2005, Effect of cruciferous vegetables on lung cancer in patients stratified by genetic status: a Mendelian randomisation approach. Lancet, 366(9496),1558–1560.

Brenner, A.V., Z. Wang, R.A. Kleinerman, L. Wang, S. Zhang, C. Metayer, K. Chen, S. Lei, H. Cui and J.H. Lubin, 2001, Previous pulmonary diseases and risk of lung cancer in Gansu Province, China. Int. J. Epidemiol., 30(1), 118–124.

Brockmoller, J., R. Kerb, N. Drakoulis, B. Staffeldt and I. Roots, 1994, Glutathione S-transferase M1 and its variants A and B as host factors of bladder cancer susceptibility: a case-control study. Cancer Res., 54(15), 4103–4111.

Cantlay, A.M., C.A. Smith, W.A. Wallace, P.L. Yap, D. Lamb and D.J. Harrison, 1994, Heterogeneous expression and polymorphic genotype of glutathione S-transferases in human lung. Thorax, 49(10), 1010–1014.

Cantlay, A.M., D. Lamb, M. Gillooly, J. Norrman, D. Morrison and C.A.D. Smith, 1995, Association between the CYP1A1 gene polymorphism and susceptibility to emphysema and lung cancer. J. Clin. Pathol. Mol. Pathol., 48, M210–M214.

Caporaso, N.E., 2002, Why have we failed to find the low penetrance genetic constituents of common cancers? Cancer Epidemiol. Biomarkers Prev., 11(12), 1544–1549.

Carbone, D.P., 2004, Lung cancer: early events, early interventions: conference summary for the–46th Annual Thomas L Petty Aspen Lung Conference. Chest, 125(5 Suppl), 167S–172S.

Cascorbi, I., S. Henning, J. Brockmoller, J. Gephart, C. Meisel, J.M. Muller, R. Loddenkemper and I. Roots, 2000, Substantially reduced risk of cancer of the aerodigestive tract in subjects with variant–463A of the myeloperoxidase gene. Cancer Res., 60(3), 644–649.

Cassidy, A., J. Myles, T. Liloglou, S.W. Duffy and J.K. Field, 2006, Defining high-risk individuals in a population-based molecular-epidemiological study of lung cancer. Int. J. Oncol., 28(5), 1295–1301.
Charloux, A., E. Quoix, N. Wolkove, D. Small, G. Pauli and H. Kreisman, 1997a, The increasing incidence of lung adenocarcinoma: reality or artefact? A review of the epidemiology of lung adenocarcinoma. Int. J. Epidemiol., 26(1), 14–23.
Charloux, A., M. Rossignol, A. Purohit, D. Small, N. Wolkove, G. Pauli, E. Quoix and H. Kreisman, 1997b, International differences in epidemiology of lung adenocarcinoma. Lung Cancer, 16(2–3), 133–143.
Chen, H., A. Lum, A. Seifried, L.R. Wilkens and L. Le Marchand, 1999, Association of the NAD(P) H:quinone oxidoreductase 609C→T polymorphism with a decreased lung cancer risk. Cancer Res., 59(13), 3045–3048.
Cheng, T.J., D.C. Christiani, X. Xu, J.C. Wain, J.K. Wiencke and K.T. Kelsey, 1995, Glutathione S-transferase mu genotype, diet, and smoking as determinants of sister chromatid exchange frequency in lymphocytes. Cancer Epidemiol. Biomarkers Prev., 4(5), 535–542.
Cheng, L., M.R. Spitz, W.K. Hong and Q. Wei, 2000, Reduced expression levels of nucleotide excision repair genes in lung cancer: a case-control analysis. Carcinogenesis, 21(8), 1527–1530.
Christensen, P.M., P.C. Gotzsche and K. Brosen, 1997, The sparteine/debrisoquine (CYP2D6) oxidation polymorphism and the risk of lung cancer: a meta-analysis. Br. J. Clin. Pharmacol., 51, 389–393.
Chyou, P.H., A.M. Nomura and G.N. Stimmermann, 1992, A prospective study of the attributable risk of cancer due to cigarette smoking. Am. J. Public Health, 82, 37–40.
Cohen, A.J., 2000, Outdoor air pollution and lung cancer. Environ. Health Perspect., 108(Suppl 4), 743–750.
Coleman, M.P., P. Babb, P. Damiecki, P. Grosclaude, S. Honjo, J. Jones, G. Knerer, A. Pitard, M.J. Quinn, A. Sloggett and B.L. de Stavola, 1998, Cancer Survival Trends in England and Wales 1971–1995: Deprivation and NHS Region, Series SMPS No. 61. The Stationary Office, London.
Coleman, M.P., B. Rachet, L.M. Woods, E. Mitry, M. Riga, N. Cooper, M.J. Quinn, H. Brenner and J. Esteve, 2004, Trends and socioeconomic inequalities in cancer survival in England and Wales up to 2001. Br. J. Cancer, 90(7), 1367–1373.
Coultas, D.B. and J.M. Samet, 1992, Occupational lung cancer clinics in chest medicine. Clin. Chest. Med., 13(2), 341–354.
Crispo, A., P. Brennan, K.H. Jockel, A. Schaffrath-Rosario, H.E. Wichmann, F. Nyberg, L. Simonato, F. Merletti, F. Forastiere, P. Boffetta and S. Darby, 2004, The cumulative risk of lung cancer among current, ex- and never-smokers in European men. Br. J. Cancer, 91(7), 1280–1286.
Darby, S., D. Hill, A. Auvinen, J.M. Barros-Dios, H. Baysson, F. Bochicchio, H. Deo, R. Falk, F. Forastiere, M. Hakama, I. Heid, L. Kreienbrock, M. Kreuzer, F. Lagarde, I. Makelainen, C. Muirhead, W. Oberaigner, G. Pershagen, A. Ruano-Ravina, E. Ruosteenoja, A.S. Rosario, M. Tirmarche, L. Tomasek, E. Whitley, H.E. Wichmann and R. Doll, 2005, Radon in homes and risk of lung cancer: collaborative analysis of individual data from 13 European case-control studies. Br. Med. J., 330(7485), 223.
Davey Smith, G., D. Leon, M.J. Shipley and G. Rose, 1991, Socioeconomic differentials among men. Int. J. Epidemiol., 20, 339–345.
de Flora, S., C. Bennicelli, F. D'Agostini, A. Izzotti and A. Camoirano, 1994, Cytosolic activation of aromatic and heterocyclic amines. Inhibition by dicoumarol and enhancement in viral hepatitis B. Environ. Health Perspect., 102(Suppl 6), 69–74.
Denissenko, M.F., A. Pao, M. Tang and G.P. Pfeifer, 1996, Preferential formation of benzo[a]pyrene adducts at lung cancer mutational hotspots in p53. Science, 274(5286), 430–432.
d'Errico, A., E. Taioli, X. Chen and P. Vineis, 1996, Genetic metabolic polymorphisms and the risk of cancer: a review of the literature. Biomarkers, 1, 149–173.
d'Errico, A., N. Malats, P. Vineis and P. Boffetta, 1999, Review of studies of selected metabolic polymorphisms and cancer. In: P. Vineis, N. Malats, M. Lang, A. d'Errico, N. Caporaso, J. Cuzick and P. Boffetta (Eds.), Metabolic Polymorphisms and Susceptibility to Cancer. IARC, Lyon. France, pp. 323–393.
Diez-Roux, A.V., 2000, Multilevel analysis in public health research. Annu. Rev. Public Health, 21, 171–192.
Dockery, D.W., C.A. Pope 3rd, X. Xu, J.D. Spengler, J.H. Ware, M.E. Fay, B.G. Ferris Jr. and F.E. Speizer, 1993, An association between air pollution and mortality in six U.S. cities. N. Engl. J. Med., 329(24), 1753–1759.
Doll, R., 1955, Mortality from lung cancer in asbestos workers. Br. J. Ind. Med., 12(2), 81–86.
Doll, R. and R. Peto, 1978, Cigarette smoking and bronchial carcinoma: dose and time relationships among regular smokers and lifelong non-smokers. J. Epidemiol. Community Health, 32(4), 303–313.

Doll, R. and R. Peto, 1981, The causes of cancer: quantitative estimates of avoidable risks of cancer in the United States today. J. Natl. Cancer Inst., 66, 1191–1308.

Dorgan, J.F., R.G. Ziegler, J.B. Schoenberg, P. Hartge, M.J. McAdams, R.T. Falk, H.B. Wilcox and G.L. Shaw, 1993, Race and sex differences in associations of vegetables, fruits, and carotenoids with lung cancer risk in New Jersey (United States). Cancer Causes Control, 4(3), 273–281.

Dosemeci, M., I. Gokmen, M. Unsal, R.B. Hayes and A. Blair, 1997, Tobacco, alcohol use, and risks of laryngeal and lung cancer by subsite and histologic type in Turkey. Cancer Causes Control, 8(5), 729–737.

Eberly, L.E., J. Ockene, R. Sherwin, L. Yang, L. Kuller and Multiple Risk Factor Intervention Trial Research Group, 2003, Pulmonary function as a predictor of lung cancer mortality in continuing cigarette smokers and in quitters. Int. J. Epidemiol., 32(4), 592–599.

Engeland, A., T. Haldorsen, A. Andersen, S. Tretli, 1996, The impact of smoking habits on lung cancer risk: 28 years' observation of 26,000 Norwegian men and women. Cancer Causes Control, 7(3), 366–376.

Etzel, C.J., C.I. Amos and M.R. Spitz, 2003, Risk for smoking-related cancer among relatives of lung cancer patients. Cancer Res., 63(23), 8531–8535.

Faggiano, F., R. Zanetti and G. Costa, 1994, Cancer risk and social inequalities in Italy. J. Epidemiol. Comm. Health, 48, 447–452.

Faggiano, F., T. Partanen, M. Kogevinas and P. Boffetta, 1997, Socioeconomic differences in cancer incidence and mortality. In: M. Kogevinas, N. Pearce, M. Susser and P. Boffetta (Eds.), Social Inequalities and Cancer. IARC Scientific Publications No. 138, IARC, Lyon, France.

Ferguson, M.K., C. Skosey, P.C. Hoffman and H.M. Golomb, 1990, Sex-associated differences in presentation and survival in patients with lung cancer. J. Clin. Oncol., 8(8), 1402–1407.

Fernandez, E. and C. Borrell, 1999, Cancer mortality by educational level in the city of Barcelona. Br. J. Cancer, 79, 684–689.

Feskanich, D., R.G. Ziegler, D.S. Michaud, E.L. Giovannucci, F.E. Speizer, W.C. Willett and G.A. Colditz, 2000, Prospective study of fruit and vegetable consumption and risk of lung cancer among men and women. J. Natl. Cancer Inst., 92(22), 1812–1823.

Feyler, A., A. Voho, C. Bouchardy, K. Kuokkanen, P. Dayer, A. Hirvonen and S. Benhamou, 2002, Point: myeloperoxidase -463G→a polymorphism and lung cancer risk. Cancer Epidemiol. Biomarkers Prev., 11(12), 1550–1554.

Field, J.K., D.L. Smith, S. Duffy and A. Cassidy, 2005, The Liverpool Lung Project research protocol. Int. J. Oncol., 27(6), 1633–1645.

Field, J.K., D. Beer, D. Carbone, E. Brambilla, E. Thunnissen, S. Duffy, R. Avila, C. Henschke, R. van Klaveren, A. Voss and J. Mulshine, A European strategy for developing lung cancer imaging and molecular diagnosis in high risk populations. Cancer, in press.

Ford, J.G., Y. Li, M.M. O'Sullivan, R. Demopoulos, S. Garte, E. Taioli and P.W. Brandt-Rauf, 2000, Glutathione S-transferase M1 polymorphism and lung cancer risk in African-Americans. Carcinogenesis, 21(11), 1971–1975.

Forey, B., J. Hamling, P. Lee and N. Wald, 2002, International Smoking Statistics, 2nd ed. Oxford University Press, Oxford.

Foote, C.S., T.E. Goyne and R.I. Lehrer, 1983, Assessment of chlorination by human neutrophils. Nature, 301, 715–716.

Friberg, L., L. Kaij, S.J. Dencker and E. Jonsson, 1959, Smoking habits of monozygotic and dizygotic twins. Br. Med. J., 46(5129), 1090–1092.

Ganti, A.K. and J.L. Mulshine, 2005, Lung cancer screening: panacea or pipe dream? Ann. Oncol., 16(Suppl 2), 215–219.

Geradts, J., K.M. Fong, P.V. Zimmerman, R. Maynard and J.D. Minna, 1999, Correlation of abnormal RB, p16ink4a, and p53 expression with 3p loss of heterozygosity, other genetic abnormalities, and clinical features in 103 primary non-small cell lung cancers. Clin. Cancer Res., 5(4), 791–800.

Ginsberg, R.J., E.E. Vokes and K. Rosenzweig, 2001, Non-small cell lung cancer. In: V.T. DeVita, S. Hellmann and S.A. Rosenberg (Eds.), Cancer: Principles and Practice of Oncology, Vol. 1, 6th ed., Lippincott Williams & Wilkins, Philadelphia pp. 925–983.

Gonzalez, F.J. and H.V. Gelboin, 1993, Role of human cytochrome P-450s in risk assessment and susceptibility to environmentally based disease. J. Toxicol. Environ. Health, 40(2–3), 289–308.

Gonzalez-Quevedo, R., P. Iniesta, A. Moran, C. de Juan, A. Sanchez-Pernaute, C. Fernandez, A. Torres, E. Diaz-Rubio, J.L. Balibrea and M. Benito, 2002, Cooperative role of telomerase activity and p16 expression in the prognosis of non-small-cell lung cancer. J. Clin. Oncol., 20(1), 254–262.

Goode, E.L., C.M. Ulrich and J.D. Potter, 2002, Polymorphisms in DNA repair genes and associations with cancer risk. Cancer Epidemiol. Biomarkers Prev., 11(12), 1513–1530.

Goodman, G.E., 2002, Lung cancer. 1: prevention of lung cancer. Thorax, 57(11), 994–999.

Grimsrud, T.K., H. Langseth, A. Engeland and A. Andersen, 1998, Lung and bladder cancer in a Norwegian municipality with iron and steel producing industry: population based case-control studies. Occup. Environ. Med., 55(6), 387–392.

Hackshaw, A.K., M.R. Law and N.J. Wald, 1997, The accumulated evidence on lung cancer and environmental tobacco smoke. Br. Med. J., 315, 980–988.

Harris, C.C. and M. Hollstein, 1993, Clinical implications of the p53 tumour-suppressor gene. N. Engl. J. Med., 329(18), 1318–1327.

Harrison, D.J., A.M. Cantlay, F. Rae, D. Lamb and C.A. Smith, 1997, Frequency of glutathione S-transferase M1 deletion in smokers with emphysema and lung cancer. Hum. Exp. Toxicol., 16(7), 356–360.

Hart, C.L., D.J. Hole, C.R. Gillis, G.D. Smith, G.C. Watt and V.M. Hawthorne, 2001, Social class differences in lung cancer mortality: risk factor explanations using two Scottish cohort studies. Int. J. Epidemiol., 30(2), 268–274.

Hayashi, S., J. Watanabe and K. Kawajiri, 1992, High susceptibility to lung cancer analysed in terms of combined genotypes of P4501A1 and Mu-class glutathione S-transferase genes. Jpn. J. Cancer Res., 83, 866–870.

Heath, C.W., 1958, Differences between smokers and nonsmokers. AMA Arch. Intern. Med., 101(2):377–388.

Hecht, S.S., 1999, Tobacco smoke carcinogens and lung cancer. J. Natl. Cancer Inst., 91(14), 1194–1210.

Hecht, S.S., 2003, Tobacco carcinogens, their biomarkers and tobacco-induced cancer. Nat. Rev. Cancer, 3(10), 733–744.

Henschke, C.I. and O.S. Miettinen, 2004, Women's susceptibility to tobacco carcinogens. Lung Cancer, 43(1), 1–5.

Henschke, C.I., D.I. McCauley, D.F. Yankelevitz, D.P. Naidich, G. McGuinness, O.S. Miettinen, D.M. Libby, M.W. Pasmantier, J. Koizumi, N.K. Altorki and J.P. Smith, 1999, Early Lung Cancer Action Project: overall design and findings from baseline screening. Lancet, 354(9173), 99–105.

Hietanen, E., K. Husgafvel-Pursiainen and H. Vainio, 1997, Interaction between dose and susceptibility to environmental cancer: a short review. Environ. Health Perspect., 105(Suppl 4), 749–754.

Hirayama, T., 1981, Non-smoking wives of heavy smokers have a higher risk of lung cancer: a study from Japan. Br. Med. J. (Clin. Res. Ed.), 282(6259), 183–185.

Hirsch, F.R. and S.M. Lippman, 2005, Advances in the biology of lung cancer chemoprevention. J. Clin. Oncol., 23(14), 3186–3197.

Hoek, G., B. Brunekreef, S. Goldbohm, P. Fischer and P.A. van den Brandt, 2002, Association between mortality and indicators of traffic-related air pollution in the Netherlands: a cohort study. Lancet, 360(9341), 1203–1209.

Holick, C.N., D.S. Michaud, R. Stolzenberg-Solomon, S.T. Mayne, P. Pietinen, P.R. Taylor, J. Virtamo and D. Albanes, 2002, Dietary carotenoids, serum beta-carotene, and retinol and risk of lung cancer in the alpha-tocopherol, beta-carotene cohort study. Am. J. Epidemiol., 156(6), 536–547.

Houlston, R.S., 1999, Glutathione S-transferase M1 status and lung cancer risk: a meta-analysis. Cancer Epidemiol. Biomarkers Prev., 8, 675–682.

Houlston, R.S., 2000, CYP1A1 polymorphisms and lung cancer risk: a meta-analysis. Pharmacogenetics, 10, 105–114.

Huber, R.M. and D.F. Stratakis, 2004, Molecular oncology—perspectives in lung cancer. Lung Cancer, 45(Suppl 2), S209–S213.

Hung, R.J., P. Boffetta, J. Brockmoller, D. Butkiewicz, I. Cascorbi, M.L. Clapper, S. Garte, A. Haugen, A. Hirvonen, S. Anttila, I. Kalina, L. Le Marchand, S.J. London, A. Rannug, M. Romkes, J. Salagovic, B. Schoket, L. Gaspari and E. Taioli, 2003, CYP1A1 and GSTM1 genetic polymorphisms and lung cancer risk in Caucasian non-smokers: a pooled analysis. Carcinogenesis, 24(5), 875–882.

Hunninghake, G.W., J.E. Gadek, O. Kawanami, V.J. Ferrans and R.G. Crystal, 1979, Inflammatory and immune processes in the human lung in health and disease: evaluation by bronchoalveolar lavage. Am. J. Pathol., 97(1), 149–206.

Hussain, S.P. and C.C. Harris, 1998, Molecular epidemiology of human cancer: contribution of mutation spectra studies of tumour suppressor genes. Cancer Res., 58(18), 4023–4037.

IARC, 1986, Tobacco Smoking. IARC Monographs on the Evaluation of Carcinogenic Risk to Humans, Vol. 38. International Agency for Research on Cancer, Lyon, France.

IARC, 2004, Tobacco Smoking and Involuntary Smoking. IARC Monographs on the Evaluation of Carcinogenic Risk to Humans, Vol. 83, International Agency for Research on Cancer, Lyon, France.

Islam, S.S. and D. Schottenfeld, 1994, Declining FEV1 and chronic productive cough in cigarette smokers: a 25-year prospective study of lung cancer incidence in Tecumseh, Michigan. Cancer Epidemiol. Biomarkers Prev., 3(4), 289–298.

Jain, M., J.D. Burch, G.R. Howe, H.A. Risch and A.B. Miller, 1990, Dietary factors and the risk of lung cancer: results from a case-control study, Toronto 1981–85. Int. J. Cancer, 45, 287–293.

Janssen-Heijnen, M.L., H.W. Nab, J. van Reek, L.H. van der Heijden, R. Schipper and J.W. Coebergh, 1995, Striking changes in smoking behaviour and lung cancer incidence by histological type in south-east Netherlands, 1960–1991. Eur. J. Cancer, 31A(6), 949–952.

Jedrychowski, W., H. Becher, J. Wahrendorf, Z. Basa-Cierpialek and K. Gomola, 1992, Effect of tobacco smoking on various histological types of lung cancer. J. Cancer Res. Clin. Oncol., 118(4), 276–282.

Jemal, A., K.C. Chu and R.E. Tarone, 2001, Recent trends in lung cancer mortality in the United States. J. Natl. Cancer Inst., 93(4), 277–283.

Jemal, A., W.D. Travis, R.E. Tarone, L. Travis and S.S. Devesa, 2003, Lung cancer rates convergence in young men and women in the United States: analysis by birth cohort and histologic type. Int. J. Cancer, 105(1), 101–107.

Jemal, A., L.X. Clegg, E. Ward, L.A. Ries, X. Wu, P.M. Jamison, P.A. Wingo, H.L. Howe, R.N. Anderson and B.K. Edwards, 2004, Annual report to the nation on the status of cancer, 1975–2001, with a special feature regarding survival. Cancer, 101(1), 3–27.

Jonsson, S., U. Thorsteinsdottir, D.F. Gudbjartsson, H.H. Jonsson, K. Kristjansson, S. Arnason, V. Gudnason, H.J. Isaksson, J. Hallgrimsson, J.R. Gulcher, L.T. Amundadottir, A. Kong and K. Stefansson, 2004, Familial risk of lung carcinoma in the Icelandic population. JAMA, 292(24), 2977–2983.

Joseph, P. and A.K. Jaiswal, 1994, NAD(P)H:quinone oxidoreductase1 (DT diaphorase) specifically prevents the formation of benzo[*a*]pyrene quinone–DNA adducts generated by cytochrome P4501A1 and P450 reductase. Proc. Natl. Acad. Sci. USA 91, 8413–8417.

Kabat, G.C., 1996, Aspects of the epidemiology of lung cancer in smokers and non-smokers in the United States. Lung Cancer, 15, 1–20.

Kamataki, T., 1993, Metabolism of xenobiotics. In: T. Omura, Y. Ishimura and Y. Fuijii-Kuriyama (Eds.), Cytochrome P-450, 2nd ed., Kodansha Ltd, Tokyo, pp. 141–158.

Kato, S., E.D. Bowman, A.M. Harrington, B. Blomeke and P.G. Sheilds, 1995, Human lung carcinogen DNA adduct levels mediated by genetic polymorphisms in vivo. J. Natl. Cancer Inst., 87(12), 902–907.

Katsouyanni, K. and G. Pershagen, 1997, Ambient air pollution exposure and cancer. Cancer Causes Control, 8(3), 284–291.

Kawajiri, K., K. Nakachi, K. Imai, S. Hayashi and J. Watanabe, 1990, Individual differences in lung cancer susceptibility in relation to polymorphisms of P-450IA1 gene and cigarette dose. Princess Takamatsu. Symp., 21, 55–61.

Keohavong, P., M.A. DeMichele, A.C. Melacrinos, R.J. Landreneau, R.J. Weyant and J.M. Siegfried, 1996, Detection of K-ras mutations in lung carcinomas: relationship to prognosis. Clin. Cancer Res., 2(2), 411–418.

Kihara, M., M. Kihara and K. Noda, 1994, Lung cancer risk of GSTM1 null genotype is dependent on the extent of tobacco smoke exposure. Carcinogenesis, 15, 415–418.

Kiyohara, C., A. Otsu, T. Shirakawa, S. Fukuda and J.M. Hopkin, 2002, Genetic polymorphisms and lung cancer susceptibility: a review. Lung Cancer, 37(3), 241–256.

Kiyohara, C., K. Yoshimasu, K. Takayama and Y. Nakanishi, 2005, NQ01, MPO, and the risk of lung cancer: a HuGE review. Genet. Med., 7(7), 463–478.

Knekt, P., R. Jarvinen, R. Seppanen, M. Hellovaara, L. Teppo, E. Pukkala and A. Aromaa, 1997, Dietary flavonoids and the risk of lung cancer and other malignant neoplasms. Am. J. Epidemiol., 146(3), 223–230.

Koo, L.C., 1988, Dietary habits and lung cancer risk among Chinese females in Hong Kong who never smoked. Nutr. Cancer, 11(3), 155–172.

Kreuzer, M., P. Boffetta, E. Whitley, W. Ahrens, V. Gaborieau, J. Heinrich, K.H. Jockel, L. Kreienbrock, S. Mallone, F. Merletti, F. Roesch, P. Zambon and L. Simonato, 2000, Gender differences in lung cancer risk by smoking: a multicentre case-control study in Germany and Italy. Br. J. Cancer, 82(1), 227–233.

Krieger, N., J.T. Chen, P.D. Waterman, D.H. Rehkopf and S.V. Subramanian, 2003, Race/ethnicity, gender, and monitoring socioeconomic gradients in health: a comparison of area-based socioeconomic measures—the public health disparities geocoding project. Am. J. Public Health, 93(10), 1655–1671.

Kure, E.H., D. Ryberg, A. Hewer, D.H. Phillips, V. Skaug, R. Baera and A. Haugen, 1996, p53 mutations in lung tumours: relationship to gender and lung DNA adduct levels. Carcinogenesis, 17(10), 2201–2205.

Kvåle, G., E. Bjelke and J.J. Gart, 1983, Dietary habits and lung cancer risk. Int. J. Cancer, 31, 397–405.

Le Marchand, L., S.P. Murphy, J.H. Hankin, L.R. Wilkens and L.N. Kolonel, 2000a, Intake of flavonoids and lung cancer. J. Natl. Cancer Inst., 92(2), 154–160.

Le Marchand, L., A. Seifried, A. Lum and L.R. Wilkens, 2000b, Association of the myeloperoxidase-463G→a polymorphism with lung cancer risk. Cancer Epidemiol. Biomarkers Prev., 9, 181–184.

Le Marchand, L., C. Guo, S. Benhamou, C. Bouchardy, I. Cascorbi, M.L. Clapper, S. Garte, A. Haugen, M. Ingelman-Sundberg, M. Kihara, A. Rannug, D. Ryberg, I. Stucker, H. Sugimura and E. Taioli, 2003, Pooled analysis of the CYP1A1 exon 7 polymorphism and lung cancer (United States). Cancer Causes Control, 14(4), 339–346.

Lemen, R.A., J.M. Dement and J.K. Wagoner, 1980, Epidemiology of asbestos-related diseases. Environ. Health Perspect., 34, 1–11.

Levi, F., E. Negri, C. LaVecchia and V.C. Te, 1998, Socioeconomic groups and cancer risk at death in the Swiss canton of Vaud. Int. J. Epidemiol., 17, 711–717.

Lewis, S.J., N.M. Cherry, R.M. Niven, P.V. Barber and A.C. Povey, 2001, Polymorphisms in the NAD(P)H: quinone oxidoreductase gene and small cell lung cancer risk in a UK population. Lung Cancer, 34(2), 177–183.

Lissowska, J., A. Bardin-Mikolajczak, T. Fletcher, D. Zaridze, N. Szeszenia-Dabrowska, P. Rudnai, E. Fabianova, A. Cassidy, D. Mates, I. Holcatova, V. Vitova, V. Janout, A. Mannetje, P. Brennan and P. Boffetta, 2005, Lung cancer and indoor pollution from heating and cooking with solid fuels: the IARC international multicentre case-control study in Eastern/Central Europe and the United Kingdom. Am. J. Epidemiol., 162(4), 326–333.

Littman, A.J., M.D. Thornquist, E. White, L.A. Jackson, G.E. Goodman and T.L. Vaughan, 2004, Prior lung disease and risk of lung cancer in a large prospective study. Cancer Causes Control, 15(8), 819–827.

Liu, B.Q., R. Peto, Z.M. Chen, J. Boreham, Y.P. Wu, J.Y. Li, T.C. Campbell and J.S. Chen, 1998, Emerging tobacco hazards in China: 1. retrospective proportional mortality study of one million deaths. Br. Med. J. 317(7170), 1411–1422.

London, S.J., A.K. Daly, J. Cooper, W.C. Navidi, C.L. Carpenter and J.R. Idle, 1997a, Polymorphism of glutathione S-transferase M1 and lung cancer risk in African-Americans and Caucasians in Los Angeles County. J. Natl. Cancer Inst., 87(16), 1246–1253.

London, S.J., A.K. Daly, J.B.S. Leahart, W.C. Navidi, C.C. Carpenter and J.R. Idle, 1997b, Genetic polymorphism of CYP2D6 and lung cancer risk in African-Americans and Caucasians in Los Angeles county. Carcinogenesis, 18, 1203–1214.

London, S.J., T. Sullivan-Klose, A.K. Daly and J.R. Idle, 1997c, Lung cancer risk in relation to the CYP2C9 genetic polymorphism among Caucasians in Los Angeles county. Pharmacogenetics, 7(5), 401–414.

London, S.J., T.A. Lehman and J.A. Taylor, 1997d, Myeloperoxidase genetic polymorphism and lung cancer risk. Cancer Res., 57(22), 5001–5003.

London, S.J., J.M. Yuan, F.L. Chung, Y.T. Gao, G.A. Coetzee, R.K. Ross and M.C. Yu, 2000, Isothiocyanates, glutathione S-transferase M1 and T1 polymorphisms, and lung-cancer risk: a prospective study of men in Shanghai, China. Lancet, 356(9231), 724–729.

Lubin, J.H., W.J. Blot, F. Berrino, R. Flamant, C.R. Gillis, M. Kunze, D. Schmahl and G. Visco, 1984, Patterns of lung cancer risk according to type of cigarette smoked. Int. J. Cancer, 33(5), 569–576.

Lubin, J.H., J.D. Boice Jr., C. Edling, R.W. Hornung, G.R. Howe, E. Kunz, R.A. Kusiak, H.I. Morrison, E.P. Radford and J.M. Samet, 1995, Lung cancer in radon-exposed miners and estimation of risk from indoor exposure. J. Natl. Cancer Inst., 87(11), 817–827.

Lynge, E., B.A. Rix, E. Vildsen, I. Andersen, M. Hink, E. Olsen, U.L. Mollar and E. Silfverberg, 1995, Cancer in printing workers in Denmark. Occup. Environ. Med., 52(11), 738–744.

Mackenbach, J.P., M. Huisman, O. Andersen, M. Bopp, J.K. Borgan, C. Borrell, G. Costa, P. Deboosere, A. Donkin, S. Gadeyne, C. Minder, E. Regidor, T. Spadea, T. Valkonen and A.E. Kunst, 2004, Inequalities in lung cancer mortality by the educational level in 10 European populations. Eur. J. Cancer, 40(1), 126–135.

Magnani, C. and M. Leporati, 1998, Mortality from lung cancer and population risk attributable to asbestos in an asbestos cement manufacturing town in Italy. Occup. Environ. Med., 55(2), 111–114.

Mallet, W.G., D.R. Mosebrook and M.A. Trush, 1991, Activation of (+/-)-trans-7,8-dihydroxy-7, 8-dihydrobenzo[a]pyrene to diolepoxides by human polymorphonuclear leukocytes or myeloperoxidase. Carcinogenesis, 12, 521–524.

Mannino, D.M., E. Ford, G.A. Giovino and M. Thun, 2001, Lung cancer mortality rates in birth cohorts in the United States from 1960 to 1994. Lung Cancer, 31(2–3), 91–99.

Mannino, D.M., A.S. Buist, T.L. Petty, P.L. Enright and S.C. Redd, 2003, Lung function and mortality in the United States: data from the First National Health and Nutrition Examination Survey follow up study. Thorax, 58(5), 388–393.

Mannisto, S., S.A. Smith-Warner, D. Spiegelman, D. Albanes, K. Anderson, P.A. van den Brandt, J.R. Cerhan, G. Colditz, D. Feskanich, J.L. Freudenheim, E. Giovannucci, R.A. Goldbohm, S. Graham, A.B. Miller, T.E. Rohan, J. Virtamo, W.C. Willett and D.J. Hunter, 2004, Dietary carotenoids and risk of lung cancer in a pooled analysis of seven cohort studies. Cancer Epidemiol. Biomarkers Prev., 13(1), 40–48.

Matakidou, A., T. Eisen and R.S. Houlston, 2005, Systematic review of the relationship between family history and lung cancer risk. Br. J. Cancer, 93(7), 825–833.

Mattson, M.E., E.S. Pollack and J.W. Cullen, 1987, What are the odds that smoking will kill you? Am. J. Public Health, 77(4), 425–431.

Mayne, S.T., J. Buenconsejo and D.T. Janerich, 1999, Previous lung disease and risk of lung cancer among men and women nonsmokers. Am. J. Epidemiol., 149(1), 13–20.

McWilliams, J.E., B.J.S. Sanderson, E.L. Harris, K.E. Richert-Boe and W.D. Henner, 1995, Glutathione S-transferase M1 deficiency is associated with a moderate increase in risk of developing lung cancer. Proc. Am. Assoc. Cancer Res., 36, 121.

Miller, A.B., H.P. Altenburg, B. Bueno-de-Mesquita, H.C. Boshuizen, A. Agudo, F. Berrino, I.T. Gram, L. Janson, J. Linseisen, K. Overvad, T. Rasmuson, P. Vineis, A. Lukanova, N. Allen, P. Amiano, A. Barricarte, G. Berglund, H. Boeing, F. Clavel-Chapelon, N.E. Day, G. Hallmans, E. Lund, C. Martinez, C. Navarro, D. Palli, S. Panico, P.H. Peeters, J.R. Quiros, A. Tjonneland, R. Tumino, A. Trichopoulou, D. Trichopoulos, N. Slimani and E. Riboli, 2004, Fruits and vegetables and lung cancer: findings from the European Prospective Investigation into Cancer and Nutrition. Int. J. Cancer, 108(2), 269–276.

Mollerup, S., D. Ryberg, A. Hewer, D.H. Phillips and A. Haugen, 1999, Sex differences in lung CYP1A1 expression and DNA adduct levels among lung cancer patients. Cancer Res., 59(14), 3317–3320.

Mooney, L.A. and F.P. Perera, 1996, Application of molecular epidemiology to lung cancer chemoprevention. J. Cell Biochem. Suppl., 25, 63–68.

Moore, S.M., D.S. Gierada, K.W. Clark, G.J. Blaine and PLCO-NLST Quality Assurance Working Group, 2005, Image quality assurance in the prostate, lung, colorectal, and ovarian cancer screening trial network of the National Lung Screening Trial. J. Digit Imaging, 18(3), 242–250.

Motulsky, A.G., 1957, Drug reactions enzymes, and biochemical genetics. J. Am. Med. Assoc., 165(7), 835–837.

Mulshine, J.L. and D.C. Sullivan, 2005, Clinical practice. Lung cancer screening. N. Engl. J. Med., 352(26), 2714–2720.

Naess, O., B. Claussen and G. Davey Smith, 2004, Relative impact of childhood and adulthood socioeconomic conditions on cause specific mortality in men. J. Epidemiol. Community Health, 58(7), 597–598.

Nafstad, P., L.L. Haheim, B. Oftedal, F. Gram, I. Holme, I. Hjermann and P. Leren, 2003, Lung cancer and air pollution: a 27 year follow up of 16 209 Norwegian men. Thorax, 58(12), 1071–1076.

Nakachi, K., K. Imai, S. Hayashi, J. Watanabe and K. Kawajiri, 1991, Genetic susceptibility to squamous cell carcinoma of the lung in relation to cigarette smoking dose. Cancer Res., 51(19), 5177–5180.

Nakachi, K., K. Imai, S. Hyashi and K. Kawajiri, 1993, Polymorphisms of the CYP1A1 and glutathione S-transferase genes associated with susceptibility to lung cancer in relation to cigarette dose in a Japanese population. Cancer Res., 53, 2994–2999.

Nelson, H.H. and K.T. Kelsey, 2002, The molecular epidemiology of asbestos and tobacco in lung cancer. Oncogene, 21(48), 7284–7288.

Neuhouser, M.L., R.E. Patterson, M.D. Thornquist, G.S. Omenn, I.B. King and G.E. Goodman, 2003, Fruits and vegetables are associated with lower lung cancer risk only in the placebo arm of the beta-carotene and retinol efficacy trial (CARET). Cancer Epidemiol. Biomarkers Prev., 12(4), 350–358.

Newhouse, M.L. and G. Berry, 1979, Patterns of mortality in asbestos factory workers in London. Ann. N.Y. Acad. Sci., 330, 53–60.

Nyberg, F., P. Gustavsson, L. Jarup, T. Bellander, N. Berglind, R. Jakobsson and G. Pershagen, 2000, Urban air pollution and lung cancer in Stockholm. Epidemiology, 11(5), 487–495.

Omoto, Y., Y. Kobayashi, K. Nishida, E. Tsuchiya, H. Eguchi, K. Nakagawa, Y. Ishikawa, T. Yamori, H. Iwase, Y. Fujii, M. Warner, J.A. Gustafsson and S.I. Hayashi, 2001, Expression, function, and clinical implications of the estrogen receptor beta in human lung cancers. Biochem. Biophys. Res. Commun., 285(2), 340–347.

Omura, T., Y. Ishimura and Y. Fujii-Kuriyama, 1993, Cytochrome P-450, 2nd Ed. Kodansha, Tokyo.

ONS, 2003, Smoking Related Behaviour and Attitudes, 2002. Office for National Statistics, London.

Osann, K.E., H. Anton-Culver, T. Kurosaki and T. Taylor, 1993, Sex differences in lung-cancer risk associated with cigarette smoking. Int. J. Cancer, 54(1), 44–48.

Osann, K.E., J.T. Lowery and M.J. Schell, 2000, Small cell lung cancer in women: risk associated with smoking, prior respiratory disease, and occupation. Lung Cancer, 28(1), 1–10.

Pages, V. and R.P. Fuchs, 2002, How DNA lesions are turned into mutations within cells? Oncogene, 21(58), 8957–8966.

Park, J., L. Chen, M.S. Tockman, A. Elahi and P. Lazarus, 2004, The human 8-oxoguanine DNA N-glycosylase 1 (hOGG1) DNA repair enzyme and its association with lung cancer risk. Pharmacogenetics, 14(2), 103–109.

Parkin, D.M., S.L. Whelan, J. Ferlay, L. Teppo and D. Thomas, 2003, Cancer incidence in Five Continents, Vol. VIII. IARC Scientific Publication No. 155, IARC Press.

Parkin, D.M., F. Bray, J. Ferlay and P. Pisani, 2005, Global cancer statistics, 2002. CA Cancer J. Clin., 55(2), 74–108.

Partanen, T. and P. Boffetta, 1994, Cancer risk in asphalt workers and roofers – review and meta-analysis of epidemiologic studies. Am. J. Ind. Med., 26(6), 721–740.

Patel, J.D., 2005, Lung cancer in women. J. Clin. Oncol., 23(14), 3212–3218.

Patrone, C., T.N. Cassel, K. Pettersson, Y.S. Piao, G. Cheng, P. Ciana, A. Maggi, M. Warner, J.A. Gustafsson and M. Nord, 2003, Regulation of postnatal lung development and homeostasis by estrogen receptor beta. Mol. Cell. Biol., 23(23), 8542–8552.

Pershagen, G. and L. Simonato, 1990, Epidemiological evidence for the carcinogeneity of air pollutants. Air pollution and human cancer. In: Tomatis, L. (Ed.), European School of Oncology Monograph. Springer-Verlag, Berlin.

Peto, J., 2001, Cancer epidemiology in the last century and the next decade. Nature, 441, 390–395.

Peto, R., A.D. Lopez, J. Boreham, M. Thun, C. Heath Jr., 1992, Mortality from tobacco in developed countries: indirect estimation from national vital statistics. Lancet, 339(8804), 1268–1278.

Peto, R., S. Darby, H. Deo, P. Silcocks, E. Whitley and R. Doll, 2000, Smoking, smoking cessation, and lung cancer in the UK since 1950: combination of national statistics with two case-control studies. Br. Med. J., 321(7257), 323–329.

Petruska, J.M., D.R. Mosebrook, G.J. Jakab and M.A. Trush, 1992, Myeloperoxidase-enhanced formation of (+/-)-trans-7,8-dihydroxy-7,8-dihydrobenzo[*a*]pyrene–DNA adducts in lung tissue in vitro: a role of pulmonary inflammation in the bioactivation of a procarcinogen. Carcinogenesis, 13, 1075–1081.

Pope 3rd, C.A., R.T. Burnett, M.J. Thun, E.E. Calle, D. Krewski, K. Ito and G.D. Thurston, 2002, Lung cancer, cardiopulmonary mortality, and long-term exposure to fine particulate air pollution. JAMA, 287(9), 1132–1141.

Prutz, W.A., 1998, Interactions of hypochlorous acid with pyrimidine nucleotides, and secondary reactions of chlorinated pyrimidines with GSH, NADH, and other substrates. Arch. Biochem. Biophys., 349, 183–191.

Qiuling, S., Z. Yuxin, Z. Suhua, X. Cheng, L. Shuguang and H. Fengsheng, 2003, Cyclin D1 gene polymorphism and susceptibility to lung cancer in a Chinese population. Carcinogenesis, 24(9), 1499–1503.

Quinones, L., D. Lucas, J. Godoy, D. Caceres, F. Berthou, N. Varela, K. Lee, C. Acevedo, L. Martinez, A.M. Aguilera and L. Gil, 2001, CYP1A1, CYP2E1 and GSTM1 genetic polymorphisms. The effect of single and combined genotypes on lung cancer susceptibility in Chilean people. Cancer Lett., 174(1), 35–44.

Radzikowska, E., P. Glaz and K. Roszkowski, 2002, Lung cancer in women: age, smoking, histology, performance status, stage, initial treatment and survival. Population-based study of 20 561 cases. Ann. Oncol., 13(7), 1087–1093.

Ratnasinghe, D., J.A. Tangrea, M.R. Andersen, M.J. Barrett, J. Virtamo, P.R. Taylor and D. Albanes, 2000, Glutathione peroxidase codon 198 polymorphism variant increases lung cancer risk. Cancer Res., 60(22), 6381–6383.

Regidor, E., J.L. Gutierrez-Fisac and C. Rodriguez, 1995, Increased socioeconomic differences in mortality in eight Spanish provinces. Soc. Sci. Med., 41, 801–807.

Richiardi, L., P. Boffetta, L. Simonato, F. Forastiere, P. Zambon, C. Fortes, V. Gaborieau and F. Merletti, 2004, Occupational risk factors for lung cancer in men and women: a population-based case-control study in Italy. Cancer Causes Control, 15(3), 285–294.

Risch, H.A., G.R. Howe, M. Jain, J.D. Burch, E.J. Holowaty and A.B. Miller, 1993, Are female smokers at higher risk for lung cancer than male smokers? A case-control analysis by histologic type. Am. J. Epidemiol., 138(5), 281–293.

Robles, A.I., N.A. Bemmels, A.B. Foraker and C.C. Harris, 2001, APAF-1 is a transcriptional target of p53 in DNA damage-induced apoptosis. Cancer Res., 61(18), 6660–6664.

Ross, J.A. and G.D. Rosen, 2002, The molecular biology of lung cancer. Curr. Opin. Pulm. Med., 8(4), 265–269.

Rostami-Hodjegan, A., M.S. Lennard, H.F. Woods and G.T. Tucker, 1998, Meta-analysis of studies of the CYP2D6 polymorphism in relation to lung cancer and Parkinson's disease. Pharmacogenetics, 8(3), 227–238.

Roth, J.A., 1995, Molecular events in lung cancer. Lung Cancer, 12(Suppl 2), S3–S15.

Saintigny, Y., D. Rouillard, B. Chaput, T. Soussi and B.S. Lopez, 1999, Mutant p53 proteins stimulate spontaneous and radiation-induced intrachromosomal homologous recombination independently of the alteration of the transactivation activity and of the G1 checkpoint. Oncogene, 18(24), 3553–3563.

Santillan, A.A., C.A. Camargo Jr. and G.A. Colditz, 2003, A meta-analysis of asthma and risk of lung cancer (United States). Cancer Causes Control, 14(4), 327–334.

Samet, J.M., C.G. Humble and D.R. Pathak, 1986, Personal and family history of respiratory disease and lung cancer risk. Am. Rev. Respir. Dis., 134(3), 466–470.

Saracci, R. and P. Boffetta, 1994, Interactions of tobacco smoking and other causes of lung cancer. In: J.M. Samet (Ed.), Epidemiology of Lung Cancer. New York, Marcel Dekker, NY, pp. 465–493.

Schabath, M.B., M.R. Spitz, W.K. Hong, G.L. Delclos, W.F. Reynolds, G.B. Gunn, L.W. Whitehead and X. Wu, 2002, A myeloperoxidase polymorphism associated with reduced risk of lung cancer. Lung Cancer, 37(1), 35–40.

Schabath, M.B., G.L. Delclos, M.M. Martynowicz, A.J. Greisinger, C. Lu, X. Wu and M.R. Spitz, 2005, Opposing effects of emphysema, hay fever, and select genetic variants on lung cancer risk. Am. J. Epidemiol., 161(5), 412–422.

Schiller, J.H., D. Harrington, C.P. Belani, C. Langer, A. Sandler, J. Krook, J. Zhu, D.H. Johnson and Eastern Cooperative Oncology Group, 2002, Comparison of four chemotherapy regimens for advanced non-small-cell lung cancer. N. Engl. J. Med., 346(2), 92–98.

Schmekel, B., Y. Hornblad, M. Linden, C. Sundstrom and P. Venge, 1990a, Myeloperoxidase in human lung lavage. II. Internalization of myeloperoxidase by alveolar macrophages. Inflammation, 14(4), 455–461.

Schmekel, B., S.E. Karlsson, M. Linden, C. Sundstrom, H. Tegner and P. Venge, 1990b, Myeloperoxidase in human lung lavage. I. A marker of local neutrophil activity. Inflammation, 14(4), 447–454.

Schwartz, A.G., 2004, Genetic predisposition to lung cancer. Chest, 125(Suppl 5.), 86S–89S.

Schwartz, K.L., H. Crossley-May, F.D. Vigneau, K. Brown and M. Banerjee, 2003, Race, socioeconomic status and stage at diagnosis for five common malignancies. Cancer Causes Control, 14(8), 761–766.

Seidegard, J., W.R. Vorachek, R.W. Pero and W.R. Pearson, 1988, Hereditary differences in the expression of the human glutathione transferase active on trans-stilbene oxide are due to a gene deletion. Proc. Natl. Acad. Sci. USA, 85(19), 7293–7297.

Selden, A.I., H.B. Westberg and O. Axelson, 1997, Cancer mortality in workers at aluminium foundries and secondary aluminium smelters. Am. J. Ind. Med., 32(5), 467–477.

Sellers, T.A., J.E. Bailey-Wilson, R.C. Elston, A.F. Wilson, G.Z. Elston, W.L. Ooi and H. Rothschild, Evidence for Mendelian inheritance in the pathogenesis of lung cancer. J. Natl. Cancer Inst., 82(15), 1272–1279.

Seow, A., C.Y. Shi, F.L. Chung, D. Jiao, J.H. Hankin, H.P. Lee, G.A. Coetzee and M.C. Yu, 1998, Urinary total isothiocyanate (ITC) in a population-based sample of middle-aged and older Chinese in Singapore: relationship with dietary total ITC and glutathione S-transferase M1/T1/P1 genotypes. Cancer Epidemiol. Biomarkers Prev., 7(9), 775–781.

Seow, A., B. Zhao, E.J. Lee, W.T. Poh, M. Teh, P. Eng, Y.T. Wang, W.C. Tan and H.P. Lee, 2001, Cytochrome P4501A2 (CYP1A2) activity and lung cancer risk: a preliminary study among Chinese women in Singapore. Carcinogenesis, 22(4), 673–677.

Sethi, T., 2002, Lung cancer. Introduction. Thorax, 57(11), 992–993.

Shoji, T., F. Tanaka, T. Takata, K. Yanagihara, Y. Otake, N. Hanaoka, R. Miyahara, T. Nakagawa, Y. Kawano, S. Ishikawa, H. Katakura and H. Wada, 2002, Clinical significance of p21 expression in non-small-cell lung cancer. J. Clin. Oncol., 20(18), 3865–3871.

Shriver, S.P., H.A. Bourdeau, C.T. Gubish, D.L. Tirpak, A.L. Davis, J.D. Luketich and J.M. Siegfried, 2000, Sex-specific expression of gastrin-releasing peptide receptor: relationship to smoking history and risk of lung cancer. J. Natl. Cancer Inst., 92(1), 24–33.

Siemiatycki, J., L. Richardson, K. Straif, B. Latreille, R. Lakhani, S. Campbell, M.C. Rousseau and P. Boffetta, 2004, Listing occupational carcinogens. Environ. Health Perspect., 112(15), 1447–1459.

Simonato, L., A. Agudo, W. Ahrens, E. Benhamou, S. Benhamou, P. Boffetta, P. Brennan, S.C. Darby, F. Forastiere, C. Fortes, V. Gaborieau, M. Gerken, C.A. Gonzales, K.H. Jockel, M. Kreuzer, F. Merletti, F. Nyberg, G. Pershagen, H. Pohlabeln, F. Rosch, E. Whitley, H.E. Wichmann and P. Zambon, 2001, Lung cancer and cigarette smoking in Europe: an update of risk estimates and an assessment of inter-country heterogeneity. Int. J. Cancer, 91(6), 876–887.

Skillrud, D.M., K.P. Offord and R.D. Miller, 1986, Higher risk of lung cancer in chronic obstructive pulmonary disease. A prospective, matched, controlled study. Ann. Intern. Med., 105(4), 503–507.

Skuladottir, H., A. Tjoenneland, K. Overvad, C. Stripp, J. Christensen, O. Raaschou-Nielsen and J.H. Olsen, 2004, Does insufficient adjustment for smoking explain the preventive effects of fruit and vegetables on lung cancer? Lung Cancer, 45(1), 1–10.

Smith, C.A. and D.J. Harrison, 1997, Association between polymorphism in gene for microsomal epoxide hydrolase and susceptibility to emphysema. Lancet, 350(9078), 630–633.

Spitz, M.R., Q. Wei, G. Li and X. Wu, 1999, Genetic susceptibility to tobacco carcinogenesis. Cancer Invest., 17(8), 645–659.

Spitz, M.R., C.M. Duphorne, M.A. Detry, P.C. Pillow, C.I. Amos, L. Lei, M. de Andrade, X. Gu, W.K. Hong and X. Wu, 2000, Dietary intake of isothiocyanates: evidence of a joint effect with glutathione S-transferase polymorphisms in lung cancer risk. Cancer Epidemiol. Biomarkers Prev., 9(10), 1017–1020.

Spitz, M.R., X. Wu, Y. Wang, L.E. Wang, S. Shete, C.I. Amos, Z. Guo, L. Lei, H. Mohrenweiser and Q. Wei, 2001, Modulation of nucleotide excision repair capacity by XPD polymorphisms in lung cancer patients. Cancer Res., 61(4), 1354–1357.

Spitz, M.R., X. Wu and G. Mills, 2005, Integrative epidemiology: from risk assessment to outcome prediction. J. Clin. Oncol., 23(2), 267–275.

Spivack, S.D., G.J. Hurteau, M.J. Fasco and L.S. Kaminsky, 2003, Phase I and II carcinogen metabolism gene expression in human lung tissue and tumours. Clin. Cancer Res., 9(16 Pt 1), 6002–6011.

Stabile, L.P., A.L. Davis, C.T. Gubish, T.M. Hopkins, J.D. Luketich, N. Christie, S. Finkelstein and J.M. Siegfried, 2002, Human non-small cell lung tumours and cells derived from normal lung express both estrogen receptor alpha and beta and show biological responses to estrogen. Cancer Res., 62(7), 2141–2150.

Steinmetz, K.A., J.D. Potter and A.R. Folsom, 1993, Vegetables, fruit, and lung cancer in the Iowa Women's Health Study. Cancer Res., 53(3), 536–543.

Steenland, K. and L. Stayner, 1997, Silica, asbestos, man-made mineral fibers, and cancer. Cancer Causes Control, 8(3), 491–503.

Strauss, G., M. Decamp, E. DiBiccaro, W. Richards, D. Harpoie, E. Healey and D. Sugarbaker, 1995, Lung cancer diagnosis is being made with increasing frequency in former cigarette smokers. Proc. Am. Soc. Clin. Oncol., 14, 362.

Sunaga, N., T. Kohno, N. Yanagitani, H. Sugimura, H. Kunitoh, T. Tamura, Y. Takei, S. Tsuchiya, R. Saito and J. Yokota, 2002, Contribution of the NQO1 and GSTT1 polymorphisms to lung adenocarcinoma susceptibility. Cancer Epidemiol Biomarkers Prev., 11(8), 730–738.

Swensen, S.J., J.R. Jett, J.A. Sloan, D.E. Midthun, T.E. Hartman, A.M. Sykes, G.L. Aughenbaugh, F.E. Zink, S.L. Hillman, G.R. Noetzel, R.S. Marks, A.C. Clayton and P.C. Pairolero, 2002, Screening for lung cancer with low-dose spiral computed tomography. Am. J. Respir. Crit. Care Med., 165(4), 508–513.

Syvanen, A.C., 2005, Toward genome-wide SNP genotyping. Nat. Genet., 37(Suppl), S5–S10.

Taioli, E. and E.L. Wynder, 1994, Endocrine factors and adenocarcinoma of the lung in women. J. Natl. Cancer Inst., 86(11), 869–870.

Taioli, E., L. Gaspari, S. Benhamou, P. Boffetta, J. Brockmoller, D. Butkiewicz, I. Cascorbi, M.L. Clapper, V. Dolzan, A. Haugen, A. Hirvonen, K. Husgafvel-Pursiainen, I. Kalina, P. Kremers, L. Le Marchand, S. London, A. Rannug, M. Romkes, B. Schoket, J. Seidegard, R.C. Strange, I. Stucker, J. To-Figueras and S. Garte, 2003, Polymorphisms in CYP1A1, GSTM1, GSTT1 and lung cancer below the age of 45 years. Int. J. Epidemiol., 32(1), 60–63.

Takata, T., F. Tanaka, T. Yamada, K. Yanagihara, Y. Otake, Y. Kawano, T. Nakagawa, R. Miyahara, H. Oyanagi, K. Inui and H. Wada, 2001, Clinical significance of caspase-3 expression in pathologic-stage I, non-small-cell lung cancer. Int. J. Cancer, 96(Suppl), 54–60.

Talbot-Smith, A., L. Fritschi, M.L. Divitini, D.F. Mallon and M.W. Knuiman, 2003, Allergy, atropy, and cancer: a prospective study of the 1981 Busselton cohort. Am. J. Epidemiol., 157(7), 606–612.
Tang, D., D.H. Phillips, M. Stampfer, L.A. Mooney, Y. Hsu, S. Cho, W.Y. Tsai, J. Ma, K.J. Cole, M.N. She and F.P. Perera, 2001, Association between carcinogen-DNA adducts in white blood cells and lung cancer risk in the physicians health study. Cancer Res., 61(18), 6708–6712.
Taylor, J.A., M.A. Watson, T.R. Devereux, R.Y. Michels, G. Saccomanno and M. Anderson, 1994, p53 mutation hotspot in radon-associated lung cancer. Lancet, 343(8889), 86–87.
Thun, M.J., C.A. Lally, J.T. Flannery, E.E. Calle, W.D. Flanders, C.W. Heath Jr., 1997, Cigarette smoking and changes in the histopathology of lung cancer. J. Natl. Cancer Inst., 89(21), 1580–1586.
Tokuhata, G.K. and A.M. Lilienfeld, 1963, Familial aggregation of lung cancer in humans. J. Natl. Cancer Inst., 30, 289–312.
Toyooka, S., T. Tsuda and A.F. Gazdar, 2003, The TP53 gene, tobacco exposure, and lung cancer. Hum. Mutat., 21(3), 229–239.
Travis, W.D., J. Lubin, L. Ries and S. Devesa, 1996, United States lung carcinoma incidence trends: declining for most histologic types among males, increasing among females. Cancer, 77(12), 2464–2470.
Trichopoulos, D., A. Kalandidi, L. Sparros and B. MacMahon, 1981, Lung cancer and passive smoking. Int. J. Cancer, 27(1), 1–4.
Trush, M.A., J.L. Seed and T.W. Kensler, 1985, Oxidant-dependent metabolic activation of polycyclic aromatic hydrocarbons by phorbol ester-stimulated human polymorphonuclear leukocytes: possible link between inflammation and cancer. Proc. Natl. Acad. Sci. USA, 82, 5194–5198.
Tsai, Y.Y., K.A. McGlynn, Y. Hu, A.B. Cassidy, J. Arnold, P.F. Engstrom and K.H. Buetow, 2003, Genetic susceptibility and dietary patterns in lung cancer. Lung Cancer, 41(3), 269–281.
Tsuruta, Y., P.D. Josephy, A.D. Rahimtula and P.J. O'Brien, 1985, Peroxidase-catalyzed benzidine binding to DNA and other macromolecules. Chem. Biol. Interact., 54, 143–158.
Tyczynski, J.E., F. Bray and D.M. Parkin, 2003, Lung cancer in Europe in 2000: epidemiology, prevention, and early detection. Lancet Oncol., 4(1), 45–55.
Tyczynski, J.E., F. Bray, T. Aareleid, M. Dalmas, J. Kurtinaitis, I. Plesko, V. Pompe-Kirn, A. Stengrevics and D.M. Parkin, 2004, Lung cancer mortality patterns in selected Central, Eastern and Southern European countries. Int. J. Cancer, 109(4), 598–610.
Vagero, D. and G. Persson, 1986, Occurrence of cancer in socioeconomic groups in Sweden. Scand. J. Soc. Med., 14, 151–160.
Vainio, H. and P. Boffetta, 1994, Mechanisms of the combined effect of asbestos and smoking in the aetiology of lung cancer. Scand. J. Work Environ. Health, 20(4), 235–242.
Vallyathan, V., F. Green, B. Ducatman and P. Schulte, 1998, Roles of epidemiology, pathology, molecular biology, and biomarkers in the investigation of occupational lung cancer. J. Toxicol. Environ. Health B Crit. Rev., 1(2), 91–116.
van Loon, A.J., R.A. Goldbohm and P.A. van den Brandt, 1995, Lung cancer: is there an association with socioeconomic status in the Netherlands? J. Epidemiol. Comm. Health, 49, 65–69.
van Loon, A.J., R.A. Goldbohm, I.J. Kant, G.M.H. Swaen, A.M. Kremer and P.A. van de Brandt, 1997, Socioeconomic status and lung cancer incidence among men in the Netherlands: is there a role for occupational exposure? J. Epidemiol. Comm. Health, 51, 24–29.
van Zandwijk, N., 2005,Chemoprevention in lung carcinogenesis – an overview. Eur. J. Cancer, 41(13), 1990–2002.
van Zandwijk, N. and F.R. Hirsch, 2003, Chemoprevention of lung cancer: current status and future prospects. Lung Cancer, 42(Suppl 1), S71–S79.
Vena, J.E., 1982, Air pollution as a risk factor in lung cancer. Am. J. Epidemiol., 116(1), 42–56.
Vineis, P., F. Veglia, S. Benhamou, D. Butkiewicz, I. Cascorbi, M.L. Clapper, V. Dolzan, A. Haugen, A. Hirvonen, M. Ingelman-Sundberg, M. Kihara, C. Kiyohara, P. Kremers, L. Le Marchand, S. Ohshima, R. Pastorelli, A. Rannug, M. Romkes, B. Schoket, P. Shields, R.C. Strange, I. Stucker, H. Sugimura, S. Garte, L. Gaspari and E. Taioli, 2003, CYP1A1 T3801 C polymorphism and lung cancer: a pooled analysis of 2451 cases and 3358 controls. Int. J. Cancer, 104(5), 650–657.
Vineis, P., M. Alavanja, P. Buffler, E. Fontham, S. Franceschi, Y.T. Gao, P.C. Gupta, A. Hackshaw, E. Matos, J. Samet, F. Sitas, J. Smith, L. Stayner, K. Straif, M.J. Thun, H.E. Wichmann, A.H. Wu, D. Zaridze, R. Peto and R. Doll, 2004a, Tobacco and cancer: recent epidemiological evidence. J. Natl. Cancer Inst., 96(2), 99–106.

Vineis, P., F. Forastiere, G. Hoek and M. Lipsett, 2004b, Outdoor air pollution and lung cancer: recent epidemiologic evidence. Int. J. Cancer, 111(5), 647–652.

Voorrips, L.E., R.A. Goldbohm, H.A. Brants, G.A. van Poppel, F. Sturmans, R.J. Hermus, P.A. van den Brandt, 2000a, A prospective cohort study on antioxidant and folate intake and male lung cancer risk. Cancer Epidemiol. Biomarkers Prev., 9(4), 357–365.

Voorrips, L.E., R.A. Goldbohm, D.T. Verhoeven, G.A. van Poppel, F. Sturmans, R.J. Hermus, P.A. van den Brandt, 2000b, Vegetable and fruit consumption and lung cancer risk in the Netherlands Cohort Study on diet and cancer. Cancer Causes Control, 11(2), 101–115.

Walaszek, Z., M. Hanausek and T.J. Slaga, 2004, Mechanisms of chemoprevention. Chest, 125(Suppl 5), 128S–133S.

Watkin, S.W., 1989, Temporal demographic and epidemiologic variation in histological subtypes of lung cancer: a literature review. Lung Cancer, 5, 69–81.

Wei, Q., L. Cheng, C.I. Amos, L.E. Wang, Z. Guo, W.K. Hong and M.R. Spitz, 2000, Repair of tobacco carcinogen-induced DNA adducts and lung cancer risk: a molecular epidemiologic study. J. Natl. Cancer Inst., 92(21), 1764–1772.

Weiland, S.K., K.A. Mundt, U. Keil, B. Kraemer, T. Birk, M. Person, A.M. Bucher, K. Straif, J. Schumann and L. Chambless, 1996, Cancer mortality among workers in the German rubber industry: 1981–91 Occup. Environ. Med., 53(5), 289–298.

Westra, W.H., R.J. Slebos, G.J. Offerhaus, S.N. Goodman, S.G. Evers, T.W. Kensler, F.B. Askin, S. Rodenhuis and R.H. Hruban, 1993, K-ras oncogene activation in lung adenocarcinomas from former smokers. Evidence that K-ras mutations are an early and irreversible event in the development of adenocarcinoma of the lung. Cancer, 72(2), 432–438.

Wiencke, J.K., M.R. Spitz, A. McMillan and K.T. Kelsey, 1997, Lung cancer in Mexican-Americans and African-Americans is associated with the wild-type genotype of the NAD(P)H: quinone oxidoreductase polymorphism. Cancer Epidemiol. Biomarkers Prev., 6(2), 87–92.

Williams, J.A., E.M. Stone, B.C. Millar, B.A. Gusterson, P.L. Grover and D.H. Phillips, 1998, Determination of the enzymes responsible for activation of the heterocyclic amine 2-amino-3-methylimidazo[4,5-f]quinoline in the human breast. Pharmacogenetics, 8(6), 519–528.

Wistuba, I.I., S. Lam, C. Behrens, A.K. Virmani, K.M. Fong, J. LeRiche, J.M. Samet, S. Srivastava, J.D. Minna and A.F. Gazdar, 1997, Molecular damage in the bronchial epithelium of current and former smokers. J. Natl. Cancer Inst., 89(18), 1366–1373.

Wogan, G.N., S.S. Hecht, J.S. Felton, A.H. Conney and L.A. Loeb, 2004, Environmental and chemical carcinogenesis. Semin. Cancer Biol., 14(6), 473–486.

Wolf, C.R., C.A.D. Smith and D. Forman, 1994, Metabolis polymorphisms in carcinogen metabolising enzymes and cancer susceptibility. Br. Med. Bulletin, 50, 718–731.

Woodson, K., C. Stewart, M. Barrett, N.K. Bhat, J. Virtamo, P.R. Taylor and D. Albanes, 1999, Effect of vitamin intervention on the relationship between GSTM1, smoking, and lung cancer risk among male smokers. Cancer Epidemiol. Biomarkers Prev., 8(11), 965–970.

Wright, M.E., S.T. Mayne, C.A. Swanson, R. Sinha and M.C. Alavanja, 2003, Dietary carotenoids, vegetables, and lung cancer risk in women: the Missouri women's health study (United States). Cancer Causes Control, 14(1), 85–96.

Wu, A.H., E.T. Fontham, P. Reynolds, R.S. Greenberg, P. Buffler, J. Liff, P. Boyd, B.E. Henderson and P. Correa, 1995, Previous lung disease and risk of lung cancer among lifetime nonsmoking women in the United States. Am. J. Epidemiol., 141(11), 1023–1032.

Wu, X., H. Zhao, C.I. Amos, S. Shete, N. Makan, W.K. Hong, F.F. Kadlubar and M.R. Spitz, 2002, p53 genotypes and haplotypes associated with lung cancer susceptibility and ethnicity. J. Natl. Cancer Inst., 94(9), 681–690.

Xu, H., M.R. Spitz, C.I. Amos and S. Shete, 2005, Complex segregation analysis reveals a multigene model for lung cancer. Hum. Genet., 116(1–2), 121–127.

Xu, L.L., J.C. Wain, D.P. Miller, S.W. Thurston, L. Su, T.J. Lynch and D.C. Christiani, 2001, The NAD(P)H: quinone oxidoreductase 1 gene polymorphism and lung cancer: differential susceptibility based on smoking behavior. Cancer Epidemiol. Biomarkers Prev., 10(4), 303–309.

Xu, L.L., G. Liu, D.P. Miller, W. Zhou, T.J. Lynch, J.C. Wain, L. Su and D.C. Christiani, 2002, Counterpoint: the myeloperoxidase -463G→a polymorphism does not decrease lung cancer susceptibility in Caucasians. Cancer Epidemiol. Biomarkers Prev., 11(12), 1555–1559.

Yang, P., A.G. Schwartz, A.E. McAllister, G.M. Swanson and C.E. Aston, 1999, Lung cancer risk in families of nonsmoking probands: heterogeneity by age at diagnosis. Genet. Epidemiol., 17(4), 253–273.

Zang, E.A. and E.L. Wynder, 1996, Differences in lung cancer risk between men and women: examination of the evidence. J. Natl. Cancer Inst., 88(3–4), 183–192.

Zhang, X., X. Miao, T. Sun, W. Tan, S. Qu, P. Xiong, Y. Zhou and D. Lin, 2005, Functional polymorphisms in cell death pathway genes FAS and FASL contribute to risk of lung cancer. J. Med. Genet., 42(6), 479–484.

Zhao, B., A. Seow, E.J. Lee, W.T. Poh, M. Teh, P. Eng, Y.T. Wang, W.C. Tan, M.C. Yu and H.P. Lee, 2001, Dietary isothiocyanates, glutathione S-transferase -M1, -T1 polymorphisms and lung cancer risk among Chinese women in Singapore. Cancer Epidemiol. Biomarkers Prev., 10(10), 1063–1067.

Zhou, W., G. Liu, S.W. Thurston, L.L. Xu, D.P. Miller, J.C. Wain, T.J. Lynch, L. Su and D.C. Christiani, 2002, Genetic polymorphisms in N-acetyltransferase-2 and microsomal epoxide hydrolase, cumulative cigarette smoking, and lung cancer. Cancer Epidemiol. Biomarkers Prev., 11(1), 15–21.

Ziegler, R.G., A.F. Subar, N.E. Craft, G. Ursin, B.H. Patterson and B.I. Graubard, 1992, Does beta-carotene explain why reduced cancer risk is associated with vegetable and fruit intake? Cancer Res., 52(Suppl 7), 2060S–2066S.

Chapter 5

Chaos, Cancer, the Cellular Operating System and the Prediction of Survival in Head and Neck Cancer

Andrew S. Jones

School of Clinical Sciences, The University of Liverpool. Surgical Departments, Third Floor, Clinical Sciences Centre, University Hospital Aintree, Liverpool L9 7AL UK
Email: orl@liv.ac.uk
Email: profasjones@beestoncastle.fsnet.co.uk

Abstract

Over the years, a large number of molecules and genes have been studied and whilst a degree of insight into the fundamental biology of the cell and oncogenesis has been obtained, our knowledge of how these molecules and genes are orchestrated into a functional living cell or carcinoma remain elusive. As yet the "operating system" that underlies life is only slightly understood but the term operating system is applied to all molecules and genes in the cell and their interaction matrix.

Biochemistry has considered cellular control as a "top-down" system from gene to phenotype each employing unique and rigid pathways. In spite of all the work on individual molecules and genes as markers of survival, loco-regional failure or response to treatment, none is as powerful as pathological staging.

Rather than rigid vertically orientated pathways, there is a system of fluid interconnections. Identical phenotypes can arise from different genotypes and the same genotype can produce a number of different phenotypes. Evidently the system is greatly more complex than first envisaged. Understanding this system presents many difficulties as the very large numbers of players interact omni-dimensionally. These interactions form a complex matrix involving and spreading through the entire cell, on to other cells and so, to a tissue. No information transfer can occur in isolation and now it is clear that the search for the cellular operating system is the most important endeavour in science. Our view is that, in terms of physics, this operating system is of complex type with multiple interactions and many possible pathways of information flow. The system is essentially non-linear with significant stochastic elements. The form the system takes is at present conjectural but our provisional concept is that it is chaotic. Such systems can be modelled successfully using artificial intelligence computer programs and given enough data, it is now theoretically possible to predict the behaviour of the system and also gain insight into how it operates.

In recent work from our group, an artificial neural network was applied to data from 1000 patients with carcinoma of the larynx seen in our institution and compared to standard regression analyses of failure. Host, tumour and treatment factors were studied. In addition, tissue for the ongoing programme investigating the role of 30 fundamental molecules and genes within the cellular system was harvested using tissue array technology. These substances are to be assayed using a variety of techniques and so far p53, pRB and mdm2 are being studied by immunohistochemistry.

So far we have demonstrated that the artificial neural network is superior to standard regression molecules at predicting survival based on a number of host, tumour and treatment parameters in laryngeal cancer.

Keywords: Modelling survival, artificial intelligence, cancer larynx, head and neck cancer, regression models.

Outcome Prediction in Cancer
Edited by A.F.G. Taktak and A.C. Fisher
© 2007 Elsevier B.V. All rights reserved

Contents

1. INTRODUCTION

In order to understand any system, adequate background knowledge of how the system operates is crucial. For example, a meteorological weather system requires a large amount of accurate data fitted to a preliminary model. This process is based on a thorough knowledge of that system. The model will require refinement as more data becomes available, but the final test is its ability to predict how the weather system develops over time. Accurate prediction is the final arbiter.

The modelling process for any complex system is the same. Thus when dealing with the fundamental biology of the cell and, in some cases, its failure as cancer develops, the same rules must apply. Therefore plentiful data are required to fit to the initial model which itself is derived from a sound understanding of fundamental biology and carcinogenesis. The model should then be refined by additional data and the model itself should be capable of identifying areas were data are weak or absent. Again, prediction is the test of the model and in the present case, is the accurate modelling of the development and course of a cancer.

The basis of the successful model and of accurate prediction involves the incorporation of as many pertinent variables as technically possible; in our case genes, molecules and pathways. Thus the first section of this chapter outlines basic cellular systems and important genes and molecules. Not only does it serve to facilitate the construction of appropriate models but it also demonstrates the limitations of the simple, linear "bio-molecular" approach to the understanding of the cell and carcinogenesis.

2. CANCER AND ITS CAUSATION

Cancer is the product of abnormalities within the genome (Cox and Sinclair, 1997). Such abnormalities are inherited or due to acquired damage, either as faults developing during cell division or defects due to physical, chemical or biological insults (DeVita et al., 1993). Almost invariably, several defects have to be present for cancer to develop, the so-called "multi-step process" (Schwab, 2001). In a few cancers for example, colonic and some breast cancers, genomic abnormalities have been linked to the phenotype and carcinogenesis with a degree of precision (DeVita et al., 1993; Cox and Sinclair, 1997; Schwab, 2001). For most cancers, however, including head and neck cancer, this is not the case and the literature provides no clear indication of any logical stepwise process, except perhaps in the vaguest terms. Although there is no algorithm that accurately describes the genesis of cancer from genome to phenotype, a number of genes and many molecules are known to be important in this process (DeVita et al., 1993; Cox and Sinclair, 1997; Schwab, 2001). One of the main difficulties in the study of carcinogenesis is the great redundancy within the genome and proteome, the vast number of interconnections between molecules, genes and receptors, and the vast number of feedback loops that must ascend and descend the connecting pathways (Lodish et al., 1999). Significantly in cancer biology very little is known about how the various fundamental elements and pathways interact. In addition, the majority of putative molecules orchestrating cell function and carcinogenesis have either not yet been identified or have uncertain function.

As we evolve, our genomes collect mutations. This can be advantageous and is one of the cornerstones of evolvability and of evolution (Basler and Struhl, 1994; Weinstein et al., 1995). Unfortunately the vast majority of such mutations are detrimental and evolution dictates that such organisms die out and with them, their genomic mutations. Nevertheless some mutations can persist and can prove particularly problematic if they are not expressed until the organism has reproduced. Examples of these to be found in man include a predisposition to cancers (vide infra), familial hyperlipidaemia and heart disease, schizophrenia, arthritis and type 2 diabetes. Central to the theories of carcinogenesis is the "multistep process" (Klein, 1998). This postulates that more than one genetic aberration must be present for cancer to develop and indeed, there are many examples of this process occurring in oncology.

The many causes of cancer all affect the genome in some disruptive way. Of the many possible scenarios the commonest include loss of a tumour suppressor gene, over expression of a proto-oncogene and damage to the DNA surveillance-repair systems. Apart from inheriting a damaged genome, such damage can be caused by errors in gene copying during life or due to environmental factors. The latter include the ingestion or inhalation of mutagens in food or in the workplace, to habits such as cigarette smoking, to infection by oncogenic viruses or to exposure to ionizing or ultraviolet radiation. In practice, endogenous and exogenous factors are likely to be present in most human cancers.

The answers to carcinogenesis and its future treatment are to be found in the genome. Thus follows a basic account of molecular biology with an emphasis on neoplasia.

3. FUNDAMENTAL CELL BIOLOGY AND ONCOLOGY

Crucial to the understanding of the cell and cancer is the study of its normal biochemistry and molecular biology. It will become evident later in this chapter that what we are missing is a coherent concept of the cellular "operating system". Thus a highly condensed description of cellular systems and the errors they may incur is presented in the following pages. The subsequent discussion of the highly complex cellular systems in health and in cancer will provide insight into why simple statistical models are inadequate to study this vast field (Maynard Smith, 1999).

The functional structure of living cells has been categorized into the genome, the proteome and recently the glyceome; the realms of genes, proteins and carbohydrates respectively. In man, the genome is thought to contain a little over 30, 000 genes, the proteome contains at least ten times this number of molecules and the glyceome possesses millions of possible molecules. Genes code for polypeptides and proteins and it was once thought that one gene coded for a single protein, however this has now been shown to be a fallacy (Cox and Sinclair, 1997; Schwab, 2001). Carbohydrates and lipids are created indirectly from genes by protein enzymes and by chemical reactions between the protein units in their tertiary and quaternary structures and available sugar and lipid molecules (Lodish et al., 1999).

Calculations suggest that each cell in our bodies (diameter 7–10 μm) contains perhaps 15 mm of DNA, and from this immense amount of genetic information, only a very small fraction is expressed (Schwab, 2001). The structure of DNA is well-known; the double helix described by Watson and Crick almost 40 years ago is formed of two strands of DNA connected by hydrogen bonds (Kornberg and Baker, 1995; Maynard Smith, 1999) (Fig. 1). The basic unit is a phosphate sugar (deoxy-ribose) and a base. The bases are of two types, a purine and a pyrimidine moiety. In turn there are two purine and two pyrimidine bases, adenine, guanidine and thymine and cytosine. Adenine always associates with thymine and guanine with cytosine. In molecular biology, the basic unit of DNA is the base pair and the

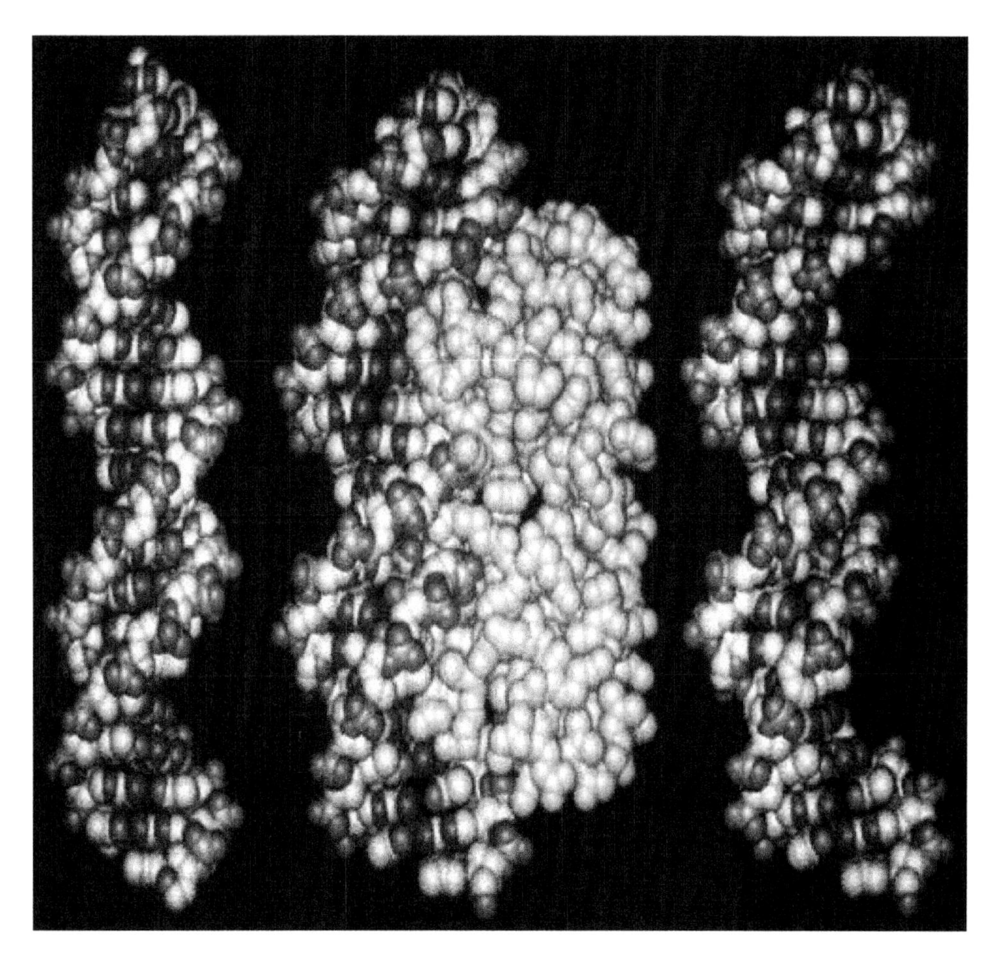

Fig. 1. Computer-generated images of DNA molecules. Note that the central one is bound by a transcription factor which is distorting the DNA molecule.

genome may contain some 3 billion base pairs. The base pairs are arranged in triplets termed codons, each usually coding for an amino acid. The natural DNA macromolecule is a right-handed β-helix (Fig. 2) although other structures are possible and can exist under certain conditions (Lodish et al., 1999).

The vast majority of base pairs in the genome are non-coding (Kornberg and Baker, 1995; Maynard Smith, 1999; Schwab, 2001). The coding fractions are termed exons and the non-coding segments, introns, with exons forming as little as 1.5% of the genome. The number of exons in a particular gene varies widely. The well-known p53 gene contains 16 exons and the retinoblastoma gene 36 exons. Each gene possesses a promotor site usually at its beginning but occasionally upstream in the DNA molecule or even elsewhere.

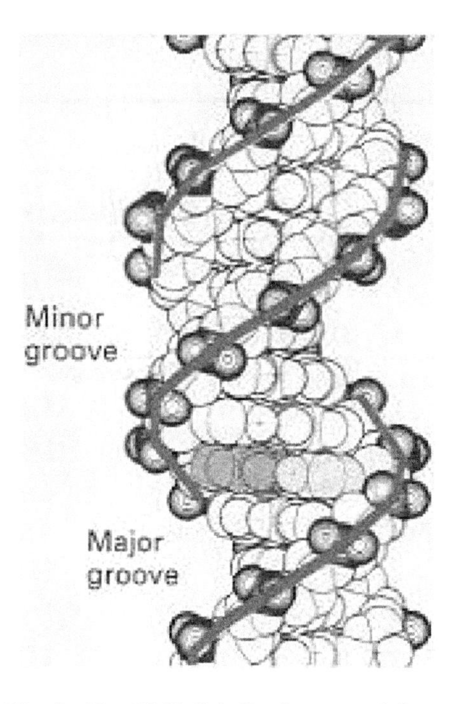

Fig. 2. The DNA β-helix, its normal form.

This promotor site has three distinct regions. These are: (1) the binding site for the transcription factor, (2) the transactivation site and (3) the transcription site. The binding site tends to be very short; in the region of 7 or 8 bp and contains highly conserved sequences. In the case of fast transactivators, the commonest is the TATA sequence (Schwab, 2001). The best-known transcription factors belong to the AP1 family, which includes fos, jun and ATF. At the transcription site RNA polymerase II forms an antisense RNA molecule. The complete length of DNA involved in producing a polypeptide chain is termed the cistron and includes not only exons and introns but also its associated upstream and downstream elements.

The exons are separated by introns and the genetic code must be interpreted by messenger RNA excluding these introns; this process is not necessarily purely linear. A hypothetical gene of three exons separated by two introns might be transferred to the messenger RNA as exon 1 + exon 2 + exon 3 but might be, for example, transferred as exon 2 and exon 3, or even exon 1, exon 1 and exon 3 (Cox and Sinclair, 1997; Lodish et al., 1999). Obviously the potential number of possibilities is great, particularly for large genes. This is one of the mechanisms by which ten times more proteins can be created than there are genes; such differences between proteins from the same gene are termed splice variants (Hertel et al., 1997). Although a large number of splice variants are possible for most genes, only a small number are actually expressed. To complicate matters further while most genes are read from "right to left" from the complimentary DNA strand, some are read in the opposite direction and a few are read from both leading and lagging strands (Cox and Sinclair, 1997; Hertel et al., 1997; Lodish et al., 1999; Schwab, 2001).

3.1. Organization of DNA

One of the problems encountered during gene transcription is in the structure of the DNA molecule itself; to contain such an immense length of DNA, the cell must adopt several strategies. One simple strategy is to break the DNA up into chromosomes, man has 46 chromosomes but the number appears fairly arbitrary as nematodes have 2, hermit crabs 254 and the chimpanzee 48. Each chromosome is then formed of a super coil of DNA which is itself coiled several times and the whole structure is twisted around a rod-like basic protein termed a histone (Fig. 3), which is able to absorb the charges on the DNA molecules. To express or copy a gene presents problems as these may be in inaccessible parts of the coil. Enzymes termed topoisomerases help untangle DNA and also reform its tertiary structure following transcription (DeVita et al., 1993; Cox and Sinclair, 1997; Lodish et al., 1999; Schwab, 2001).

3.2. Telomeres

In cell division, a difficult problem arises when a chromosome is being transcribed. Each end of a chromosome has a region termed a telomere (Autexier and Greider, 1996) containing repeating units of 6 base pairs. Each time a chromosome divides, these telomeres gradually reduce in length. This is a function of the "end replication problem". When DNA polymerase copies the two strands of DNA in a chromosome it must recognize

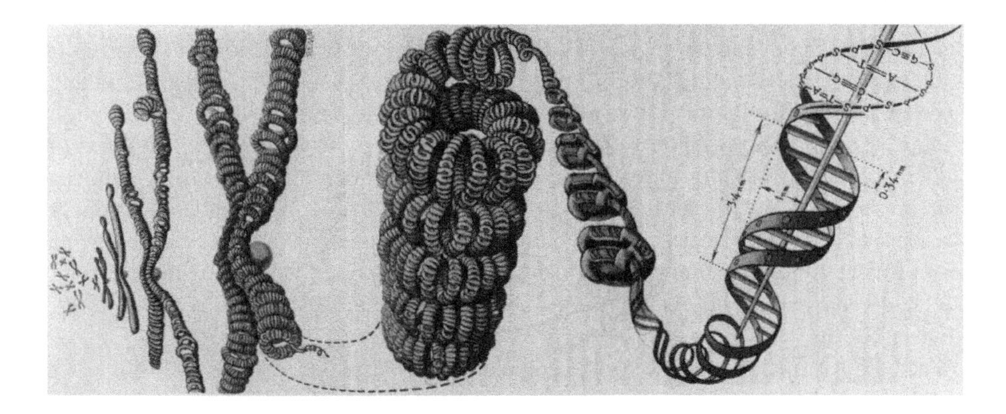

Fig. 3. The supercoiling of DNA.

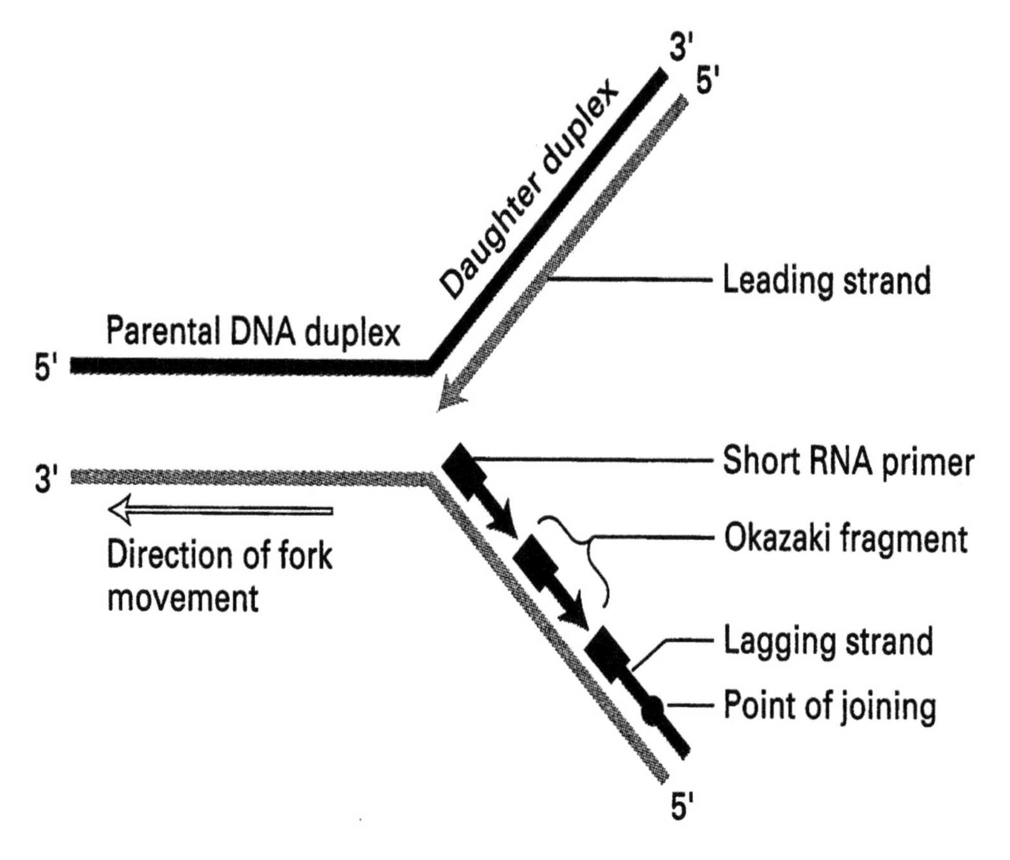

Fig. 4. The retreating "fork" of DNA as it undergoes replication.

a length of bases beyond the region to be copied (Fig. 4). The mechanism for the replication of the two DNA strands is different. One strand is termed the leading strand and the other the lagging strand. The leading strand is copied continuously in the direction of the receding DNA "fork". For the lagging strand, a new RNA primer is required to initiate synthesis forward of each specific DNA fragment. As the "fork" moves upstream, a new RNA primer must be laid down near the "fork" as each DNA segment is copied and the new pieces of DNA joined by a ligase enzyme. This is at least one reason for the finite life of normal animal cells, which have a theoretical limit of about 70 cell divisions (DeVita et al., 1993; Cox and Sinclair, 1997; Lodish et al., 1999; Schwab, 2001).

When the termination of code for the lagging strand is reached, there is no distal DNA for the primer to attach to. Thus the end of the strand cannot be copied unless an additional piece of DNA is present and hence, the importance of the telomere. The telomere is therefore a piece of DNA, which can be sacrificed during DNA synthesis.

3.3. Non-coding RNAs and RNA interference

An as yet unknown number of genes code for messenger RNA that are not translated into proteins (DeVita et al., 1993; Cox and Sinclair, 1997; Schwab, 2001). One such large RNA molecule is termed XIST and effectively blocks the X-chromosome in a male embryo allowing the male phenotype to develop. Other large RNA molecules occur some of which become oncogenic in certain conditions including some viral infections. Similar are the micro-RNAs that are relatively short stretches of RNA, which again do not code for a protein. These micro-RNAs have been said to form the basis of the "operating system" of the genome. Because genes are essentially a linear construct, communication between genes has been difficult to understand. Micro-RNAs may provide at least one solution to the problem; at least 20 have been discovered in human beings and 50 in yeast. It is likely that many more will yet be identified.

A recent concept is of RNA interference (Cox and Sinclair, 1997; Lodish et al., 1999; Schwab, 2001). Here a section of RNA present in the nucleus interferes with the expression of a gene. In some cases the interfering RNA is quite long but it is often short and quite specifically binds with a crucial sequence of the mRNA gene transcript, effectively inactivating the gene. Finally certain molecules such as the enzyme telomerase contain both protein and RNA.

3.4. Recombination

The basic concept of genetics is the interchange of genomic material between two organisms (DeVita et al., 1993; Kornberg and Baker, 1995; Stahl, 1996; Cox and Sinclair, 1997; Sachs et al., 1997; Lodish et al., 1999; Maynard Smith, 1999; Schwab, 2001). Central to this process is meiosis where the diploid set of 46 chromosomes is reduced to the haploid number (23). During fertilization of the ovum by a spermatozoon, the diploid number of chromosomes is regained, one set from each parent. Once an embryo is formed, only mitosis occurs. Here the relatively simple copying of genetic material from cell to daughter cell occurs. By this means, the skin and the aero-digestive tract mucosa are maintained as an intact layer. Unfortunately, by this method, cancer cells also divide. The above is true except for the sex-cell-producing organs, the testes and the ovaries. Although meiosis appears fairly straightforward, the molecular processes involved are complex but essential for the preservation of the species. Perhaps the most important phenomenon is termed recombination (DeVita et al., 1993; Cox and Sinclair, 1997; Schwab, 2001). In this process, genetic material is swapped between chromosome pairs at cross over points termed chiasmata. Some of the offspring will inherit a "vigorous" genome that allows a more successful adaptation to the environment into which they are born. This mechanism ensures that the most appropriate genes survive and allows the species to thrive (Whitfield, 1993). It is not only crucial for selecting the most beneficial genes but also for, perhaps, a more sinister reason. Not only does the genome gradually accumulate mutations but it is also becomes "infected" with ancient virus-like self-replicating regions termed repetitive elements and the genome has systems to "quarantine" these. Some of these regions will inevitably be discarded by recombination to a weaker genome and ultimately lost during evolution.

3.5. Transcription

The nuclear membrane possesses pores and it is through these that protein-coding messenger RNAs (type 2 RNA) are transported to the ribosome (Latchman, 1996; Hertel et al., 1997; Sachs et al., 1997). The ribosome contains two RNA-based structures, one larger than the other; termed ribosomal RNA (type 1 RNA) and here the messenger RNA is converted into proteins by transfer RNA (type 3 RNA). Each molecule of transfer RNA contains three coding bases and each code for one amino acid. Until recently only 20 amino acids were known, a 21st was then added and very recently a 22nd. This latter transfer RNA interestingly utilizes a triplet usually reserved as a stop signal. Gradually the transfer RNAs build up amino acids into long chains (Fig. 5). These building block amino acids become polypeptides and then proteins. This linear protein construct then undergoes structural (but not linear) modification into a secondary, tertiary and quaternary structure. Once synthesized these proteins are frequently modified in the Golgi apparatus and endoplasmic reticulum forming glycoproteins, lipoproteins etc. The possible structures of proteins are infinite and the primary structure and function of the protein very often dictates its shape (Fig. 6). Apart from the DNA in the nucleus, a cell also contains some DNA within the mitochondria. These are mainly concerned with the generation of adenosine triphosphate (ATP) from glucose oxygen phosphates. The ATP molecule forms the basic energy unit of the cell. Other mitochondrial genes are present and participate in the control of the various biochemical pathways of cellular respiration and metabolism. Such genes are amongst the most ancient, also being present in primitive organisms.

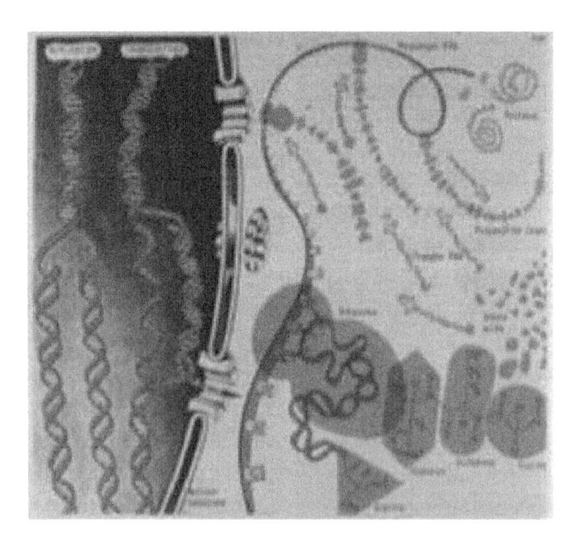

Fig. 5. A diagram summarizing the role of the RNAs in transcription.

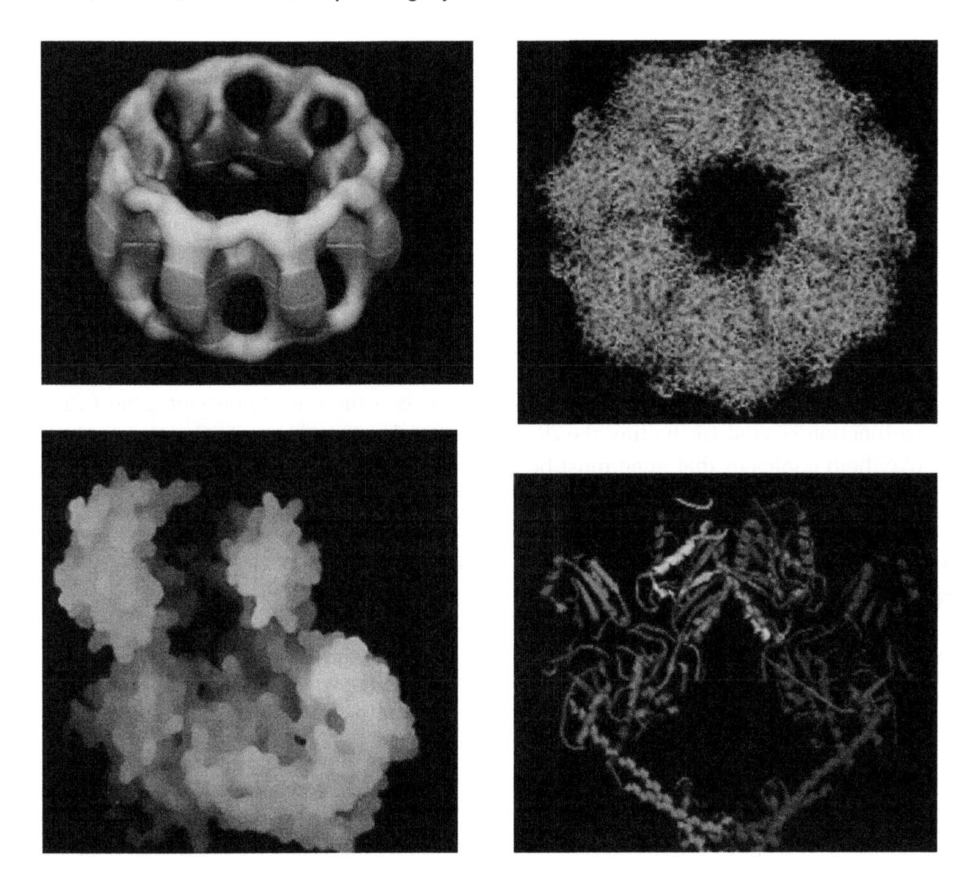

Fig. 6. Examples of protein structures. Their shape frequently suggests their purpose. For example, the structure on the top left is a membrane pore.

3.6. Gene expression

Only a small proportion of our genes are expressed and even then, only some on rare occasions. The sonic hedgehog gene has very powerful effects during development of the embryo. It is very well conserved and a member of the homeobox group of genes. Another member of this group, the HOX gene is responsible for the organization of the embryo into a head, thorax and abdomen (Spiers et al., 2000; Schwab, 2001). Evidently cells from different tissues express different groups of genes. The expression of genes is related to various factors most primitively to stress, whether this is from heat, toxins, osmolarity or desiccation. In normal physiology, gene expression is largely controlled by cell surface receptors and their respective ligands. Genes can be switched on artificially. For example introducing β- FGF (fibroblast growth factor) into a duck embryo leads to the hatching of a duck with teeth and thus simple molecules and environmental changes can switch on genes. Ancient mechanisms for controlling gene expression include RNA interference (Maynard Smith, 1999; Schwab, 2001) and the binding of a potentially active gene product to a cellular protein such as a heat shock protein.

Recently described is the phenomenon of cis-regulation. Here a gene has a detached regulatory segment located some distance from the gene itself but on the same strand of DNA.

3.7. Epigenetic inheritance

This term describes the inheritance of certain traits which are not within the genetic code. Perhaps the commonest and certainly the most studied is hypermethylation of a gene (Cavalli and Paro, 1998). The retinoblastoma gene is a tumour suppressor gene (TSG) whose function is vital for halting the development of cancer. For a TSG to be rendered inactive, both copies of that gene must be deleted. This can be detected by the technique of loss of heterozygosity (LOH). In some tumours, the retinoblastoma gene product is found to be non-functioning even though there is no associated LOH (normal). A closer study will frequently demonstrate that the gene has been inactivated by hypermethylation.

3.8. Evolution

At this stage, I have dealt with and briefly discussed the genome, its expression as cellular molecules and its control. The genome is very ancient and yet is continually undergoing modification (Whitfield, 1993; Doolittle, 1997). Life developed on Earth around three billion years ago. The early organisms may well have been like modern bacteria but probably did not use oxygen for respiration but rather other gases such as hydrogen sulphide. It is suspected that such organisms developed near volcanoes, such as pools of hot, mineral rich, water or undersea hydrothermal vents. Evolution is driven by a number of crucial genetic events. The first is sexual reproduction where two genomes are merged, the second is recombination and the third is spontaneous or inherited genetic mutation. These processes are continually injecting new genetic material and new combinations of material into the common genome of a living colony. The outside factor is natural selection where only the fittest (and the best genome) will survive. Thus from hydrothermal vents to mankind but in a timescale that is difficult to comprehend.

3.9. Proto-oncogenes

Oncogenes comprise a disparate group of genes potentially capable of stimulating cell growth and division (Sachs et al., 1997; Rafferty et al., 2001). They include transcription factors, regulators of the cell cycle or growth factor receptors or their ligands. Originally the term was applied specifically to transforming genes identified in RNA tumour viruses and have the prefix *v*-. It was soon realized that *v*-oncogenes were, in fact derived from the host cell, captured by the viral genome soon after infection by a mechanism termed as transduction. Examples of such capture are often ancient. The cellular counterparts of *v*-oncogenes are *c*-oncogenes or proto-oncogenes and comprise a highly conserved part of the genome. In retroviral infection, the RNA viral genetic code must be translated into the appropriate DNA sequence by viral reverse transcriptase and then inserted into the host genome. If this insertion occurs near a proto-oncogene, the latter may be rendered oncogenic. As discussed elsewhere the supercoiling of DNA and, indeed the organization of the β-helix itself makes a large proportion of our DNA inaccessible without the appropriate actions of topoisomerases and other enzymes. Thus a retrovirus may not insert itself randomly within the genome, but rather may insert in an uncoiled, active area of the genome. The risk of a proto-oncogene being active at any given time is high. If a foreign gene is semi-randomly inserted near the promotor region of such a gene, enhanced transcription is a likely sequel. Indeed there are a number of theoretical ways in which an inserted active gene may permanently switch on an oncogene. There is also evidence to suggest that retroviruses may specifically target certain regions and sequences of a host's genome and at least some of these regions would juxtapose proto-oncogene sites.

Proto-oncogenes may be rendered oncogenic in four ways:

- Deregulation of expression;
- Gene mutation;
- Translocation;
- Amplification.

Viruses only rarely cause human cancers although they are involved in several including tonsillar, nasopharyngeal and cervical carcinoma; but other mutagenic events are common. Examples are inhaled carcinogens, dietary mutagens, low intake of free radical scavengers and antioxidants, ionizing and ultraviolet radiation, reduced immune surveillance and DNA copying errors during cell division.

3.10. Tumour suppressor genes

The tumour suppressor genes (TSGs) are complimentary to proto-oncogenes and, as implied by their name, are "safety" genes that counterbalance the growth and mitotic potential of proto-oncogenes (Jones and Field, 1999; Rafferty et al., 2001). They are recessive genes that negatively regulate cell proliferation and promote apoptosis and differentiation. According to the hypothesis of Knudson, both copies of a TSG must be non-functional for a cancer to supervene and in familial retinoblastoma both gene copies are missing. If only one copy is absent, which is the most common scenario, tumours will not develop unless the remaining copy also becomes damaged. Such an event, although unusual, does occur and puts such a patient at risk of developing a malignancy. Unlike oncogenes, TSGs were first noted as genomic deletions in human cancers. One of the best-known and first discovered is the RB1 gene and if absent, half the individuals will develop familial retinoblastoma, this tumour otherwise being extremely rare as a sporadic event. Most researchers now suspect that multiple losses or failures of TSGs occur in most cancers. The TSGs are biochemically diverse including phosphatases, kinases, cyclin-dependant kinase inhibitors, transcription factors, cell adhesion molecules, protein degradation proteins and DNA repair molecules.

3.11. Genes controlling the function of the nucleus

The mechanisms involved in gene expression are immensely complex and incompletely understood (Latchman, 1996; Nasmyth, 1996; Sachs et al., 1997; Jones and Field, 1999; Rafferty et al., 2001). One of the most studied areas involves a transcription factor termed AP-1 (activating protein-1). It is a member of the jun and fos (ATF) family of proto-oncogenes involved in the normal functioning of the cell including cell division and differentiation and response to growth factors and cytokines. They are also important in the cells' response to stress, mitogens and ionizing radiation. Finally, as proto-oncogenes, they can become oncogenic leading to neoplasia.

Some transcription factors are powerful transactivators of gene expression whereas others are weak. Strong transactivators include c-jun, c-fos. Those with weak activity such as JunB and Fra-1 may act as suppressors of transactivation by competitively blocking a specific DNA binding domain.

3.12. The cell cycle

Normal cell division is central to the survival of mankind; this is a normal and essential part of physiology (DeVita et al., 1993; Kornberg & Baker, 1995; DePamphilis, 1996; Nasmyth, 1996; Cox and Sinclair, 1997; Lodish et al., 1999; Schwab, 2001). We lose vast quantities of cells from our aero-digestive tracts and from our skin every day as well as very large numbers of lymphocytes and other immune cells. In the mature mammal one type of cell may only divide into a similar cell; thus an osteoblast will only make bone. There are exceptions and these are called stem cells, these cells are totipotent, that is they can mature into a variety of tissues. Stem cells exist in the basal layers of the epidermis and in the base of the crypts in intestinal mucosa. They are also known to exist in bone marrow. Traditionally, some cells such as muscle cells and brain cells have been considered not to divide although it is becoming increasingly likely that this view is incorrect. Certainly stem cells for these tissues exist.

To replace cells that have died and for normal growth, cells must undergo cell division termed mitosis. Essentially mitosis is the process where one cell divides into two identical cells and during this process, the nuclear material must split into two with the copying of chromosome pairs; the process being termed the cell cycle (Fig. 7). The stages of mitosis as seen by light and electron microscopy are well-known to students of biology. In interphase, the cell is in the resting state or has become differentiated. However, on initiation of the cell cycle, although there is no visible change, at the molecular level G1, S and early G2 phases of the cell cycle are completed. Thus, long before morphological changes occur, most of the cell cycle is complete. Regulation of the cell cycle takes place mainly at G1 (gap) but also at G2 and DNA synthesis occurs in S phase.

Towards the end of G1 phase is a critical point, the restriction point (R), once the cell cycle has passed this it will continue to cycle even without the presence of growth factors. The time taken by this complex process is short being over in a day, although it does vary between cell types. G1 is the longest and most complex phase and lasts 14 hours or so, mitosis itself is of only two hours duration. Most of the following discussion will deal with

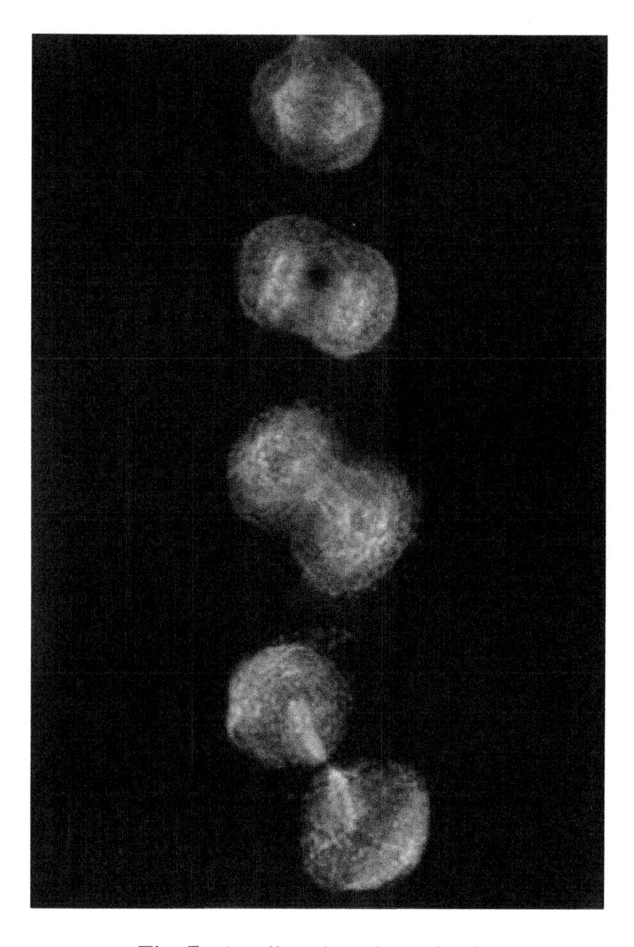

Fig. 7. A cell undergoing mitosis.

control of the cell cycle and in particular G1. G2 occurs between S phase and mitosis and it may be convenient to discuss first.

If G2 is passed successfully, the cell will undergo mitosis. On microscopy, the dramatic morphological changes of mitosis occur here. Before a cell may enter mitosis, several criteria must be met. Most important is that S phase has been completed successfully with accurate copying of the genome. Morphologically the first event is the condensation of the chromatin and dissolution of the nuclear envelope. Microtubules increase in number by a factor of 10 and focus on the centrosomes (Baas, 1996) leading to the formation of the spindle. In metaphase the chromosomes line up equatorially on the spindle (Fig. 8), the two pairs of chromosomes separate and in anaphase move to opposite poles of the spindle, the process culminating with the final division of the cell in telophase. On the molecular level the cyclin B1/CDK1 complex controls the G2 checkpoint, although other cyclins are also involved to a lesser extent. The above complex gradually accumulates during S phase

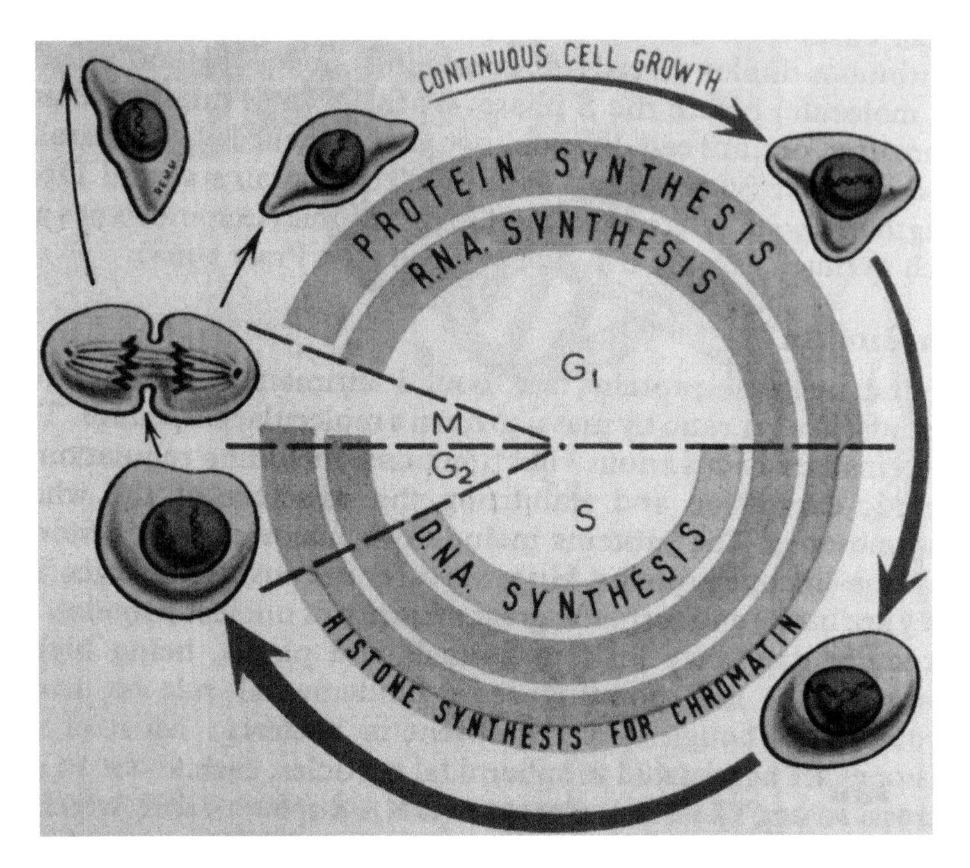

Fig. 8. The cell cycle with the various organelles shown.

and early G2 but then is abruptly released allowing the cell through G2. The storage and quick release of the complex is accomplished by the sequestration of CDK1 by inhibitory phosphorylation. The process is under the control of two kinases: Wec1 (nuclear) and Myt1 (cytoplasmic). For mitosis to occur, the CyclinB1/CDK1 phosphorylation must be reversed by Cdc25C a member of the Cdc25 family that includes not only Cdc25C but also Cdc25B and Cdc25p among others. If DNA damage or miscopy is recognized, phosphorylation of Cdc25C occurs creating a 14-3-3 protein-binding site. This when bound to Cdc25p blocks the CyclinB1/CDK1 complex by inhibiting its dephosphorylation.

The term growth fraction is used to define the proportion of cells in a tissue that are proliferating and typically, in head and neck cancer, is about 30%. The signals for appropriate mitosis to start are usually growth factors that bind to cell receptors. Cell adhesion molecules also have a role, as does the mere contact between one cell and another and between cells and the basement membrane. A typical sign of neoplasia in cell culture is the loss of "contact inhibition" where cells start to grow over each other.

3.13. Cell cycle control, G1, p53 and RB

The cell cycle is controlled primarily by a group of proteins termed cyclins which are numbered A, B, D1, D2, D3 and E and have one thing common; they are all serine threonine kinases (Whitmarsh et al., 1995; Nasmyth, 1996; Cox and Sinclair, 1997; Jones and Field, 1999; Lodish et al., 1999; Maynard Smith, 1999; Rafferty et al., 2001). They operate via cyclin-dependant kinases, the enzymatic activity of the cyclin only becoming active when associated with a specific CDK protein (cyclin-dependant kinase). The genes coding for cyclins are themselves under the control of other genes, perhaps the most important of which is p53 (Jones and Field, 1999). This protein is so important it has been called the "guardian of the genome". p53 constantly surveys the genome and if any aberrations are apparent, the repair system will come into operation. If this is not possible p53 will induce a process that ends in apoptosis, otherwise known as programmed cell death (Vaux and Korsmeyer, 1999). The anti-cancer importance of this process can hardly be emphasized enough as over half of human cancers have damage to the p53 locus to the extent that the p53 protein product cannot function. In addition, p53 itself is sensitive to DNA damaging agents for example cytotoxic drugs and also to ionizing irradiation. p53 exerts its effect on the cell cycle in a complex fashion by causing production of p16, p21 and p27 all of which inhibit some or all of the cyclins thus forming a negative feedback loop where irreparable damage to the genome detected by p53 causes cessation of the cell cycle. A positive feedback loop also exists where p53 causes production of mdm2, which in turn inhibits further p53 activity.

3.13.1. p53

As discussed above the p53 gene, crucially important in the life cycle of the cell is located on chromosome 17 (Fig. 9). The gene is highly conserved being present almost universally in the animal kingdom (Jones and Field, 1999). Germ line mutations of p53 cause the Li–Fraumeni syndrome leading to various cancers (Cox and Sinclair, 1997). It binds several cellular proteins including mdm2 and several viral proteins including the adenovirus E1B protein. This mdm2 stabilizes p53 effectively inhibiting it whereas other proteins (TAFIID, TF11H) are required to initiate transcript activation. The next domain following the acidic terminus is involved in apoptosis whereas the central region, which is almost identical from man through to insects, contains the DNA-binding domains. This is central to the function of p53 and unfortunately most mutations occur in this region. The carboxyl terminus has three very important biochemical functions, first it binds to damaged DNA, second it negatively regulates the specific DNA-binding activity of p53 and third it can repair complementary single stranded DNA. As discussed earlier, the p53 gene is capable of causing apoptosis, should the genome be severely enough damaged. Repair is, however, often possible and this involves proteins such as Ercc2 and Ercc3 which are components of the TF11H DNA repair system. p53 itself can activate a number of other genes including p21(waf1), GADD45, Bax, Btg2, Pig3, IGF-BP3 to mention a few. The feedback loop described between p53 and mdm2 (the latter inhibiting transcription of the former) is extremely important as p53 function is otherwise regulated entirely within the cell not at the level of transcription.

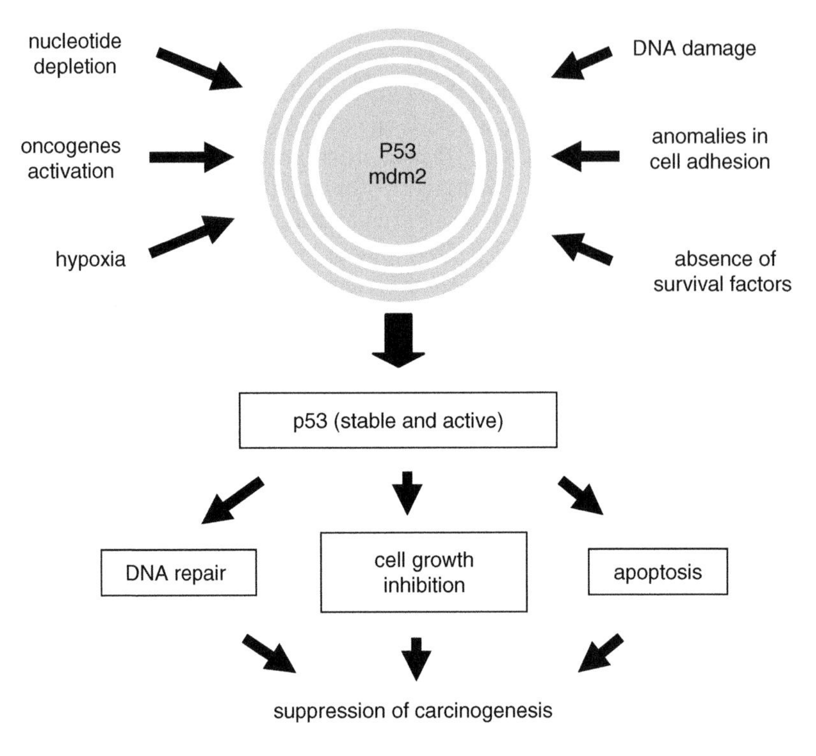

Fig. 9. A summary of the actions and interactions of p53.

3.13.2. The retinoblastoma gene

This gene (RB1) is located on chromosome 13 (Jones and Field, 1999). Certain oncogenic viral proteins can affect this gene for example the viral onco-proteins such as the SV40 large T antigen, the adenovirus E1A and the E7 protein of human papilloma virus. Unlike p53, pRB is inactivated by phosphorylation. Inactivation of pRB allows the cell cycle to enter S-phase but can also facilitate apoptosis. PRB allows mdm2 to inhibit p53 thus inhibiting one of the apoptotic pathways but facilitating cell cycle entry. Active (un-phosphorylated) pRB causes expression of the all important transcription factor, AP1 allowing differentiation of the cell (Fig. 10).

3.14. Apoptosis and cell death

At the present time, the dogma is that cell death that is programmed to occur in tissues for the purposes of remodelling is due to apoptosis (Vaux and Korsmeyer, 1999). Apoptosis is considered to be the main process by which cancer cells die, for whatever reason (DeVita and Sinclair, 1997; Lodish et al., 1999; Schwab, 2001). Apoptosis, however, is by no means the only mechanism of cell death. Cells can also die by necrosis, which usually

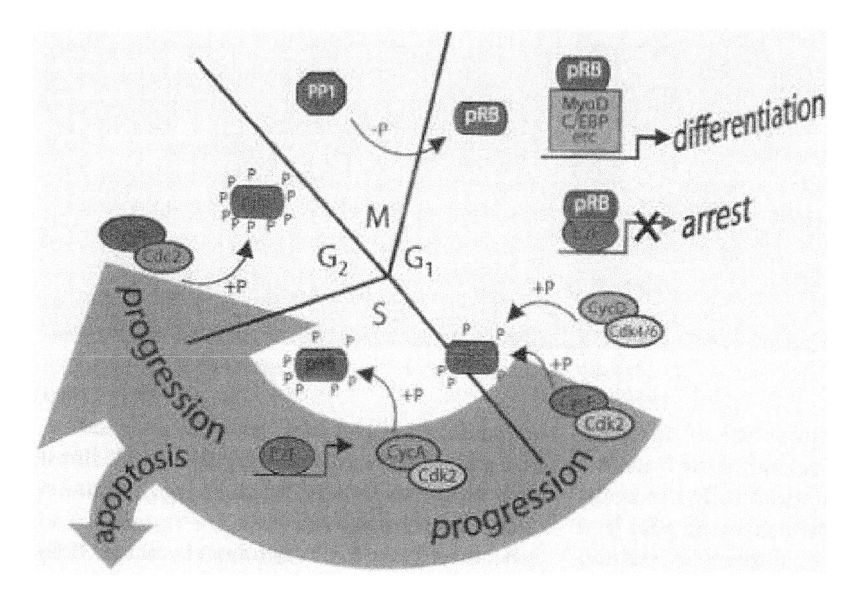

Fig. 10. A summary of the functions of pRB.

occurs in disease, by cellular catastrophe during mitosis (e.g. after ionizing radiation) by paraptosis or by being lost, for example from epithelial surfaces.

In the repair and remodelling of tissues, apoptosis is as important as the creation of new cells and is the physiological process by which unwanted cells are removed. A pathognomic feature of apoptosis is the formation of dense short fragments of chromosomal DNA termed nucleosomes and the presence of enzymes termed caspases. Evidently, in a tissue where cells are not lost by any other process and which is stable, the growth and apoptotic fractions must be equal. Perhaps up to one third of cells in the mucous membranes of the head and neck are undergoing proliferation. Estimates of the proportion of cells undergoing apoptosis vary from 5 to 10%. This discrepancy is partly explained by the fact that apoptosis is a quick process and also because cells are being continuously lost.

Arguably the most important role of apoptosis is the precipitation of programmed cell death in a cell whose genome is irreversibly damaged. This occurs during mitosis and may indicate a faulty genome or inaccurate DNA replication.

Cytokine death factors when liberated bind to a trans-membrane protein termed fas. An intracellular death domain of fas, via an intermediate, causes production of active caspase 8. Two things can then happen, caspase 8 can activate caspase 3 as occurs in geno-toxic-induced apoptosis, or caspase 8 can be produced which via an intermediate, stimulates mitochondria to produce bcl-2. This, via several intermediates leads to the production of caspase 9 then caspase 3, which again causes cell death as described earlier. Finally, a lack of growth factors can signal apoptosis.

As with nearly all biological systems, there are positive and negative feedback loops. To make matters somewhat more complicated, bcl-2 is not a single gene product but is a member of a gene family. There are three sub-groups, the first includes bcl-2 that is anti-apoptotic and can rescue the cell from apoptosis. The second group include the pro-apoptotic bax, which is a heterodimer of bcl-2 and directs the cell towards apoptosis. An example of the final group is bad which again is pro-apoptotic.

3.15. Cell membrane and receptors

In this discussion, it will become apparent just how complex the signalling pathways of the cell are, even when only described superficially. In practice, pathways overlap and no pathway works alone. Such complexity allows the cell great adaptability but also renders its mechanisms difficult to explore (DeVita et al., 1993; Cox and Sinclair, 1997; Lodish et al., 1999; Schwab, 2001).

The bi-lipid cell membrane effectively isolates the inside of the cell from the outside and this is true for extra-cellular ligands including agonists and antagonists (Cross and Mercer, 1993). Many consider that the cell membrane must have evolved first, before life on earth could begin, perhaps developing as simple liposomes. The membrane is formed of a phospholipid bi-layer. The hydrophilic phosphate groups are aligned to the membrane's surface. The hydrophobic lipid termini face each other in the interior of the membrane. Various proteins float in this lipid bi-layer including Na^+/K^+ ATPase pumps (Higgins, 1995), Ca^{++} channels, receptors (Figs. 11–13) and adhesion molecules to name but a few. Parts of these protein molecules are outside the membrane (the receptor itself), part is within the membrane and the remainder is within the cytoplasm. In the case of receptors this moiety is usually a receptor tyrosine kinase initiating signal transduction. The cell membrane itself is not spherical but very extensively invaginated, providing a huge surface area. This structure is termed the endoplasmic reticulum (ER) and can be rough or smooth (Cross and Mercer, 1993) (Figs. 13 and 14).

Specific damage to receptors signalling cell division can make them oncogenic – always switched on; a gene that codes for such a damaged receptor is an oncogene and a gene, which can be converted to the latter, is a proto-oncogene. The whole family of tyrosine kinase receptors are growth factor receptors and bind to polypeptide ligands. Examples of these receptors are the epidermal growth factor receptor (EGFR) (Figs. 11 and 12) and the closely related erb-B receptors, the platelet derived growth factor receptor and the insulin receptor. The extra-cellular domains frequently include immunoglobulins and fibronectin type 3 binding regions (Higgins, 1995; Rafferty et al., 2001).

When a receptor binds a ligand, the receptor molecule undergoes dimerization and activation of its intrinsic tyrosine kinase activity that in turn leads to phosphorylation of the receptor (Rafferty et al., 2001) (Fig. 11). The receptor is now active in its intra-cellular domain (Barrit, 1992) (Fig. 11) where cytoplasmic signalling molecules containing certain domain sequences, such as the phospho-tyrosine binding domain, recognize the phospho-tyrosine residues on the activated receptor. A complex signalling mechanism cascade then ensues which usually involves heterotrimeric GTP-binding proteins (guanine triphosphate). These G proteins bind and hydrolyse GTP, and subsequently regulation of the activity of serine/threonine kinases occurs. Finally, the nuclear transcription factors are activated via the process of phosphorylation.

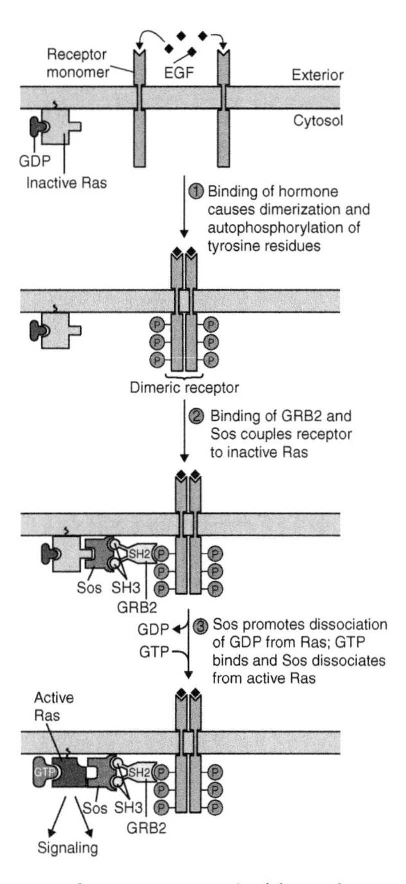

Fig. 11. A cell transmembrane receptor (epidermal growth factor receptor).

CLINICALLY IMPORTANT GROWTH FACTOR RECEPTORS

The Ret oncogene is associated with medullary thyroid cancer and papillary thyroid cancer. The mechanism of activation in the former is a point mutation and in the latter, is a fusion of genes.

Trk is associated with papillary thyroid carcinoma by a mechanism of gene fusion.

Met is associated with thyroid, gastric and colorectal cancer and the mechanism of activation is gene amplification or over expression.

Kit is associated with gastric cancers and haematopoietic malignancy; the mechanism is by point mutation.

HER 2 is associated with breast and ovarian cancer and is caused by gene amplification or over expression.

EGF-R (Figs. 10 and 11) is associated with brain tumours due to over expression of the gene.

PDGF-R is associated with dermatofibrosarcoma protuberans and with chronic myelo-monocytic leukaemia and the mechanism of increased activity is by gene fusion.

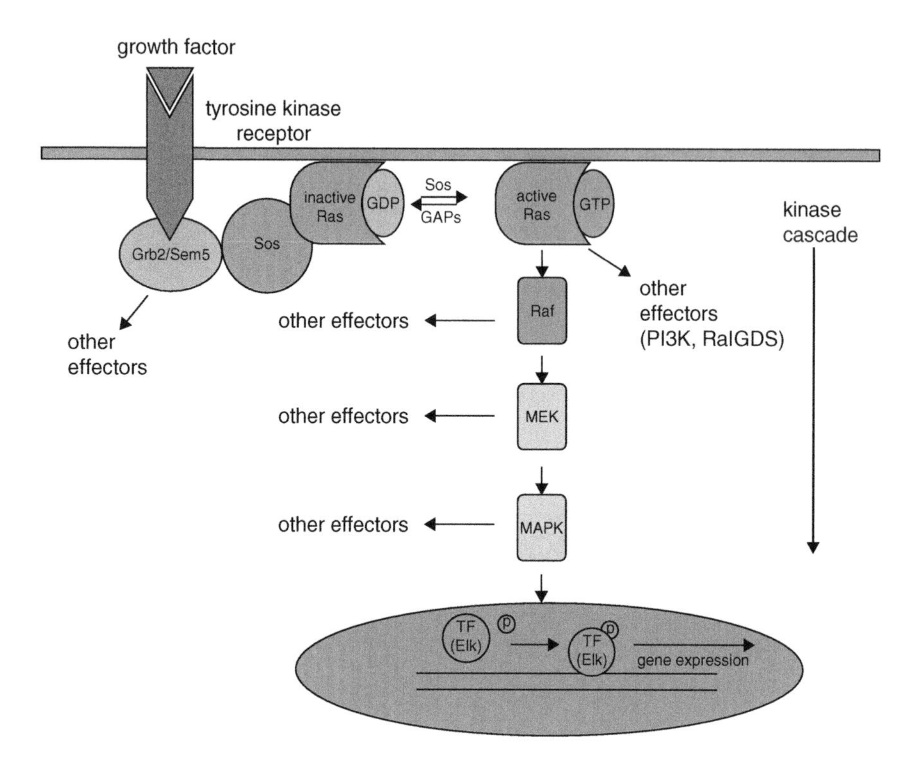

Fig. 12. A further example of a receptor.

3.16. Cell adhesion molecules

Cancer cells lose adhesion to the matrix early on in the oncogenic process; normally cells attach to the matrix and this signals the cells not to grow further (Cross and Mercer, 1993). Other factors also inhibit cell growth including contact inhibition. These molecules, all trans-membrane, are of five types (Gumbiner, 1996; Chothia and Jones, 1997):

The cadherins are calcium dependant, transmembrane proteins. They typically possess five cadherin repeats which bind to other cadherins on adjacent cells.

The integrins are heterodimers consisting of an α- and a β- sub-unit. They interact with members of the immunoglobulin super family, which may also be receptors themselves. Very importantly, the integrins interact with the extra-cellular matrix, for example the macromolecules fibronectin and lamenin.

The immunoglobulin-like adhesion molecules have a variable number of immunoglobulin-like sub-units, and fibronectin-like molecules may also be present. They bind to integrins or to members of the immunoglobulin family.

Selectins contain a calcium-dependant selectin domain that binds to carbohydrates.

The proteoglycans are macromolecules possessing a small protein core to which are attached long chains of negatively charged glycosaminoglycans. These receptors combine with a variety of other receptors but most importantly, with the extra-cellular matrix (ECM).

3.17. The cyto-skeleton and extra-cellular matrix

The cyto-skeleton is a complex matrix of structures including microfilaments, intermediate filaments and microtubules (Cross and Mercer, 1993; Welch et al., 1997) (Figs. 13 and 14). They give the cell its shape, allow movement and spindle formation and give attachment to transmural cell adhesion molecules. The skeleton is built of various proteins. The microfilaments are formed of the motile protein, actin and the microtubules from tubulin. Other proteins of great importance are cytokeratin, vimentin and desmin.

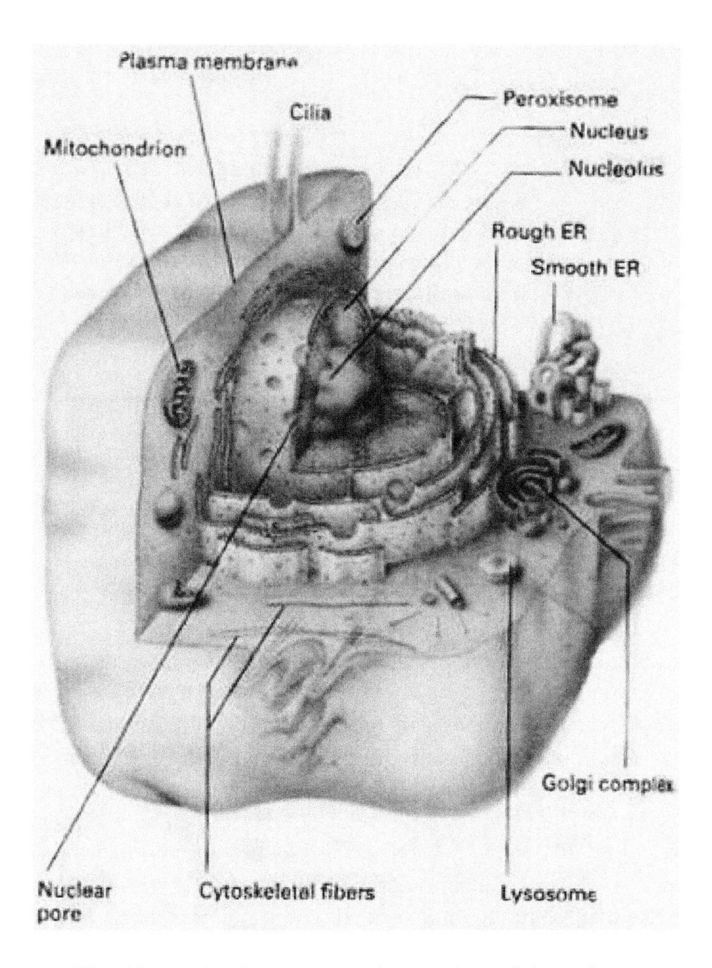

Fig. 13. A detailed cutaway impression of the cell.

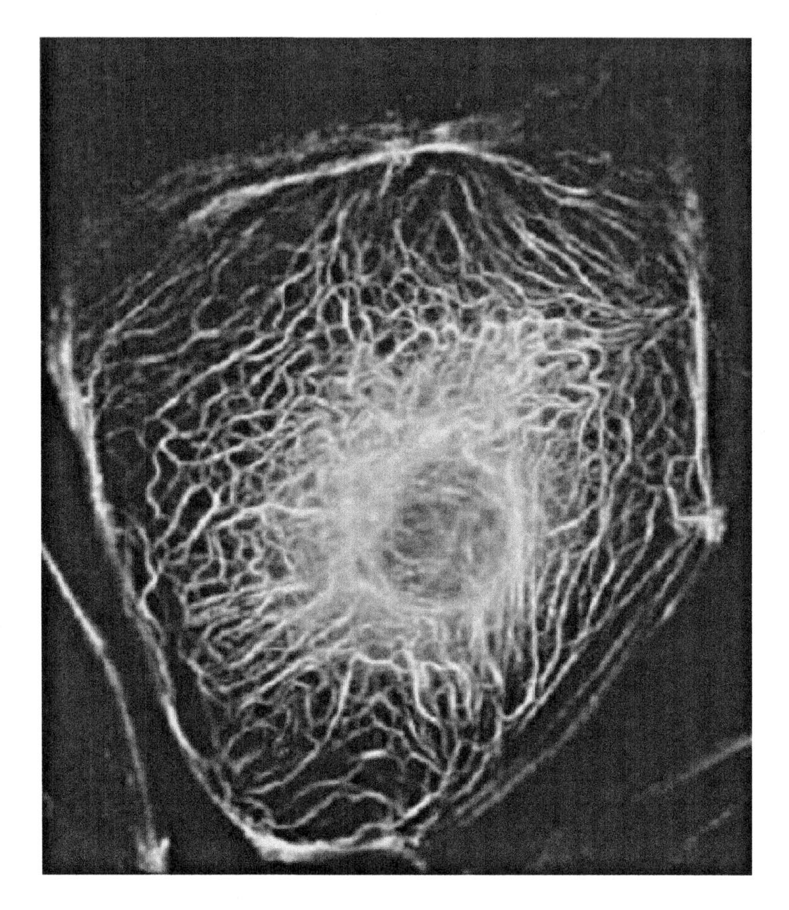

Fig. 14. Cellular microfilaments seen on electron microscopy.

4. A NEW DIRECTION FOR FUNDAMENTAL CELL BIOLOGY AND ONCOLOGY

4.1. Non-linearity, complex systems theory and analysis

Molecular biologists, cell scientists and fundamental oncologists are all involved in the study, in minute detail, of various genes, molecules and pathways. There is no doubt that this work has to be done and that, without it, our ultimate goal of understanding the cell, cancer and indeed life itself can never be achieved. Nevertheless, one must conclude that fundamental oncology like many other sciences has become too focused. There is now a bewildering array of genes, molecules and pathways but little concept of the basic organizational concepts that make the cell work. In Liverpool, our group has worked on both fundamental and clinical oncological research for over fifteen years. No gene, protein, receptor, adhesion molecule, marker or pathway, so far studied, has proved better than simple clinico-pathological data for prognostication or even providing an estimate of tumour aggressiveness.

It is, perhaps, not so surprising. One thing that the human genome project has shown is that there is massive redundancy within the genome. The function of many genes overlap and even more genes have, little understood, close homologues. Paul Rainey, in his experiments on *Pseudomonas fluorescens*, has demonstrated very elegantly that the pathways from genome to phenotype also show great redundancy (Spiers et al., 2000; Hodgson et al., 2002). He has also shown that organisms with very similar or identical genomes can produce widely different phenotypes in response to environmental stimuli. Whilst the standard textbook descriptions of gene expression in response to environmental factors appear elegant, they are also simplistic. Even if all the details of all the transcription factors were understood, gene expression could still not be predicted accurately. As discussed, there are the unpredictable problems of genomic and proteomic duplicity, of which genes are transcribed and which are not and of recombination. If these where not difficulties enough, we also have the practically unquantifiable problems of RNA interference, cis-regulation, micro-RNAs, splice variants, heat-shock protein sequestration of gene products and many more. No doubt there are many stories yet to be told regarding these "alternative" systems, most of which are ancient and highly conserved.

John Maynard Smith proposes that more than enough data on fundamental biology has been collected to provide a good understanding of how the cell functions (Maynard Smith, 1999). He suggests that information or game theory be applied to all the detailed information we know and perhaps a simple basic concept of life could then emerge. The massive emphasis placed by the big research institutions, the Universities and the grant awarding bodies on focused research has diverted research effort in a direction that is unlikely to uncover the underlying basic organizational systems that must be behind life. In many ways, biology has gone the way of high-energy particle physics. Expensive research has produced a virtual zoo of particles but no "Grand Unification Theory" that links the quantum world with cosmology and all four basic forces of modern physics. At least physics is not short of theorists and mathematicians to trawl through experimental results searching for a fundamental truth. Regrettably fundamental biology, with only a few exceptions, is not so fortunate.

4.2. The cellular operating system

The simplistic view that derangement of a single molecule, such as p53, or even a suite of molecules, as the answer to carcinogenesis has been proven unrealistic (Barritt, 1992) not least by over a decade of work by our own group (Basler and Struhl, 1994; Kornberg and Baker, 1995; Autexier and Greider, 1996; Doolittle, 1997; Hertel et al., 1997; Sachs et al., 1997; Klein, 1998; Maynard Smith, 1999). Many investigators have long argued that a number of processes must work together for carcinogenisis to proceed (Schwab, 2001). The great majority of fundamental oncological research analyses data very simplistically. Even those studies that do perform some type of mathematical modelling rely on regression models that assume linearity in the data and also assume normality of distribution. As yet, no group has been able to shed much light on the fundamentals of overall cellular function. Whilst cameos of cellular function such as biochemical pathways, some pathways from genome through to proteome, and occasionally through to phenotype may behave in a quasi-linear fashion (Barrit, 1992; Spiers et al., 2000), the broader concept of overall cellular function does not, being instead characterized by non-linearity and chaotic and stochastic processes.

It seems inevitable that to decipher the overall workings of the cell the fundamental, and generally held, concept of linearity requires reappraisal. In the natural world, systems are not exclusively linear or random, they frequently chaotic (Glerick, 1998). Pilot studies modelling our group's data supports this view, with dysfunctions occurring in at least ten crucial elements, including key genes and proteins before carcinomas of the head and neck are initiated. In addition, the relationship between key elements in cellular systems is not constant. It seems evident that for every dysfunctional crucial molecule, other related systems will also be thrown into disarray. Such complex dysfunctions operating bidirectionally on various levels of the molecular hierarchy, between these levels and also between pathways are likely to behave chaotically. Chaotic systems, including oncogenesis, are characteristically unstable and exquisitely sensitive to the initial conditions, as in cancer, with probably a relatively small number of genomic aberrations. Such systems can be modelled, as in meteorology, but require highly sophisticated analysis of large numbers of observations (variables) using techniques derived from higher and computational mathematics.

Paul Rainey has concluded from his work on *Pseudomonas fluorescens*, that pathways involving certain genotypes through to phenotypes are modular, but with "loose linkages" between components (Spiers et al., 2000; Hodgson et al., 2002). In addition, he has found that different pathways from genotype to phenotype frequently result in the same phenotype. He has also noted that even organisms with identical genotypes are able to exhibit different phenotypes in response to different environmental factors. These findings support the view that single, specific pathways are not necessary for a particular event to occur and single specific genes are not necessary for a single specific phenotype. Thus, gene expression is very dependant on cell receptor status and also lends support to the concept that proteins of major functional importance can be sequestered in the cell. This is known to be possible by binding to, for example, heat shock proteins. The late Stephen Jay Gould felt that such a mechanism could allow relatively sudden, major phenotypic changes in evolution to appear in the absence of linear changes in the genome (Gould, 1998).

John Maynard Smith (1999) has suggested that the fundamental biology of the cell could follow some basic principles. He has postulated that these rules may be more in the form of an algorithm or "computer program" representing a complex series of interacting instructions. In carcinogenesis this system is likely to be even more complex with a number of dysfunctional genes operating and interacting simultaneously (Maynard Smith, 1999). Of course these instructions also operate at the cytoplasmic level, below the genome. Even this view is probably an over simplification as we know that the behaviour of a cell is highly dependant on its environment (Spiers et al., 2000; Hodgson et al., 2002) and its neighbouring cells and interactions via ligands and their receptors facilitate or inhibit the expression of a vast number of genes. Smith went on to say that pure mathematics was unlikely to be the key to understanding the operating system of the cell but rather something more akin to information theory. It is in the analysis of precisely such a

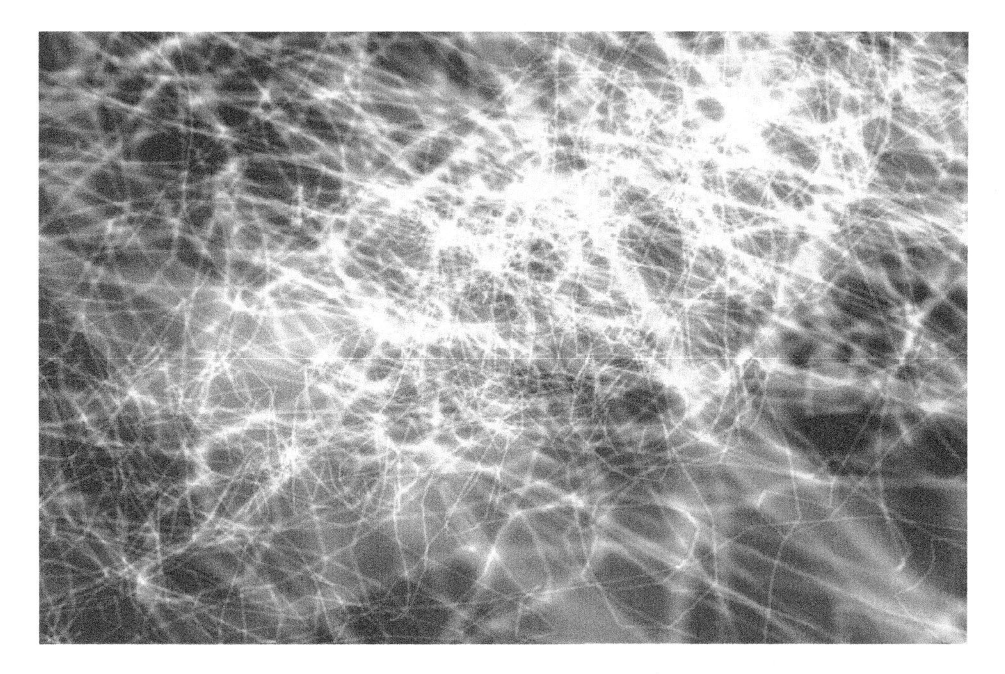

Fig. 15. A "biological" matrix which gives an idea of what structure the cellular operating system may take.

system with a vast array of bidirectional information exchanges that artificial intelligence programming including neural networks and the evolutionary algorithms should excel.

The "anatomy" of cellular systems may be regarded, in terms of mathematics and physics, as a complex multiplaner matrix (Fig. 15). Although many biologists feel that ultimately simple fundamental laws will underlie "life", as they do in all other branches of science (Doolittle, 1997; Gould, 1998; Maynard Smith, 1999) the evidence for such laws is likely to be concealed within the immense complexity of the system being studied. In addition, a stage in fundamental biology and oncology has been reached where a very large amount of carefully collected data has been accrued but no satisfactory unifying theory proposed. Maynard Smith agrees and suggests that enough information has already been identified, in terms of molecules, genes and pathways, for the fundamental operation of the cell to be understood, if only it were analysed appropriately.

4.3. The concept of non-linearity in systems in fundamental biology and oncology

In recent years, a number of systems governed by deterministic laws have, on more critical examination, been found to contain a substantial proportion of stochastic processes. Typically the equations that exist to describe these complex systems are non-linear and involve a large number of input variables. Such systems are characteristically unstable and very sensitive to initial conditions and the final resolution of such systems tends, on analysis, to involve more than one possible solution. Thus small genetic derangements may produce very large phenotypic changes or, conversely, may have no effect at all on the phenotype. The systems described above may be considered as chaotic. Natural systems fall into three main categories, linear, chaotic and random. Since we are evidently not dealing with a random system, neither is it linear, chaos would seem the logical category. Thus to extend the knowledge of fundamental biology, it would be reasonable and, perhaps essential, to regard the ultimate functioning of the cell and carcinogenesis as representing a chaotic system. In defence of this view, the following arguments are presented:

- The movement of information from genome to phenotype is clearly not entirely linear and flows in both directions.
- The movement of information down pathways is complex, multidirectional and includes lateral flow to parallel pathways. The system of information flow may best be described as a multiplex.
- Genotypic changes produce unpredictable changes in phenotype.
- Changes in phenotype can occur in the absence of genomic alterations.
- Linear models are unable to predict reliably these effects whereas empirical models may.
- There are no known equations that describe accurately the functioning of the cell, information flow through the cell or oncogenesis.
- Provisional analysis of our own data on fundamental biology and oncology suggests that they can be modelled by multiple iterations of one of the characteristic formulae identified in chaotic systems:

$$f(x) = \frac{1}{2}\left(x - \frac{1}{x}\right)$$

4.4. The pragmatic approach

Whether cellular function and oncogenesis take the form of an essentially linear system but in the complex form of a multiplanar matrix (Fig. 15) or whether they are chaotic is open to debate. It is true that in simple laboratory studies, some linear elements exist. In addition, the failure of fundamental oncology to define any type of operating system points to, at the very least, some stochastic elements within the system. Such mixtures of elements almost always occur in chaotic systems. However, whatever the final outcome of such a debate, there is no doubt that these two elements exist in the cell, are represented in its overall function and contribute to its overwhelming complexity.

In practice, the basic system category is unimportant from the analytical point of view. It is evident that the system is highly complex, has large numbers of "nodal" molecules and a very large number of shifting interconnections. Additionally, a large number of measurements of many variables would be necessary to describe the overall cellular "operating system" and oncogenesis. Regression models are not suited to systems where non-linearity is, at least, common, or to very large numbers of measurements related to each other in a complex and frequently temporary way. Finally it seems very apparent that simple standard mathematical formulae are incapable of describing this "operating" system.

Whilst the above arguments would appear to rule out the use of regression models, self-learning, highly interconnected analytical systems are ideal. One such system is the artificial neural network and this is used extensively by our group. In addition to the above discussion, the neural network assumes no underlying mathematical formulae relating the data. If the cellular "operating system" turns out to be chaotic, then the network is a good method of analysis of such systems. Recently, we have applied an evolutionary algorithm to our own tumour data and have so far found the results very encouraging.

5. COMPLEX SYSTEMS ANALYSIS AS APPLIED TO BIOLOGICAL SYSTEMS AND SURVIVAL ANALYSIS

The analysis of complex systems essentially falls into three distinct categories: classification, explanation and prediction. For explanation and prediction, various types of regression analysis are used (Altman, 1991). These include multiple linear regression, multiple logistic regression, proportional hazards modelling and generalized linear interactive modelling. All these methods assume a mathematical relationship between "input" and "output" variables (Hair et al., 1988). In addition, they assume some sort of linearity in the system under study, even in the case of proportional hazards models (SAS Institute, 1995). In many ways, neural networks can be considered a logical development from generalized linear interactive models. Indeed the latter models may be considered as a simple neural network with only two layers: an input and an output layer.

Neural networks have been in common use in medical research for the past 20 years. They have been used for classification and for prediction of hazard or failure and have found their most extensive use in oncology. However, even now, they are still not widely used for explanation or prediction. Although neural networks can address various multivariate problems, including complex multivariate regression, they have been criticized by statisticians for not being rigorous. In response, a duly statistical technique has been applied and incorporated into artificial neural networks, greatly enhancing their use in the biological sciences. In addition the (of necessity) binary output can be modified by, for example, adding a Bayesian function to the output stage so that survival probabilities can be given.

Whilst they are effective at classification and in facilitating decision making (Prismatic Project Management Team, 1999; Gerstle et al., 2000; Le Goff et al., 2000) they have so far appeared less effective at prognostication (DeLaurentis and Ravdin, 1994; Liestol et al., 1994; Faraggi and Simon, 1995; Burke et al., 1997; Biganzoli et al., 1998a,b; Bryce et al., 1998; Kattan et al., 1998; Anand et al., 1999; Lundin et al., 1999; Snow et al., 2001; Lisboa et al., 2003) with only half of the published studies claiming networks to be superior to statistically based regression methods. Most studies, however, are flawed technically, mathematically or methodologically.

In most studies on survival prediction, the neural network has been compared to the survival results computed by multiple logistic regression. Unfortunately, this method is not the analysis of choice for survival data. Simplistically it may be regarded as a multivariate extension analogous to the X^2 analysis. In practice, an estimation of the number of patients alive after a particular time interval is computed and compared with the output of an artificial neural network. This lacks the subtleties of accepted, conventional survival analysis and is very wasteful of data. Only two papers deal with the comparison of results from neural networks and Cox's model (Lundin et al., 1992; Kattan et al., 1998). Both studies, one dealing with breast cancer and the other with leukaemia, found that the neural network was superior to Cox's model at predicting survival.

Only one study on survival in head and neck cancer is reported (Bryce et al., 1998). Here neural networks were compared with multiple logistic regression and the network was found to be superior.

It should be emphasized that not all researchers feel that neural networks are appropriate for analysing survival data and feel that the currently used regression models are superior (Liestol et al., 1994). This view ignores the fact that regression models are very limited in dealing with interactions (DeLaurentiis and Ravdin, 1994) and almost useless for lending insight into the functioning of complex systems.

6. METHODS OF ANALYSING FAILURE IN BIOLOGICAL SYSTEMS

6.1. Descriptive methods–univariate

By convention, survival data are depicted on an *x–y* plot giving a survival curve with the proportion surviving (0–1 or 0–100%) on the *y* axis and the survival time on the x axis (Fig. 16). The scale of survival time varies with the scenario being studied but in head and neck, squamous carcinoma is generally taken as five years as index tumour deaths or recurrences do not occur after this time.

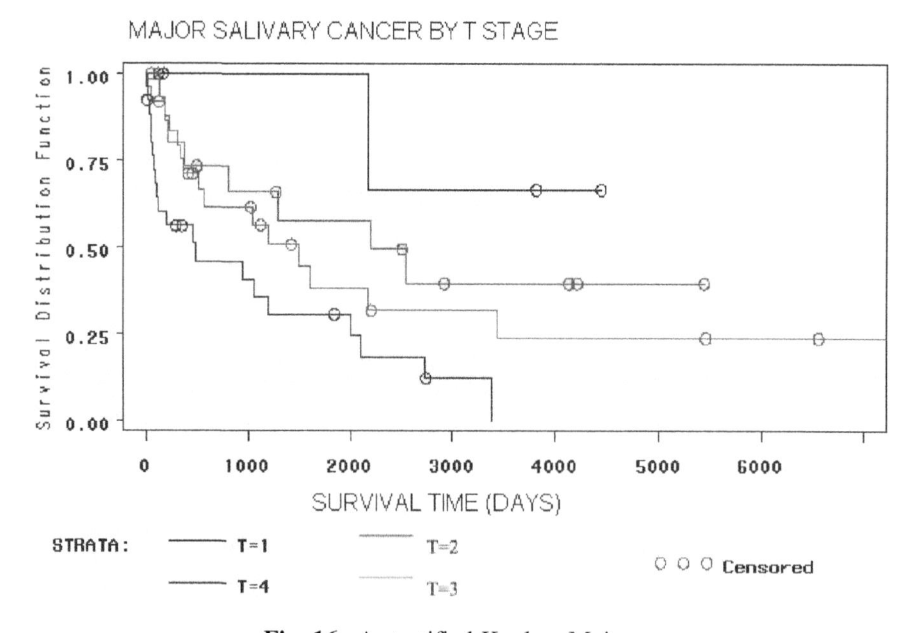

Fig. 16. A stratified Kaplan–Meier curve.

There are two basic methods that give equivalent results (Altman, 1991):

- The Life-Table method. First described by Edmund Halley, it is the method traditionally used by actuaries and is often termed actuarial survival. The technique is simple. The time-period of interest is divided into discrete and equal intervals (usually months) and the number of, say, patients dying every month tabulated and a graph drawn. A little more involved is the concept of adjusted or specific survival. In the case of cancer, tumour-specific survival is most commonly studied. In this case, in the life-table, only deaths from the index tumour are counted and deaths from any other cause adjusted for, so that they do not appear on the subsequent plot. This technique is termed censoring and the data are thus censored.
- The Kaplan–Meier Product Limit Estimator (Altman, 1991; SAS Institute, 1995). In principle this method is very similar. However the timescale is not divided into discrete periods and the plot falls abruptly every time an event such as death occurs, the completed plot showing as a series of steps. Adjustment for tumour-specific survival or whatever is made in the same way as for life-table analysis. Mathematically, the technique takes the product of all the surviving proportions ensuring that the resultant overall probability falls between zero and one.

6.1.1. Stratification and significance testing

More than one survival curve is usually drawn on a single graph representing discrete categories of the same patient population and this is termed stratification. In head and neck cancer, survival is frequently stratified by size of tumour (T-stage) or by the presence or absence of regional metastases (N-stage). Differences between these curves can be tested for statistical significance. There are two tests in common use and both take account of the whole curve and not merely the survival at, say five years.

- The Log-Rank test. Attributed to Julian Peto is a non-parametric test related to the X^2 test (Altman, 1991; SAS Institute, 1995). The principle is to divide survival time into discrete intervals. When comparing a number of groups, the test produces an observed and an expected number of events. The square of observed minus expected events divided by the expected is calculated (X^2) and the results summed. The statistic is then compared with the X^2 distribution with n–1 degrees of freedom and the significance level obtained. A variation of this test can be used to give a log-rank test for trend.
- The Wilcoxon (survival) Test. This is not in routine use and relies on a ranking technique (SAS Institute, 1995). It is more sensitive to early differences between survival curves than the log-rank test but otherwise yields similar results.

6.2. Prediction using the proportional hazards models–multivariate (after Cox)

The general principles behind Cox's proportional hazards model are well known and generally accepted. This model is the "standard" method for the multivariate regression analysis of failure in oncology to which any new method must be compared.

Although the fundamental mathematics is complex, the basic principles are relatively straightforward and are given in Altman and the SAS handbook (Altman, 1991; SAS Institute, 1995).

The proportional hazards model uses a baseline hazard derived from the data and is summarized below:

$$\left(\frac{h_{\mathrm{p}}(t)}{1-h_{\mathrm{p}}(t)}\right)=\left(\frac{h_{\mathrm{o}}(t)}{1-h_{\mathrm{o}}(t)}\right)\exp(\beta\times p)$$

The model fits data to a distribution. In the case of Cox this is almost always the Weibull. The fit of the model to this curve is imperfect (Fig. 17) although accurate enough for most purposes.

Because of the mathematics of Cox's regression a statistic is calculated that is equal to $e^{\exp(x)}$, if all other covariates are set to 0. Prognosis may then be calculated for these covariates. The survival fraction at a given time [S(t)] can then be calculated simply by referring to the baseline survival fraction at that time [$S_0(t)$] (Fig. 18):

$$S(t) = S_0(t)^{\exp(x)}$$

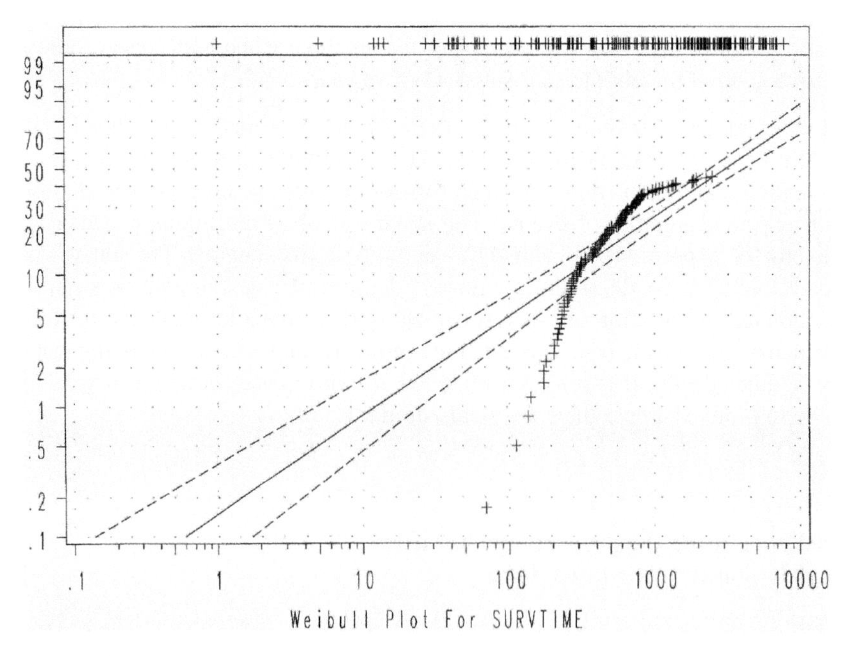

Fig. 17. A printout of the goodness of fit between the Cox survival versus time curve with the Weibull distribution.

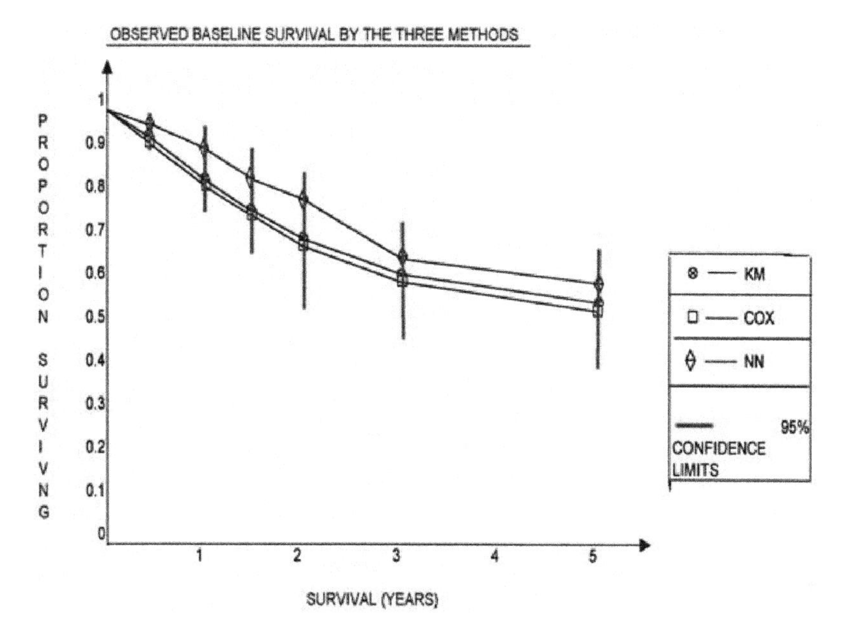

Fig. 18. The baseline Cox survival plot.

6.3. Prediction using neural networks

The basic methodology is given by Biganzoli et al. (1998 a,b), Lisboa et al. (2003) and others (SAS Institute, 1995; Demuth and Beale, 2001). It should be emphasized that the neural network does not use the background hazard described above but rather generates a hazard function illustrated by the general equation below:

$$\frac{h_{\mathrm{p}}(t)}{1-h_{\mathrm{o}}(p)} = \exp\left(\sum_{h} w_{h} g\left(\sum_{i} w_{ih} x_{pi} + b_{h}\right) + b\right)$$

where w are the weights, x the covariates, b the biases and g the sigmoid transfer function.

Much confusion overlies the terminology and types of neural network and thus some discussion of this is necessary. The crucial characteristic of an artificial neural network is that simple computing elements are incorporated into a highly interconnected matrix, which is capable of investigating complex phenomena and generating appropriate predictions. In recent years, methods from statistics and numerical analysis have been incorporated, thus allowing neural networks to be developed into probabilistic and invaluable "statistical" modelling systems. A feed forward neural network may be considered as a class of flexible non-linear regression, common discriminant and data-reducing models. There are three precepts to be considered of neural networks. First, when large quantities of data are available for training, the first half of a data set may be used to train a network. If insufficient data is available for the above method to be feasible, recourse must be made to other techniques. These involve some type of over sampling such as the 'bootstrap' technique.

In the case of survival analysis, prediction is more important than explanation although the latter can be explored by interrogation of the hidden layer. Finally, mathematical formulae are not assumed relating data points to one another in the system being studied and also do not directly apply between the related input and its output. However there are formulae and weights defining the connections and relations between layers and nodes.

A neural network is organized into nodes and layers. The first are the input nodes and the last the output nodes, in the middle there are a number of hidden layers consisting of a number of nodes. It has been demonstrated that a single hidden layer, usually containing three nodes provides the best compromise in terms of accurate results in a specific context, but also allowing for generalization. The greater the number of hidden layers, the greater the number of hidden nodes and the more complex and time consuming the analysis. More importantly the risk of over-fitting is greatly increased with loss of general applicability.

The number of input nodes is dependant on the data. A metric variable will use only one node but a non-metric variable must be processed into several variables for the purposes of logical input and will require more nodes. When putting in data, care must be taken to ensure that they are equivalently scaled and highly skewed data will require transformation or other manipulation before input. Types of input data may be interval, ordinal or nominal. For nominal or ordinal data of C categories, the network automatically generates $C-1$ dummy variables, which may be displayed in a table, so familiar when analysing nominal data. Ordinal data is, in addition, coded prior to input using the "bathtub" method. Interval data is accepted without modification (vide supra).

The multiplanar perceptron network has a linear combination function and a hyperbolic activation function. Usually it has only a single default hidden layer. An example of the activation function of a hidden unit is:

$$h_j = \tanh\left\{b_j + \sum_i w_{ij} x_{ij}\right\}$$

where: h_j = The activation of the jth hidden unit
b_j = The bias or inverse width of the jth hidden unit
i = The input state shared by all hidden units
w_{ij} = The weight connecting the ith input to the jth hidden unit
x_i = The ith hidden value

Neural networks produce one output node for each nominal and each categorical target variable and one node (only) for all interval variables. More than one output layer can be created. The three types of data have different activation functions:

- Interval = Identity;
- Ordinal = Logistic, (0,1), $^{1}/_{1+\exp(-g)}$; and
- Nominal = Softmax, (0,1), $^{\exp(g)}/_{\Sigma \text{ exponentials}}$.

6.4. Refinements

There are two important refinements to the neural network that should be considered when predicting survival.

First, there is the method of Bayesian inference based on the concept of prior and posterior probabilities. Evidently the first output from the network represents an early posterior probability and is fed back to the input so that the survival estimate may be refined. The method of empirical prior probability is usually chosen where the data are used to inform the prior. Care must be taken to ensure that both the prior and the posterior probability distributions were from the same "family" of distributions; that is the method of conjugate priors.

Second, the binary output of a neural network must be converted to a survival probability distribution by generating a ROC curve. The Receiver Operator Characteristic curve was originally developed to train and calibrate RADAR devices and operators and is used, typically when data cut-off points are not obvious. For a "test" situation, such as correctly identifying an aeroplane on a RADAR screen, it is merely the plot of sensitivity versus 1-specificity. It is particularly valuable when there are many possible cut-off points as in survival prediction. Essentially the method allows the determination of a continuous survival probability of between 0 and 1 from the binary inputs to the neural network.

7. A COMPARISON OF A NEURAL NETWORK WITH COX'S REGRESSION IN PREDICTING SURVIVAL IN OVER 800 PATIENTS WITH SQUAMOUS CELL CARCINOMA OF THE LARYNX (ORIGINAL WORK PERFORMED BY OUR GROUP)

This study illustrates the actual findings of a neural network and gives indications as to why differences between it and Cox's regression occur and what they may imply.

- The findings of this study are summarized thus;
- The neural network can be used to generate survival curves;
- The network demonstrates a significant difference in survival for dichotomous variables;
- The network duplicates the qualitative findings of Cox's regression in nearly all cases (Fig. 20) (see case of age);
- The network behaves as a "multivariate" analysis (see case of age);
- The network gives different quantitative findings to Cox's regression (and to the univariate Kaplan–Meier plots); and
- In all cases the network shows significant enhanced dichotomy compared with the other two techniques of plotting and predicting survival (Figs. 19 and 20).

The null hypotheses that neural networks compute equivalent results to Cox's model and simple Kaplan–Meier plots was refuted. Although the network produced qualitatively similar survival predictions to Cox's model, these predictions were significantly different quantitatively.

7.1. Why the disparity?

Much of this disparity may lie with the methodologies of the different techniques. The method of Kaplan and Meier is a simple univariate technique plotting observed survival

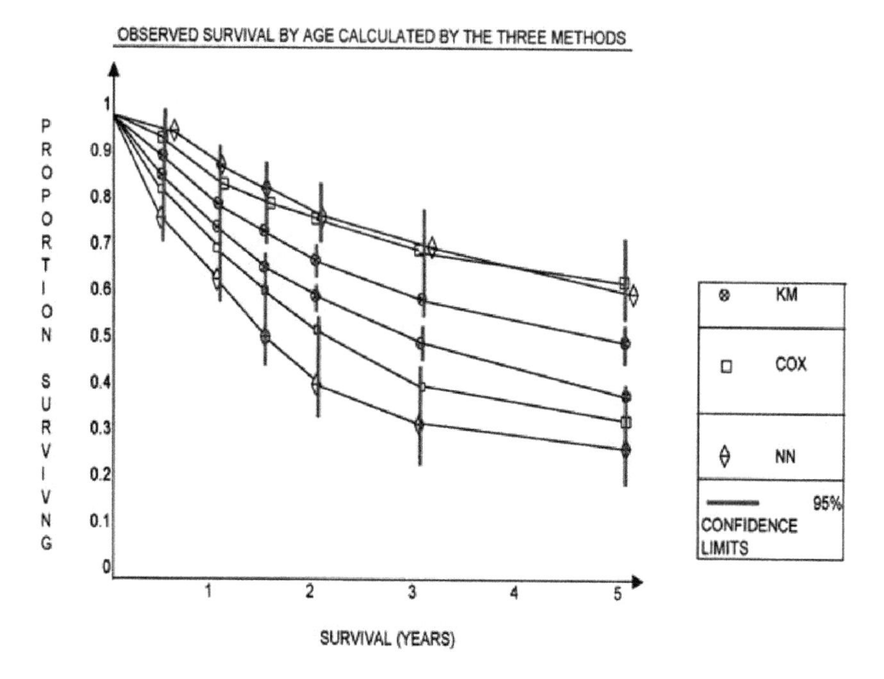

Fig. 19. The plot of the survival predictions of Cox's regression and a neural network. On the same axes is drawn the Kaplan–Meier curve. The data are for age of the patient. Significane testing showed that only the neural network found that advanced age adversely affected survival (the expected finding).

directly from the data. It is only descriptive not predictive. If we take the example of the stage of disease (Sobin and Wittekind, 1997) at the primary site (T-stage) and plot early (T1–2) against advanced (T3–4) disease, a dichotomous result will be obtained with early disease having a good prognosis and advanced disease a poor one. In a univariate technique such as this, no account is taken of confounding factors. T1–2 disease will include a whole group of covariates including the effects due to age, sex, general condition, subsite, histology, and N stage. Evidently the same will be true for T3–4 disease but the covariates will be in different proportions and have different values. It is impossible for a univariate survival plot to give a true picture of the survival of say T3–4 disease. Even with extensive stratification, no true picture will emerge. For example if a group of patients with T3–4 disease were identified with no neck node metastases (N0) this would not be representative of T3–4 disease as it would indeed be a very unusual subset of advanced disease at the primary site that was not associated with neck node metastases.

Thus to obtain a true picture of the behaviour of a particular pattern of disease, we must move on to multivariate techniques. Typically these are based on the concepts of multiple regression, but with time as the dependant variable. The method used, almost universally, is Cox's proportional hazards model almost always fitted to the Weibull distribution and is briefly described in the methods section. With such an analysis, the model will consider all

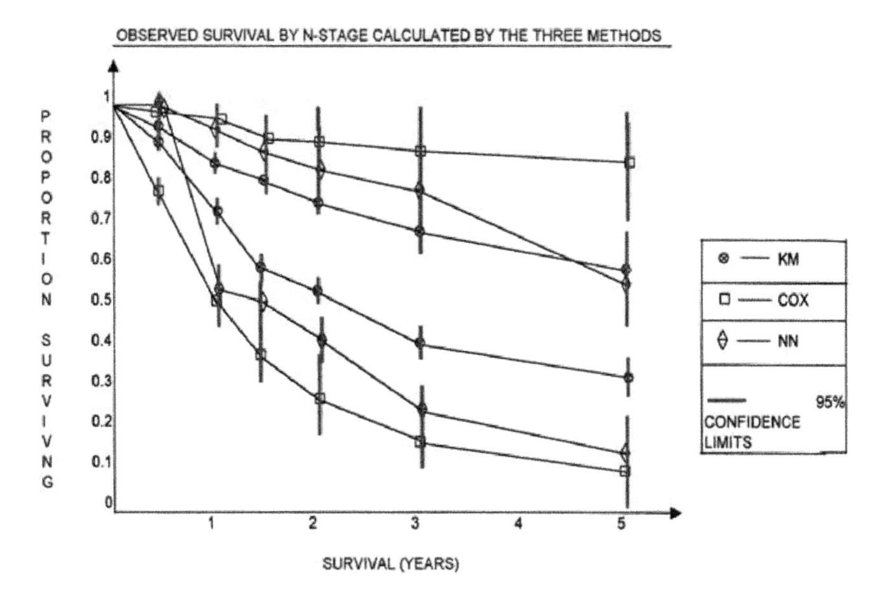

Fig. 20. The plot of the survival predictions of Cox's regression and a neural network. On the same axes is drawn the Kaplan–Meier curve. The data are stratified by the extent of neck node metastases.

covariates (variables) incorporated in the equation from a dataset and the relative effect of each covariate will be computed and assigned a significance level. Those covariates with very low *p* values are considered particularly important for the survival of patients within that dataset whereas non-significant covariates are unlikely to have any bearing on survival.

7.2. The problems with Cox's model

This model has several, potentially severe, conceptual and mathematical limitations (Altman, 1991; SAS Institute, 1995; Kattan et al., 1998). It must be emphasized, however, that for several decades it has been the most successful, most accurate and almost universally employed technique for the multivariate analysis of biological failure and survival. Although it is non-parametric with regard to survival time, it is parametric with regard to covariates. This is a serious problem in theory, although in practice, it appears less of a limitation. Most covariates, with the exception of age are non-parametric and some are only nominal. A second incorrect assumption is that the relative contributions of the various covariates to the hazard remain constant over time. They do not. The hazard is initially very high and gradually reduces over a period of two years following which the hazard rapidly declines. As this process proceeds the relative contributions of each covariate to the hazard will vary with some being important early, and others later, over the time-period of interest. Another area of concern when using Cox's model as a tool for prognostication is that it employs the concept of baseline hazard derived from the raw data. In this regard Cox's model is used for explanation and not prediction. This baseline hazard is that plot derived when all covariates are set to zero is almost identical with the overall, non-stratified, Kaplan–Meier plot of the observed data. Because, in prediction, this background hazard is usually taken from the data to be explored, there is a serious limit as to how much genuine prognostication is possible. In the present study using a training set of data to provide the background hazard from which survival was predicted in the study group is likely to have greatly reduced this effect as the "training" and "study" datasets were very well matched being drawn from the same population. Finally Cox's model is basically one of a family of linear regression techniques but where linearity is imposed on the curvilinear function of survival time. This, it is usually able to do successfully. The reason the model works at all is because the period of interest, say 6 months to 4 years usually falls within the 95% confidence interval of the linearized survival plot.

The present context was to employ Cox's regression to calculate a predicted survival curve based on a particular covariate. To achieve this, all other covariates must be set to zero (see methods section for a discussion of this point). In many ways this is imposing on a multivariate technique, a number of the disadvantages of a univariate one. Thus it is unlikely that neither Kaplan–Meier nor Cox's model can be relied upon to give a "true" set of predicted survival curves with which to compare the neural network.

7.3. The neural network

In our group's experience, the network gave similar qualitative results as Cox's model but in all cases, are a significantly greater dichotomy. This has also been noted elsewhere (Kattan et al., 1998; Lundin et al., 1999). In complex analyses in physics and natural systems in general, the technique producing the largest data separation tends, ultimately, to be correct (Reisman, 1996). Why the neural network exhibits this phenomenon in our study is conjectural. From the foregoing discussion of Kaplan–Meier plots and Cox's model, it is evident that the network is the only technique that can take realistic account of the other variables considered in the system examined. In the present case, it may be regarded as the only true "multivariate" technique. When the network considers the effect of the dichotomous variable, T stage, the other 6 variables are also included in the model. Thus for patients with early primary site disease (T1–2) the effect of confounding variables such as neck node metastases (*N* stage) will be reduced giving an improved overall survival. Conversely, for those patients with adverse primary site disease (T3–4) not only will this be assessed but also the "true" effect of such advanced cancers. Whilst such disease will naturally include some effect from significant neck node metastases it will, more importantly, indicate the true biological behaviour of the advanced primary tumour. Thus the reason for the increased dichotomy with the predictive neural network can be, at least partly, explained. No doubt other, subtler, reasons will come to light as experience with the technique increases.

7.4. Cox's model and the neural network

One clear reason why Cox's proportional hazards model and the network produce different results is in the way the background hazard is derived. With Cox's model it is that residual survival curve when all covariates are set to zero. The neural network does not use the background hazard data *per se* but computes background hazard as detailed in the methods section. Because the two predictive methods use different concepts to derive the background hazard function, it would seem unlikely that this divergence is merely anomalous. Most likely it represents a true effect.

The findings discussed above show that the survival differences obtained for binary covariates is considerably and significantly greater when calculated by the neural network than when calculated by Cox's proportional hazards model. This is particularly relevant because the neural network does not use a constant hazard term nor does it use the baseline hazard derived from the data. It thus appears highly probable that the increased divergence of binary variables calculated by the prognostic methods represents a true finding (Faraggi and Simon, 1995; Burke et al., 1997; Anand et al., 1999).

8. THE NEURAL NETWORK AND FUNDAMENTAL BIOLOGY AND ONCOLOGY

As alluded to earlier the standard concept of the functioning of the cell and oncogenesis is based on the premise that very complex, fluid interactions underpin the functioning of the cell. The "top-down" approach from genome through to phenotype has proved useful in the past but is now tending to retard progress in the understanding of the dynamic systems of fundamental cell biology. Indeed a growing body of robust evidence now lends support to this view (Gould, 1998; Maynard Smith, 1999; Spiers et al., 2000; Hodgson et al., 2002).

If we accept that the systems involved in cell biology and oncogenesis to exhibit significant non-linearity, then artificial neural networks are an excellent method of analysis and have already been used for various studies in the field of oncology. Neural networks have been used in various studies dealing with the classification of tumours at various sites as diverse as prostate, breast, cervix, bladder, oesophagus, thyroid and lymphomas and leukemia. They have also, rarely, been applied to head and neck cancer (Prismatic Project Management Team, 1999; Drago et al., 2002).

8.1. Prognostication and the neural network

Here I am concerned with the ability of neural networks to prognosticate accurately in patients with head and neck cancer. A number of papers deal with cancers of various sites including breast, colon, lung and prostate and, quite reasonably, compare neural networks with standard regression procedures, usually multiple logistic regression (Faraggi and Simon, 1995; Burke et al., 1997; Biganzoli et al., 1998a,b; Bryce et al., 1998; Kattan et al., 1998). Some publications only compared the networks prognostic performance with staging systems (e.g. TNM) or with survival plots from the dataset. Of the papers quoted, 44% found the performance of the neural networks to be equivocal and of those that tested a network against some type of regression, 60% found the network no better than the standard statistical technique.

Unquestionably, the standard multivariate method of assessing the impact of prognostic factors on survival and of predicting survival itself is the proportional hazards model (Cox, 1972; Hair et al., 1988; Altman, 1991) and thus must be the method to which the neural network is compared. Two papers address this problem quite properly comparing the results of a network with those of the proportional hazards model (Kattan et al., 1998; Anand et al., 1999). Anand, studying bowel cancer found that neural networks performed better than the proportional hazards model as long as the network was a hybrid containing some type of statistically based output system. Kattan, studying leukaemia, found the network to be superior to the proportional hazards model. Finally in Bryce's study of survival in head and neck cancer (part of a randomized control trial of chemo-radiation versus radiation alone for advanced head and neck cancer), neural networks were clearly superior to multiple logistic regression (Bryce, 1998).

8.2. Difficulties and deficiencies with Cox's model

A summary of the reasons why a substitute for Cox's proportional hazards model is urgently required is given below:

- Cox's model is limited to analysing only a small number of covariates.
- It is limited as to the complexity of the system to be studied.
- It cannot deal with non-linearity and stochastic elements within a system.
- It is unable to deal with chaotic systems.
- There are mathematical limitations to Cox's model:
  (a) It is parametric with regard to covariates;
  (b) It assumes that the relative contributions of the covariates to hazard is constant over time; and
  (c) It does not fit the prognostic index well to the survival versus survival time curve.

9. THE DIRECTION OF FUTURE WORK

The long-term aim of the application of neural networks, evolutionary algorithms and other self-learning computational modelling techniques, must be to attempt to gain greater understanding of the complex, highly fluid, "operating system" of both normal and cancer cells. Statistically based regression models are unable to deal with the very large number of possible interactions that must inevitably underlie cellular function and oncogenesis. Neural networks are the next step in the development of the analysis of such systems. Indeed many consider that when analysing data with many input parameters, neural networks are essential as no regression-based method is suitable (Biganzoli et al., 1998b; Lisboa et al., 2003). This is particularly applicable when large numbers of biological markers are involved and with the advent of tissue and DNA microarrays. Again when data is characterized by many complex interconnections many consider neural networks mandatory (DeLaurentis and Ravdin, 1994). While many researchers have felt that neural networks were neither designed nor equipped to carry out survival analysis this, as we have shown, is not the case. Indeed Biganzoli et al. (1998b) states that using the "feed forward network with logistic activation and entropy error function [it is] possible to estimate smoothed discreet hazards as conditional probabilities of failure".

Whilst artificial neural networks are powerful modelling tools, they are not a panacea and other methods exist. The neural network is only one of the species of self-learning computer-based algorithms. We have some experience of evolutionary or genetic algorithms which have described only fairly recently. It harnesses the three driving forces of evolution: recombination, mutation, and natural selection and expresses them mathematically. The provisional model is treated as the emergence of a new species which will succeed or die depending on its "fitness". New ideas are introduced as mutations and useful "inherited" traits are passed on, and sometimes shuffled by the process of recombination.

Evolutionary algorithms are an elegant and satisfying concept but their true place in modelling complex biological systems has yet to be proven.

10. SUMMARY

In this chapter, the immense complexity of the cell and its progression to cancer has been outlined. Classically the cellular systems have been considered in an "anatomical" fashion with the various structures operating more or less separately and independently. Similarly, biochemistry has tended to consider the cell as a maze of mostly independent pathways. This chapter has attempted to dispel this view and to concentrate on the cellular "operating system" as a very highly interconnected, highly complex structure allowing a vast range of possible response patterns to various stimuli. The chapter has put forward the concept of cellular systems adopting the form of a three-dimensional matrix with fluid multi-directional interactions with the whole functioning as a chaotic system.

The chapter has also dealt with the techniques available to model and predict cellular function and in particular, failure. The standard statistically based regression model of Cox (1972) has been considered unsuitable for modelling such a complex and chaotic system as the cell and, indeed, the entire organism. Because of the well-known physics of chaotic systems, modelling and prediction is only possible if large numbers of observations are incorporated into the model. This cannot be done with regression models but is not a problem for self-learning programmes including an artificial neural network. Neural networks are also designed for pattern recognition and thus, modelling the whole cellular matrix. As the network is self-learning for each run of the programme, the model continues to improve.

Thus for successfully modelling the cell and colonies of cells, artificial intelligence programming is mandatory and cannot be performed by regression-based systems burdened as they are by so many assumptions and limitations. Using self-learning programmes with large amounts of data on large numbers of cells/organisms/patients a clearer picture of not only the cellular "operating system" will emerge but also a greater understanding of cancer and indeed diseases in general.

In the near future it should not only be possible to predict accurately an individual patient's prognosis but also plan the optimum treatment for a particular patient with a particular cancer.

REFERENCES

Altman, D.G., 1991, Practical Statistics for Medical Research. Chapman & Hall, London, pp. 387–395.

Anand, S.S., A.E. Smith, P.W. Hamilton, J.S. Anand, J.G. Hughes and Bartels, 1999, An evaluation of intelligent prognostic systems for colorectal cancer. Artif. Intell. Med., 15(2), 193–214.

Autexier, C. and C.W. Greider, 1996, Telomerase and cancer: revisiting the telomere hypothesis. Trends Biochem., 21, 387–391.

Baas, P.W., 1996, The neuronal centrosome as a generator of microtubules for the axon. Curr. Topics Dev. Biol., 33, 281–296.

Barritt, G.J., 1992, Communication within Animal Cells. Oxford Science Publications, Oxford, pp. 1–243.

Basler, K. and G. Struhl, 1994, Compartment boundaries and the control of Drosophila limb pattern by Hedgehog protein. Nature, 368, 208–214.

Biganzoli, E., P. Boracchi, M.G. Diadone, M. Gion and E. Marubini, 1998a, Flexible modelling in survival analysis. Structuring biological complexity from the information provided by tumour markers. Int. J. Biol. Markers, 13(3), 107–123.

Biganzoli, E., P. Boracchi, L. Mariani and E. Marubini, 1998b, Feed forward neural networks for the analysis of censored data: a partial logistic regression approach. Stat. Med., 17(10), 1169–86.

Bryce, T.J., M.W. Dewhirst, C.E. Floyd Jr., V. Hars and D.M. Brizel, 1998, Artificial neural network model of survival in patients treated with irradiation with and without concurrent chemotherapy advanced carcinoma of the head and neck. Int. J. Radiat. Oncol. Biol. Phys., 41(2), 339–45

Burke, H.B., P.H. Goodman, D.B. Rosen, D.E. Henson, J.N. Weinstein, F.E. Har Jr., J.R. Marks, D.P. Winchester and D.G. Bostwick, 1997, Artificial neural networks improve the accuracy of cancer survival prediction. Cancer, 79(4), 857–62

Cavalli, G. and R. Paro, 1998, Chromo-domain proteins: linking chromatin structure to epigenetic regulation. Curr. Opin. Cell Biol., 10, 354–360.

Chothia, C. and E.Y. Jones, 1997, The molecular structure of cell adhesion molecules. Ann. Rev. Biochem., 66, 823–862.

Cox, D.R., 1972, Regression models & life tables. J. Roy. Stat. Soc. B., 34, 187–220.

Cox, T.M. and J. Sinclair, 1997, Molecular Biology in Medicine. Blackwell Science, Oxford, pp. 1–340.

Cross, P.A. and K.L. Mercer, 1993, Cell and Tissue Ultrastructure: A Functional Perspective. WH Freeman & Co, New York, pp. 1–528.

Demuth, H. and M. Beale, 2001, Neural Networks Toolbox: User's Guide, version 4. Natick: The Math Works Inc., pp. 41–42.

DePamphilis, M., 1996, DNA Replication in Eukaryotic Cells. Cold Spring Harbour Laboratory Press, Cold Spring Harbour, pp. 1–327.

DeVita, V.T., S. Hellman and S.A. Rosenberg (Eds.), 1993, Cancer – Principles and Practice of Oncology 4th ed., 2 Vols., Lippincott, Philadelphia, pp. 1–2747.

Doolittle, W.F., 1997, Archaea and the origins of DNA synthesis. Cell, 87, 995–998.

Faraggi. D. and R. Simon, 1995, A neural network model for survival data. Stat. Med. 14(1), 73–82

Gerstle, R.J., S.R. Aylward, S. Kromhout-Schiro and S.K. Mukherji, 2000, The role of neural networks in improving the accuracy of MR spectroscopy for the diagnosis of head and neck squamous cell carcinoma. Am. J. Neuroradiol., 21(6), 1133–1138.

Gould, S.J. 1998, Gulliver's further travels: the necessity and difficulty of a hierarchical theory of selection. Philos. Trans. Ray. Soc. Lond. B Biol. Sci., 353, 307–314.

Gumbiner, B.M., 1996, Cell adhesion: the molecular basis of tissue architecture and morphogenesis. Cell, 84, 345–357.

Hair Jr., J.F., R.E. Anderson, R.L. Tatham and W.C. Black, 1988, Multivariate Data Analysis, 5th ed., Pearson Education, New Jersey, pp. 387–395.

Hertel, K.J., K.W. Lynch and T. Maniatis, 1997, Common themes in the function of transcription and splicing enhancers. Curr. Opin. Cell. Biol. 9, 350–357.

Higgins, C.F., 1995, The ABC of channel regulation. Cell, 82, 693–696.

Hodgson, D.J., P.B. Rainey and A. Buckling, 2002, Mechanisms linking diversity, productivity and invisibility in experimental bacterial communities. Proc. Ray. Soc. Lond. B Biol. Sci., 269(1506), 2277–2283

Imreh, S., 1999, Genetic alterations in solid Tumours, Cary (NC), Seminars in Cancer Biology Inc., pp. 54–69.

Jones, A.S. and J.K. Field 1999, Tumour suppressor genes in head and neck cancer. Gen. Otolaryngol., 56, 249–260.

Kattan, M.W., K.R. Hess and J.R. Beck, 1998, Experiments to determine whether recursive partitioning (CART) or an artificial neural network overcomes theoretical limitations of Cox proportional hazards regression. Comput. Biomed. Res., 31(5), 363–373

Klein, G., 1998, Foulds' dangerous idea revisited: the multistep development of tumours 40 years later. Adv. Cancer Res., 72, 1–23.

Kornberg, A. and T.A. Baker, 1995, DNA Replication, 2nd ed., WH Freeman & Co, New York, pp. 1–395.

Latchman, D.S., 1996, Transcription–factor mutations and disease. N. Engl. J. Med, 334, 28–33.

De Laurentiis, M. and P.M. Ravdin, 1994, Survival analysis of censored data: neural network analysis detection of complex interactions between variables. Breast Cancer Res. Treat., 32(1), 113–118.

Le Goff, J.M., L. Lavayssiere, J. Rouesse and F. Spyratos, 2000, Non-linear discriminant analysis and prognostic factor classification in node-negative primary breast cancer using probabilistic neural networks. Anticancer Res., 20(3B), 2213–2218.

Liestol, K., P.K. Andersen and U. Andersen, 1994, Survival analysis and neural nets. Stat. Med. 13(12), 1189–1200.

Lisboa, P.J., H. Wong, P. Harris and R. Swindell, 2003, A Bayesian neural network approach for modelling censored data with an application to progress after surgery for breast cancer. Artif. Intell. Med., 28, 1–25.

Lodish, H., A. Berk, S.L. Zipursky, P. Matsudaira, D. Baltimore and J. Darnell, 1999, Molecular Cell Biology, 4th ed., WH Freeman, New York, pp. 1–1084.

Lundin, M., J. Lundin, H.B. Burke, S. Toikkanen, L. Pylkkanen and Joensuu, 1999, Artificial neural networks applied to survival prediction in breast cancer. Oncology, 57(4), 281–286.

Maynard Smith J. 1999, The 1999 Crafoord Prize Lecture. The idea of information in biology. Q. Rev. Biol., 74, 395–400.

Nasmyth, K., 1996, Viewpoint: putting the cell cycle in order. Science, 274, 1643–1645.

Prismatic Project Management Team, 1999, Assessment of automated primary screening on PAPNET of cervical smears in the PRISMATIC trial. Lancet, 353(9162), 1381–1385 [Erratum in 353(9169), 2078].

Rafferty, M.A., J.E. Fenton and A.S. Jones, 2001, An overview of the role and interrelationship of epidermal growth factor receptor, cyclin D and retinoblastoma protein on the carcinogenisis of squamous cell carcinoma of the larynx. Clin. Otolaryngol., 26, 317–320.

Reisman, Y., 1996, Computer-based clinical decision aids. A review of methods and assessment of systems. Med. Inform., 21, 179–197.

Sachs, A.B., P. Sarnow and M.W. Hentze, 1997, Starting at the beginning, middle, and end: translation initiation in eukaryotes. Cell, 89, 831–838.

SAS Institute Inc, 1995, User's Guide: Statistics Version,5th ed., Cary (NC), SAS Institute, pp. 1–859.

Schwab, M. (Ed.), 2001, Cancer. Springer, Berlin, pp. 1–992.

Snow, P.B., D.J. Kerr, J.M. Brandt, D.M. Rodvold, 2001, Neural network and regression predictions of 5 year survival after colon carcinoma treatment. Cancer, 91(8 Suppl), 1673–1678

Sobin, L.H. and C.H. Wittekind, 1997, TNM Classification of Malignant Tumours, 5th ed., John Wiley & Sons, New York, pp. 17–50.

Spiers, A.J., A. Buckling, B. Paul and Rainey, 2000, The cause of Pseudomonas diversity. Microbiology, 146, 2345–2350.

Stahl, F., 1996, Meiotic recombination in yeast: coronation of the double-strand break repair model. Cell, 87, 965–968.

Vaux, D.L. and S.J. Korsmeyer, 1999, Cell death in development. Cell, 96, 245–254.

Weinstein, I.B., A.M. Carothers, R.M. Santella and F.P. Perera, 1995, Molecular mechanisms of mutagenesis and multistage carcinogenesis. In: J. Mendelsohn, P.M. Howley, M.A. Isreal and L.A. Liotta (Eds.), The Molecular Basis of Cancer. WB Saunders, Philadelphia, pp. 59–85.

Welch, M.D., A. Mallavarapu, J. Rosenblatt and T.J. Mitchison, 1997, Actin dynamics in vivo. Curr. Opin. Cell. Biol. 9, 54–61.

Whitfield, P., 1993, Evolution. Marshall, London, pp. 1–219.

Whitmarsh, A.J., P. Shore, A.D. Sharrocks and R.J. Davis, 1995, Integration of the MAP kinase signal transduction pathways at the serum response element. Science, 269, 403–407.

Section 3

Mathematical Background of Prognostic Models

Chapter 6

Flexible Hazard Modelling for Outcome Prediction in Cancer: Perspectives for the Use of Bioinformatics Knowledge

Elia Biganzoli[1] and Patrizia Boracchi[2]

[1]*Unità di Statistica Medica e Biometria, Istituto Nazionale per lo Studio e la Cura dei Tumori, Milano, Italy*
Email: elia.biganzoli@istitututmori.mi.it
[2]*Istituto di Statistica Medica e Biometria, Università degli Studi di Milano, Milano, Italy*
Email: patrizia.boracchi@unimi.it

Abstract

Biological tumour markers are expected to improve outcome prediction and response to tailored therapies. However, complex effects could be underlying the dependence of the outcome from several variables measured on a continuous scale. Such a problem is of increasing importance since the advent of high throughput genomic/proteomic bioassay techniques.

Linear and non-linear flexible regression analysis techniques, such as those based on splines and feed forward artificial neural networks (FFANN), have been proposed for the statistical analysis of censored survival time data, to account for the presence of non-linear effects of predictors. Among survival functions, the hazard has a biological interest for the study of the disease dynamics, moreover it allows for the estimation of cumulative incidence functions for predicting outcome probabilities over follow-up. Therefore, specific error functions and data representation have been introduced for FFANN extensions of generalized linear models, in the perspective of modelling the hazard function of censored survival data. These techniques can be exploited for the assessment of the prognostic contribution of new biological markers, investigated by means of genomic/proteomic techniques. The application of suitable measures of prognostic accuracy will allow for the evaluation of the real improvement in outcome prediction due to the addition of the new molecular markers to the traditional clinical ones.

List of Acronyms. ANN – artificial neural networks, CR – competing risks, CSH – cause-specific hazard, DFS – disease-free survival, DM – distant metastasis, ER – oestrogen receptors, FF – feed forward, GLM – generalized linear models, HR – hazard ratio, IBTR – intra-breast tumour recurrence, IDC – infiltrating ductal carcinoma, ILC – infiltrating lobular carcinoma, MCA – multiple correspondence analysis, MLP – multi-layer perceptron, PgR – progesteron receptors, PLANN – partial logistic artificial neural networks, RBF – radial basis function, r.v. – random variable,

Acknowledgement

Partly supported by EU *Biopattern* project FP6–2002–IST–1 N°508803.

Keywords: Hazard function, outcome prediction, flexible regression modelling, artificial neural networks.

Contents

Outcome Prediction in Cancer
Edited by A.F.G. Taktak and A.C. Fisher

© 2007 Elsevier B.V. All rights reserved

1. INTRODUCTION

In biomedicine, modelling the time to occurrence of a specific event (failure time) is relevant to build decision support systems for the prediction of patients outcome with the aim of treatment planning. As an example, in clinical oncology, the study of prognostic factors has acquired a growing interest to identify groups of patients with different risks of unfavourable events (death, distant metastases, local recurrences, etc.). Two decades ago interest was focused on the effects of a few clinical variables only, measured mainly on a qualitative basis, such as tumour stage or histologic type. Relatively simple statistical models were able to process these data. Complexity of cancer biology prompted the investigation of an increasing number of tumour features; for this reason, the use of traditional clinical prognostic factors has been integrated by biological variables measured with quantitative analytical techniques in blood or tumour tissue. Moreover, recent high-throughput genomic/proteomic bioassay techniques allowed for the simultaneous measurement of the expression of thousands of genes. Due to the large number of putative prognostic factors to be investigated and to the presence of possibly complex prognostic relationships (non-linear and non-additive effects), feed forward artificial neural networks (FFANN) have been advocated for outcome analysis in oncology (Baxt, 1995). In such a context, multi-layer perceptron (MLP) and radial basis function (RBF) networks are flexible alternatives to traditional statistical tools. The benefits of the integration of FFANN with traditional methods for outcome prediction are still to be exploited; however, some reviews (Ripley and Ripley, 1998; Schwarzer et al., 2000; Lisboa, 2002) have pointed out the advantages and the possible limitations caused by the adoption of heuristic approaches, without a full account of the specific features of censored failure time data.

Conventional parametric models for survival analysis are based on strict assumptions on failure time distributions and the effect of covariates on the distribution parameters. However, such assumptions are not tenable in most applied situations. To overcome the problem, piecewise and discrete (grouped) time models have been proposed, based on the partition of the time axis into intervals, each with a specific time distribution (Elandt-Johnson and Johnson, 1980; Kalbfliesch and Prentice, 1980). As an alternative, semiparametric regression models like the Cox's model (Cox, 1972), are not constrained to specific time distributions, implying only assumptions on the relative effect of covariates. Semiparametric models are useful when the interest is focused on the effects of prognostic factors, but they do not allow direct estimate of the distribution functions. Articles merging survival analysis theory with artificial neural networks methodology in a discrete multiple classification framework were first published by Liestol et al. (1994), whereas a FFANN extension of the Cox's model was proposed by Faraggi and Simon (1995) and applied by Mariani et al. (1997) after some modifications.

Among the different survival distributions, the hazard function (i.e. the instantaneous relative failure rate) has a key role in investigating the disease dynamics. Estimation of the hazard as a conditional function of time and covariates is a difficult problem, possibly characterized by non-monotonic behaviours and high-order interactions between time and covariates; for this problem, FFANNs could provide substantial advantages with respect to linear methodologies. Starting from the relationships between generalized linear models (GLMs) with Poisson or binomial errors and piecewise parametric or grouped time models, respectively (Efron, 1988; Aitkin et al., 1989), their extension with MLPs and RBFs has been recently proposed for flexible modelling of the hazard function, allowing for non-linear and non-proportional effects of covariates (Biganzoli et al., 1998, 2002; Boracchi and Biganzoli, 2002).

Quite often the clinical course of a disease is characterized by different possible events that represent the "failure causes" of the therapeutic intervention. In oncology, typically local–regional relapses, distant metastases, new primary tumours or death, may occur. From a statistical point of view, model suited to assess the dependence of the risk of each event (*cause-specific hazard* (CSH)) on the measured covariates are needed (Marubini and Valsecchi, 1995).

Flexible linear approaches based on spline functions have been proposed for competing estimation of risks, through the extension of GLMs with Poisson error (Boracchi et al., 2001). However, when the a priori knowledge is limited, linear models may be difficult to implement, being at risk of a possible overparameterization. As previously mentioned, an alternative is represented by artificial neural networks (ANNs) models, which implicitly account for non-linear and non-additive effects of covariates (Biganzoli et al., 1998).

The aim of this chapter is to present a general framework to define FFANN models on survival data, based on the relationship between GLM and piecewise parametric and grouped time models. To this aim the peculiar features of survival data are presented and the extension of GLM with MLPs and RBFs for survival data processing is subsequently illustrated. Two application examples are discussed and final considerations are provided.

2. FAILURE TIME DATA

Let Z be the random variable (r.v.) of time elapsed from the beginning of the observation (e.g. date of the surgical intervention) to the appearance of a specific event (e.g. death or relapse of the disease). The following functions of Z can be defined:

- *survival*

$$S(z) = P(Z > z) = 1 - \int_0^z f(u)\mathrm{d}u = \int_z^\infty f(u)\mathrm{d}u,$$

where $f(u)$ is the *probability density function*

- *hazard*

$$h(z) = \lim_{\Delta z \to 0^+} \frac{P(z < Z \leq z + \Delta z \mid Z > z)}{\Delta z} = \frac{f(z)}{S(z)}$$

A feature of failure time (survival) data is the possible incomplete observation. The time of the considered event may be unknown for the ($i = 1, 2, \ldots, N$) experimental unit. This situation is known as censorship, and it may happen because of time limits in follow-up or other possible restrictions that depend on the nature of the study. Different types of censorship are possible and they have to be considered in an appropriate way in the statistic models (Klein and Moeschberger, 1997). In the present section, only the right censoring will be considered which verifies if the event is not observed before the term of the study or of a competitive event that causes the interruption of the individual sequence of visits (follow-up). For the ith subject, who will be characterized by the vector of covariates $\mathbf{x}_i$, the existence of a time of event (Z_i) and one of censors (C_i) are assumed; then the time observed t_i is the realization of the r.v. $T_i = \min(Z_i, C_i)$. Right-censored data are represented by two random variables (T_i, δ_i), where δ_i has actual value $d_i = 1$ if the event is observed ($T_i = Z_i$) and $d_i = 0$ if $T_i = C_i$.

The general expression of the function of likelihood for survival data in the presence of tight censoring, conditionally to x_i is given by

$$L = \prod_{i=1}^{N} f(t_i, \mathbf{x}_i)^{d_i} \cdot S(t_i, \mathbf{x}_i)^{1-d_i} = \prod_{i=1}^{N} h(t_i, \mathbf{x}_i)^{d_i} \cdot S(t_i, \mathbf{x}_i)$$

3. PARTITION AND GROUPING OF FAILURE TIMES

Given the continuous r.v. T, piecewise models derive from the partition of the time axis into $l = 1, 2, \ldots, L$ disjoint intervals $A_l = (\tau_{l-1}, \tau_l)$, with $\tau_0 = 0$. For the ith subject and the lth interval, T follows a distribution $f_l(t, \mathbf{x}_i)$ with a hazard function $h_l(t, \mathbf{x}_i)$.

Since the density functions are allowed to change in different intervals, the *piecewise survival* function for the ith subject on l intervals is

$$S(t, x_i) = \left[\prod_{v=1}^{l=1} \frac{S_v(\tau_v, \mathbf{x}_i)}{S_v(\tau_{v-1}, \mathbf{x}_i)} \right] \cdot \frac{S_l(t, \mathbf{x}_i)}{S_l(\tau_{l-1}, \mathbf{x}_i)} \tag{1}$$

For simplicity in Eq. (1) and in the following calculations concerning products on the intervals it is assumed that the quantity [•] is equal to 1 for $l < 2$.

Discrete time models are obtained by grouping the observed times on a point of each interval, for example τ_l. For the ith subject and the lth interval, the event probability is $\tilde{f}_l(\mathbf{x}_i)$ and the conditional event probability (*discrete hazard*) is

$$\tilde{h}_l(\mathbf{x}_i) = P(Z \in A_l \mid Z > \tau_{l-1}, \mathbf{x}_i) = \frac{\tilde{f}_l(\mathbf{x}_i)}{S(\tau_{l-1}, \mathbf{x}_i)}, \tag{2}$$

where $S(\tau_{l-1}, \mathbf{x}_i) = \Sigma_{v>l-1} \tilde{f}_w(\mathbf{x}_i)$.

The survival function can be written as a function of discrete hazards

$$S(\tau_l, \mathbf{x}_i) = \prod_{v=1}^{l} [1 - \tilde{h}_v(\mathbf{x}_i)] \tag{3}$$

The general expression of the likelihood function for the piecewise model for continuous time data with right censorship is given by

$$L_C = \prod_{i=1}^{N} \left\{ h_{l_i}(t_i, \mathbf{x}_i)^{d_i} \cdot \left[\prod_{v=1}^{l_i-1} \frac{S_v(\tau_v, \mathbf{x}_i)}{S_v(\tau_{v-1}, \mathbf{x}_i)} \right] \right\} \cdot \frac{S_{l_i}(t_i, \mathbf{x}_i)}{S_{l_i}(\tau_{l_i-1}, \mathbf{x}_i)}, \tag{4}$$

where l_i is the last interval in which the ith subject is observed. For grouped data, Eqs. (2) and (3) allow to express the likelihood function as

$$L_G = \prod_{i=1}^{N} \left\{ \tilde{h}_{l_i}^{d_i} \cdot (1 - \tilde{h}_{l_i})^{1-d_i} \cdot \left[\prod_{v=1}^{l_i-1} (1 - \tilde{h}_v) \right] \right\} \tag{5}$$

3.1. Piecewise and grouped times parametric models

Piecewise and grouped times parametric models provide a flexible alternative to the traditional ones (Aitkin et al., 1989). Concerning the piecewise model, when $h_l(t, \mathbf{x}_i)$ is assumed to be constant in each interval l, then $\mathbf{Z}$ will follow the exponential distribution with parameter $h_l(\mathbf{x}_i)$. The piecewise exponential is obtained and, according to Eq. (1), for the ith subject

$$S(t, \mathbf{x}_i) = \left[\prod_{v=1}^{l=1} \exp(-h_v(\mathbf{x}_i) \cdot (\tau_v - \tau_{v-1})) \right] \cdot \exp[-h_l(\mathbf{x}_i) \cdot (t - \tau_{l-1})]$$

Begining from Eq. (4), after defining: (i) the indicator variable d_{li} which is equal to 1 if, for the ith subject, the event of interest happens in the interval A_l, or 0 otherwise and (ii) the risk exposure time $U_{il} = I(t_i > \tau_{l-1}) \cdot [\min(t_i, \tau_l) - (\tau_{l-1})]$, the conditional likelihood function can be expressed as

$$L_P = \prod_{i=1}^{N} \prod_{l=1}^{l_i} \left\{ h_l(\mathbf{x}_i)^{\gamma il} \cdot \exp(-h_l(\mathbf{x}_i)) \right\}^{U_{il}}, \tag{6}$$

where $\gamma_{il} = d_{il}/U_{il}$. Equation (6) is proportional to the likelihood of $N \cdot l_i$ Poisson random variables. If the subjects can be grouped into K cells having equal covariate vectors $\mathbf{x}$, a further version of Eq. (6) is given by

$$L_{PK} = \prod_{k=1}^{K} \prod_{l=1}^{L} \left\{ h_l(\mathbf{x}_k)^{\gamma_{kl}} \cdot \exp[-h_l(\mathbf{x}_k)] \right\}^{U_{kl}}, \tag{7}$$

where $\gamma_{kl} = d_{kl}/U_{kl}$ *(empirical rates)*, $d_{kl} = \sum_{i \in k} d_{il}$ and $U_{kl} = \sum_{i \in k} U_{il}$. Equation (7) is proportional to the likelihood of $K \cdot L$ Poisson r.v.

Concerning grouped data, the conditional likelihood function can be obtained from Eq. (5) as

$$L_B = \prod_{i=1}^{N} \prod_{l=1}^{l_i} \left\{ \tilde{h}_l(\mathbf{x}_i)^{d_{il}} \cdot \left[1 - \tilde{h}_l(\mathbf{x}_i)\right]^{1-d_{il}} \right\} \tag{8}$$

which results from the product of Bernoulli likelihoods, one for each ith individual in the lth interval in which he/she is observed. Grouping over K cells, the likelihood

$$L_{BK} = \prod_{k=1}^{K} \prod_{l=1}^{L} \left\{ \tilde{h}_l(\mathbf{x}_k)^{p_{kl}} \cdot \left[1 - \tilde{h}_l(\mathbf{x}_k)\right]^{1-p_{kl}} \right\}^{n_{kl}} \tag{9}$$

is obtained, with $p_{kl} = d_{kl}/n_{kl}$ (*empirical risks*), d_{kl} and n_{kl} are the number of events and observed subjects in the kth cell, respectively. Equation (9) is proportional to the likelihood of $K \cdot L$ independent binomial r.v.

4. COMPETING RISKS

In the presence of R different types of events ($r = 1, \ldots, R$) with potential occurrence times $Z^1, \ldots, Z^R$, data may be represented by the realization of the random variables (T_i, δ_i, $\delta_i \rho_i$), where $T_i = \min(C_i, Z_i^1, \ldots, Z_i^R)$, $\delta_i = 0$ if $T_i = C_i$ and it is equal to 1 otherwise, and ρ_i is the type of failure corresponding to T_i. For T continuous, the CSH functions are the instantaneous hazard rate for the rth event, in the presence of other failure causes, given the absence of events before t;

$$h_r(t, \mathbf{x}_i) = \lim_{\Delta t \to 0} \frac{P(t < T \leq t + \Delta t, \rho = r \mid T \geq t, \mathbf{x}_i)}{\Delta t} \tag{10}$$

The survival function can be expressed as a function of the CSHs

$$S(t, \mathbf{x}_i) = \exp\left(-\int_0^t h(., u, \mathbf{x}_i)\,\mathrm{d}u \right), \tag{11}$$

where

$$h(., u, \mathbf{x}_i) = \sum_{r=1}^{R} h_r(u, \mathbf{x}_i)$$

Concerning the piecewise exponential model for competing risks (Larson, 1984; Kramar et al., 1987); the CSH functions are assumed constant in each lth interval and will be indicated by $h_{lr}(\mathbf{x}_i)$.

Introducing the indicator variable d_{ilr}, equal to 1 if the ith patient, in the lth time interval, had the rth event and equal to 0 otherwise, the extension of Eq. (6) is

$$L_{PR} = \prod_{i=1}^{N} \prod_{l=1}^{l_i} \prod_{r=1}^{R} \{h_{lr}(\mathbf{x}_i)^{\gamma_{ilr}} \cdot \exp(-h_{lr}(\mathbf{x}_i))\}^{U_{il}},$$

where $\gamma_{ilr} = d_{ilr}/U_{il}$.

Grouping subjects in K cells, the extension of Eq. (7) is

$$L_{PKR} = \prod_{k=1}^{K} \prod_{l=1}^{L} \prod_{r=1}^{R} \{h_{lr}(\mathbf{x}_k)^{\gamma_{klr}} \cdot \exp(-h_{lr}(\mathbf{x}_k))\}^{U_{kl}}, \tag{12}$$

where $d_{klr} = \sum_{i \in k} d_{ilr}$ and $\gamma_{klr} = d_{klr}/U_{kl}$.

Concerning grouped time models, the extension of Eq. (8) becomes

$$\begin{aligned} L_{BR} &= \prod_{i=1}^{N} \prod_{l=1}^{l_i} \left\{ \prod_{r=1}^{R} [\tilde{h}_{lr}(\mathbf{x}_i)]^{d_{ilr}} \cdot [1-\tilde{h}_l(\mathbf{x}_i)]^{1-d_{il}} \right\} \\ &= \prod_{i=1}^{N} \prod_{l=1}^{l_i} \left\{ \prod_{r=1}^{R} \left[\tilde{h}_{lr}(\mathbf{x}_i)\right]^{d_{ilr}} \cdot \left[1-\sum_{r'=1}^{R} \tilde{h}_{lr'}(\mathbf{x}_i)\right]^{1-\sum_{r'=1}^{R} d_{ilr}} \right\} \end{aligned} \tag{13}$$

since $d_{il} = \Sigma_{r'=1}^{R} d_{ilr}$.

Grouping subjects into K cells, the extension of Eq. (9) can be written as

$$L_{\mathrm{BKR}} = \prod_{k=1}^{N} \prod_{l=1}^{L} \left\{ \prod_{r=1}^{R} \left[\tilde{h}_{lr}(\mathbf{x}_k)\right]^{e_{klr}} \cdot \left[1-\sum_{r'=1}^{R} \tilde{h}_{lr}(\mathbf{x}_k)\right]^{n_{kl}-\sum_{r'=1}^{R} e_{klr}} \right\} \tag{14}$$

with $e_{klr} = \Sigma_{i \in k} d_{ilr}$ and n_{kl} the number of subjects "at risk" for each kth cell in each lth time interval. If a $R + 1$ additional "at risk" indicator $d_{il(R+1)}$ is introduced, equal to 1 in the interval A_l in which the subjects are observed without failure, and equal to 0 otherwise, $e_{kl(R+1)} = \Sigma_{i \in k} d_{il(R+1)} = n_{kl} - \Sigma_{i=1}^{R} e_{klr}$, Eq. (14) is simplified as

$$L_{BKR} = \prod_{k=1}^{K} \prod_{l=1}^{L} \prod_{r=1}^{R+1} \left[\tilde{h}_{lr}(\mathbf{x}_k)\right]^{e_{klr}} \tag{15}$$

Equation (14) is proportional to the likelihood of $K \cdot L$ independent multinomial distributions. Under the constraint

$$\sum_{r=1}^{R+1} \tilde{h}_{lr}(\mathbf{x}_k) = 1 \tag{16}$$

the quantity $\tilde{h}_{l(R+1)}(\mathbf{x}_k)$ represents the conditional probability of being censored in the lth time interval.

5. GLMs AND FFANNs

A general framework for the development of FFANNs for survival data is that of the GLMs (McCullagh and Nelder, 1989). For such models, it is assumed that each component of the r.v. **Y** has a distribution $f(y;\ \theta,\ \phi)$ in the exponential family, whose log-likelihood function is given by

$$l(\theta,\phi;y)=\log[f(y;\theta,\phi)]=[y\theta-b(\theta)]/a(\phi)+c(y,\phi)$$

If ϕ is known, $f(y;\theta,\phi)$ is an exponential family model with the *canonical parameter* θ. It can be shown that $E(Y)=\mu=b'(\theta)$ and $\mathrm{Var}(Y)=b''(\theta)\,a(\phi)$. Typically, $a(\phi)=\phi/w$, where ϕ is a constant *dispersion parameter* and w is a *prior weight* that varies from observation to observation. In a GLM, μ is related to the systematic part of the model η (*predictor*) by the *link function* $g(\mu)=\eta$. The predictor η has a linear additive form $\eta=\beta_0+\boldsymbol{\beta}^{\mathrm{T}}\mathbf{x}$, with β_0 intercept and $\boldsymbol{\beta}$ the vector of regression coefficients. FFANNs can be considered as GLMs with a non-linear predictor (Biganzoli et al., 2002) as a multi-layer perceptron (MLP)

$$\eta=\beta_0+\sum_{v=1}^{H}\beta_v^{\alpha}\cdot\alpha_v(\beta_{0v}+\beta_v^{\mathrm{T}}\mathbf{x}) \tag{17}$$

or a RBF network

$$\eta=\beta_0+\sum_{v=1}^{H}\beta_v^{\varphi}\cdot\varphi_v(\|\mathbf{x}-\mathbf{c}_v\|) \tag{18}$$

con $v = 1, \ldots, H$ *hidden units*, α_v, φ_v *activation functions* and $\mathbf{c}_v$ the centre of the vth radial basis (Bishop, 1995). Equations (17) and (18) could be called *neural predictors*. The network output values will be

$$O(\mathbf{x},\beta)=\mu=\alpha_0(\eta)$$

whereas the output activation function will be the inverse link function: $\alpha_0(\eta)=g^{-1}(\eta)$. In general, the following relationships hold

$$\frac{\partial l}{\partial\eta}=\frac{\partial l}{\partial\theta}\frac{\partial\theta}{\partial\eta}=[y-b'(\theta)]/a(\phi)\cdot\frac{\partial\theta}{\partial\eta}$$

$$\frac{\partial l}{\partial\beta}=\frac{\partial l}{\partial\theta}\frac{\partial\theta}{\partial\mu}\frac{\partial\mu}{\partial\beta}=\frac{(y-\mu)}{b''(\theta)a(\phi)}\mathbf{x}\frac{\partial\mu}{\partial\eta}$$

By fixing $\eta=\theta(\mu)$, a *canonical link* function is obtained. It follows that $\mu=g^{-1}(\eta)=b'(\eta)$ and for each ith observation

$$\frac{\partial l_i}{\partial\beta}=\mathbf{x}_i[y_i-\mu_i]/a(\phi)$$

It is an alternative way to obtain the *delta rule* of the *backpropagation* algorithm, which, for a model with a linear predictor η, is

$$\Delta_i \beta = v \frac{\partial l_i}{\partial \beta} = v[y_i - g^{-1}(\eta_i)]\mathbf{x}_i = v[y_i - O(\mathbf{x}_i, \beta)]\mathbf{x}_i,$$

where v is a suitable coefficient (*learning rate*). The result can be directly extended to MLP or RBFN network structures. If α_0 is chosen to coincide with the canonical link, the *delta rule* will provide maximum likelihood estimates. The property corresponds to the "natural pairing" of error functions and activation functions reported by Bishop (1995, p. 240).

5.1. Regression models for survival data

Following the preceding considerations, GLMs may be adopted for studying the dependence of the hazard function with the covariates **x**. Without loss of generality, models for subjects grouped into K cells will be considered. For fitting the piecewise exponential and grouped time models, distributions from the exponential family are adopted, namely the Poisson for the *empirical rates* γ_{kl} and the binomial for *empirical proportions* p_{kl}.

The terms $c(y,\phi)$ in Table 1 correspond to the logarithm of the aforementioned proportionality constants of the likelihood function. To fit the two models, it is useful to minimize the distance function given by the difference between the maximum log-likelihood achieved by the perfect fit of each observation $l(\mathbf{y}, \phi; \mathbf{y})$ and that achieved for the model under investigation $l(\hat{\boldsymbol{\mu}}, \phi; \mathbf{y})$, with estimates of the canonical parameter denoted by $\breve{\boldsymbol{\theta}} = \boldsymbol{\theta}(\mathbf{y})$ and $\hat{\theta} = \theta(\hat{\mu})$ respectively. Thus:

$$E = \sum_{k=1}^{K} \sum_{l=1}^{L} \left[y_{kl}(\breve{\theta}_{kl} - \hat{\theta}_{kl}) - b(\breve{\theta}_{kl}) + b(\hat{\theta}_{kl}) \right] \cdot w_{kl} / \phi$$

which amounts to half the (scaled) *deviance* of the model (McCullagh and Nelder, 1989). This statistic allows to define in a general way error functions for generalized regression models to be fitted with ANNs. The corresponding error functions for the piecewise exponential and the grouped time models for a single and competing risks, grouping subjects in cells, are respectively

$$E_{PK} = \sum_{k=1}^{K} \sum_{l=1}^{L} \left\{ \gamma_{kl} \log \left[\frac{\gamma_{kl}}{h_{l(\mathbf{x}_k)}} \right] - \gamma_{kl} + h_l(\mathbf{x}_k) \right\} \cdot U_{kl} \quad (19)$$

$$E_{PKR} = \sum_{k=1}^{K} \sum_{l=1}^{L} \sum_{r=1}^{R} \left\{ \gamma_{krl} \log \left(\frac{\gamma_{klr}}{h_{lr}(\mathbf{x}_k)} \right) - (\gamma_{klr} - h_{lr}(\mathbf{x}_k)) \right\} \cdot U_{kl} \quad (20)$$

and

$$E_{BK} = \sum_{k=1}^{K} \sum_{l=1}^{L} \left\{ p_{kl} \log \left[\frac{p_{kl}}{\tilde{h}_l(\mathbf{x}_k)} \right] + (1 - p_{kl}) \log \left[\frac{1 - p_{kl}}{1 - \tilde{h}_l(\mathbf{x}_k)} \right] \right\} \cdot n_{kl} \quad (21)$$

Table 1 Binomial and multinomial distributions (for single and competing risk GLMs)

	Poisson		Binomial	Multinomial
	Single	Competing	Single	Competing
y	γ_{kl}	γ_{klr}	p_{kl}	p_{klr}
$a(\phi)=\phi / w$	$1/U_{kl}$	$1/U_{kl}$	$1/n_{kl}$	$1/n_{kl}$
$\theta(\mu)$	$\log[h_l(\mathbf{x}_k)]$	$\log[h_{lr}(\mathbf{x}_k)]$	$\log\left[\frac{\tilde{h}_l(\mathbf{x}_k)}{1-\tilde{h}_l(\mathbf{x}_k)}\right]$	$\log\left[\frac{\tilde{h}_{lr}(\mathbf{x}_k)}{\tilde{h}_{l(R+1)}(\mathbf{x}_k)}\right]$
$b(\theta)$	$h_l(\mathbf{x}_k)=\exp(\theta)$	$h_{lr}(\mathbf{x}_k)=\exp(\theta)$	$-\log[1-\tilde{h}_l(\mathbf{x}_k)]$ $=\log[1+\exp(\theta)]$	$-\log\left[1-\sum_{r=1}^{R}\tilde{h}_{lr}(\mathbf{x}_k)\right]$ $=\log\left[1+\sum_{r=1}^{R}\exp(\theta)\right]$
$b'(\theta)=E(Y;\theta)$	$\exp(\theta)$	$\exp(\theta)$	$\frac{\exp(\theta)}{1+\exp(\theta)}$	$\frac{\exp(\theta)}{1+\sum_{r=1}^{R}\exp(\theta)}$
$c(y,\phi)$	$\gamma_{kl}U_{kl}\log(U_{kl})+$ $-\log[(\gamma_{kl}U_{kl})!]$	$\gamma_{klr}U_{kl}\log(U_{kl})+$ $-\log[(\gamma_{klr}U_{kl})!]$	$\log\binom{n_{kl}}{d_{kl}}$	$\log\left(\frac{n_{kl}}{\prod_{r=1}^{R+1}e_{ilr!}}\right)$

Models are member of the exponential family, $f(y;\theta,\phi)=\exp\{[y\theta-b(\theta)]\,a(\phi)+c(y,\phi)\}$

$$E_{BKR} = \sum_{k=1}^{K} \sum_{l=1}^{L} \sum_{r=1}^{R+1} \left\{ p_{klr} \log\left[\frac{p_{klr}}{\tilde{h}_{lr}(\mathbf{x}_k)} \right] \right\} \cdot n_{kl}, \tag{22}$$

where U_{kl} and n_{kl} have the role of prior weights.

For a single risk in the discrete context, a proportional odds model with the *logit* link, canonical with respect to Eq. (8), was proposed by Cox (1972) as

$$\log\left[\frac{\tilde{h}_l(\mathbf{x}_k)}{1 - \tilde{h}_l(\mathbf{x}_k)} \right] = \beta_l^0 + \boldsymbol{\beta}^{\mathrm{T}} \mathbf{x}_k \tag{23}$$

where $\beta_l^0 = \log[(\tilde{h}_l(0))/(1 - \tilde{h}_l(0))]$. It is analogous to ANN models (without hidden units) for classification problems with error function Eq. (21), since the logit link is the inverse of the logistic activation function. The partial logistic artificial neural network (PLANN), proposed by Biganzoli et al. (1998), follows such an approach to provide smoothed discrete hazard estimates by adopting a neural predictor Eq. (17) for model Eq. (23) and relaxing additivity constraints. The resulting MLP model is parameterized as follows:

$$\tilde{h}_l(\mathbf{x}_k) = \frac{\exp\left\{ \beta_0 + \sum_{v=1}^{H} \beta_v^{\alpha} \cdot \alpha_v(\beta_{0v} + \boldsymbol{\beta}_v^{\mathrm{T}} \mathbf{v}_{kl}) \right\}}{1 + \exp\left\{ \beta_0 + \sum_{v=1}^{H} \beta_v^{\alpha} \cdot \alpha_v(\beta_{0v} + \boldsymbol{\beta}_v^{\mathrm{T}} \mathbf{v}_{kl}) \right\}}$$

corresponding to the well-known regression model for binary classification, with the logistic activation function $\alpha_v(u) = \exp(u)/(1 + \exp(u))$ the additional input for the time interval is included in $\mathbf{v}_{kl} = (\mathbf{x}_k, \tau_l)$. In the Poisson model for competing risks, an input vector $\mathbf{v}_{klr} = (\mathbf{x}_k, \tau_l, r)$ is used, with a further input for the specific cause of failure.

The discrete time model for competing risks can be fitted by modelling the e_{klr} with GLM with multinomial error and the *canonical* inverse multinomial logit link.

$$\tilde{h}_{lr}(\mathbf{x}_k) = \frac{\exp[\eta_{lr}(\mathbf{x}_k)]}{\sum_{r=1}^{R+1} \exp[\eta_{lr}(\mathbf{x}_k)]}, \tag{24}$$

where $\eta_{lr}(\mathbf{x}_k)$ is the model predictor, which can be either linear or neural as

$$\eta_{lr}(\mathbf{x}_k, \boldsymbol{\beta}) = \beta_0 + \sum_{v=1}^{H} \beta_r^{\alpha} \alpha_v(\beta_{0v} + \boldsymbol{\beta}_v^{\mathrm{T}} \mathbf{v}_{kl})$$

Therefore, the single risk model has a logistic output activation function, whereas for competing risks, Eq. (24) is used considering $R + 1$ outputs. Such a function, called *softmax* in the ANN jargon, corresponds to the multinomial generalization of the logistic function.

It can also be considered that in such models, though approximate, the assumption of independence of the contribution to the likelihood for each individual across time intervals leads to reasonable results, extending arguments for the binomial model provided by Efron (1988). Since the grouped time competing risk model can also be viewed as an extension of PLANN (Biganzoli et al., 1998, 2002) to multiple failure causes in a competing risks framework, it is denoted by the acronym PLANNCR (Biganzoli et al., 2006).

The models can be implemented using conventional back-propagation as a training algorithm, but in the original proposal (Biganzoli et al., 1998), model optimization has been performed with a quasi-Newton algorithm, namely the *nnet* function of the S-plus software, provided by Venablc and Ripley (1999). Regularization is applied to control model complexity in the form of *weight decay*; to this aim, a penalty term is added to the error function (Eq. (21)) obtaining

$$E_G^* = E_G + \lambda \sum \beta^2 .$$

In an analogous way, the log-linear piecewise exponential models with canonical link $\log[h_l(\mathbf{x}_i)]$ can be considered (Larson, 1984). An advancement of the approach was proposed in the competing risks framework (Boracchi and Biganzoli, 2002), by considering the RBF expansion (Eq. (18)) as a model predictor and the error function (Eq. (19)).

For a single event, the resulting RBF model has the following structure:

$$h_l(\mathbf{x}_k) = \exp\left\{ \beta_0 + \sum_{v=1}^{H} \beta_v^{\varphi} . \varphi_v (\| \mathbf{v}_{kl} - \mathbf{c}_v \|) \right\}$$

where the H localized radially symmetric basis functions have centres $\mathbf{c}_v$. The Euclidean distance and Gaussian function are adopted giving

$$\varphi_v (\| \mathbf{v}_{kl} - \mathbf{c}_v \|) = \exp\left[-\frac{1}{2} (\mathbf{v}_{kl} - \mathbf{c}_v)^{\mathrm{T}} \sum\nolimits_v^{-1} (\mathbf{v}_{kl} - \mathbf{c}_v) \right]$$

where Σ_v, in the simplest form, is a diagonal matrix with equal terms $\sigma_j = \sigma$.

Two step procedures can be adopted for model optimization (Bishop, 1995); namely, in step 1 (*unsupervised*) the parameters of the hidden units, $\mathbf{c}_v$ and σ_j, are determined by clustering or sampling methods which only use input vectors $\mathbf{v}_{kl}$, whereas in step 2 (*supervised*), optimization techniques for GLMs like *iterative reweighted least squares*, are applied.

6. APPLICATIONS TO CANCER DATA

In this section, three examples on real data, already analysed by Biganzoli et al. (1998, 2003) and Boracchi et al. (2001) are presented. The first example concerns the survival of head and neck cancer patients. Grouped failure times have been analysed with a linear spline regression model by Efron (1988) to obtain a flexible interpolation of the discrete hazards. A comparison between the results of the flexible linear model and the PLANN model is considered. The second example concerns the analysis of individual risk profiles in node-negative primary breast cancers. PLANN model was used to estimate discrete hazards of tumour relapses. The covariate effects were then visualized by three-dimensional surface plots of estimated conditional discrete hazard as a function of time and covariates. Multiple correspondence analysis (MCA) was finally adopted to visualize the relationship between model predictions of 5-year relapse probabilities and covariate patterns. In the third example, a problem of competing risks in breast cancer is considered. The risk of local relapses intra-breast tumour recurrence (IBTR) and distant metastasis (DM) has been studied according to the patient age at surgery, tumour size, histological type, number of axillary metastatic lymph nodes and site of the tumour. RBF model was used and the covariate effects on CSHs of the two events were visualized by three-dimensional surface plots of estimated conditional CSHs as a function of time and covariates.

6.1. Head and neck cancer study

A two-arms (different treatments) clinical trial is considered, details on the data set are reported in Efron (1988) and Biganzoli et al. (1998). Efron (1988) provided smoothed estimates of the discrete hazard function, separately for the two arms, with a logistic regression model for grouped failure times. To this aim, he adopted a cubic–linear spline function on follow-up time grouped into months. A dynamic logistic model with linear predictor was then applied by Fahrmeir (1994). A PLANN model was then adopted to assess the conditional discrete hazard, as a joint function of time and therapy. Different configurations have been evaluated, with 12 hidden units and a penalty value of $\lambda = 0.075$. The effective number of estimated free parameters, having adopted a penalized estimation, was about 6.

The spline function adopted by Efron (1988) considered four linear coefficients for each of the two arms of the study (excluding the position of the spline knot); hence, in this case the PLANN model and the linear one would have a comparable number of estimated parameters. Figure 1A reports the results of the PLANN model: the continuous lines are the predicted risks from the neural network. The cubic–linear spline function estimates are reported in the same figure as broken lines. The estimated shapes of the two models are similar. Figure 1B reports the estimated survival functions with the PLANN model, the cubic–linear spline and the non-parametric Kaplan–Meier estimator. Adopting the same number of hidden units, but with a lower penalty ($\lambda = 0.025$) less smoothed estimates have been achieved (please compare Fig. 2(A and B). The hazard function displayed in Fig. 3A has similar behaviour to that estimated by Fahrmeir (1994).

The application of spline functions requires prior information for the choice of the number and location of the knots; moreover, a joint model for the two treatment arms, should use additional terms for the main effect of the treatment for the interaction with time. In this example, the application of FFANN model has allowed the joint evaluation

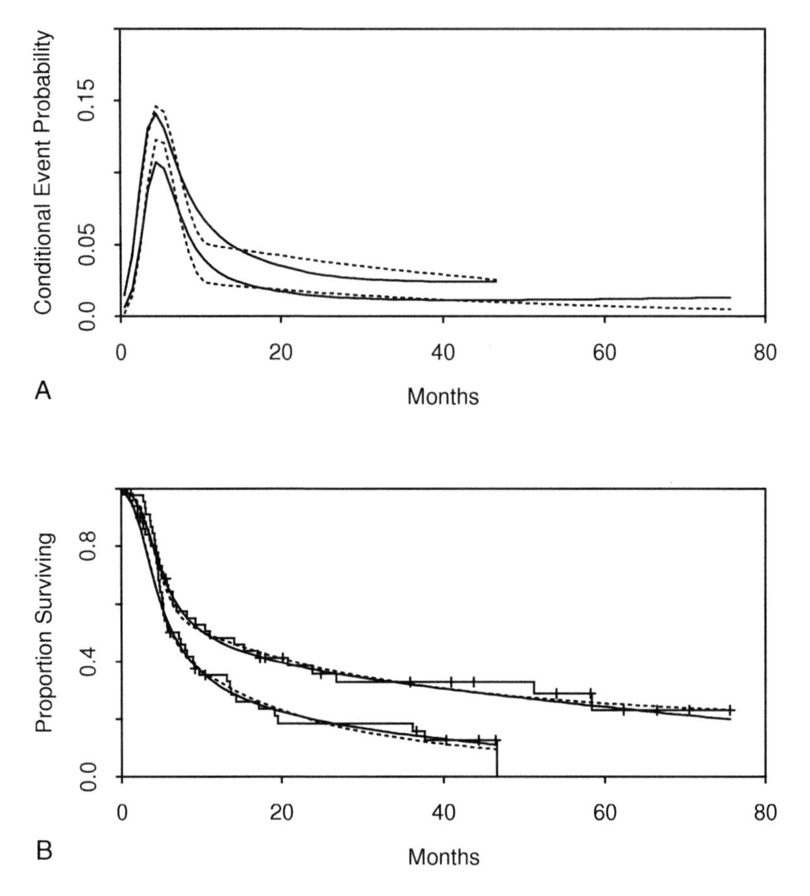

Fig. 1. (A) Estimated event conditional probability obtained by the optimal PLANN configuration ($H = 12$, $\lambda = 0.075$, continuous line) and the linear cubic spline proposed by Efron (1988) (dotted line). (B) Corresponding estimates of survival functions (continuous and dotted lines, respectively) and Kaplan–Meier estimates (step function).

of the effects of time and of therapy on the hazard function, without any assumption on the structure of the dependence relationships. Moreover, modulating the degree of smoothing for the penalized estimation, possible complex patterns underlying data have been explored.

6.2. Analysis of individual risk profiles in node-negative primary breast cancers

In the traditional clinical setting, only a few standardized and routinely assessed factors have recognized prognostic relevance in primary breast cancer. However, studies on

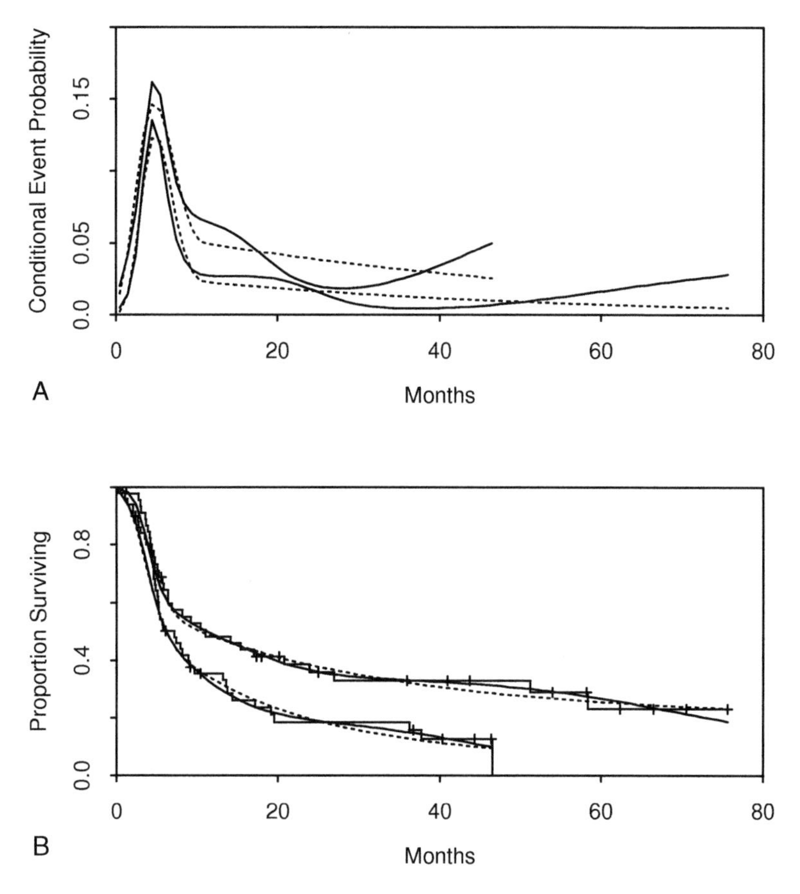

Fig. 2. (A) Estimated event conditional probability obtained by a suboptimal PLANN configuration ($H = 12$, $\lambda = 0.025$, continuous line) and the linear cubic spline proposed by Efron (1988) (dotted line). (B) Corresponding estimates of survival functions (continuous and dotted lines, respectively) and Kaplan–Meier estimates (step function).

genomic markers have shown that prognostic criteria based on few conventional markers could be improved by the joint evaluation of the differential expression of genes, related to tumour aggressiveness or response to adjuvant therapies, among patients with different outcomes. To this aim, a critical issue is the additional contribution of genomic markers to the information provided by the traditional ones. Moreover, improvements to current practice might be achieved by accounting for the modulation of the effects of the considered tumour and patient features on the rate of disease recurrence in the course of follow-up. It is also evident that, so far, the predictive role of such features was suboptimally investigated in oversimplified statistical models, like the widespread Cox regression model under the assumption of linear and proportional hazards effects. The use of suitable flexible

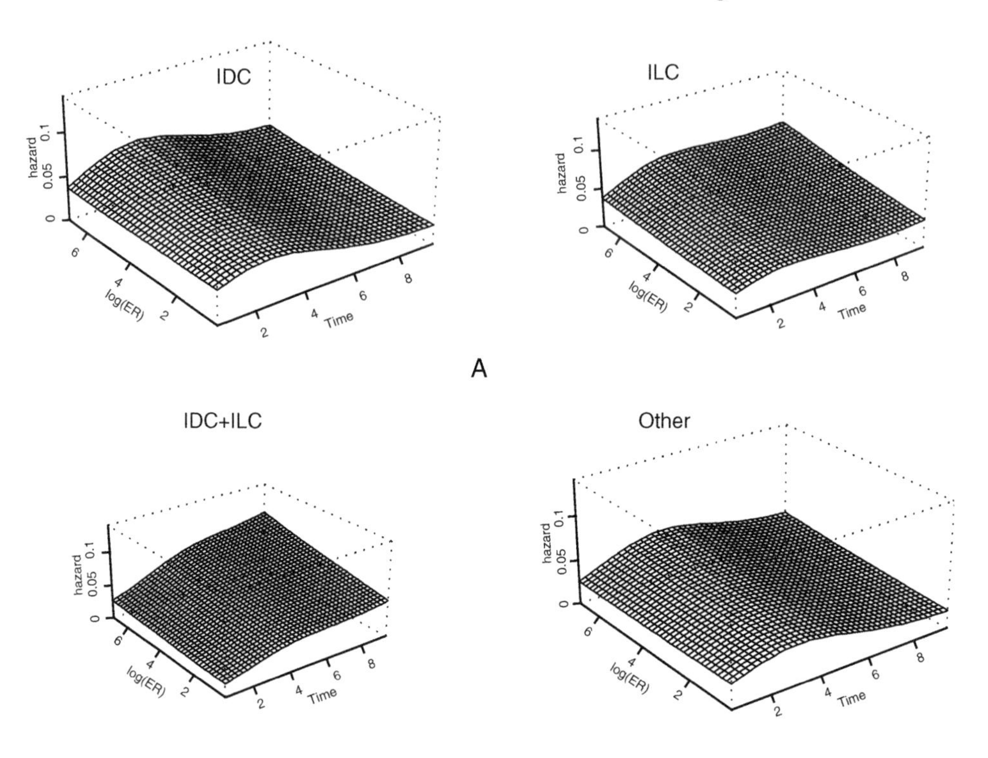

Fig. 3. Surface plots of PLANN model results for (A) logarithm of oestrogen receptors log(ER) and (B) tumour size. Estimated conditional hazards are plotted as a function of follow-up time (years) for each histology type.

statistical models like ANNs, tailored for survival data analysis, could substantially improve the analysis of traditional markers, providing a benchmark for the assessment of predictive contribution of the genomic ones.

Statistical models on the hazard function (i.e. the instantaneous risk of disease recurrence) are suited for this task, having an exploratory role in the "knowledge phase" of the disease dynamics. Relevant effects, discovered within this phase, support the development of prognostic classification schemes for the subsequent "decision phase".

For example, although prior knowledge about the time-dependent prognostic relevance of steroid receptors was available, it was not investigated jointly with other prognostic factors and no information on the shape of the hazard, as a function of time and features, was available from the Cox model.

The aim of the present study (Biganzoli et al., 2003) was to investigate the joint role of oestrogen and progesterone (ER, PgR) receptors and other clinically relevant patient and tumour characteristics (age, tumour size, histology) on the risk of cancer recurrence during follow-up after surgery of N patients. ER, PgR, age and tumour size were analysed

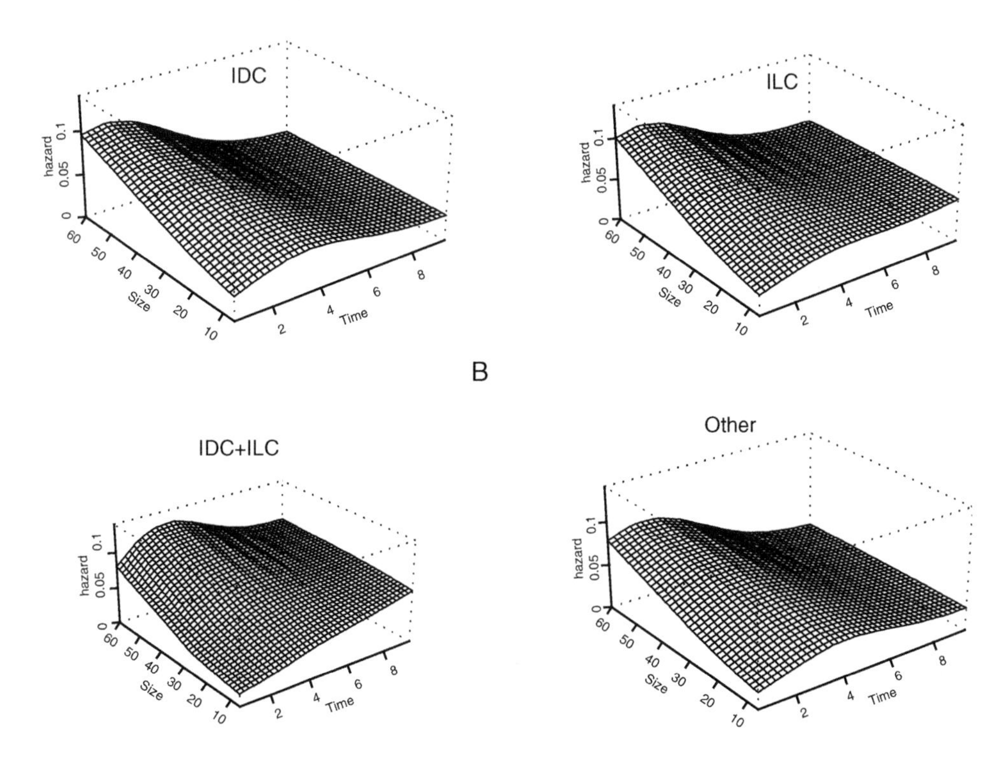

Fig. 3. Cont'd.

accounting for their original scale of measurement, in order to improve the accuracy of the picture of their effects on the hazard function and individual risk profiling.

The case series consisted of 1793 women with primary resectable invasive breast cancer who had no axillary lymph node involvement and no radiologic or clinical evidence of DM, a synchronous bilateral tumour, or a second primary tumour. Cases with these clinicopathologic features and with a minimal potential follow-up of 10 years (i.e. the time elapsed from the date of surgery to the last update of the patient records) were selected from about 7000 women with an operable tumour, consecutive with respect to ER and PgR determination, who underwent surgery at the Istituto Nazionale Tumori of Milan between January 1981 and December 1986.

The first documented evidence of local recurrence or regional axillary relapse (183 cases), DM (225 cases), contralateral breast cancer (119 cases) or other second primary cancer (75 cases) was considered as endpoint for disease-free survival (DFS). Local, regional, contralateral and distant failures were accurately assessed by clinical, radiologic and, whenever possible, histopathologic examination. The median follow-up was 127 months (25th percentile, 79; 75th percentile, 148).

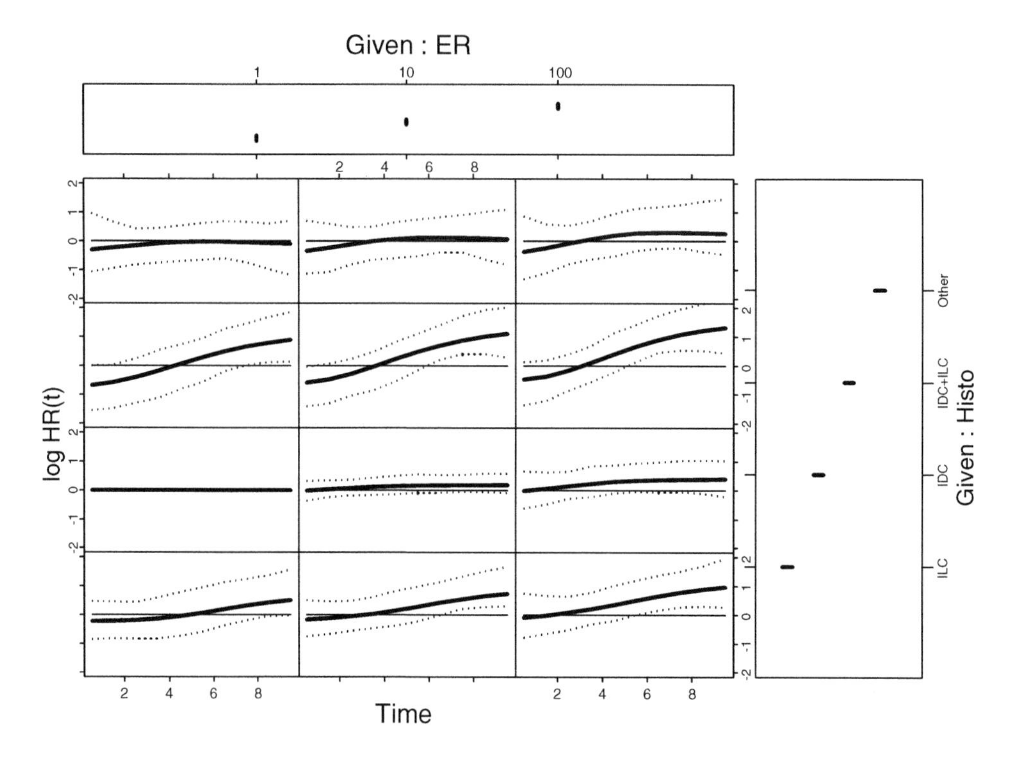

Fig. 4. Multipanel conditioning plot of PLANN model results for histology and oestrogen (ER) receptors. Estimated log relative hazards are plotted as a function of follow-up time (years) for selected ER and PgR values.

To visualize the effect of the continuous covariate (ER, PgR, age, tumour size) and the categorical one (histology: IDC, ILC, IDC+ILC, other), model results were represented by three-dimensional surface plots of estimated conditional discrete hazard as a function of time and of the continuous covariate for each type of histology, after fixing other continuous covariates to their median values. To investigate possible high-order interactions, multipanel conditioning plots were adopted. These plots display the joint effect of two covariates and follow-up time on the logarithm of the relative hazard (log (HR)), fixing other continuous covariates to their median values. Confidence intervals were estimated by means of a non-parametric bootstrap procedure. Multiple correspondence analysis (MCA) was finally adopted to visualize the relationship between model predictions and covariate patterns.

The plots of the PLANN-estimated hazards as a function of follow-up time and log (ER), and tumour size are reported for different histologies, in Fig. 3(A and B), respectively. Overall, the plots show that the shape of the hazard function changes according to histology. A marked non-monotonic shape over time is observed for IDC and for the class "other" histology, whereas for ILC such behaviour is attenuated and for IDC + ILC the

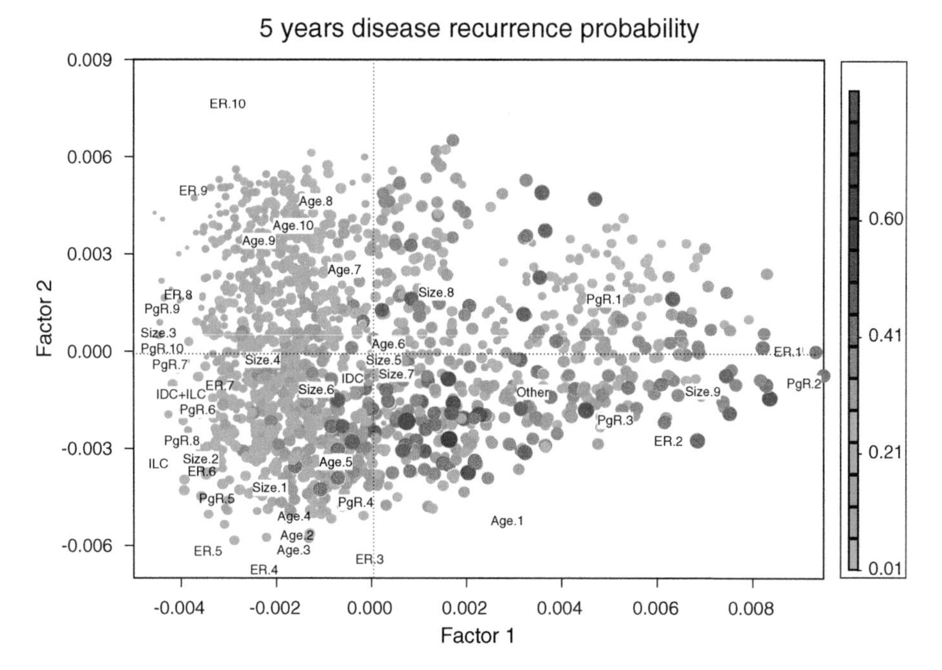

Fig. 5. Visualization of five-year predicted disease recurrence probabilities and covariate patterns by means of multiple correspondence analysis (MCA) on the plane identified by the first two factorial axes (Factors 1 and 2). Point coordinates are factorial scores. Dots identify subjects, dot size and colour level are proportional to the predicted probability of disease recurrence. The corresponding colour scale is reported on the right of each panel. The labels in the plot correspond to the class in which the specific covariate has been grouped.

hazard appears to be steadily increasing, this pattern confirms the time-dependent role of histology. Concerning ER, small or no effect on the hazard is present early during follow-up, whereas after about 3 years increasing log(ER) values have an unfavourable prognostic effect. Such behaviour seems different according to histology, suggesting the presence of a high-order interaction with follow-up time, which would be difficult to detect with conventional statistical approaches.

The time-dependent prognostic role of tumour size is also evident: the risk of recurrence is the greatest for early follow-up time and large tumour size, it increases with increasing tumour size, but this effect lessen after about five years of follow-up with the decrease of the hazard.

The joint effects of histology and ER have been further investigated in Fig. 4, resorting to multipanel conditioning plots of the PLANN-estimated log HR for different combinations of the above two variables. Point estimates (solid lines) with 95% bootstrap confidence intervals (dotted lines) are reported, considering as reference low ER (1 fmol/mg) and IDC histology. The long-term risk effect of ILC and IDC + ILC is much more evident for intermediate (10 fmol/mg) to high (100 fmol/mg) ER values. Increasing ER values appear to be associated with a slight increase of the log HR at long follow-up, however this time-dependent effect is lower than that of histology.

Finally, in Fig. 5, PLANN-predicted disease recurrence probabilities for each subject were jointly projected with covariate categories onto a plane defined by the first two factorial axes of MCA. For a dynamic view of the evolution of the risk of disease recurrence, predictions at different follow-up times can be plotted, but in the figure only that at five years are reported.

According to the general trend, high-risk predictions are mainly concentrated in the lower right corner of the graph, being associated with intermediate to large tumour size, low ER and PgR levels, young age. Conversely, low-risk predictions appear to be well separated, being mainly concentrated in the upper left corner and associated with older age, high ER and high PgR levels.

6.3. Study of competing events after conservative surgery of the breast cancer

The study includes 2233 patients hospitalized at the Istituto Nazionale per Studio e la Cura dei Tumori di Milano between 1970 and 1987. Details on the study and on the strategy adopted for the evaluation of the artificial neural network RBF models have been reported in the article of Boracchi et al. (2001). Globally, non-monotonic patterns of the CSH functions in time and different covariate effects have been observed for the two considered events: IBTR and DM. The prognostic impact of age, tumour size and histology on IBTR appears more evident than that of the number of axillary metastatic lymph nodes and tumour site. The CSH for IBTR decreases with the increase in age (Fig. 6A), increases with the increasing tumour size (Fig. 6B) and tends to decrease with the increase in the number of axillary metastatic lymph nodes (Fig. 6C). The effects of interaction between variables and time have been explored resorting to multiple conditioning panel graphs; for example, the effect of the metastatic lymph nodes on IBTR appears more evident in the youngest patients, with highest CSH in the absence of metastatic axillary lymph nodes. Concerning DM, the pattern of risk in time appears markedly non-monotonic and the maximum value is observed at about two and a half years of follow-up (Fig. 7). The impact of the tumour size and the metastatic lymph nodes on DM appears to be more marked than that of the age, histology and tumour site. CSH weakly decreases as age increases, increases as tumour size and the number of axillary metastatic lymph nodes increase. The effect of the tumour size decreases with follow-up time, pointing out the possible time-dependent role of this prognostic variable, in agreement with the findings in other case series.

7. CONCLUSIONS

Building a multiple regression model for outcome prediction is a problem of approximation of an unknown multivariate dependence relationship. In the presence of non-linear

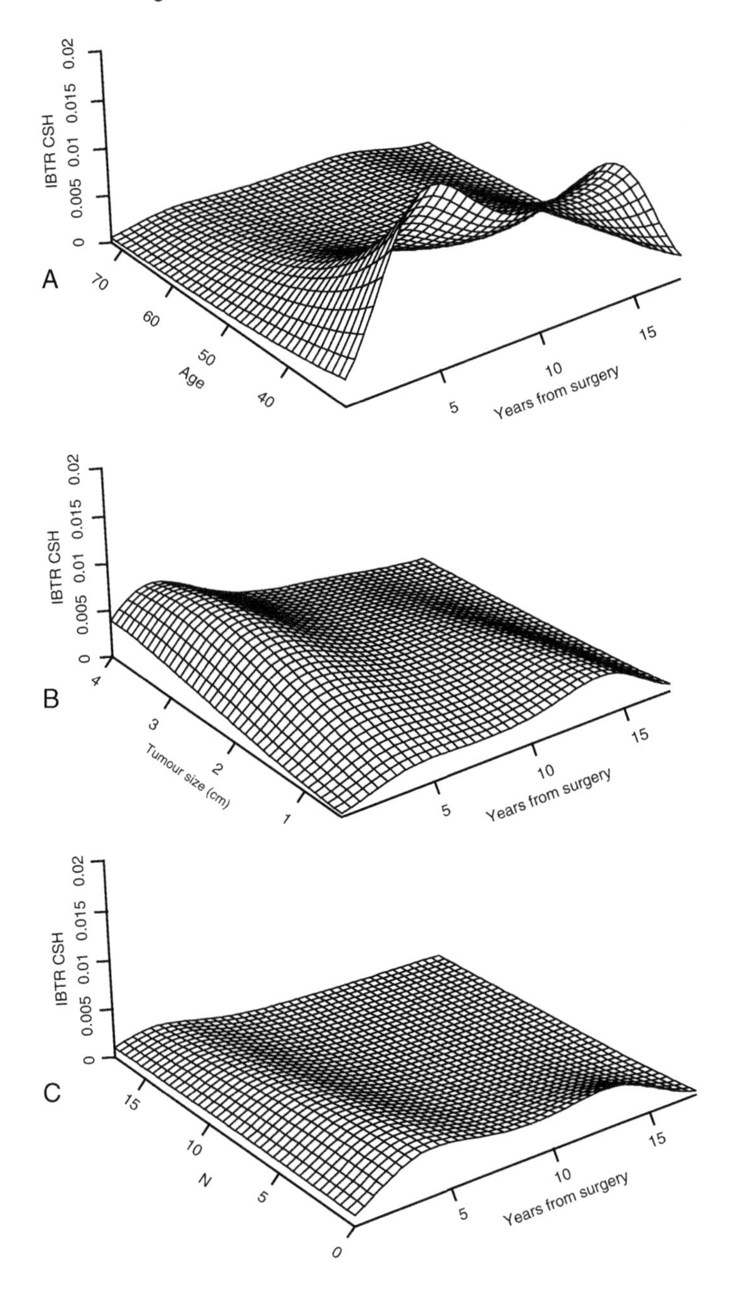

Fig. 6. Graph of the conditioned surface of the CSHs for IBTR as a function of age (A), tumour size (B) and number of metastatic axillary lymph nodes (C). Other covariates are fixed to the median values for age and tumour size and to modal categories for tumour site and histological type.

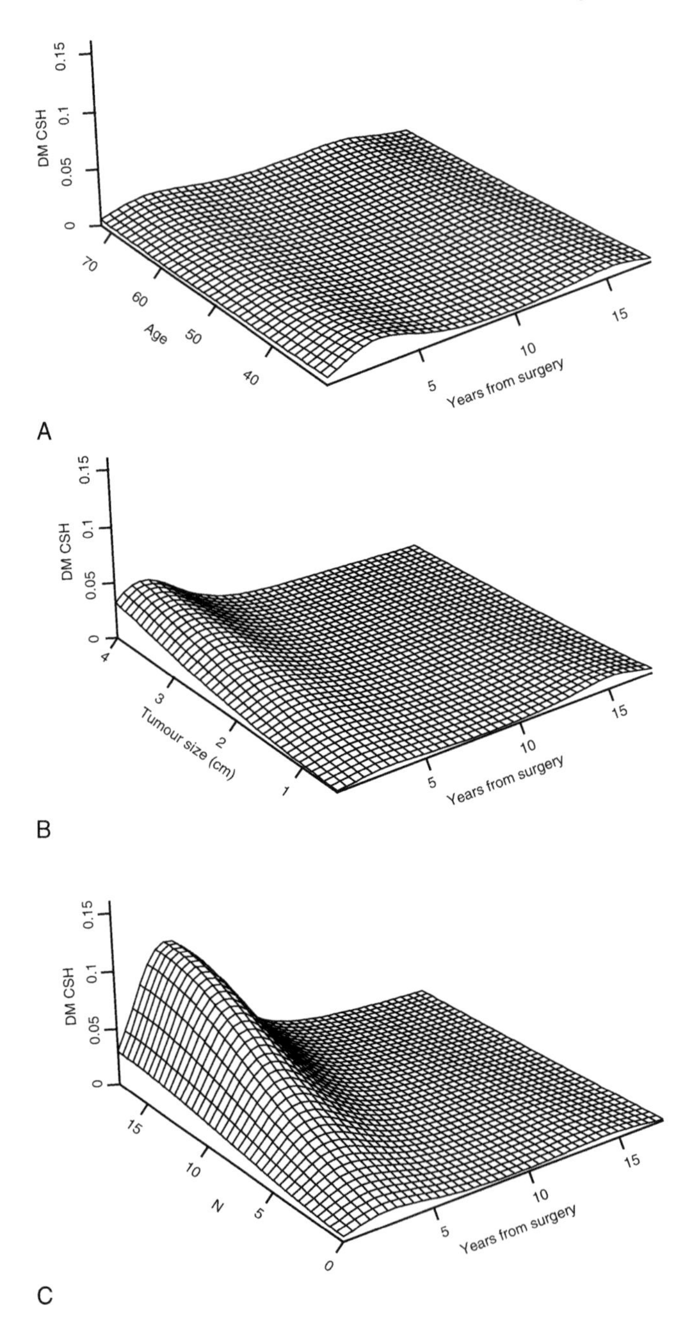

Fig. 7. Graph of the conditioned surface of the CSHs for DM as a function of age (A), tumour size (B) and number of metastatic axillary lymph nodes (C). Other covariates are fixed to the median values for age and tumour size and to modal categories for tumour site and histological type.

effects and/or non-additive effects, an approach commonly assumed as "natural" is that of including in the model (Schwarzer et al., 2000) polynomial terms and their cross-products. However, this approach is not necessarily optimal if less a priori knowledge of the phenomenon is available. FFNN and RBF models offer an alternative model parameterization not constrained to strong assumptions on the effect of the covariates. Therefore, the use of neural network models for outcome prediction could be mostly relevant for exploratory analyses and as a benchmark for assessing the performances of other concurrent models. The PLANN(CR) model can provide relevant indications on the underlying patterns to the prognostic problem under evaluation, thus substantially contributing to the individual risk bioprofiling. Moreover the Bayesian extension of PLANN proposed by Lisboa et al. (2003), faces the aspect of optimal control of model complexity in a principled way.

ANN-based models rely on inductive inference. They attempt to discover biologically and clinically relevant prognostic relationships directly from patient and tumour data, thereby avoiding too restrictive a priori assumptions. In their conventional application to outcome prediction, ANNs have been adopted according to this principle, even though they are essentially used as "black boxes". In fact, although they may improve the accuracy of prediction, they consist of a statistical model not immediately accessible to clinicians and investigators. As we are aware of the need to increase the knowledge of the dynamics of breast cancer recurrence, the PLANN(CR) model is not exploited as a black box in the above applications; namely: (i) multivariate visualization techniques are adopted for exploring covariate effects on the hazard function over time, and (ii) patient profiles are displayed with the corresponding model-predicted disease recurrence probabilities at different follow-up times. According to this strategy, prognostic relationships underlying data are identified, in order to understand how the model predicts outcomes before further clinical application. To this aim, the identification of time-dependent risk profiles can be useful to improve follow-up and/or therapy planning.

In recent research studies, there was a specific interest in the application of advanced regression techniques such as neural networks for the analysis of genomic/proteomic data. Overall, a critical aspect is related to the evaluation of the model performance to assess the true gain from such approaches when applied on noisy data from microarray analyses (Biganzoli and Boracchi, 2004). Several applications considered outcome prediction, but most of them failed to account for censored survival data. The latter situation is partly motivated by study design issues (Biganzoli et al., 2005).

In the light of the continuous improvement in genomic/proteomic techniques for increasing the signal-to-noise ratio of such measurements, it should be expected a relevant contribution of flexible regression techniques for joint exploratory modelling of the effect of several gene expression measures, accounting for their non-linear/non-additive effects on the outcome of interest.

Nevertheless, waiting for the refinement of the proteomic/genomic techniques, neural networks techniques for censored failure data can now play a critical role (Biganzoli et al., 2003) in substantially improving outcome prediction strategies in cancer, based on traditional and/or new clinical and biological markers.

REFERENCES

Aitkin, M., D. Anderson, B. Francis and J. Hinde, 1989, Statistical Modelling in GLIM. Oxford University Press, New York.

Baxt, W.G., 1995, Application of artificial neural networks to clinical medicine. Lancet, 346, 1135–1138.

Biganzoli, E. and D. Boracchi, 2004, Old and new markers for breast cancer prognosis: the need for integrated research on quantitative issues. Eur. J. Cancer, 40, 1803–1806.

Biganzoli, E., P. Boracchi, L. Mariani and E. Marubini, 1998, Feed forward neural networks for the analysis of censored survival data: a partial logistic regression approach. Stat. Med., 17, 1169–1186.

Biganzoli, E., P. Boracchi and E. Marubini, 2002, A general framework for neural network models on censored survival data. Neural Netw., 15, 209–218.

Biganzoli, E., P. Boracchi, D. Coradini, M.G. Daidone and E. Marubini, 2003, Prognosis in node-negative primary breast cancer: a neural network analysis of risk profiles using routinely assessed factors. Ann. Oncol., 14, 1484–1493.

Biganzoli, E., N. Lama, F. Ambrogi, L. Antolini and P. Boracchi, 2005, Prediction of cancer outcome with microarrays (letter). The Lancet, 365, 1683.

Biganzoli, E., P. Boracchi, F. Ambrogi and E. Marubini, 2006, Artificial neural network for the joint modelling of discrete cause-specific hazards. Artif. Intell. Med., 37, 119–130.

Bishop, C.M., 1995, Neural networks for pattern recognition. Oxford University Press, New York.

Boracchi, P. and E. Biganzoli, 2002, Radial basis function neural networks for the analysis of survival data. Metron, 60, 191–210.

Boracchi, P., E. Biganzoli and E. Marubini, 2001, Modelling cause-specific hazards with radial basis function artificial neural networks: application to 2233 breast cancer patients. Stat. Med., 20, 3677–3694.

Cox, D.R., 1972, Regression models and life-tables (with discussion). J. Roy. Stat. Soc. Series B, 34, 187–220.

Efron, B., 1988, Logistic regression, survival analysis, and the Kaplan-Meier curve. J. Am. Stat. Assoc., 83, 414–425.

Fahrmeir, L., 1994, Dynamic modelling and penalized likelihood estimation for discrete time survival data. Biometrika, 81, 317–330.

Faraggi, D. and R. Simon, 1995, A neural network model for survival data. Stat. Med., 14, 73–82.

Elandt-Johnson, R.C. and N.L. Johnson, 1980, Survival Models and Data Analysis. John Wiley & Sons, New York.

Klein, J.P. and M.L. Moeschberger, 1997, Survival Analysis. Techniques for Censored and Truncated Data. Springer-Verlag, New York.

Kramar, A., M.H. Pejovic and D. Chassagne, 1987, A method of analysis taking into account competing events: application to the study of digestive complications following irradiation for cervical cancer. Stat. Med., 6, 785–794.

Larson, M.G., 1984, Covariate analysis of competing-risks data with log-linear models. Biometrics, 40, 459–468.

Liestol, K., P.K. Andersen and U. Andersen, 1994, Survival analysis and neural nets. Stat. Med., 13, 1189–1200.

Lisboa, P.J., 2002, A review of evidence of health benefit from artificial neural networks in medical intervention. Neural Netw., 15, 11–39.

Lisboa, P.J., H. Wong, P. Harris and R. Swindell, 2003, A Bayesian neural network approach for modelling censored data with an application to prognosis after surgery for breast cancer. Artif. intell. Med., 28, 1–25.

Mariani, L., D. Coradini, E. Biganzoli, P. Boracchi, E. Marubini, S. Pilotti, B. Salvadori, R. Silvestrini, U. Veronesi, R. Zucali and F. Rilke, 1997, Prognostic factors for metathronous contralateral breast cancer: a comparison of the linear Cox regression model and its artificial neural network extension. Breast Cancer Res. Treat., 44, 167–178.

Marubini, E. and M.G. Valseccbi, 1995, Analysing Survival Data from Clinical Trials and Observational Studies. John Wiley & Sons, Chichester.

McCullagh, P. and J.A. Nelder, 1989, Generalized Linear Models, 2nd ed. Chapman & Hall, London, UK.

Ripley, B.D. and R.M. Ripley, 1998, Neural networks as statistical methods in survival analysis. In: R. Dybowski and V. Cant (Eds.), Artificial Neural Networks: Prospects for Medicine. Cambridge University Press, Cambridge, UK, in press.

Schwarzer, G., W. Vach and M. Schumacher, 2000, On the misuses of artificial neural networks for prognostic and diagnostic classification in oncology. Stat. Med., 19, 541–561.

Venable, W.N. and B.D. Ripley, 1999, Modern Applied Statistics with S-Plus, 3rd ed. Springer-Verlag, New York.

Chapter 7

Information Geometry for Survival Analysis and Feature Selection by Neural Networks

Antonio Eleuteri[1,2], Roberto Tagliaferri[2,3], Leopoldo Milano[1,2] and Michele de Laurentiis[4]

[1]*Dipartimento di Scienze Fisiche, Università degli Studi di Napoli "Federico II", Italy*
[2]*NFN sez. Napoli, Italy*
[3]*DMI, Università degli Studi di Salerno, Italy*
[4]*Dipartimento di Endocrinologia ed Oncologia Molecolare e Clinica, Università degli Studi di Napoli "Federico II", Italy*

Abstract

In this chapter, an information geometric approach to survival analysis is described. It is shown how a neural network can be used to model the probability of failure of a system, and how it can be trained by minimizing a suitable divergence functional in a Bayesian framework. By using the trained network, minimization of the same divergence functional allows for fast, efficient and exact feature selection. Finally, the performance of the algorithms is illustrated on some datasets.

Keywords: Information geometry, feature selection, neural networks, Bayesian inference, survival analysis.

Contents

Outcome Prediction in Cancer
Edited by A.F.G. Taktak and A.C. Fisher
© 2007 Elsevier B.V. All rights reserved

1. INTRODUCTION

In the literature, we can find different modelling approaches to survival analysis. Conventional parametric models may involve overly strict assumptions on the distributions of failure times and on the form of the influence of the system features on the survival time, assumptions which usually simplify the experimental evidence, particularly in the case of medical data (Kalbfleisch and Prentice, 1980). In contrast, semi-parametric models do not make assumptions on the distributions of failures, but instead make assumptions on how the system features influence the survival time: furthermore, usually these models do not allow for direct estimation of survival times. Finally, non-parametric models allow only for a qualitative description of the data.

Neural networks (NNs) have been recently used for survival analysis with many reported successes but with some caution (Liestøl et al., 1994; Faraggi and Simon, 1995; Burke et al., 1997; de Laurentiis et al., 1999; Wong et al., 1999; Lisboa and Wong, 2001; Biganzoli et al., 2002; Eleuteri et al., 2003). One of the problems in many neural network approaches is that they do not take into account censoring, since the common modelling approaches by using Multilayer Perceptron networks only allow regression and classification problems. For a critical survey on the current use (and misuse) of neural networks we refer to Ripley and Ripley (1998) and Schwarzer et al. (2000).

A fundamental issue in survival analysis is feature selection. Often the phenomenon we are trying to model is very complex, and there is no prior knowledge which can be used to select the input variables which are relevant to modelling the survival function. Hence, the usual approach is to use all the available inputs, as is common in the analysis of cancer data. The inclusion of many variables, however, has many drawbacks: interpreting the model is difficult, irrelevant variables act as noise worsening the generalization capability of the model, data gathering can be much more costly and small data sets become less appealing because of the overhead of high dimensionality.

In this chapter, we describe a neural network architecture, a generalization of the model proposed in Eleuteri et al. (2003), which overcomes some of the limitations of currently available neural network models without making assumptions on the underlying survival distribution. This network belongs to a class of models aimed at conditional probability estimation (Eleuteri, 2003).

In this case, the network models the survival function and the density of failure of a system which is conditioned on descriptive variables. Furthermore, the model takes into account relevant censoring information explicitly.

The network is trained by using the information geometric concept of divergence (Amari, 2000). Training corresponds to minimization of the divergence function in a Bayesian framework (Robert, 2001). Use of Bayesian methods in survival analysis was first advocated by Raftery et al. (1994), since it helps taking into account model uncertainty and improves the predictive performance of a model. It is worth noting that the only neural network architectures aimed at survival analysis and trained in a Bayesian framework are described by Bakker and Heskes (1999), Neal (2001) and Eleuteri et al. (2003).

The common approach to feature selection is to use suboptimal search criteria, like forward and backward substitution (Fukunaga, 1990), coupled with retraining of the model. Instead, we again make use of information geometry, by using the *only* trained model, and by minimizing the same divergence functional used in training, but with a different optimization procedure, which can be coupled with an efficient and exact "branch and bound" (Fukunaga, 1990) search in feature space.

We apply the model to synthetic and real data, and show how it can outperform classical Cox analysis and naive neural network models.

2. SURVIVAL FUNCTIONS

Let $T(\mathbf{x})$ denote an absolutely continuous random variable (rv) describing the failure time of a system defined by a vector of features $\mathbf{x}$. If $fT\ (t|\mathbf{x})$ is the density of failure, then we can define the *survival function*:

$$S(t\,|\,\mathbf{x}) = P(T(\mathbf{x}) > t) = 1 - \int_0^t f_T(u\,|\,\mathbf{x})\mathrm{d}u \tag{1}$$

which is the probability that the failure occurs after time t.

In many studies (e.g. in medical statistics and in quality control), we do not observe realizations of the rv $T(\mathbf{x})$. Rather, this variable is associated with some other rv $Y \sim r$ such that the observation is a realization of the rv $Z = q(\mathrm{T}, Y)$, where $q(\ )$ is a function which depends on the kind of survival problem. In this case, we say that the observation of the time of the event is *censored*. If Y is independent from T, we say that censoring is *uninformative*. In this chapter, we consider survival problems with *right censoring*, where $q \equiv \min(.,.)$.

We can define the sampling density $p(t\,|\,y, \mathbf{x})$ of a survival process (assuming, e.g. right censoring) by noting that, if we observe an event ($y = 1$), it directly contributes to the evaluation of the sample density; if we do not observe the event ($y = 0$), the best contribution is to evaluate $P(T > Y)$ (i.e. $S(t|\mathbf{x})$).

We have then:

$$p(t\,|\,\mathbf{x}, y) = S(t\,|\,\mathbf{x})^{1-y} f_T(t\,|\,\mathbf{x})^y \tag{2}$$

The joint sample density for a set of independent observations $D = \{(t_k, \mathbf{x}_k, y_k)\}$ can then be written as:

$$L = \prod_k p(t_k | y_k, \mathbf{x}_k). \tag{3}$$

Since the censoring is supposed to be uninformative, it does not influence inference on the failure density, but gives contribution to the sample density.

3. STANDARD MODELS FOR SURVIVAL ANALYSIS

In the next section, some of the most commonly used models are described, for both homogeneous (time-only) and heterogeneous modelling.

3.1. The Kaplan–Meier non-parametric estimator

The Kaplan–Meier (KM) estimator is a non-parametric maximum likelihood estimator of the survival function (Kalbfleisch and Prentice, 1980). It is piecewise constant, and can be thought of as an empirical survival function for censored data. It is only homogeneous.

Let k be the number of events in the sample, $t_1, t_2, \ldots, t_k$ the event times (supposed to be unique and ordered), e_i the number of events at time t_i and r_i the number of times (events or censoring) greater than or equal to t_i. The estimator is given by the formula:

$$S_{\mathrm{KM}}(t) = \prod_{i:t_i<t} \frac{r_i - e_i}{r_i}. \tag{4}$$

It should be noted that the estimator is noisy when the data are few, in particular when the events are rare, since it is a piecewise constant. Despite its restrictions, this is the most widely used tool for analysing survival data, because its estimation is very fast and it allows qualitative inference on the data. In the following section, we use it to assess the performance of our model.

3.2. Proportional hazards model

The most used survival specification which takes into account system features is to allow the hazard function to have the form:

$$\lambda(t|\mathbf{x}) = \lambda(t)\exp(\theta^{\mathrm{T}}\mathbf{x}), \tag{5}$$

where $\lambda(t)$ is some homogeneous hazard function (called the *baseline hazard*) and θ are the feature-dependent parameters of the model. This is called a *proportional hazards* (PH) model. The two most used approaches for this kind of model are:

- Choose a parameterized functional form for the baseline hazard, then use Maximum Likelihood (ML) techniques to find values for the parameters of the model; and
- Do not fix the baseline hazard, but make an ML estimation of the feature-dependent part of the model, and a non-parametric estimation of the baseline hazard. This is called Cox's model (Kalbfleisch and Prentice, 1980).

Also, neural network models have been applied to estimate the feature-dependent part of the model: however, the main drawback remains, which is the assumption of proportionality between the time-dependent and feature-dependent parts of the model.

4. THE NEURAL NETWORK MODEL

In this section, we define a neural network which, given a data set of system features and times, provides a model for the survival function (and implicitly, by suitable transforms, of the other functions of interest).

Let us consider a parameterized function of the form:

$$P(t \mid \mathbf{x},\theta) = s(a(\theta)), \tag{6}$$

where:

$$\theta = (\mathbf{v}, c, \tau, \mathbf{d}, (\mathbf{w}_i), \mathbf{b}, \mathbf{u}), \quad a_i = \mathbf{w}_i \cdot \mathbf{x} + b_i + u_i t$$

$$a = \sum_i^H v_i g(a_i) + c + \tau h(t) + \mathbf{d} \cdot \mathbf{x}$$

and s and g are logistic sigmoids. Equation (6) defines a fully connected, one-hidden-layer network with parameter vector θ. We call the resulting model the Conditional Probability Estimating Neural Network (CPENN).

It should be noted that both the time t and the vector $\mathbf{x}$ are presented as inputs to the network. We call these *predictive input* and *conditioning input*, respectively. We call the unit whose activation is the h function a *predictive hidden unit*. The following two propositions, as proven in Eleuteri (2003), characterize the CPENN model:

Proposition 4.1.
Sufficient conditions for the CPENN model to define the conditional Cumulative Distribution Function (CDF) of failure are:

(1) $h(t) \equiv \log t$

(2) $v_i \geq 0, u_i \geq 0, \tau \geq 0 \, \forall i \in \{1, \ldots, H\}$

Proposition 4.2.
The CPENN model can predict a nonlinear process in the deterministic limit.

A theorem (Hornik et al., 1990) ensures that a network which enjoys the universal approximation capability can approximate both a function and its derivatives of any order. By applying this theorem to the CPENN model, we find that it is a universal approximator for conditional cdfs of failure and for the corresponding densities.

5. LEARNING IN THE CPENN MODEL

As shown, the CPENN model output defines a conditional cdf. This implies that we do not have targets which we can use for learning. In fact, the CPENN model uses the targets (seen as realizations of the random variable of which we want to model the distribution law) as inputs. So, how can we solve the problem?

Since the CPENN family of densities defines a manifold (Eleuteri, 2003), we can use the information geometric concept of divergence (Amari, 2000) to derive a cost functional suitable for learning. There are other theoretical reasons to defend the use of the divergence: these range from decision theory and information theory, to the relevance of the logarithmic score rule and to the location-scale invariance of the distance (Robert, 2001).

Let $p^*(t, x, y)$ be the sampling density of a survival process, and $p(t, x, y|\theta)$ a parametric density. The divergence is:

$$\mathrm{D}(p^* \| p) = \iint p^* \log \frac{p^*}{p} \mathrm{d}x \, \mathrm{d}t \, \mathrm{d}y \geq 0. \tag{7}$$

It can be shown by a simple application of Jensen's inequality that the functional D has zero minimum if and only if the two densities are equal. We can factorize the two densities as:

$$\begin{aligned} p^*(t,x,y) &= p^*(t \mid x,y) p^*(x,y) \\ p(t,x,y \mid \theta) &= p(t \mid x,y,\theta) p^*(x,y), \end{aligned} \tag{8}$$

where the last step follows from the fact that we use the parameters to only model the conditional density by the CPENN model, since $p(x, y)$ is not modelled by the network. It can then be shown (Eleuteri, 2003) that we can find the density which minimizes the divergence by minimizing the following function of the parameter vector θ (a Monte Carlo estimator of Eq. (7):

$$E_N(\theta) = -\frac{1}{N} \sum_i^N \log p(t_i \mid x_i, y_i, \theta), \tag{9}$$

where $p(t_i|x_i, y_i, \theta) = S(t_i|\mathbf{x}_i, \theta)^{1-yi} f_T (t_i|\mathbf{x}_i, \theta)^{yi}$ and f_T (and S) are modelled by the CPENN model. We can also derive the likelihood function of the data as $L(\theta) = -NE_N(\theta)$ + constant.

6. THE BAYESIAN APPROACH TO MODELLING

In the conventional maximum-likelihood approach to training, a single weight vector is found which minimizes an error function: in contrast, the Bayesian scheme considers a probability distribution over the parameters. We build a *Hierarchical Bayes model*, which is comprised of a parametric statistical model (the likelihood), a parameterized prior distribution over the parameters and a *hyperprior* over the *hyperparameters*.

The learning process in this case is described by a prior distribution $p(\theta|\alpha)$ which is modified when we observe the data D through the likelihood $p(D|\theta)$. This process can be expressed by Bayes' theorem:

$$p(\theta, \alpha \mid D) = \frac{p(D \mid \theta) p(\theta \mid \alpha) p(\alpha)}{\int p(D \mid \theta) p(\theta \mid \alpha) p(\alpha) \mathrm{d}\theta \mathrm{d}\alpha}. \tag{10}$$

The prior over parameters should reflect any knowledge we have about the mapping we want to build. For the CPENN model, we must then take into account the fact that we want a smooth mapping and that we have both constrained and unconstrained parameters: furthermore, we should take into account the specialized role the parameters have in the network depending on their position.

For the unconstrained parameters we can choose a Gaussian prior:

$$p(\theta_u \mid \alpha_u) \propto \sum_{k \in \mathcal{G}u} \frac{\alpha_k}{2} \sum_{i_k=1}^{W_k} \theta_{i_k}^2 \tag{11}$$

where θ_u is the vector of unconstrained parameters, $\mathcal{G}_u$ is the set of the unconstrained parameter groups, W_k is the cardinality of the kth group and α_u is the vector of hyperparameters (inverse variances) whose components are the α_k coefficients.

For the constrained parameters we choose a *stable* (Feller, 1971) Lévy density:

$$p(\theta_c \mid \alpha_c) \propto \exp\left(\sum_{k \in G_c} \sum_{i_k=1}^{W_k} \left(\frac{3}{2} \log \theta_{i_k} + \frac{\alpha_k}{2\theta_{i_k}} \right) \right) \mathbb{I}(\theta_c), \tag{12}$$

where θ_c is the vector of constrained parameters, G_c is the set of the constrained parameter groups, W_k is the cardinality of the kth group, α_c is the vector of hyperparameters (scale factors) and $\mathbb{I}(.)$ is the set indicator function.

It can be shown that an appropriate noninformative hyperprior over the hyperparameters is the so-called *improper* density (Robert, 2001), $p(\alpha) \sim 1/\alpha$, and that this choice does not lead to marginalization paradoxes (Eleuteri, 2003).

6.1. Gibbs sampling

Given the posterior and the data, we are interested in sampling *predictive densities* for a test pattern:

$$P(t_{N+1} \mid x_{N+1}, D) = \int P(t_{N+1} \mid x_{N+1}, \theta) p(\theta, \alpha \mid D) \mathrm{d}\theta \mathrm{d}\alpha \tag{13}$$

This can be seen as an evaluation of the expectation of the network function with respect to the posterior distribution of the network parameters. In our case the integral cannot be solved analytically, so we must approximate the integral with the following Monte Carlo estimator (using M samples from the posterior):

$$P(t_{N+1} \mid x_{N+1}, D) \approx \frac{1}{M} \sum_{i=1}^{M} P(t_{N+1} \mid x_{N+1}, \theta_i) \tag{14}$$

which is guaranteed to converge by the Ergodic Theorem to the true value of the integral, as M goes to infinity (Robert and Casella, 1999), provided the samples form a Markov chain which, assuming ergodicity, converges to the posterior.

Although we are interested in evaluating the parameters $\{\theta_i\}$ to estimate Eq. (14), we must also generate samples of hyperparameters $\{\alpha_j\}$. Sampling from the full posterior follows an iterative process known as *Gibbs sampling*:

- Sample the distribution $p(\theta|\hat{\alpha}, D)$ by using the *slice sampling* algorithm (Neal, 2000); and
- Sample the distribution $p(\alpha|\hat{\theta}, D) \sim p(\hat{\theta}|\alpha)\, p(\alpha)$. This last step can be efficiently done in our case, since it can be shown that $p(\alpha|\hat{\theta},D)$ is a gamma density (Eleuteri, 2003).

7. VARIABLE SELECTION

Given a set of observations D, and a model of these observations $M(\theta|D)$, the goal is to reduce the dimension of the conditioning input vector $\mathbf{x}$ while preserving as much as possible the prediction capability of the model. Correspondingly, we obtain a new model $M(\xi|D)$. We would like the new model to be as "near" as possible to the starting one.

Removal of a set of inputs $\{x_k\}$ is equivalent to fixing the respective input nodes at zero. If we view the parameters as coordinates of some space, then from a geometric viewpoint, setting them to zero can be seen as a projection of the original space onto a lower dimensional space. To make this projection, however, we must take into account the nature of the space and its geometric structure, and some kind of distance must be defined.

The neural network which models the data is deterministic: however, it may be convenient to consider a stochastic extension of the network, such that the output of the deterministic network is the expectation of the stochastic one.

In the case of the CPENN network, we can build a simple (virtual) Bernoulli noise model by taking into account that the output is a probability. We can denote by y and $\mathbf{x}$ the output noise and the input (both conditioning and predictive), respectively.

We can consider the joint distribution of model and data, and evaluate the divergence from the starting model $p(\mathbf{x}, y|\theta)$ to a reduced model $p(\mathbf{x}, y|\xi)$, in analogy with Eq. (7):

$$\begin{aligned} D(p \| q) &= \mathrm{E}_x\left[D(p(y \mid \mathbf{x}, \theta)p(\mathbf{x}) \| p(y \mid \mathbf{x}, \xi)p(\mathbf{x}))\right] \\ &= \mathrm{E}_x\left[D(p(y \mid \mathbf{x}, \theta) \| p(y \mid \mathbf{x}, \xi))\right]. \end{aligned} \tag{15}$$

The parameters of the projected density can be found by minimizing the above function. However, the solution may be hard to find and there is no guarantee that it is unique; furthermore, there are also constraints on the parameter space.

In a Bayesian framework, we can calculate the divergence by evaluating the posterior expectation of Eq. (15) with respect to the posterior distribution of network parameters by a Monte Carlo approximation using a sample of parameters from the posterior. For each parameter vector, we can then solve a minimization problem to find the corresponding projected parameter vector.

In the next section, we show how to find a solution to this problem in an efficient way.

8. THE LAYERED PROJECTION ALGORITHM

Let us consider a further stochastic extension, in which each hidden unit activation has a noise model whose probability (density) is $p(z_i|\mathbf{x}, \zeta_i^{(1)})$, where $\zeta_i^{(1)}$ is the vector of first layer parameters feeding the ith unit. Given a noise model on the outputs, $p(y|\mathbf{z}, \zeta_i^{(2)})$, where $\zeta_i^{(2)}$ is the vector of second layer parameters, we can then define the joint model of output and hidden activations $g(\cdot)$, where the noise models for the hidden units are assumed independent:

$$\begin{aligned} p(y,\{z_i\}\,|\,\mathbf{x},\boldsymbol{\zeta}^{(1)},\boldsymbol{\zeta}^{(2)}) &= p(y\,|\,\{z_i\}\,|\,\boldsymbol{\zeta}^{(2)})\prod_i^H p(z_i\,|\,\mathbf{x},\boldsymbol{\zeta}_i^{(1)}) \\ &= p(y\,|\,\mathbf{z},\boldsymbol{\zeta}^{(2)})p(\mathbf{z}\,|\,\mathbf{x},\boldsymbol{\zeta}^{(1)}). \end{aligned} \tag{16}$$

This factorization is possible due to the information flow in the MLP, in fact the output depends on the first layer parameters through the hidden activations, which do not depend on the second layer parameters.

Exact evaluation of the expectations w.r.t. $\mathbf{x}$ is not possible, since the input density cannot be assumed to be known. Furthermore, we work with a finite data set. It is therefore necessary to use a finite-sample approximation (Robert and Casella, 1999), so that the divergence can be written in the form:

$$\begin{aligned} D_N &= \frac{1}{N}\sum_k^N \int p(\mathbf{z}\,|\,\mathbf{x}_k,\theta^{(1)})\log\frac{p(\mathbf{z}\,|\,\mathbf{x}_k,\theta^{(1)})}{p(\mathbf{z}\,|\,\mathbf{x}_k,\xi^{(1)})}d\mathbf{z} \\ &+ \frac{1}{N}\sum_k^N \int p(y\,|\,\mathbf{z}_k,\theta^{(2)})\log\frac{p(y\,|\,\mathbf{z}_k,\theta^{(2)})}{p(y\,|\,\mathbf{z}_k,\xi^{(2)})}dy \\ &= D_N^1 + D_N^2. \end{aligned} \tag{17}$$

It should be noted that, if the variables we integrate over are not continuous, then the integrals become sums (this happens if the models are described in terms of probability distributions instead of densities).

The structure of Eq. (17) reflects the layered structure of the CPENN model, and the chain of dependencies between parameters and activations implied by Eq. (16) suggests that the two terms can be minimized in sequence (Eleuteri, 2003):

(1) Minimize the first term, with respect to $\theta^{(1)}$, using information from:

- inputs,
- first layer weights of the starting network, and
- hidden activations of the starting network;

(2) Minimize the second term, with respect to $\theta^{(2)}$, using information from:

- projected first layer weights $\theta^{(1)}$,
- hidden activations evaluated using projected $\theta^{(1)}$,
- second layer weights of the starting network, and
- output activation of the starting network.

In practice, the first stage "prunes" the weights corresponding to some removed inputs. The second stage is then used to adapt the second layer weights so that their values reflect the new overall input–output mapping induced by the removal of some first layer weights, and the modification of others. It is worth noting that the second layer weights cannot remain unaltered, since their values were originally adapted to a different network structure with a greater number of inputs. We have thus obtained the following result:

Proposition 8.1.
Divergence projection for variable selection in CPENN models only requires solving a sequence of single-layer minimization problems.

We call the resulting algorithm *Layered Projection*.

8.1. Hidden noise model

If, without loss of generality for the approximation capabilities of the model, we assume that the hidden activation functions are logistic sigmoids, then a simple noise model is given by a Bernoulli distribution for each hidden activation. In this case, since each hidden unit activation can be seen as a probability, the resulting activation model is:

$$p(z_i \mid \mathbf{x}, \zeta_i^{(1)}) = g(\zeta_i^{(1)} \cdot \mathbf{x})^{z_i} (1 - g(\zeta_i^{(1)} \cdot \mathbf{x}))^{1-z_i}. \tag{18}$$

Note that the hidden activation of the deterministic CPENN is just the expectation of the activation of the stochastic CPENN. This choice of noise model is not restrictive, since we just create a stochastic model of a deterministic network.

The activation for each hidden unit can be put in an exponential family form:

$$p(r_i \mid \omega(\mathbf{x}, \zeta_i^{(1)})) = \exp\left(\omega(\mathbf{x}, \zeta_i^{(1)}) r_i - \psi(\omega(\mathbf{x}, \zeta_1^{(1)}))\right), \tag{19}$$

where $\omega(f) = \log(f/(1 - f))$, $\psi = \log(1 + \exp(\omega))$, $r = \delta(z - 1)$. For a set of N independent observations, the activation is still an exponential family of larger dimension:

$$\begin{aligned} p(\{z_{i,k}\}_k \mid \{\mathbf{x}_k\}, \zeta_i^{(1)}) &= \prod_{k=1}^{N} p(r_{i,k} \mid \omega(\mathbf{x}_k, \zeta_i^{(1)})) \\ &= \exp(\boldsymbol{\omega}^*_{i,N} \cdot \mathbf{r}^*_{i,N} - \psi_N), \end{aligned} \tag{20}$$

where

$$\begin{aligned} \mathbf{r}^*_{i,N} &= (r_{i,1}, \ldots, r_{i,N}), \quad \psi_N = \sum_k \psi(\omega(\mathbf{x}_k, \zeta_i^{(1)})) \\ \boldsymbol{\omega}^*_{i,N} &= (\omega(\mathbf{x}_1, \zeta_i^{(1)}), \ldots, \omega(\mathbf{x}_N, \zeta_i^{(1)})). \end{aligned} \tag{21}$$

If we denote by $S_{i,k} = \{p(r_{i,k} \mid \omega(\mathbf{x}_k, \zeta_i^{(1)}))\}$ the manifold of distributions corresponding to the kth pattern, then the joint distribution of Eq. (20) is an element of the product manifold $S^*_{i,N} = S_{i,1} \times S_{i,2} \times \cdots \times S_{i,N}$.

Since $\omega^*_{i,N}$ is a function of $\zeta_i^{(1)}$, it cannot take arbitrary values, and is therefore restricted to a region of $S^*_{i,N}$. This region is called a *curved exponential family* (Amari, 2000) in $S^*_{i,N}$, with inner coordinate system $\zeta_i^{(1)}$.

8.2. Properties of the projections

The dualistic structure of the manifold induces a divergence which is equal to the Kullback divergence. This fact gives a justification for the use of the Kullback divergence as a distance between models (Amari, 2000; Eleuteri, 2003).

The projection corresponds to a maximum likelihood estimation of the coordinates of the projected sub-manifold, which can be carried out by solving a sequence of likelihood equations $\nabla \xi_i (k) D_N^k = 0$ for each layer k. These can be seen as the maximum likelihood equations for a Generalised Linear Model (GLM) with logistic canonical link (McCullagh and Nelder, 1989), to which the Iteratively Reweighted Least Squares (IRLS) algorithm (McCullagh and Nelder, 1989) can be applied to solve the problem in a very fast and efficient way.

The dualistic structure of the manifold also ensures that the divergence has two properties: transitivity and additivity. These two properties are fundamental, because they ensure that the order in which we select the variables is not relevant, and that embedded models are always at a greater "distance" from the starting model than embedding models. These properties ensure the monotonicity of the divergence, which implies that fast, exact search algorithms (e.g. "branch and bound" (Fukunaga, 1990)) can be applied without having to explore the full feature space.

This implies that the complexity of our algorithm strongly depends on the computational complexity of the adopted search algorithm. For optimal search methods, in which we are interested, the effective complexity for a given problem instance cannot be predicted in advance, since it depends on how "relevant" the inputs are to the problem at hand (and we are searching for precisely this information!) However, some optimal search methods can be more efficient than others. In the sample applications in the chapter, we used the "improved branch and bound" algorithm (Fukunaga, 1990) just for the sake of simplicity, but it should be noted that it surely is not the most efficient to date (Yu and Yuan, 1993, Kittler et al., 2004).

9. A SEARCH STRATEGY

The divergence evaluated from the projection operation is used as a criterion in a "branch and bound" search of the input space. This is possible because of the additivity, transitivity and monotonicity properties of the Layered Projection criterion.

For a complete exploration, the search is repeated for each possible reduced dimension of the input space (i.e. for n inputs, the search is run $n-1$ times). The kth search gives the network with k inputs, nearest to the starting one. It should be noted that each search is independent of the others, which opens the possibility of an efficient parallel implementation. Furthermore, we are not forced to search for all possible dimensions: we are interested in selecting a restricted number of inputs.

After the search, we have to rank the different alternatives, since we want the network which best describes our data, but with the smallest input dimension. In fact it should be noted that the distance from the starting model is not related to the "prediction quality" of the projected models (some inputs could be acting as noise, worsening the prediction capability of the network), so the model "nearest" to the starting one is not necessarily the one with the best prediction capabilities. As shown in Fig. 1, a projected model which is near the starting one can be far from the true density, and conversely, a projected model which is far from the starting one can be near the true density.

To solve the problem, we evaluate the posterior model probabilities by Bayes' Theorem (Robert, 2001), and retain the models with the highest posterior probabilities:

$$P(M_i \mid D) = \frac{p(D \mid M_i)P(M_i)}{\sum_{j \in \Xi} p(D \mid M_j)P(M_j)} = \frac{p(M_i)\int_{\chi_i} p_i(D \mid \chi_i)p_i(\chi_i)\mathrm{d}\chi_i}{\sum_{j \in \Xi} P(M_j)\int_{\chi_i} p_j(D \mid \chi_j)p_j(\chi_j)\mathrm{d}\chi_j}, \tag{22}$$

where D is the data, Ξ is the set of model indicators (we also consider the "full" model for reference), M_i is the model under evaluation, and the integrals are the normalization constants (also termed *marginal likelihoods*) of the posterior distributions on the model parameters.

To evaluate the posterior in Eq. (22), we need to assign a prior probability to each model. A possible prior which embodies our prior lack of preference for any model is the discrete uniform distribution $P(M_i) = 1/K$, where K is the cardinality of Ξ (for a complete

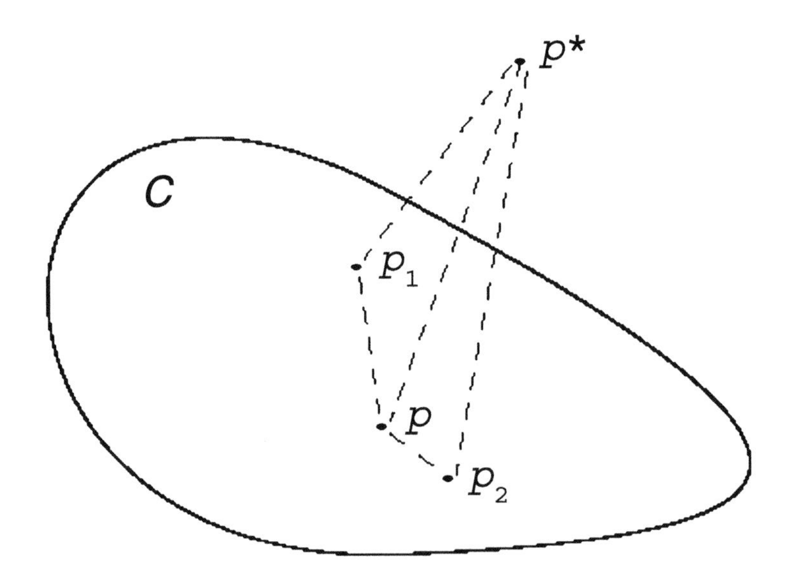

Fig. 1. Distances between the starting CPENN model density p and two model projections p_1 (with one residual input) and p_2 (with two residual inputs) in a CPENN manifold C. Their distances from p are due to the monotonicity property of the projection criterion. The true survival process density is p. The distances have been traced as line segments for illustration purposes only. In general, the metric is not Euclidean, so the distances must be considered as evaluated on geodesics.

search, $K = n$). With this choice, models can be ranked simply by evaluation of the marginal likelihoods.

It then follows that, to select a model, we must simply *look for the network with the least number of variables and lowest posterior error on the data D.* We note that, since to each posterior error evaluation we can assign some credibility intervals, we may obtain solutions which are within the bounds of each other, and therefore are statistically equivalent.

Finally, it should be noted that the use of the Bayesian framework to train the networks is fundamental, since otherwise such a selection procedure could always result in the choice of the most complex models due to overfitting.

9.1. Evaluation of the marginal likelihoods

We may use a set of samples $\{\theta_1, \dots, \theta_M\}$ from the posterior $p(\theta|D)$ (which we obtained during the training phase) to get a Monte Carlo approximation of the negative logarithm of marginal likelihood (posterior marginal error) (Eleuteri, 2003):

$$E(D) \equiv -\log p(D) = \log \sum_{k}^{M} \frac{1}{p(D \mid \theta_k)} - \log M \tag{23}$$

This estimator is consistent but may have infinite variance (Robert and Casella, 1999; Robert, 2001), which appears as very large jumps in the cumulative estimate of the harmonic mean. While we cannot formally verify that CPENN model likelihoods give rise to this kind of behaviour, we have experimentally seen that the cumulative harmonic mean does not show jumps, so the estimates of the marginal likelihood seem to be stable.

Our selection criterion will then be to choose models with the least number of variables and lowest posterior error.

10. EXPERIMENTS

In this section, we show the performance of the CPENN model on two data sets, a synthetic heterogeneous problem and a real heterogeneous medical problem.

All the software for the simulations has been written by the authors in the Matlab® (Mathworks Inc.) language. In each experiment two models were fitted: a Cox PH model and a CPENN model with 20 hidden units. KM estimates were then evaluated for each model.

The Cox PH model was trained using standard ML estimation while the CPENN model was trained with the MCMC slice sampling algorithm with Gibbs sampling of the hyperparameters. The first 400 samples were omitted from the chain. Then, 700 samples were generated by alternating between normal and over relaxed steps. Finally, the last 100 samples were used to obtain the Monte Carlo estimator of the CPENN output, based on an inspection of the energies of the chain. Note that in a real use of the algorithm, a simple inspection of the energies might not be sufficient to assess convergence; instead, a formal test of convergence, like the *Estimated Potential Scale Reduction* diagnostic (Robert and Casella, 1999) should be used.

10.1. Synthetic heterogeneous data

In this section, we show the performance of the CPENN model and the Layered Projection algorithm on a synthetic heterogeneous problem. We considered a mixture of Weibull and gamma densities with parameters dependent on the variables x_1, x_2:

$$\begin{aligned} f_T(t \mid \mathbf{x}) = x_2 \mathcal{W}e(x_1^2, \sin(x_1)^3 + 2) \\ + (1 - x_2)\mathcal{G}a((x_1 + 1)^2, \exp(\cos(x_1) + 2)) \end{aligned} \tag{24}$$

The covariates x_1 and x_2 were first sampled from a bivariate Gaussian with mean vector $(0, 0)$ and full covariance matrix such that the correlation coefficient of the variables was –0.71. Next, the variable x_2 was transformed to a binary indicator: values greater than or equal to 0 were set to 1, values less than 0 were set to 0. After the transformation the correlation coefficient was –0.57. Then, 2000 samples were generated from the mixture,

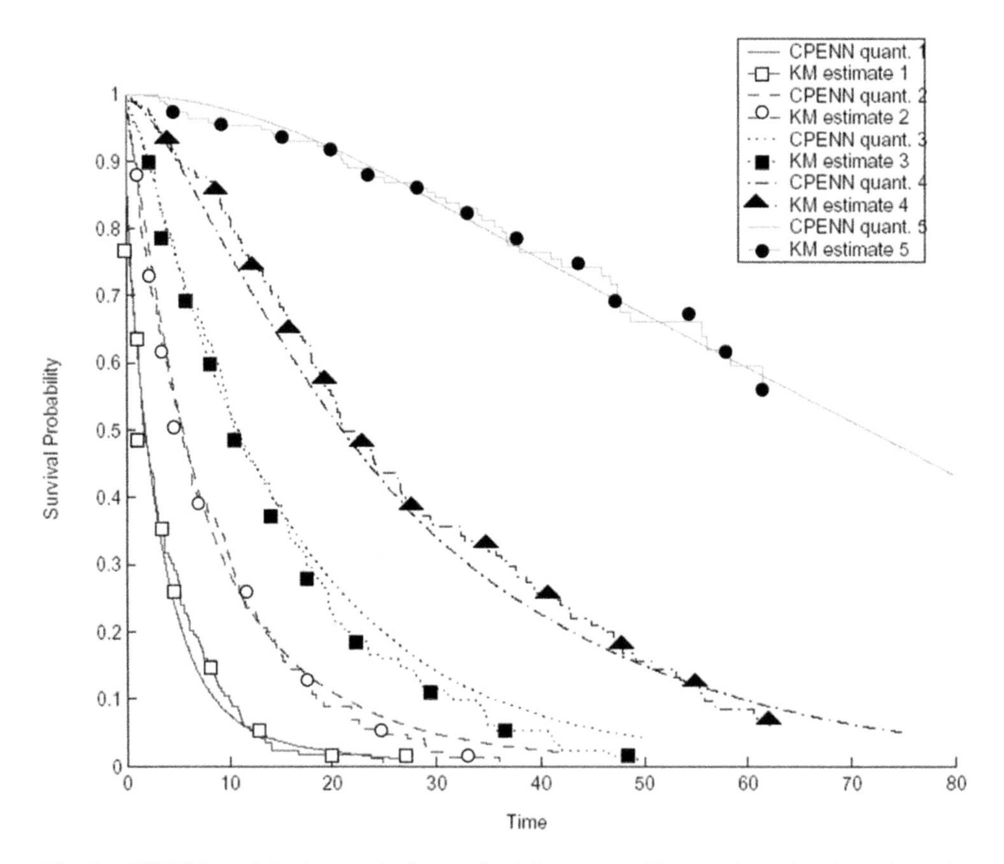

Fig. 2. CPENN model of a synthetic survival function with covariates (evaluated on the test set).

with about 30% uniformly right censored data in the interval [0, 70]. The data were then uniformly split into two disjoint data sets: a training set of 1000 samples and a testing set of 1000 samples (with the same proportion of censored data in each set). Two irrelevant features were added to the training data set; $x_3 \sim N(0, 1)$, $x_4 = 3(x_3 - 1)$. This data set was built to test the CPENN model in the case in which the proportional hazards assumption is not verified.

To get an intuitive understanding of how well the CPENN model is capturing the behaviour of the censored data, we made a comparison with KM estimates. The test data was stratified into 3 quantiles based on the survival estimates of the models at $t = 7.4$ (median time). Then, the mean (with respect to the covariates) survival probabilities were estimated, together with KM estimates of the quantiles induced by the models. If a model is able to capture the distribution of the data we expect the output of the model and KM estimates to be similar. As shown in Fig. 2, the CPENN model shows good performance on all quantiles despite the presence of irrelevant input features, while the Cox PH model in Fig. 3, as was to be expected, shows good performance only on bad prognosis quantiles.

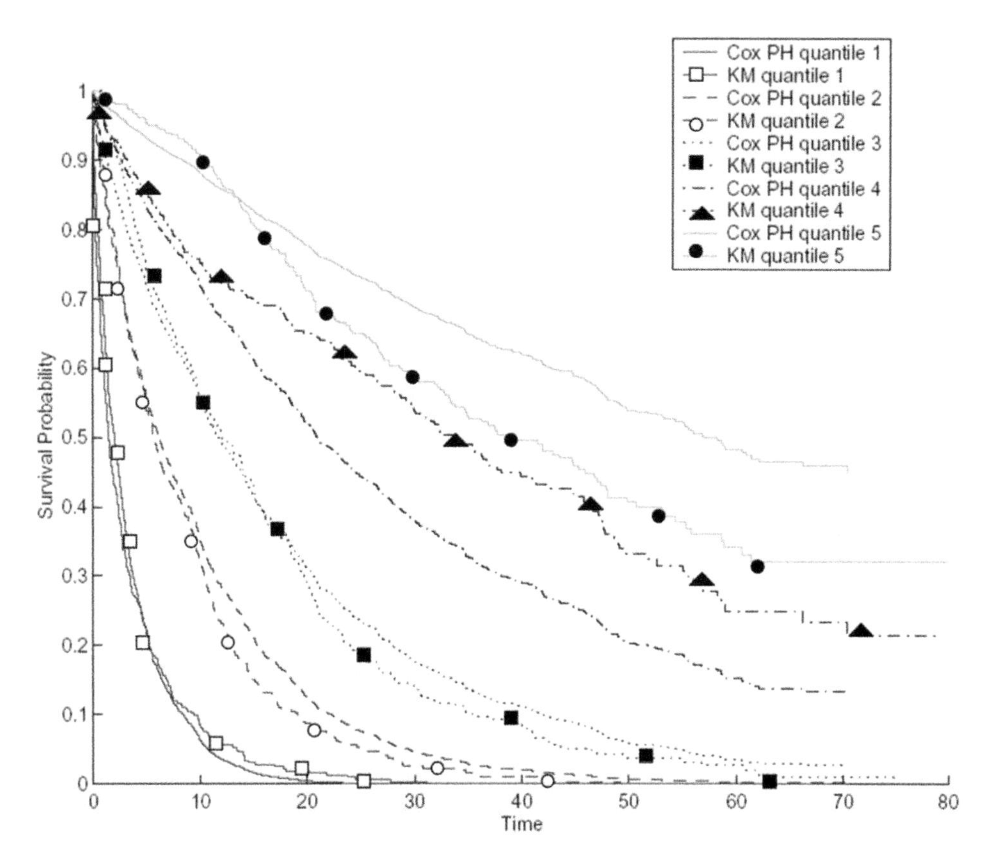

Fig. 3. Cox PH model of a synthetic survival function with covariates (evaluated on the test set).

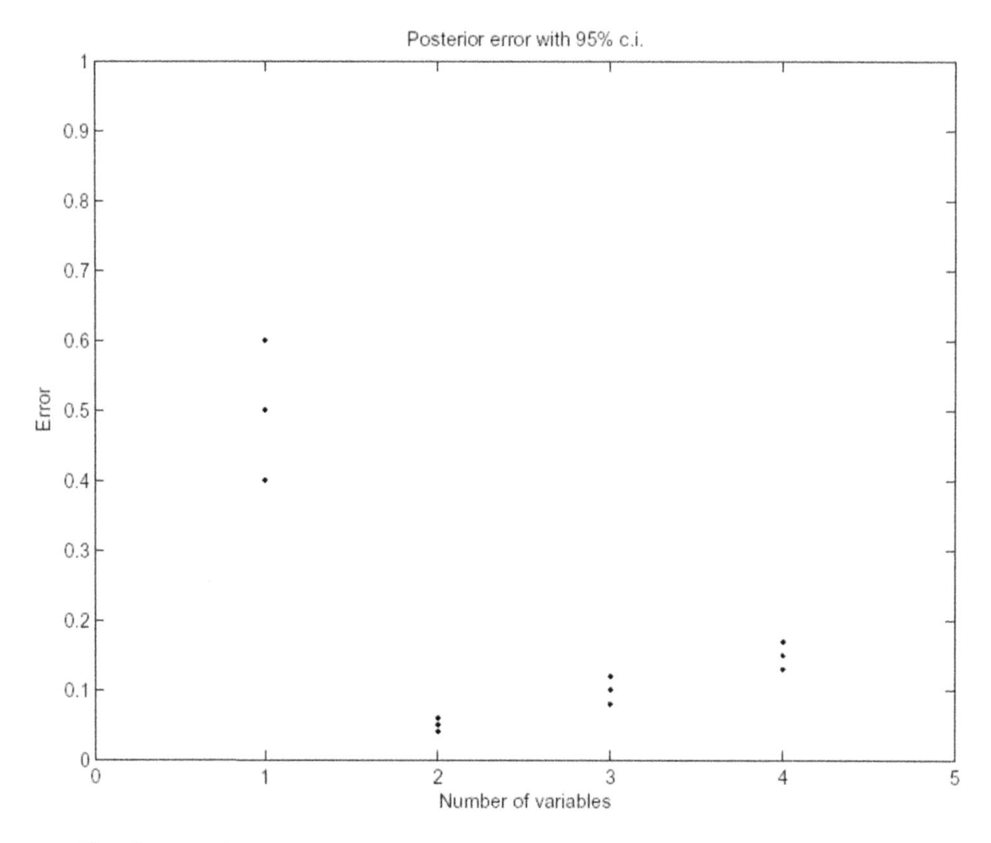

Fig. 4. Posterior error with 95% credibility intervals versus number of variables.

In Fig. 4, it can be seen that the CPENN model with two variables has the lowest posterior error, so we should choose it. The two variables selected by the algorithm are x_1 and x_2, the correct ones.

10.2. Real heterogeneous data

These data are taken from the trials of chemotherapy for stage B/C colon cancer (http://www.r-project.org). It comprises of 1776 samples, with 12 covariates. The data set was split into a training set of 1076 samples, and a test set of 700 samples. About 49% of the data are censored, which makes the analysis of the data a complex task.

The test data were stratified in three quantiles based on the survival estimates of the models at $t = 217$ weeks. Then, the mean (with respect to the covariates) survival probabilities were estimated, together with KM estimates of the quantiles induced by the models. If the model can capture the distribution of the data we expect the output of the model and KM estimates to be similar.

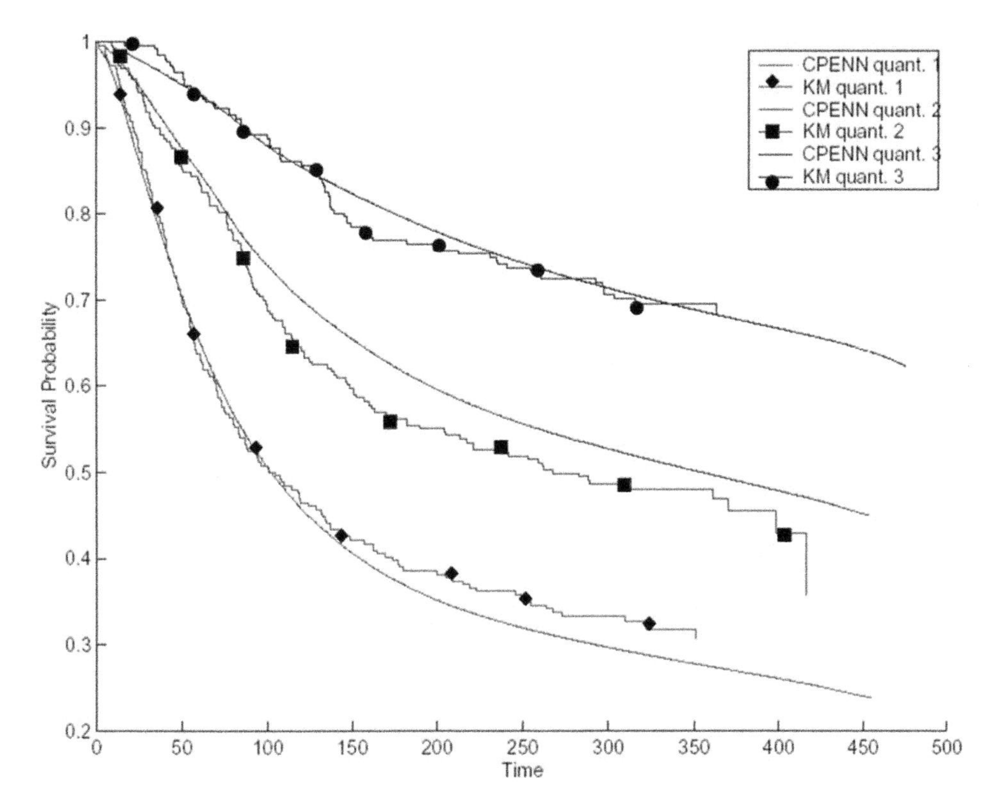

Fig. 5. CPENN model of a real survival function with covariates (evaluated on the test set).

As shown in Figs. 5 and 6, both the CPENN and Cox PH models exhibit good discriminatory powers, even if the Cox estimate is noisy, since it is a piecewise constant. This test shows that the CPENN model is able to work with real-world data for which the proportional hazards assumption is roughly verified.

11. CONCLUSION

In this chapter, we have described a novel approach to survival analysis. A neural network architecture is defined and trained according to information geometric principles. These same concepts are applied to exploit the geometric structure of the network and an algorithm is formulated which efficiently solves the feature selection problem.

The proposed approach does not make any assumption on the form of the survival process, and does not use discretizations or piecewise approximations as other neural network approaches to survival analysis do. Furthermore, the feature selection step makes full use of the information obtained in the training phase, and does not need retraining of the network,

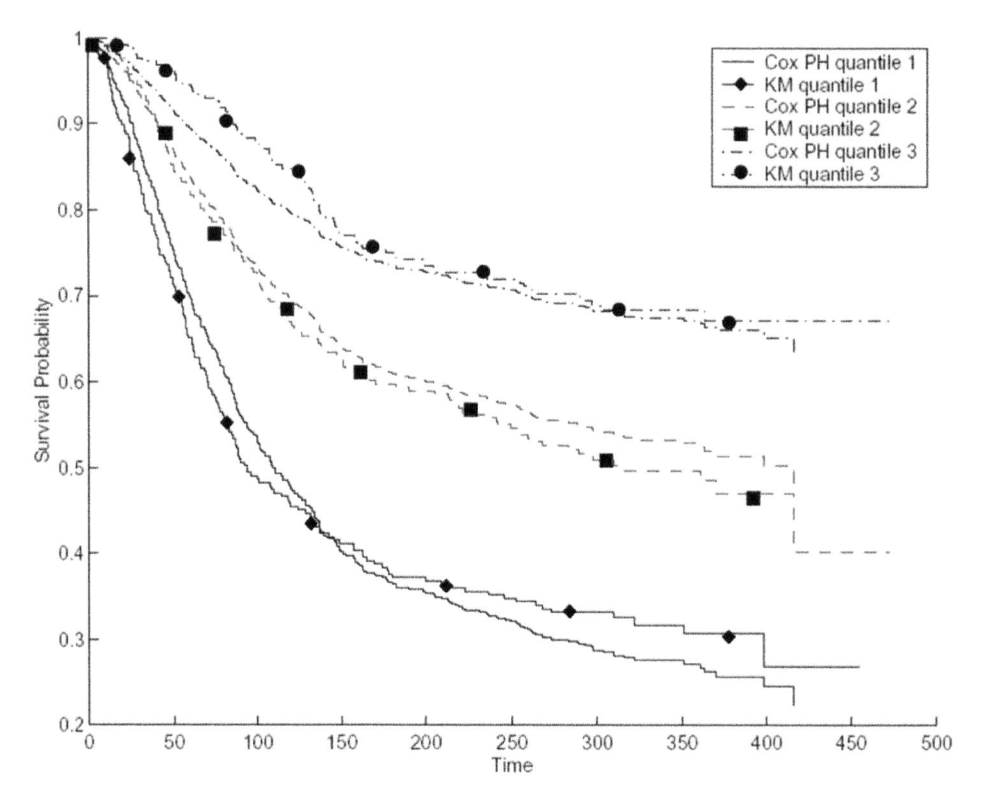

Fig. 6. Cox PH model of a real survival function with covariates (evaluated on the test set).

nor the full exploration of the feature space. Instead, the monotonicity of the proposed selection criterion allows for a fast and "clever" exploration of the input space.

Sample experiments on synthetic and real survival data show that the CPENN model can approximate complex survival functions: these approximations closely follow the time evolution of the KM nonparametric estimator.

Furthermore, we have shown how the Layered Projection algorithm is able to identify the relevant features in a problem.

REFERENCES

Amari, S., 2000, Methods of Information Geometry. Translations of Mathematical Monographs 191, Oxford University Press, Oxford.

Bakker, B. and T. Heskes, 1999, A neural-Bayesian approach to survival analysis. Proceedings ICANN '99, pp. 832–837.

Biganzoli, E., P. Boracchi and E. Marubini, 2002, A general framework for neural network models on censored survival data. Neural Netw., 15, 209–218.

Bishop, C.M., 1996, Neural Networks for Pattern Recognition. Clarendon Press, Oxford.

Burke, H.B., P.H. Goodman, D.B. Rosen, D.E. Henson, J.N. Weinstein, F.E. Harrell, J.R. Marks, D.P. Winchester and D.G. Bostwick, 1997, Artificial neural networks improve the accuracy of cancer survival prediction. Cancer, 79(4), 857–862.

de Laurentiis, M., S. de Placido, A.R. Bianco, G.M. Clark and P.M. Ravdin, 1999, A prognostic model that makes quantitative estimates of probability of relapse for breast cancer patients. Clin. Cancer Res., 19, 4133–4139.

Eleuteri, A., 2003, On a novel neural computation approach to conditional probability estimation and variable selection. Ph.D. Thesis, DMA "R. Caccioppoli", Universit`a degli Studi di Napoli "Federico II". Available at: http://people.na.infn.it/~eleuteri.

Eleuteri, A., R. Tagliaferri, L. Milano, S. de Placido and M. de Laurentiis, 2003, A novel neural network-based survival analysis model. Neural Netw. 16, 855–864.

Faraggi, D. and R. Simon, 1995, A neural network model for survival data. Stat. Med., 14, 73–82.

Fukunaga, K., 1990, Introduction to Statistical Pattern Recognition, 2nd Ed. Academic Press.

Feller, W., 1971, An Introduction to Probability Theory and its Applications, Vol. II, 2nd Ed. John Wiley, New York.

Hornik, K., M. Stinchcombe and H. White, 1990, Universal approximation of an unknown mapping and its derivatives using multilayer feedforward networks. Neural Netw., 3, 551–560.

Kalbfleisch, J.D. and R.L. Prentice, 1980, The Statistical Analysis of Failure Time Data. John Wiley, New York.

Kittler, J., P. Somol and P. Pudil, 2004, Fast branch & bound algorithms for optimal feature selection. IEEE Trans. Pattern Anal. Mach. Intell., 26(7), 900–912.

Liestøl, K., P.K. Andersen and U. Andersen, 1994, Survival analysis and neural nets. Stat. Med., 13, 1189–1200.

Lisboa, P.J.G. and H. Wong, 2001, Are neural networks best used to help logistic regression? An example from breast cancer survival analysis. Proceedings International Joint Conference on Neural Networks, 2001, Washington D.C., paper 577, 2472–2477.

MacKay, D.J.C., 1992, A practical Bayesian framework for backpropagation networks. Neural Comput., 4(3), 448–472.

McCullagh, P. and J. Nelder, 1989, Generalised Linear Models. Chapman and Hall, London.

Neal, R.M., 1996, Bayesian Learning for Neural Networks. Springer, New York.

Neal, R.M., 2000, Slice Sampling. Technical Report No. 2005, Department of Statistics, University of Toronto.

Neal, R.M., 2001, Survival Analysis Using a Bayesian Neural Network. Joint Statistical Meetings Report, Atlanta.

Raftery, A.E., D. Madigan and C.T. Volinsky, 1996, Accounting for model uncertainty in survival analysis improves predictive performance. Bayesian Statistics, 5, J.M. Bernardo, J.O. Berger, A.P. Dawid and A.F.M. Smith (Eds.), Oxford University Press, pp. 323–349.

Ripley, B.D. and R.M. Ripley, 1998, Neural Networks as Statistical Methods in Survival Analysis. In: R. Dybowsky and V. Gant (Eds.), Artificial Neural Networks: Prospects for Medicine. Landes Biosciences Publishers.

Robert, C.P. and G. Casella, 1999, Markov Chain Monte Carlo Methods. Springer, New York.

Robert, C.P., 2001, The Bayesian Choice, 2nd Ed. Springer, New York.

Samorodnitsky, G. and M.S. Taqqu, 1994, Stable Non-Gaussian Random Processes: Stochastic Models with Infinite Variance. Chapman & Hall, New York.

Schwarzer, G., W. Vach and M. Schumacher, 2000, On the misuses of artificial neural networks for prognostic and diagnostic classification in oncology. Stat. Med., 19, 541–561.

Watanabe, S., 2001, Learning Efficiency of Redundant Neural Networks in Bayesian Estimation. Technical Report No. 687, Precision and Intelligence Laboratory, Tokyo Institute of Technology.

Wong, H., P. Harris, P.J.G. Lisboa, S.P.J. Kirby and R. Swindell, 1999, Dealing with censorship in neural network models. IEEE Trans. Neural Netw., 3702–3706.

Yu, B. and B. Yuan, 1993, A more efficient branch and bound algorithm for feature selection. Pattern Recognition, 26, 883–889.

Chapter 8

Artificial Neural Networks Used in the Survival Analysis of Breast Cancer Patients: A Node-Negative Study

C.T.C. Arsene and P.J.G. Lisboa

School of Computing and Mathematical Sciences, Liverpool John Moores University, Byrom Street, Liverpool L3 3AF, UK
C.Arsene@ljmu.ac.uk
P.J.Lisboa@ljmu.ac.uk

Abstract

Artificial neural networks have been shown to be effective as general non-linear models with applications to medical diagnosis, prognosis and survival analysis. This chapter begins with a review of artificial neural networks used as non-linear regression models in the survival analysis of breast cancer patients. These techniques are of much interest because they allow modelling of time-dependent hazards in the presence of complex non-linear and non-additive effects between covariates. First, the role of neural networks is introduced within the context of statistical methods and parametric techniques for prognosis of survival in breast cancer. Second, these methods are applied in a study comprising node-negative breast cancer patients in order to evaluate the evidence for improved models or combination of prognostic indices to be used in a clinical environment. In particular, node-negative breast cancer is an early form of breast cancer in which cancer cells have not yet spread to the regional lymph nodes. There is much interest in determining the relevant prognostic factors that can allocate node-negative patients into prognostic groups correlating with the risk of disease relapse and mortality following surgery. This risk index can then be used to inform the choice of therapy. The Cox regression model and Artificial Neural Networks (ANN), a Partial Logistic Artificial Neural Network with Automatic Relevance Determination (PLANN-ARD) are used in order to identify and interpret the prognostic group allocation. A monthly retrospective cohort study with 5-year follow-up is conducted in pathologically node-negative patients selected from two datasets collected from Manchester Christie Hospital, UK.

Acknowledgments

The authors are grateful to Mr. Ric Swindell from Manchester Christie Hospital (UK) who provided the datasets and Dr. Pete Harris who reviewed the modelling techniques used in this chapter. The authors would like to thank the BIOPATTERN Network of Excellence (EU) who funded this work.

Keywords: Artificial neural networks, survival analysis, breast cancer, node-negative breast cancer, treatment options.

Contents

Outcome Prediction in Cancer
Edited by A.F.G. Taktak and A.C. Fisher
© 2007 Elsevier B.V. All rights reserved

1. INTRODUCTION

Survival analysis is an important part of medical statistics, frequently used to define prognostic indices for mortality or recurrence of a disease, and to study the outcome of treatment. The books by Kalbfleisch and Prentice (1980), Lawless (1982) together with the more recent ones by Lee (1992), Collett (1994), and Marubini and Valsecchi (1995) illustrate the methodology of survival analysis using biological and medical data.

It has been recognized in the medical literature that ANNs have much to contribute to the clinical functions of prognosis and survival analysis, in the medical domains of oncology (Bugliosi et al., 1994; Bryce et al., 1998; Glass and Reddick, 1998; Kothari et al., 1996; Ravdin, 2001), critical care (Stock et al., 1994; Si et al., 1998; Zernikow et al., 1999) and cardiovascular medicine (Baxt and White, 1995; Georgiadis et al., 1995; Selker et al., 1995; Smith et al., 1996; Ellenius et al., 1997; Goodenday et al., 1997; Polak et al., 1997; Lindahl et al., 2000). Lisboa (2002) presented a comprehensive survey of the neural networks applied in various medical applications within the context of advances in medical decision support (Campbell et al., 2000) arising from parallel developments in statistics and artificial intelligence (Bishop, 1995; MacKay, 1995). The chapter covers the domains of artificial intelligence, neural networks, statistics and medical decision support, and proposes a blueprint for the design of medical decision systems incorporating neural networks.

While ANN methods can be used in several medical domains, applications of particular interest are in oncology and in this chapter a review of these methods applied in the prognosis of survival of breast cancer patients is addressed.

ANNs have been used in the non-linear modelling of survival data since they allow for the detection of complex non-linear and non-additive effects from several input variables on the outcome, which can represent the mortality rate or recurrence of the disease (Burke et al., 1997; Biganzoli et al., 2002; Lisboa et al., 2003). Furthermore, usually in breast cancer patients, there can be a number of events which can be considered as the outputs of the artificial neural network and act in a competitive way when considered as first failure, intra-breast tumour recurrence and distant metastases. Therefore two situations can be delimited in this context: (i) only one of the possible events can be observed (Biganzoli et al., 1998; Lisboa et al., 2003; Jerez-Aragones et al., 2003); (ii) more events can be observed subsequently but only the first is of interest to evaluate the effect of first-line treatment because the patient maybe subsequently submitted to further treatments that alter the subsequent event history (Boracchi et al., 2003).

First, in this chapter the statistical methods and the ANN techniques used in the survival analysis of breast cancer patients are reviewed and second, these methods are applied to a class of breast cancer patients characterized by the number of cancer cells in the regional lymph nodes equal to zero, group of patients that are called node-negative breast cancer patients.

2. BREAST CANCER

Breast cancer is the most common cancer among women other than skin cancer as the figures stand at the beginning of the twentieth-first century. More than 1 000 000 new cases of breast cancer are reported worldwide annually and the risk of a woman developing breast cancer during her lifetime is approximately 11% (about one in nine of all women worldwide). In the EU countries, 191 000 new cases will be diagnosed, while in the US, more than 215 000 American women will be diagnosed with breast cancer this year, according to ACOR (2004). In the UK, each year there are 40 000 new cases of breast cancer reported (Breast Cancer Care, 2005; Cancer Research UK, 2005). However, the good news is that the incidence of disease relapse and mortality has decreased constantly in these areas because of advances in treatment options and the introduction of breast cancer screening programmes since the beginning of 1990s in countries like UK or Sweden. These screening programmes consist of mammography (i.e. X-ray examination of the breast) with or without clinical breast examination, which can decrease breast cancer mortality because early detection of breast cancer increases the chances of successful treatment. The National Cancer Institute in US has a set of recommendations with regard to the women with a higher risk of developing breast cancer that should present regularly to the screening programmes:

- Women in their 40s should be screened every one to two years with mammography.
- Women aged 50s should be screened every one to two years with mammography.
- Women who are at a higher than average risk of breast cancer should seek medical advice about whether screening should begin before the age of 40 and the frequency of screening.

Several well-established factors have been associated with an increased risk of breast cancer such as older age, family history, nulliparity, early menarche, advanced age and a personal history of breast cancer (in situ or invasive).

Given the extension of breast cancer in some regions of the world, pathologists have focused on identifying histological and immunohistochemical markers that have a direct bearing on both the treatment and the behaviour of breast cancer: activated Akt kinase (Schmitz et al., 2004), age (Marcus et al., 1994), angiogenesis (Dales et al., 2004), bilateral cancers (Regitnig et al., 2004), biopsy effect (Wiley et al., 2003), CD105 (Dales et al., 2003), chromosomal abnormalities (Farabegoli et al., 2004), cyclooxygenase-2 (Shim et al., 2003), DNA ploidy (Wenger et al., 1993), DCIS associated (Jacquemier et al., 1990), fibrotic focus (Hasebe et al., 1996), glutathione *S*-transferase (Huang et al., 2003), hormone receptor status (Nicholas et al., 2003), lobular carcinoma in situ (Abner et al., 2000), lymph node status (Goldstein et al., 1999), lymphovascular invasion (Hasebe et al., 2004), mast cells (Dabiri et al., 2004), metalloproteinase (Nakopoulou et al., 2002) and another few dozen such as microarray gene expression, mitotic figure count, myxoid change, neuroendocrine differentiation, nuclear features, oncogenes (e.g. *EGFR* or *HER-1*, *HER-2/neu*, *HER-3*, *HER-4*, *BRCA-1* and *BRCA-2*), *p53* (i.e. tumour-suppressor gene), pregnancy associated, pregnancy concurrent, pregnancy subsequent in breast cancer survivors, race, second primary breast cancer, size of tumour, stromelysin-3, topoisomerase, treatment inadequacies, tumour-associated antigens and vascular endothelial growth factor. Obviously, the variety of prognostic factors for breast cancer disease and the number of publications addressing one or a combination of these factors is by far very large. In general, the prognostic factors that are most used are as follows: size of primary tumour, age of patient, lymph node involvement, histological type and grade of tumour, oestrogen and progesterone receptor status, proliferative rate of tumour, amplified oncogenes, degree of angiogenesis and lymphovascular invasion.

The figures presented before, show that breast cancer is potentially a very serious condition and can be life threatening. Therefore, early detection of breast cancer is vital as it increases the chances of successful treatment (Andersen et al., 1988; National Institutes of Health Consensus Development Conference, 2000; Wait et al., 2000; NHS Breast Screening Programme, 2005).

The decisions with regard to the chosen type of treatment are formulated according to the prognostic factors enumerated before, upon which a staging system is applied in order to group the patients with respect to prognosis. The TNM classification (T = tumour, N = node, M = metastasis) is most widely used (Beahrs et al., 1992; Greene et al., 2002).

For lymph node status, the TNM is N0 – no regional lymph nodes metastasis, N1 – metastasis to movable ipsilateral axillary lymph nodes, N2 – metastasis to ipsilateral axillary lymph nodes fixed or mated, or in ipsilateral internal mammary nodes in the absence of clinically evident lymph node metastasis, N3 – metastasis in ipsilateral infraclavicular lymph nodes with or without node involvement, or metastasis in ipsilateral supraclavicular lymph nodes with or without axillary or internal mammary lymph nodes, or metastasis in internal mammary lymph nodes and in the presence of clinically evident axillary lymph node metastasis.

Our analysis is focused on the survival and the prognostic factors for patients with node-negative breast cancer. This is an early form of cancer with no cancer cells from the breast having been found in the lymph nodes in the armpit area, which corresponds to regional lymph nodes N0.

In addition to the TNM staging system, which is a clinical procedure carried out by a medical specialist (i.e. oncologist), usually the breast cancer datasets include also the number of nodes involved for a patient. Number of nodes involved equal to zero describes the node-negative breast cancer patients and corresponds to regional lymph nodes N0 in the TNM staging. However, in some breast cancer datasets, patients with N0 in the TNM staging, the number of nodes involved is different from zero. This is because the TNM staging is a clinical procedure in which the oncologist may use only radiological (i.e. mammography) and physical investigations to estimate the stage, while the number of nodes involved may be obtained by using additional tests (e.g. cyst aspiration, biopsy, ultrasonography, Magnetic Resonance Imaging (MRI), Computed Tomography (CT)). For example, the mammography is able to detect over 90% of breast cancer cases but declines significantly with increasing breast density in young women. The investigations from this study address node-negative breast cancer patients with the number of nodes involved equal to zero and the TNM staging N0.

Some recent studies have shown a general benefit in giving adjuvant systemic therapy including chemotherapy (e.g. cyclophosphamide, methotrexate and 5-fluorouracil) hormonal therapy (e.g. tamoxifen) and radiation therapy to all operable breast cancer patients regardless of axillary lymph node status (Early Breast Cancer Trialists' Collaborative Group, 1998a,b). However, only 25–30% of node-negative breast cancer patients are expected to relapse following surgery. Therefore, a great effort has been made in recent years to identify the proportion of patients that needs adjuvant therapy, thus sparing toxicity to those node-negative patients who could be considered cured by surgery alone (Fisher et al., 2001a; Goldhirsch et al., 2001; Castiglione-Gertsch, 2002; Jagsi et al., 2003).

The prognostic effect of tumour size (O'Reilly et al., 1990), oestrogen receptor (ER) status, tumour ploidy, S-phase fraction (SPF) (Lundin et al., 2001) and other several biological parameters, including oncogenes, growth factors and growth factor receptors, tumour suppressor genes, and cancer cell proliferation markers (Clark et al., 1989; Sigurdsson et al., 1990; Clark and McGuire, 1991; Gasparini et al., 1992; Thor et al., 1992; Toikkanen et al., 1992; Ross and Fletcher, 1998; de Placido et al., 1999; van der Wal et al., 2002; Cody et al., 2004) have been investigated in node-negative breast cancer patients to identify those at high risk of relapse following surgery. These prognostic groupings can help to identify the patients that are most suitable for adjuvant therapy.

Disease recurrence (Huseby et al., 1988; Medri et al., 2000; Biganzoli et al., 2003; Fisher et al., 2004) and survivorship (Camp et al., 2000; Lisboa et al., 2003; Noguchi et al., 2005) are usually followed for this type of breast cancer. An important conclusion draws Ferrero et al. (2000) that for node-negative breast cancer patients, in order to assess the prognostic value of various biological factors, the cohorts of patients should be followed over periods in excess of ten years.

3. STATISTICAL METHODS IN SURVIVAL ANALYSIS FOR BREAST CANCER CENSORED DATA

Statistical methods have been adopted as modelling and analysing tools for breast cancer datasets. Let t be the actual survival time of an individual, which can be regarded as representing the time elapsed from some particular recruitment date (e.g. date of surgery) to the occurrence of a specific event (i.e. death or disease recurrence such as intra-breast tumour recurrence) and can also be considered as a single non-negative random variable (T). The different values that T can take have a *probability distribution* in which case T is the *random variable* associated with the survival time. The random variable T has a probability distribution with underlying *probability density function* $f(t)$. The *distribution function* of T represents the probability that the survival time is less than some value t and is given by

$$F(t) = P(T < t) = \int_0^t f(u)\,du \tag{1}$$

The survivor function $S(t)$ is the probability that the survival time is greater than or equal to t

$$S(t) = P(T \geq t) = 1 - F(t) \tag{2}$$

The survivorship function is a monotonic decreasing continuous function with $S(0) = 1$ and $S(\infty) = \lim_{t\to\infty} S(t) = 0$.

The hazard function $h(t)$ is the probability that an event happens between time t and $t + \delta t$. This is defined as

$$h(t) = \lim_{\delta t \to 0} \frac{P(t \le T < t + \delta t \mid t \le T)}{\delta t}. \tag{3}$$

The hazard rate can also be written as (Lawless, 1982; Collett, 1994)

$$h(t) = \frac{f(t)}{S(t)}. \tag{4}$$

It then follows that

$$h(t) = -\frac{d}{dt}\{\log S(t)\}. \tag{5}$$

The cumulative hazard function can be defined as

$$H(t) = \int_0^t h(u)du \tag{6}$$

from where the survivor function can be written as

$$S(t) = \exp\left(-\int_0^t h(u)du\right) = \exp\{-H(t)\} \tag{7}$$

For survival data, some of the observations may be incomplete over the study time. Moreover, the time of occurrence of the considered event may not be known for every patient. These groups of patients are usually omitted for the subsequent study time and this is known as *censoring* (Lawless, 1982; Collett, 1994). In discrete time modelling, time is split into several time intervals and each time interval includes at least one event case. The time intervals are not necessarily uniformly distributed. There could be more than one individual observed to experience the event of interest at any particular event time. At the end of some of these time intervals, a number of patients may be left out for the remaining study time because the information with regard to their status (e.g. death or alive, recurrence of disease or cured from disease) is missing.

There are three types of censoring that need to be carefully considered when dealing with breast cancer datasets (Collett, 1994; Klein and Moeschberger, 1997; Biganzoli et al., 2002): right censoring, left censoring or interval censoring. It is possible also to have two types of censoring combined (double censoring). Right censoring is when the event of interest does not happen before a predefined time interval or some other competing event, in which case for each individual the observed time t is calculated as the minimum between the time to event and a censoring time. Left censoring is when the observed time t is located before the time of the beginning of the observation for the patient and t is equal with the maximum between the time to event and the censoring time. Interval censoring occurs when the time to event is not known but it is known that it falls in an interval. The most common type of censoring is right censoring which was also applied to the breast cancer datasets described later in this chapter.

Suppose there are n individuals observed with observed times $t_1, t_2, t_3, \ldots, t_n$. There are r event times in total, $r \leq n$, so the ordered event times are $t_{(1)} \leq t_{(2)} \leq t_{(3)} \leq \cdots \leq t_{(j)}$, where $j = 1, 2, \ldots, r$ and d_j denotes the number of events (e.g. deaths, recurrence of disease, distant metastasis) at the jth time interval. The probability of an individual experiencing the event at that time interval is given by the hazard rate which is

$$h(t_j) = \frac{d_j}{n_j}, \tag{8}$$

where d_j represents the number of failures at time t_j, and n_j is the number of individuals at risk at that time. The Kaplan–Meier estimate (Kaplan and Meier, 1958) is a non-parametric method used to describe the survival function to time t for discrete survival data

$$S(t) = \prod_{j=1}^{k} \left(\frac{n_j - d_j}{n_j} \right) \tag{9}$$

for $t_{(k)} \leq t \leq t_{(k+1)}$, where $k = 1, 2, \ldots, t_{k+1}$.

Examples of Kaplan–Meier survival curves for breast cancer data can be found in Galea et al. (1992), Marubini and Valsecchi (1995), Wong (2001), and Lisboa et al. (2003). An approximation for the estimated standard error of the Kaplan–Meier estimate of the survivorship function is given by Greenwood formula (Collett, 1994; Marubini and Valsecchi, 1995). Once the standard error of the estimated survivorship function is calculated, confidence intervals for the estimated survivorship function can also be obtained. The confidence intervals is a range of values around the estimate which gives a percentage level that the true underlying survivorship function is included within the interval (Marubini and Valsecchi, 1995; Wong, 2001).

Predictive models (i.e. prognostic indexes) can be obtained by pooling together similar patients into a grouped Kaplan–Meier curve which can also act as a prognostic score associated with the respective group of patients. In order to obtain such grouping, the log-rank test is usually used (Peto and Peto, 1972). The log-rank test determines, at a given significance level, whether the population comprise of two subgroups with different survivorship. The null hypothesis is that there is no difference in the survivorship of the individuals in the two groups. This hypothesis is tested by considering the difference between the observed number of surviving individuals in the two groups at each time points and the number expected under the null hypothesis. Examples of log-rank test applied to breast cancer datasets collected from Manchester Christie Hospital in UK between 1983 and 1989 and 1990–1993 can be found in Wong (2001) and Lisboa et al. (2003). Efficace et al. (2004) used the log-rank test in order to determine the most important clinical prognostic factors in a dataset of 275 female patients with metastatic breast cancer.

Their dataset was from the European Organization for Research and Treatment of Cancer (EORTC, http://www.eortc.be).

However, these predictive models are most commonly estimated on the basis of the maximum likelihood principle (Lawless, 1982; Gray, 1996; Saphner et al., 1996; Kleinbaum, 1997; Hilsenbeck et al., 1998; Hosmer and Lemeshow, 2000) as shown in Section 4. The contributions to the likelihood function are coming from the uncensored observations, right-censored observations, left-censored observations and interval-censored observations. In the case of non-parametric situation where there is no covariate (i.e. no prognostic factor) and no other assumptions are made, the maximum likelihood estimate coincide with the Kaplan–Meier estimate of the survival function shown in Eq. (9).

3.1. Clinically used prognostic algorithms

Although statistical modelling can be a complex process resulting in data models that are elaborate and detailed, it is also the case that much simpler algorithms have been abstracted from statistical analysis, in particular with regard to prognostic indices, such as Nottingham Prognostic Index (NPI). The NPI (Haybittle et al., 1982; Galea et al., 1992), which was developed in UK, is based on three traditional prognostic factors, tumour diameter, lymph node status and histological grade:

$$\text{NPI} = \text{tumour size (cm)} \times 0.2 + \text{histological grade} + \text{lymph node status} \tag{10}$$

Galea et al. (1992) applied NPI index for an operable breast cancer dataset of 1629 female patients for which they used the log-rank test in order to compare different prognostic groups. Seshadri et al. (1997) developed Adelaide Prognostic Index (API), subsequently modified by Lockwood et al. (1999), which was based on a single traditional morphological factor, tumour diameter, and two biopathological factors, the oestrogen factor receptor (ER) status and cell kinetics according to the Ki67/MIB-1 antibody. Sidoni et al. (2004) compared the NPI and API prognostic indexes for 82 cases of breast cancer gathered between 1987 and 1990 in Italy with a minimum follow-up of 5 years. Log-rank test identified three prognostic groups with respect to the overall survival with NPI as opposed to the API. NPI could discriminate between the three prognostic factors at an early stage and maintained this capacity during the entire period of follow-up of 10 years. This is important, since it allows early discrimination of the more aggressive tumours (D'Eredita et al., 2001). The performances of NPI were augmented by the addition of the progesterone receptor (PGR) status (Collett et al., 1998), angiogenesis (Hausen et al., 2000) and vascular endothelial growth factor (VEFG) status (Coradini et al., 2001) to the classical parameters of NPI.

4. PARAMETRIC MODELS AND COX REGRESSION FOR BREAST CANCER DATA

Parametric models have been frequently used in survival analysis by defining a functional form of the hazard function $h(t)$ from which the functions $S(t)$ and $f(t)$ can be derived

(Lawless, 1982; Marubini and Valsecchi, 1995). In the exponential model, the probability of failure (hazard rate) is assumed constant in a time interval t

$$h(t) = \lambda \tag{11}$$

The survival function becomes

$$S(t) = \exp(-\lambda t) \tag{12}$$

The probability density function $f(t)$ of the random variable T associated with the survival time is

$$f(t) = -\frac{dS(t)}{dt} = \lambda \exp(-\lambda t) \tag{13}$$

The exponential distribution is a particular case of the Weibull distribution (Weibull, 1951) which is very frequently used in survival analysis. The hazard function for Weibull distribution is

$$h(t) = \lambda \ p(\lambda t)^{p-1}, \tag{14}$$

where $\lambda > 0$ and $p > 0$ are parameters. For $p = 1$, the Weibull distribution becomes the exponential distribution from Eq. (11).

For the exponential model from Eq. (12) and no censored data, the likelihood function L is proportional to the joint probability of the n outcomes of the random variable T consisting of $t_1, t_2, t_3, \ldots, t_n$ times to the event of interest (e.g. recurrence of disease).

$$L(\lambda; t_1, t_2, t_3, \ldots, t_n) = \prod_{i=1}^{n} f(t_i; \lambda) = \prod_{i=1}^{n} \lambda \exp(-\lambda t_i) \tag{15}$$

The aim is to find the value of λ which maximizes the likelihood function from the previous equation or its logarithm.

$$\log L(\lambda; t) = \sum_{i=1}^{n} \log[\lambda \exp(-\lambda t_i)] = n \log \lambda - \lambda \sum_{i-1}^{n} t_i \tag{16}$$

The likelihood function can be modified so that to include censored data. For each patient a pair of variables (t_i, δ_i) is introduced. A patient who fails at t_i ($\delta_i = 1$) has the contribution to the likelihood function given by $f(t_i)$, while a patient who is censored at t_i ($\delta_i = 0$) has the contribution to the likelihood given by the probability of survival beyond that point in time $S(t_i)$. The likelihood function in the presence of right-censored data is

$$L(\lambda; t) = \prod_{i=1}^{n} [f(t_i)]^{\delta_i} [S(t_i)]^{1-\delta_i} \tag{17}$$

The likelihood function is usually extended to account for left-censored data or interval censored data (Lawless, 1982) as well as to include modelling of the expectation of time to failure $E(T)$ by factors of clinical concerns by introducing a vector of covariates x for each patient.

Ripley and Ripley (1998) obtained the survivorship function for a dataset of 500 breast cancer patients assuming a Weibull parametric model for the hazard function. The same

Weibull parametric model was used to estimate the survivorship for a second dataset of 300 breast cancer patients, which was in turn compared with the survivorship calculated from other regression models (i.e. proportional hazards, log-logistic regression model, binary classification). In Marubini and Valsecchi (1995), a comparison is made in terms of the estimates of the regression coefficients and their standard errors between the Weibull model and the Cox model, the log-logistic model and the log-normal model for a breast cancer dataset of 716 patients. The last three models were preferred to the Weibull model following an analysis based on the estimated hazard functions and the graphical analysis of results.

Such parametric models for survival analysis are based on the strict assumption of the time distributions of the event of interest and the effect of covariates on the distribution parameters λ or p that are not tenable in many situations. Therefore, the refinement of the parametric models brought the *piecewise* parametric models which consist of the partition of the time axis into $l = 1, 2, \ldots, L$ intervals with a specific hazard rate h on each interval (Elandt-Johnson and Johnson, 1980). The case with an exponential distribution on each time interval forms the piecewise exponential model (Aitkin et al., 1989; Biganzoli et al., 2002).

A *grouped* time model (Kalbfleisch and Prentice, 1980; Ripley and Ripley, 1998; Biganzoli et al., 1998) is obtained if all the observations within a time interval $(t_{l\text{-}1}, t_l]$ are grouped on a single point of each time interval which is usually taken as the midpoint of the time interval. The survival function and the likelihood function for the piecewise exponential model and the grouped time model are shown in Biganzoli et al. (2002) for multiple time intervals $l \geq 2$.

A general framework for regression models on survival data is the Generalized Linear Model (GLM) (McCullagh and Nelder, 1989). For such models, it is assumed that each component of a vector of random variables independently distributed has a distribution in the exponential family. If Y is the vector of random variables, it has a vector of expected values (means) $E(Y)$ noted with μ and a variance vector Var(Y) (Biganzoli et al., 2002). The relationship between the regression model η (predictor) and the expected values μ is given by the link function g

$$\eta = g(\mu) \tag{18}$$

Usually, in a GLM, η has a linear additive form $\eta = \beta_0 + \beta^{\mathrm{T}}x$, where β_0 is called the intercept term and β is the vector of regression coefficients. An example of GLM is the linear model for which the link function g is the identity function and Y has a normal distribution. Given $x_1, x_2, x_3, \ldots, x_p$ covariates with known values, then β_j are the parameters whose values are estimated from data with the log-likelihood function.

GLMs can be adopted to model the dependence of the hazard function from the covariates. Link functions other than the identity function, are used such as the logit link function (g) and an example is the proportional hazards model also called Cox regression (Cox, 1972). This model is a multiple linear regression of the hazard function, under the assumption that all time dependence is specified by a reference group of patients called the baseline population. It is possible to introduce time dependence via interaction terms, but this adds considerable complexity to the model design and is generally a heuristic procedure reliant on the statistical expertise of the user.

For discrete time intervals t_k, the proportional hazards model parameterises the odds of survival in proportion to a baseline, as follows:

$$\frac{h_i(t_k, x_i)}{1-h_i(t_k, x_i)} = \frac{h_0(t_k)}{1-h_0(t_k)}\exp(\beta^{\mathrm{T}} x_i), \tag{19}$$

where i denotes the individual patient record and x_i is a static covariate vector containing a set of explanatory variables extracted from the patient record.

The Cox model is not a fully parametric model since it does not specify the form of $h_0(t_k)$. A baseline population must be selected to establish the time dependence of the hazards. Its covariate vector will contain all zero. The dependence on the covariates is aggregated into the scalar $\beta^{\mathrm{T}}x_i$, which represents a risk score or prognostic index (PI). As described in Section 3, the log-rank test can be used to allocate patients into prognostic groups as a function of their prognostic indexes. In the limit of infinitely short time intervals, the discrete time model in Eq. (19) converged to the familiar parameterization of proportional hazards in continuous time given by

$$h_i(x_i, t) = \exp(\beta^{\mathrm{T}} x_i) h_0(t) \tag{20}$$

The survival function for the ith individual is calculated as follows:

$$S_i(t) = (S_0(t))^{\exp(\beta^{\mathrm{T}} x_i)} \tag{21}$$

Cox regression has been widely used for survival analysis in breast cancer (Lisboa et al., 2003). There are also models which extend the Cox regression for competing risks in breast cancer (Larson, 1984; Klein et al., 1989; Wohlfahrt et al., 1999; Boracchi et al., 2001). The Cox regression is preferable when the interest is focused on the effects of prognostic factors. When the interest is on the dependence on time and covariates of the shape of the hazard functions then a smoothing estimation procedure should be taken in to consideration. Such a procedure is the ANNs, which can be used as non-linear regression models suitable to model non-linear and non-additive interactions between covariates. In this case, the linear predictor η from GLM becomes a non-linear neural predictor given by

$$\eta = \phi(\beta_0 + \beta^{\mathrm{T}} x), \tag{22}$$

where ϕ can be a non-linear function such as the sigmoid function. In this case, the output activation function ϕ_0 of the ANN will be the inverse of the link function from Eq. (18)

$$\phi_0(\eta) = g^{-1}(\eta) \tag{23}$$

The vector of expected values μ, represented here by the recurrence time of disease or other type of event (e.g. distant metastasis, death), equals the prediction of the ANN which is $\phi_0(\eta)$

$$\mu = \phi_0(\eta) \tag{24}$$

GLM can be seen as a particular case of feed forward ANN with a linear predictor η. When the hazard functions are expected to behave in a non-proportional way, covariate effects change during the follow-up or there may be interactions between covariate's effects, then ANNs for single and competing risks can deal with these problems. An example of non-proportional hazards is the mortality of patients from a low-risk cohort group estimated as the output of a neural network (Wong, 2001; Lisboa et al., 2003). In Gore et al. (1984) it was shown on a breast cancer dataset that if the time to peak hazard is earlier in some prognostic groups than in others, then the proportional hazard assumption is no longer sustained.

5. ARTIFICIAL NEURAL NETWORKS FOR CENSORED SURVIVAL DATA

ANNs are non-linear, semiparametric models that have been considered as alternative models for survival analysis in the presence of censorship. An ANN used for survival analysis can be viewed as a GLM with a non-linear predictor (Biganzoli et al., 2002) such as a Multi-Layer Perceptron (MLP) (Biganzoli et al., 1998; Lisboa et al., 2003) or a Radial Basis Function (RBF) network (Boracchi et al., 2001).

A general ANN model has an input layer, one or more intermediate hidden layers and the output layer. Let $j = 1, 2, \ldots, J$ and $k = 1, 2, \ldots, K$ be the input and output nodes ($k = 1$ for single output, $k > 1$ for multiple outputs), respectively, x_{ij} will be the input values and y_{ki} the observed responses (targets) for each subject $i = 1, 2, \ldots, n$. The model will compute the outputs $\hat{y}_{ki}$ to approximate the y_{ki}. Each node in the hidden layer computes a weighted sum of the inputs x_{ij} with weights w_{jh}, adds a constant α_h (bias), and applies an activation function ϕ_h to obtain its output a. The outputs of the hidden layer become the inputs of the output layer nodes; their outputs are computed in the same way as the hidden layer with weights w_{hk} and the activation ϕ_0. The presence of the hidden nodes provides a non-linear dependence of the outputs on the input variables. The mathematical representation of an ANN with a single hidden layer is given below (Biganzoli et al., 1998; Lisboa et al., 2003):

$$\hat{y}_k(x_i, w) = \phi_0\left(\alpha_k + \sum_{h=1}^{H} w_{hk}\phi_h\left(\alpha_h + \sum_{j=1}^{J} w_{jh}x_{ij}\right)\right) \tag{25}$$

The activation function ϕ_h used for hidden nodes is generally the logistic function:

$$\phi_h(u) = \frac{1}{1+\exp(-u)} \tag{26}$$

The same activation function can be used for the output node

$$\phi_0(a) = \frac{1}{1+\exp(-a)} \tag{27}$$

The estimates of the weights w, parameters of the model and the outputs $\hat{y}_{ki}(x_i, w)$ are obtained by minimizing an appropriate error function. Several error functions can be used, one of them is the quadratic error

$$E = \sum_{k=1}^{K}\sum_{i=1}^{n}(\hat{y}_k(x_i, w) - y_{ki})^2 \tag{28}$$

while for binary classification problems the appropriate function is the cross-entropy error (Bishop, 1995) given by

$$E = -\sum_{k=1}^{K}\sum_{i=1}^{n}\{y_{ki}\log\hat{y}_k(x_i, w) + (1 - y_{ki})\log(1 - \hat{y}_k(x_i, w))\} \tag{29}$$

Biganzoli et al. (1998) proposed a Partial Logistic regression model based on a feed forward ANN (PLANN), which has one input node j for each covariate and the vectors x_i for each of n patients are replicated for all the time intervals in which the patient is observed. The target vector y_{ki} is zero or one if the ith patient is observed alive, or when the event of interest happened in that time interval, but is removed from the study when the outcome for that time interval is not observed. For k equals 1, y_{ki} corresponds to an ANN with single output.

The cross-entropy error function from Eq. (29) becomes in the context of breast cancer survival analysis (Wong, 2001; Lisboa et al., 2003) as follows:

$$E = -\sum_{p=1}^{\text{no. of patient}}\sum_{k=1}^{t}\{d_{pk}\log h_p(x_i, t_k) + (1 - d_{pk})\log(1 - \log h_p(x_i, t_k))\}, \tag{30}$$

where d_{pk} is the target vector y_{ki} from Eq. (29), $h_p(x_i, t_k)$ is the single output of the neural network and represents the hazard rate (probability of survival) for patient p during t_k time interval. The time interval is introduced as a separate variable represented by the midpoint of the interval. What is important is that this model does not require proportionality of the hazards over time as in the Cox regression model and it implicitly models interactions between the explanatory variables and time. Moreover, it predicts a smooth hazard function that is independent of the baseline population. The single output of ANN, which is the hazard rate $h_p(x_i, t_k)$ and the activation function for the output node from Eq. (27) gives the analytical expression of the ANN, which resembles the odds of survival from Eq. (19) for the Cox regression model

$$\frac{h_p(x_p, t_k)}{1 - h_p(x_p, t_k)} = \exp\left(\sum_{h=1}^{N_h} w_h g\left(\sum_{i=1}^{N_i} w_{ih}x_{pi} + wt_k + b_h\right) + b\right), \tag{31}$$

where the indices i and h denote the input and hidden node layers, respectively, and the non-linear function g has the form from Eq. (27).

Once the network weights w are estimated, the survivorship is calculated from the estimated discrete time hazard by multiplying the conditionals for survival over successive time intervals, treated as independent events, to give

$$S(t_k) = \prod_{l=1}^{k} P(t > t_l \mid t > t_{l-1}) = \prod_{l=1}^{k}(1 - h(t_l)) \tag{32}$$

However, neural networks are prone to over-fitting unless careful regularization is applied. The Bayesian neural network approach (MacKay, 1992a,b) is commonly used to regularize binary classification problems including soft model selection through Automatic Relevance Determination (ARD) where the hyperparameters regularizing the objective function suppress irrelevant variables.

In prognosis after surgery in breast cancer for censored data, an extension of PLANN with the Bayesian framework for ARD was developed in Lisboa et al. (2003) and Wong (2001). In this case, the weights are estimated by an iterative training process that optimizes the evidence for the weight set $\{w\}$ given the data D, the penalty parameters α, and the model hypothesis H

$$P(w \mid D,\alpha,H) = \frac{P(D \mid w,\alpha,H)P(w \mid \alpha,H)}{P(D \mid \alpha,H)} \tag{33}$$

The numerator consists of the likelihood that the model fits the data

$$P(D \mid w,\alpha,H) = \mathrm{e}^{-E} \tag{34}$$

multiplied by the prior distribution of the weights, which is normally assumed to be centred at zero with variance $1/\alpha$

$$P(w \mid \alpha,H) = \frac{\mathrm{e}^{-G(w,\,\alpha)}}{Z_w(\alpha)}, \tag{35}$$

where $G(w,\alpha) = (1/2)\Sigma_{m=1}^{N_\alpha}\alpha_m\Sigma_{n=1}^{N_m}w_{mn}^2$. The index n indicates a group of weights w_{mn} sharing a common regularization parameter α_m of which there are N_m. These weights correspond to attributes from a single field, or variable. As the training progresses, the α_m for variables with little predictive power increase in size, forcing the corresponding weights towards zero, hence, the term “weight decay” commonly used for this regularization method. This is the main mechanism for complexity control in the neural network, and it has a key role later during model selection. The normalization constant is readily calculated from a product of univariate normal distributions, giving $Z_w(\alpha) = \Pi_{m=1}^{N\alpha}(2\pi/\alpha_m)^{N_m/2}$. Finally, the weights are estimated by an iterative “training” process that optimizes

$$P(w \mid D,\alpha,H) \propto \mathrm{e}^{-E}\mathrm{e}^{-G(w,\,\alpha)} = \mathrm{e}^{-S(w,\,\alpha)} \tag{36}$$

by minimizing the penalized objective function $S(w,\alpha) = E + G(w,\alpha)$. For this ANN, the optimization of the objective function was carried out by scaled-conjugate gradients optimization, implemented in the Matlab code Netlab (Nabney, 2001).

In Wong (2001), Lisboa et al. (2003), and Arsene and Lisboa (2005), the Bayesian framework for the regularization of hyperparameters was also applied. The hyperparameters controlled the influence of each input covariate (time, size of tumour, etc.) on the prediction of survival. There are separate hyperparameters for each input covariate each shared among multiple attributes. The hyperparameters are calculated by maximizing the Bayesian expression

$$P(\alpha \mid D,H) = \frac{P(D \mid \alpha,H)P(\alpha \mid H)}{P(D \mid H)} \tag{37}$$

The first-term in the numerator is the normalizing constant in Eq. (33) and it can be written as

$$P(D \mid \alpha,H) = \int P(D \mid w,\alpha,H)P(w \mid \alpha,H)dw = \int \frac{\mathrm{e}^{-S(w,\,\alpha)}}{Z_W(\alpha)}dw \tag{38}$$

The integral is solved by using a Taylor expansion around the "most probable" weights w^{MP} of $S(w, \alpha)$

$$S^*(w,\alpha) \approx S(w^{\mathrm{MP}},\alpha) + \frac{1}{2}(w - w^{\mathrm{MP}})^{\mathrm{T}}A(w - w^{\mathrm{MP}}), \tag{39}$$

where the matrix A is the Hessian of S with respect to the weights. The evidence for the hyperparameters becomes

$$P(\alpha \mid D, H) \propto \frac{\exp(-S(w^{\mathrm{MP}},\alpha))}{Z_w(\alpha)}(2\pi)^{N_w/2}\det(A)^{-1/2} \tag{40}$$

Maximizing Eq. (39) results in a closed form solution for the hyperparameters

$$\gamma_m = N_m - \alpha_m \mathrm{Tr}_m(A^{-1}) = \frac{N_m \sum_{n=1}^{N_m}(W_{mn}^{\mathrm{MP}})^2}{\sum_{n=1}^{N_m}(W_{mn}^{\mathrm{MP}})^2 + \mathrm{Tr}_m(A^{-1})}$$

$$\frac{1}{\alpha_m} = \frac{\sum_{n=1}^{N_m}(W_{mn}^{\mathrm{MP}})^2}{\gamma_m} = \frac{\sum_{n=1}^{N_m}(W_{mn}^{\mathrm{MP}})^2 + \mathrm{Tr}_m(A^{-1})}{N_m}, \tag{41}$$

where $\mathrm{Tr}_m(A^{-1})$ is the trace of the inverse Hessian taken over the weights sharing α_m. This trace term is a measure of the uncertainty in the estimation of the weights, therefore, it follows from Eq. (41) that the intermediate parameter γ_m is positive and reaches its upper limit only when all of the N_m weights associated with α_m have zero error bars. The interpretation of γ_m is that it represents the number of well-determined parameters in the group of m weights. There are separate (α_m, γ_m) hyperparameters for each input covariate, each shared among multiple attributes; for the time covariate; for the bias terms in the hidden units; for the weights to the single output unit; and for the output node bias.

To remain in the area of Bayesian neural networks, Moore and Hoang (2002) have presented a Bayesian neural network and compared it with the standard neural network model and the logistic regression model for the prediction of survival on a breast cancer dataset from the National Cancer Institute, United States. They found that their Bayesian model performs better than the other models tested and offers the possibility of explaining the causal relationships among the variables. Eleuteri et al. (2003) presented an ANN based on the Bayesian framework for the estimation of the weights together with the regularization of the hyperparameters. They do not adopt the standard form of the output and hidden activation functions from Eqs. (26) and (27), and their model does not make any assumption on the form of the survival process such as piecewise approximations (Boracchi et al., 2001) or discretizations. Furthermore, their Survival Neural Network (SNN) consists of a hierarchical Bayesian model (Neal, 1996, 2001; Robert, 2001). First, the posterior density of the weights is sampled by using Markov chain Monte Carlo (MCMC) method (Neal, 2000) that generates a sequence of weight vectors, which is then used to approximate the output of SNN with a Monte Carlo estimator. In the same time, the optimization of the hyperparameters is carried out by using Gibbs sampling from a specific distribution for the hyperparameters. Hence, the hierarchical Bayesian modelling of the learning process is developed for SNN. The results showed that SNN can approximate complex survival functions, and in addition it had similar performance to the Cox model, demonstrating the capability of modelling the proportional hazards.

The ANNs presented so far have been applied in single risk cases. When competing risks are taken into consideration, such as intra-breast tumour recurrence and distant metastases, the PLANN suffers modifications. For the output nodes the activation function is softmax function (Bishop, 1995):

$$\phi_0(a_k) = \frac{\exp(a_k)}{\sum_{k'} \exp(a_{k'})}. \tag{42}$$

where the summation at the denominator is taken over all the outputs k'. The objective function from Eq. (43) is taken now over the number of risks R, patients and number of time intervals t as

$$E = -\sum_{r=1}^{R} \sum_{p=1}^{\text{no. of patients}} \sum_{l=1}^{t} \left\{ d_{rpl} \log\left(\frac{h_p(x_i, t_k, r)}{d_{rpl}} \right) \right\}, \tag{43}$$

where the indicator d_{rpl} equals 1 for the pth patient when the event of interest happened on the lth time interval, and otherwise 0.

The extension of the PLANN (Biganzoli et al., 1998) for competing risks and applied to a node-negative breast cancer dataset of 1793 who underwent surgery at the Milan Cancer Institute in Italy between 1981 and 1986 is shown in Biganzoli et al. (2002).

Ripley et al. (1998) proposed an MLP extension of the proportional hazards model, which was applied to prognosis of survival for patients suffering from breast cancer. Jerez-Aragones et al. (2003) developed a decision tool for the prognosis of breast cancer relapse, which uses an algorithm called Control of Induction by Sample Division Method (CISDM) (Ruiz-Gomez et al., 1999; Ramos-Jimenez et al., 2000) for improving the selection of the attributes that would better explain the patient dataset. This allowed them to develop decision trees smaller than those obtained with other algorithms (Quinlan, 1979, 1983, 1986, 1993) and therefore to perform the selection of the most important attributes for the inputs of their neural network system. This system consisted of specific topologies of MLP networks for different time intervals during the follow-up of the patients, considering the events occurring in different intervals as different problems. A method for the estimate of Bayes' optimal error using the neural network paradigm is also proposed. The decision tool was applied on a dataset of 1035 patients with breast cancer from the Medical Oncology Service of the Hospital Clinico Universitario of Malaga collected and recorded during the period 1990 and 2000.

Burke et al. (1997) have used a 3-layer neural network with backpropagation training, the maximum likelihood criterion function and gradient descent optimization method, for prognosis of survival on 3 datasets of breast cancer patients from the National Cancer Institute's Surveillance, Epidemiology, and End Results (SEER), Commission on Cancer's breast and colorectal carcinoma Patient Care Evaluation (PCE) and from the American College of Surgeons (ACS) – accredited hospital tumour registries in the United States. They compared the predictive accuracy of their ANN with the TNM staging system (Beahrs et al., 1992). Their study concluded that the ANNs are more accurate than the TNM staging system and in addition the ANNs can be expanded to include any number of prognostic factors, can accommodate continuous variables and can be extended to provide more insight into presurgery and postsurgery treatment predictions.

Another example of ANN model applied in regression problems is the Radial Basis Function Neural networks (RBFNs) in which case Eq. (25) becomes:

$$\hat{y}_k(x_i, w) = \phi_0\left(\alpha_k + \sum_{h=1}^{H} w_{hk}\varphi_h\left(\| x_{ij} - c_j \|\right)\right), \tag{44}$$

where c_j are the centres of the J localized Radially symmetric Basis Functions (RBFs), $\|x_{ij} - c_j\|$ is the Euclidian distance and the Gaussian transform is adopted for ϕ_0.

Ripley (1996) proposed an RBF neural network for the prediction of survival in breast cancer with a single event of interest. Boracchi et al. (2001) developed a RBFN approach for the joint modelling of cause-specific hazards as a function of several continuous and discrete covariates within the framework of competing risks. The RBFN approach for competing risks was applied on a dataset of 2233 breast cancer patients (Veronesi et al., 1995). The results obtained for competing risks have confirmed that the RBFNs provide flexible non-additive parameterization regression model for joint modelling of cause-specific hazard functions, which can provide additional information on the disease dynamics than the standard Cox regression models. Non-linear and time-dependence effects of clinical relevance were identified for the covariates (number of metastatic axillary nodes, histology, tumour site) with effect on the competing risks of interest (intra-breast tumour recurrence and distant metastases) which were not identified with other existing regression models.

Other machine learning techniques (Etchells and Lisboa, 2003) have been applied to survival analysis in breast cancer. Wolberg et al. (1993, 1994) used decision trees for breast cancer prognosis while Mangarisan et al. (1995) have applied linear programming-based machine learning techniques to improve the accuracy of breast cancer prognosis on a dataset of 569 patients from the University of Wisconsin Hospital. Choong et al. (1996) and Pantel (1998) have applied entropy maximization networks for survival prediction in breast cancer.

We should also mention the cubic spline interpolation data which although does not belong to the class of neural networks, it provides a powerful tool for smoothing of the hazard function (Kooperberg et al., 1995; Kooperberg and Clarkson, 1997) or the cause-specific hazard functions, as a joint function of time and of discrete and continuous covariates.

Boracchi et al. (2003) applied cubic splines with truncated power (TP) bases (Eubank, 1984) to study the effect of different prognostic factors on the cause-specific hazard functions for intra-breast tumour recurrences and distant metastases from a case series of 2233 breast cancer patients who underwent conservative surgery at the Milan Cancer Institute between 1970 and 1987 (Veronesi et al., 1995). Their method consisted of two steps: first, the exploration of the cause-specific hazard functions was jointly conducted without allowing for covariate effects and the estimates of cumulative Cause Specific Hazards (CSHs) show similarity with the Aelen–Nelson non-parametric estimates. At the next step, covariates were introduced in the model and the analyses were carried out again.

5.1. Model selection with the neural network

The Bayesian framework can be utilized to carry out model selection once the PLANN parameters have been estimated with ARD regularization to soft-prune irrelevant variables in the model. From previous studies with PLANN-ARD, it was shown that careful identification of the explanatory variables is the single major determinant of the accuracy and generality of predictive models.

In this study, model selection is carried out with a time step of one month. Once a preferred model is established, the predictive modelling is carried out. The results obtained with PLANN-ARD are obtained by cross-validation so that, for each individual, they represent an out-of-sample prediction. A five-fold cross-validation was used during the training/testing of PLANN-ARD with the node-negative cohort.

The evidence in support of a particular model hypothesis H requires a third level in the ARD methodology, beyond the estimation of the evidence for the weight parameters and regularization of hyperparameters by using Bayes theorem

$$P(H \mid D) = \frac{P(D \mid H)P(H)}{P(D)} \tag{45}$$

Assuming a flat prior for the space of possible models, considered here as the available set of explanatory variables, the evidence for a particular model selection is given by

$$P(H \mid D) \propto P(D \mid H) = \int P(D \mid \alpha, H)P(\alpha \mid H)d\alpha \tag{46}$$

which is the analytical expression for the normalizing constant in the evidence for the hyperparameters, just as its numerator required an estimation of the denominator in the evidence calculation for the weights, Eq. (37).

Assuming a log-normal distribution for the hyperparameter priors $P(\alpha|H)$, the variance of the distribution of $\log(\alpha_m)$~$2/\gamma_m$ (Bishop, 1995). Approximating the integral in Eq. (46)

by its mode multiplied by the width of the prior, we obtain an analytical approximation to the evidence in support of candidate PLANN model, given by

$$\log(P(D\,|\,H)) \approx -S(w^{\mathrm{MP}}, \alpha) - \frac{1}{2}\log(\det(A)) + \frac{1}{2}\sum_{m=1}^{N_\alpha}(N_m \log(\alpha_m)) + \frac{1}{2}\sum_{m=1}^{N_\alpha}\log\left(\frac{2}{\gamma_m}\right) + \frac{N_\alpha}{2}\log(2\pi) + \log\left(N_h!N_h^2\right) \tag{47}$$

The evidence is calculated using the most probable values of the network outputs. The accurate evaluation of the evidence can be difficult on real examples. Since the Hessian matrix is given by the product of the eigenvalues, the determinant of the Hessian, which measures the volume of the posterior distribution, will be dominated by the small eigenvalues. These small values correspond to directions in which the distribution is relatively broad. Some approaches to avoid such problems are presented in Bishop (1995). For example, the calculation of α depends on the sum of the eigenvalues and so is less sensitive to errors in the small eigenvalues.

In this chapter, for the input variables with prognostic significance, the hyperparameters α are lower in size while for the less important input variables, the hyperparameters have higher values. The model selection to be performed herein is based on the values of the hyperparameters.

5.2. Marginalization of the network predictions in the Bayesian neural networks

In survival modelling, the distribution of the binary indicator label, or target, is heavily skewed due to scarcity of events and the large number of time steps used in the analysis. Skewed target distributions need to be regularized to equal numbers of "zeros" and "ones". Moreover, the posterior distribution for the network parameters in the Bayesian framework requires a modulation of the network outputs towards what is called the guessing line in the Receiver Operating Characteristic framework, which corresponds to assigning the output to the prevalence (MacKay, 1995; Lisboa, 2002) when the weights have large error bars. For the PLANN-ARD with a single output and sigmoid activation function, the marginalization of the network predictions was applied for a breast cancer dataset of 1616 female patients, which was used as training/test data for the PLANN-ARD (Wong, 2001; Lisboa et al., 2003).

The predicted hazard is the mean calculated from the distribution of the activation $a(.)$ which is the argument of the exponential in the right-hand side of Eq. (31), $h(x, t) = g(a)$, giving

$$h_g(x,t) = \int g(a)P(a\,|\,x_p,t,D)da \tag{48}$$

In this expression, D represents the target distribution contained in the training data. This integral is not analytical, but it can be evaluated when the activation is expanded as a linear function of the weights

$$a^*(x_p,t,w) \approx a^{\mathrm{MP}}(x,t,w) + g^{\mathrm{T}}(x_p,t,w^{\mathrm{MP}})\,(w - w^{\mathrm{MP}}) \tag{49}$$

The distribution of the activation is found by integrating over the posterior distribution for the weights, Eq. (36), using the Taylor expansion of the objective function, Eq. (38), variance s^2 (Bishop, 1995), resulting in

$$P(a \mid x_p, t, D) \propto \exp\left(-\frac{\left(a - a^{\mathrm{MP}}\right)^2}{2g^{\mathrm{T}} A^{-1} g} \right) \tag{50}$$

Having obtained the variance of the activation values, the predicted hazards is now well approximated (Bishop, 1995) by

$$h_g(x,t) \approx g\left(\frac{a^{\mathrm{MP}}(x,t)}{\sqrt{1 + (\pi/8) g^{\mathrm{T}} A^{-1} g}} \right) \tag{51}$$

Therefore, the inherent uncertainty in the network predictions may be described by marginalizing over the activation and thus moderating the network output towards the guessing line. However, $h_g(\cdot) \to_{s \to o} 1/2$, therefore, the prevalence of the binary targets assumed in Eq. (48) is 50%.

In order to update the standard regularization framework to take account of the prevalence $P_d = P(d_{pk} = 1)$ by re-scaling the log-likelihood, together with the calculation of the gradient and the Hessian (Lisboa et al., 2003) as follows:

$$E = -\sum_{p=1}^{\text{no. of patients}} \sum_{k=1}^{t} \left\{ \frac{1}{2P_d} d_{pk} \log h_p(x_i, t_k) + \frac{1}{2(1-P_d)} (1 - d_{pk}) \log\left(1 - \log h_p(x_i, t_k)\right) \right\} \tag{52}$$

and compensating the resulting marginalized network prediction $\tilde{h}_g(x_p, t)$

$$h_g(x_p, t) = \frac{\tilde{h}_g(x_p, t) P_d}{\tilde{h}_g(x_p, t) P_d + (1 - \tilde{h}_g(x_p, t))(1 - P_d)} \tag{53}$$

6. DATA DESCRIPTION

In this section, two datasets, previously reported in Wong (2001), Lisboa et al. (2003) and Jarman and Lisboa (2004), are discussed in order to illustrate the reviewed techniques on node-negative breast cancer patients. The selection criteria in our study is tumour stage either 1 or 2, TNM node stage N0, number of node involved 1 and metastasis stage 0 which corresponds to node-negative breast cancer patients.

The first dataset consists of 917 records (Lisboa et al., 2003) referred to Manchester Christie Hospital between 1983 and 1989. The event of interest is defined to be death attributed to breast cancer and other causes of death and losses to follow-up were regarded as censorship. All surviving patients were censored after 5 years. The selection criterion is tumour stage either 1 or 2, node stage 0, number of nodes involved 1 or 5 (unknown) and metastasis stage 0. This selection criterion reduced the initial dataset to 615 patients. The distribution of patients with respect to the number of nodes involved is 164 patients in group 1 and 451 in group 5.

The second dataset in this study consists of the records of a low-risk group of 932 female patients referred to the Manchester Christie Hospital between 1990 and 1993. The same as the previous dataset, this is a 5-year study from the date of surgery, the event of interest is again defined to be death attributed to breast cancer with all other causes of death and losses to follow-up being regarded as censorship, and all surviving patients were censored after 5 years. The same selection criterion is applied consisting of tumour stage either 1 or 2, node stage 0, metastasis stage 0 and number of nodes involved 1 or 5 which resulted in a dataset of 588 female patients. There were 408 patients with the number of nodes involved in group 1 and 180 patients with the number of nodes involved unknown.

The two datasets were collected at the same hospital during different time intervals. Besides the performances of the reviewed ANNs and semiparametric regression techniques in terms of the accuracy of the estimated hazard rate and survivorship function, there is also interest in exploring any changes in the dependence of the hazard rate and survivorship function on the key prognostic factors in relation to the different times when the two datasets were gathered at the same hospital on the same type of node-negative breast cancer patients. Examples of such changes might be found in the treatment options for patients with similar pathological characteristics due to the introduction of breast cancer screening programmes and early detection of disease or advances in prevention and treatment of breast cancer (Fisher et al., 2001a,b).

The 18 categorical variables that describe the two datasets are summarized in Table 1. For the model selection there were records with missing variables. Previous analysis on these datasets suggested that missing variables might be informative. Therefore, any missing values in the 18 categories were coded as a separate attribute (variables affected – pathological size, nodes involved, nodes ratio, histology and ER status).

7. NODE-NEGATIVE BREAST CANCER PROGNOSIS

The Cox regression model was implemented in SPSS (SPSS, 1999) with stepwise model selection using the Akaike Information Criterion (AIC) (Collett, 1994). This procedure begins by searching for the most significant univariate model. At any stage in the selection process, each remaining variable is added to the model and the most significant multivariate model is selected. Each variable is then dropped from the model, in turn, to test whether there is evidence that any of the existing variables has become redundant. The procedure then continues by iteration, using a significance measure based on

$$\mathrm{AIC} = -2\log(\hat{L}) + \alpha N_{\beta}, \tag{54}$$

where $\hat{L}$ is the optimized log-likelihood function for the proportional hazards model, N_{β} the number of degrees of freedom which is the same as the number of attributes excluding those for the baseline population and α is a predetermined constant that took the

Table 1. Variables recorded in two UK national breast cancer datasets

Variable	Categories	Coded attributes
Menopausal status	Pre-menopausal	1
	Peri-menopausal	2
	Post-menopausal	3
Age group	20–39	1
	40–59	2
	60+	3
Predominant site	Upper outer	1
	Lower outer	2
	Upper inner	3
	Lower inner	4
	Subareolar	5
Side	Right	1
	Left	2
Maximum tumour diameter (cm)	<2	1
	2–5	2
	5+	3
	Unknown	9
Clinical stage tumour	T0 (No tumour)	0
	T1 (Tumour <2 cm)	1
	T2 (2–5 cm)	2
	T3 (5+ cm)	3
	T4 (any size but fixed on the rib cage)	4
Clinical stage nodes	N0 (no nodes found clinically, or node negative by histology)	0
	N1 (ipsilateral and mobile axillary nodes)	1
	N2 (nodes fixed)	2
	N3 (nodes fixed and cannot be removed)	3
Clinical stage metastasis	M0 (no distant metastasis)	0
	M1 (positive)	1
Clinical stage (TNM)	0	1
	1	2
	2	3
	3	4
	4	5
Radiotherapy	No	1
	Yes	2
Histology	Infiltrating ductal	1
	Infiltrating lobular	2

Table 1. cont'd

Variable	Categories	Coded attributes
	In situ/mixed/medullary/ucoid/ papillary/tubular/other mixed in situ	3
	Unknown	9
Surgery	None	1
	Incision biopsy	2
	Excision biopsy	3
	Simple mastectomy	4
	Radical mastectomy	5
	Wide local excision and axillary clearance	6
	Radial mast and axillary clearance	7
	Surgery after neo adjuvant chemotherapy	8
	Not known	9
Number of nodes involved	0	1
	1–3	2
	4+	3
	98 (too many to count)	4
	Unknown	5
Adjuvant treatment	None	1
	Chemotherapy (CMF)	2
	Melphalan (MELPH)	3
	Tamoxifen (TAM)	4
	XRAM	5
	OOPH	6
	Cyclo-phosphamide (CYCLO)	7
	TAM + CYC	8
	TAM + PRED	9
	ZOLADEX	10
	TAM + ZOL	11
	Megestrol acetate (MEGACE)	12
	ZOL + TAM + CMF	13
	NEO ADJ-PRE SURG	14
	CMF + TAM	15
	FAC chemotherapy	16
Number of nodes removed	0–9	1
	10–19	2
	20+	3

Continued

Table 1. cont'd

Variable	Categories	Coded attributes
	98 (too many to count)	4
	Unknown	5
Node ratio (%)	0–20	1
	20–40	2
	40–60	3
	60+	4
	Unknown	5
Pathological size (cm)	<2	1
	2–5	2
	5+	3
	Unknown	4
ER status (oestrogen level)	0–10	1
	10+	2
	8888 (high positive value)	3
	Unknown	4

recommended value of 3 which is roughly equivalent to a 5% significance level to distinguish between nested models with few variables (Collett, 1994). This parameter may be adjusted upwards if the resulting models are judged to generalize poorly.

The model for the first dataset comprised three variables with a total of six degrees of freedom, namely, histology, pathological size and oestrogen. In Fig. 1, the prognostic group with the lowest survival is denoted first followed in order by the prognostic groups with higher survival. This notation is hold throughout the chapter.

There are 369 patients in the prognostic group 1 and 246 patients in the prognostic group 2. The Kaplan–Meier curve is also shown for the two prognostic groups. The attribute histograms are of interest for PI1 and PI2 and they are shown in Fig. 2.

The comparison of attribute profile of risk group PI2 with risk group PI1, shows that patients with histology attribute 1 (infiltrating ductal carcinoma) and pathological size 2 (2–5 cm) have smaller 5-year survivorship than patients with histology attribute 2 (infiltrating lobular carcinoma) or histology attribute 3 (in situ and mixed/medullary/tubular micro invasive carcinoma) and pathological size 1 (0–2 cm).

The attribute profile of 12 variables (menopausal status, age group, side of tumour, tumour diameter, predominant site, histology, pathological size, number of nodes involved, numbed of nodes removed, nodes ratio and oestrogen) is shown in Fig. 3 for risk groups PI1 and PI2. The differences between the two prognostic groups are mainly from histology, pathological size and oestrogen factor.

The adjuvant treatment, surgery and radiotherapy received by the node-negative patients from the two risk groups are shown in Fig. 4. The attributes for adjuvant treatment corresponds to the first 11 attribute from Table 1: 1 – no treatment, 2 – CMF, 3 – MELPH, 4 – TAM, 5 – XRAM, 6 – OOPH, 7 – CYCLO, 8 – TAM + CYC, 9 – TAM + PRED, 10 – ZOLADEX, 11 – TAM + ZOL, 12 – MEGACE, 13 –ZOL + TAM + CMF, 14 – NEO ADJ-PRE SURG, 15 – CMF + TAM, 16 – FAC.

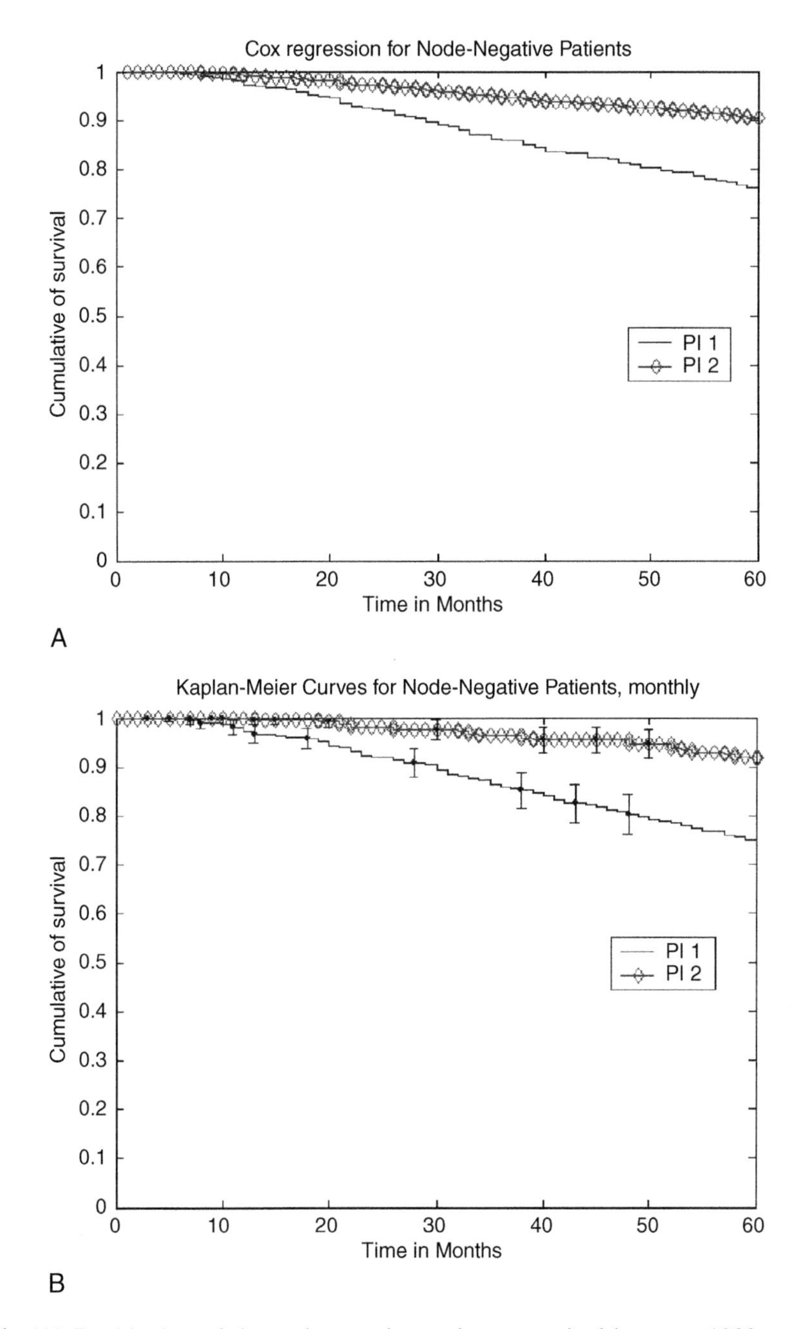

Fig. 1. (A) Partitioning of the node-negative patients recruited between 1983 and 1989 using Cox regression and log-rank test into two prognostic groups, with 369 patients in the prognostic group 1 and 246 patients in the prognostic group 2, respectively and (B) the corresponding grouped Kaplan–Meier curves.

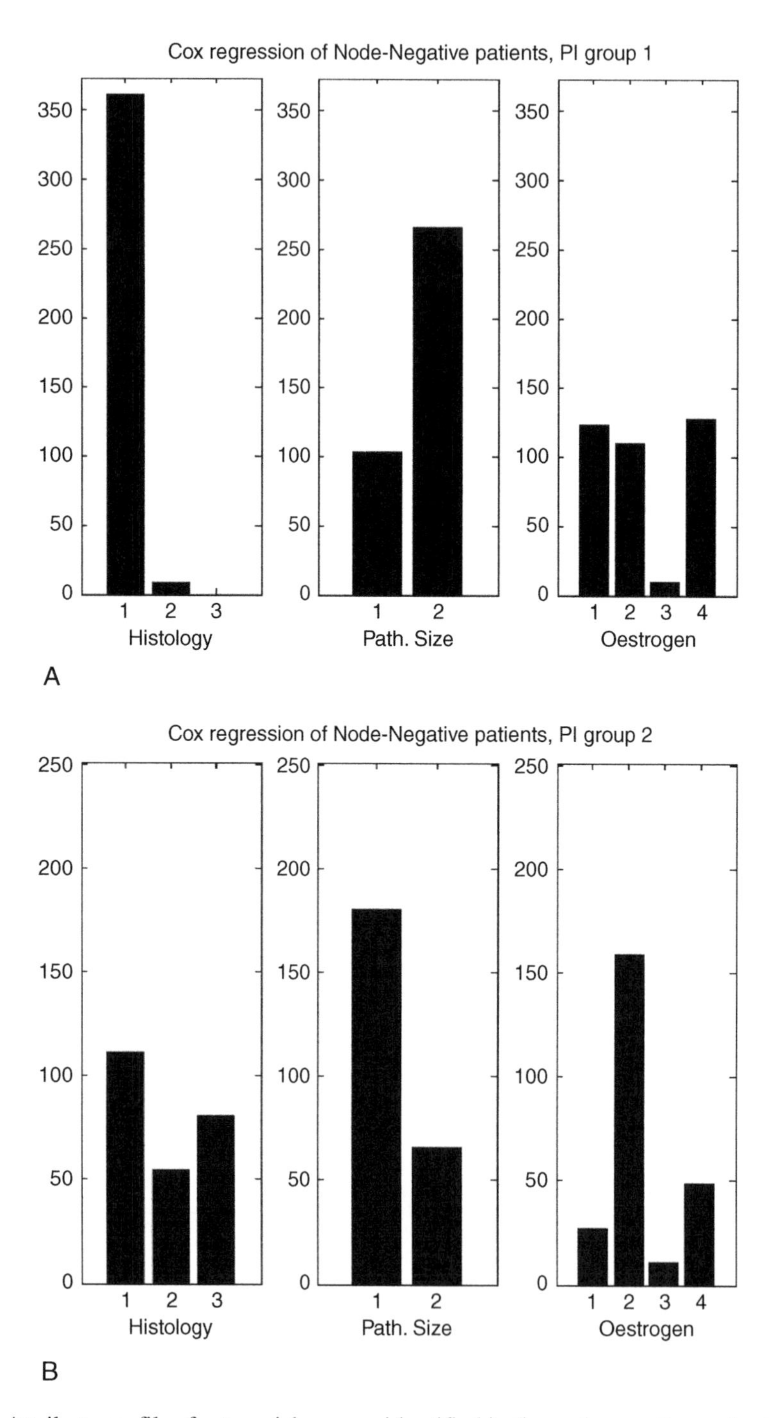

Fig. 2. Attribute profiles for two risk groups identified in the node-negative patients by the proportional hazards model for the dataset collected between 1983 and 1989.

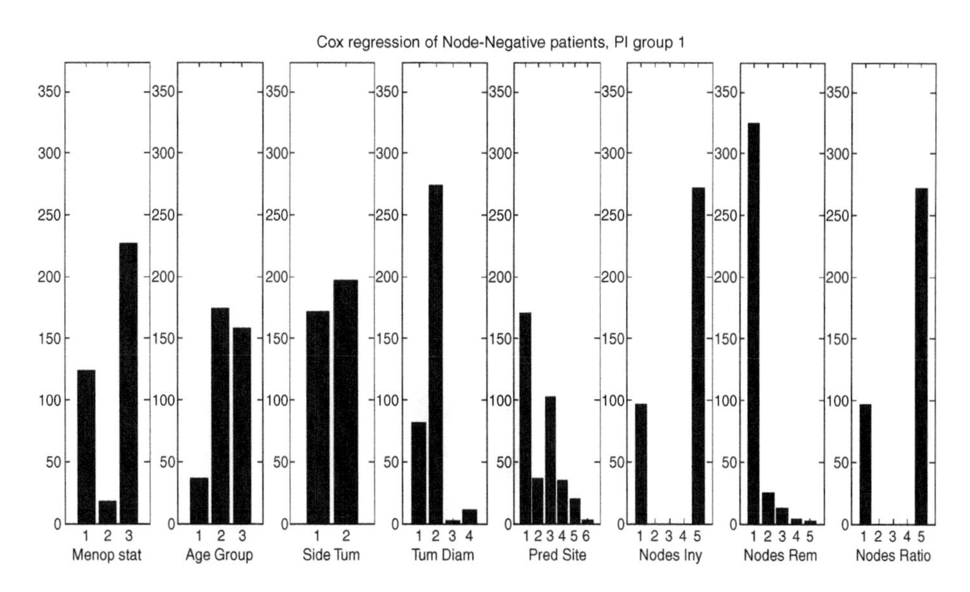

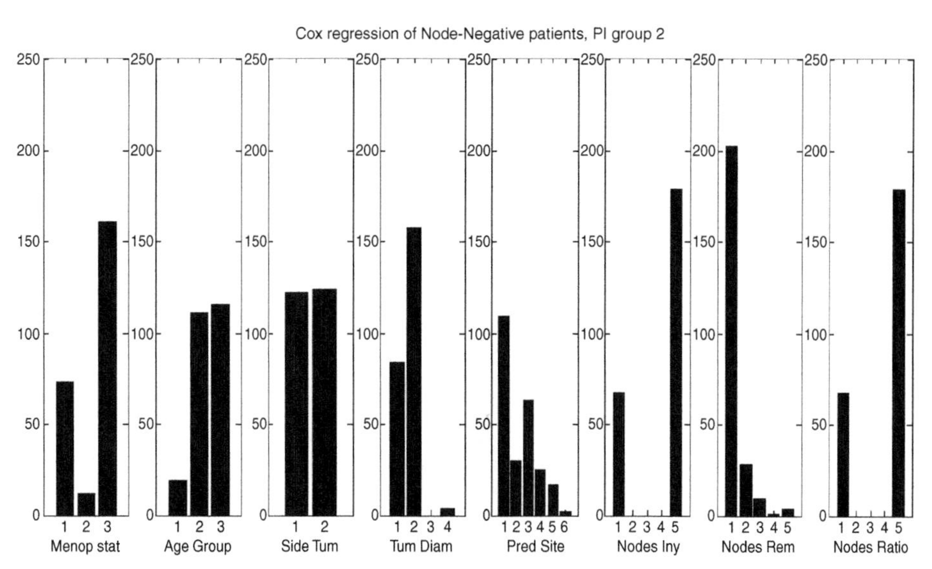

Fig. 3. The complete attribute profiles for two risk groups identified in the node-negative patients by the proportional hazards model for the dataset collected between 1983 and 1989.

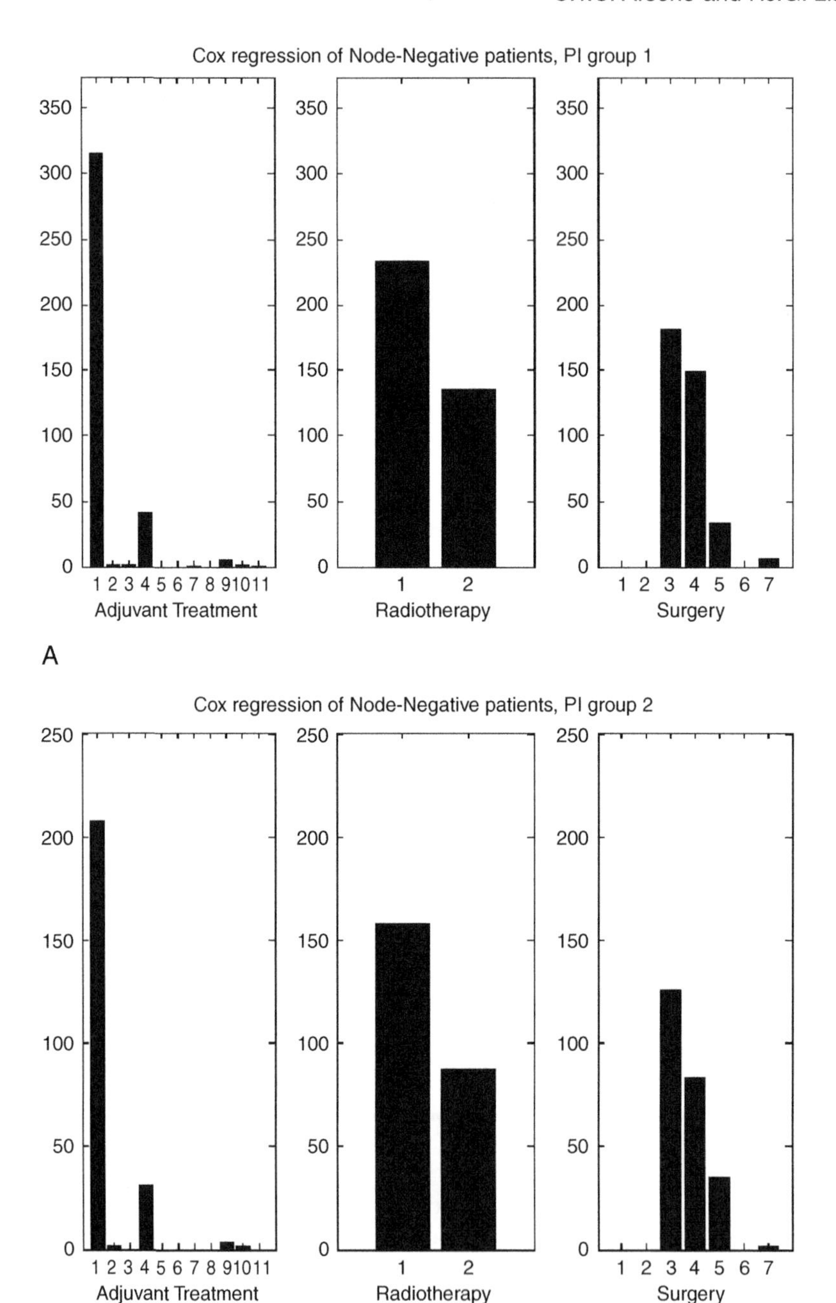

Fig. 4. Attribute profiles for adjuvant treatment, radiotherapy and surgery for two risk groups (A, B) identified in the node-negative patients by the proportional hazards model for the dataset collected between 1983 and 1989.

The model for the second dataset of 588 female patients comprises three variables, namely, histology, pathological size and number of nodes involved.

There is a similarity between the variables selected for this dataset with AIC and the ones selected for the dataset 1990 and 1993. The difference is made by the number of nodes involved instead of oestrogen factor. Three risk groups (risk group PI1 – 11 patients, risk group PI2 – 160 patients, risk group PI3 – 417 patients) have been identified from the prognostic index $\beta^T x_p$ with the log-rank test, and the corresponding survivorship functions are shown in Fig. 5B. There is a good match between predicted and observed survivorship shown in Fig. 5(A and B). The attribute histogram for these three risk groups is shown in Fig. 6.

The attribute histograms show a pathological pattern which is strongly correlated with the histological grade: patients from PI1 risk group with histological grade 1 (infiltrating ductal carcinoma), pathological size 2 and number of nodes involved unknown have lower 5-year survivorship. There are 160 patients in the PI2 risk group who have pathological size 1 and number of nodes involved unknown or pathological size 2 and number of nodes involved 1. There are 190 patients in the PI3 risk group with infiltrating ductal carcinoma who had pathological size 1 and number of nodes involved 1. The remaining 227 patients from the PI3 risk group have infiltrating lobular carcinoma or in situ/mixed/medullary/tubular micro invasive carcinoma with pathological size 1.

In comparison with the dataset from Manchester Christie hospital gathered between 1983 and 1989, it can be observed that the patients from the risk groups PI2 and PI3 in the dataset collected between 1990 and 1993 (Fig. 5) have higher survivorship than the patients from the risk groups PI1 and PI2 in the dataset gathered between 1983 and 1989 (Fig. 1).

Figure 7 suggests a relationship between the hormone receptor status (oestrogen variable) and hormone therapy. Medical doctors take the decision of whether to recommend adjuvant hormone therapy based on the presence of hormone receptors, as assessed by immunohistochemical staining of breast cancer tissue. Hormone therapy seeks to prevent breast cancer cells from receiving stimulation from oestrogen. Such stimulation occurs primarily in tumours that contain hormone receptor protein, so tumours that contain this protein may respond to hormone therapy. Depriving the breast cancer cells of oestrogen may be achieved by blocking the receptor via the most commonly used hormone therapy, i.e. tamoxifen. It is usually used alone or in combination with chemotherapy.

Adjuvant chemotherapy corresponds to the second column in the adjuvant treatment and hormone therapy to the third column, respectively. The three attributes for radiotherapy are 1 – no radiotherapy, 2 – patients with radiotherapy (identical with adjuvant radiotherapy) and 3 – unknown. By using the Nottingham Prognostic Index (NPI), patients can be allocated into three risk groups with *high*, *medium* and *low* survival, as a function of the value of NPI, that is high survival $NPI < 3.4$, medium survival $3.4 < NPI < 5.4$ and low survival $NPI > 5.4$. Usually patients with NPI score smaller than 3.4 do not need adjuvant chemotherapy, patients with NPI score between 3.4 and 5.4 may benefit from adjuvant chemotherapy and for the low survival group the adjuvant chemotherapy is needed.

The PI2 risk group contains 7 patients out of 160 who received adjuvant chemotherapy while the PI3 group has 4 patients out of 417 patients. This gives 4% of patients in PI2 risk group that received adjuvant chemotherapy compared to 1% of patients in PI3 risk group.

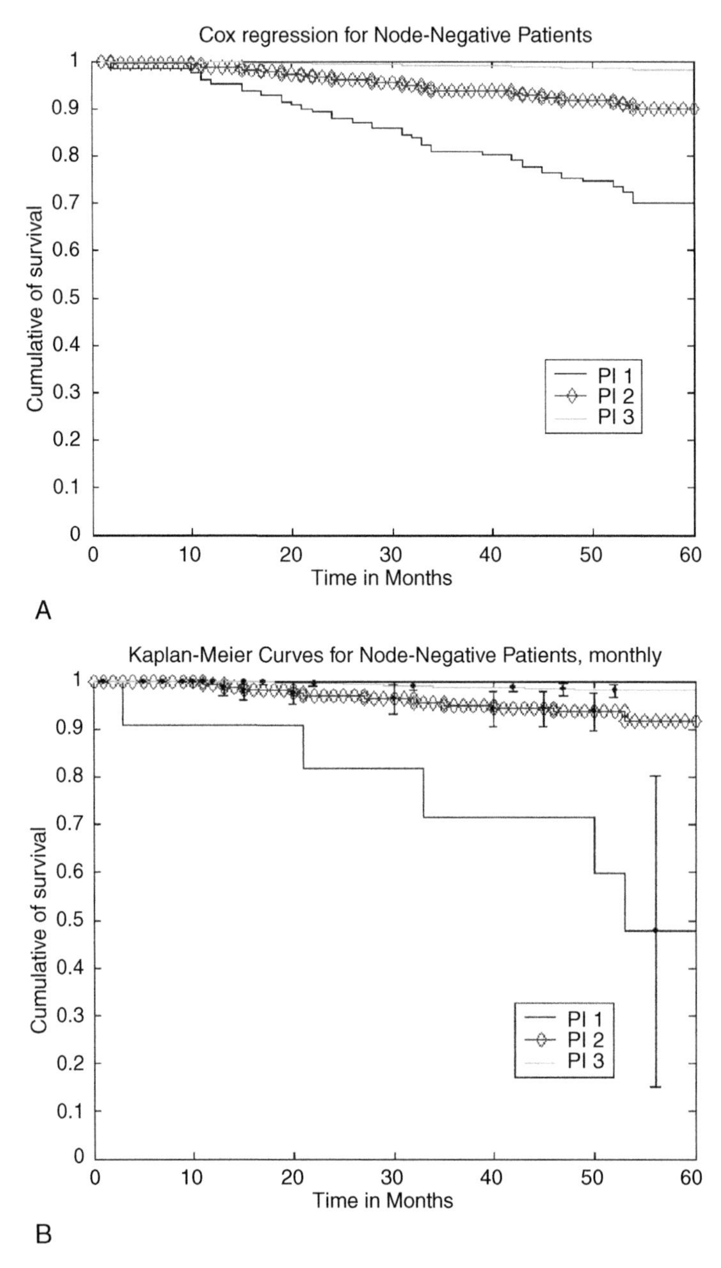

Fig. 5. (A) Partitioning of node-negative patients with log-rank test into three prognostic groups with 417 patients in the prognostic group 3, 160 patients in the prognostic group 2 and 11 patients in the prognostic group 1; (B) the corresponding grouped Kaplan–Meier curves for groups 3 and 2, while group 1 is left out because it comprises a low number of patients (model selection did not include surgery, hormone therapy and adjuvant treatment).

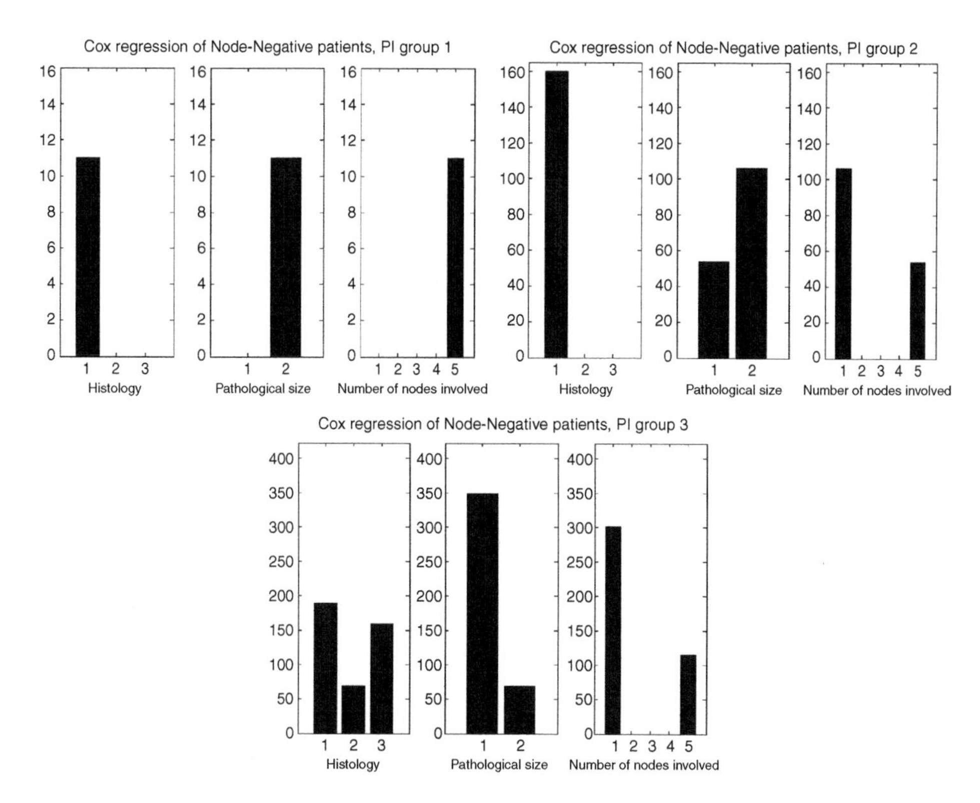

Fig. 6. Attribute profile for risk groups PI1, PI2 and PI3 identified in the node-negative patients by the proportional hazards model and the log-rank test for the dataset 1990–1993.

The question arises whether the 1% patients in PI3 risk group do really need adjuvant chemotherapy or were they over treated.

There are 4 node-negative patients in the risk group PI3 that received adjuvant chemotherapy and have high 5-year survivorship. The contribution of the node-negative patients to the NPI score is 1 which is true for these 4 patients (i.e. Eq. (10)). With regard to the histological grade, one patient had in situ breast cancer and tumour size between 2 and 5 cm (i.e. NPI score equals 3). Two patients had infiltrating lobular carcinoma with NPI score equal to 4 and one patient had infiltrating ductal carcinoma with NPI score equal to 5. The patient with NPI score 3 is in the high survival group for which the adjuvant chemotherapy is usually not needed and was potentially over treated (Desch et al., 1993). This patient had post-menopausal status and was more than 60 years old.

The second question is whether more than 1 patient in the risk group PI1 out of 11 patients would benefit from adjuvant chemotherapy. It is usual that node-negative patients with oestrogen receptor-negative should receive chemotherapy while oestrogen receptor-positive should receive chemotherapy and tamoxifen. All patients in the risk group

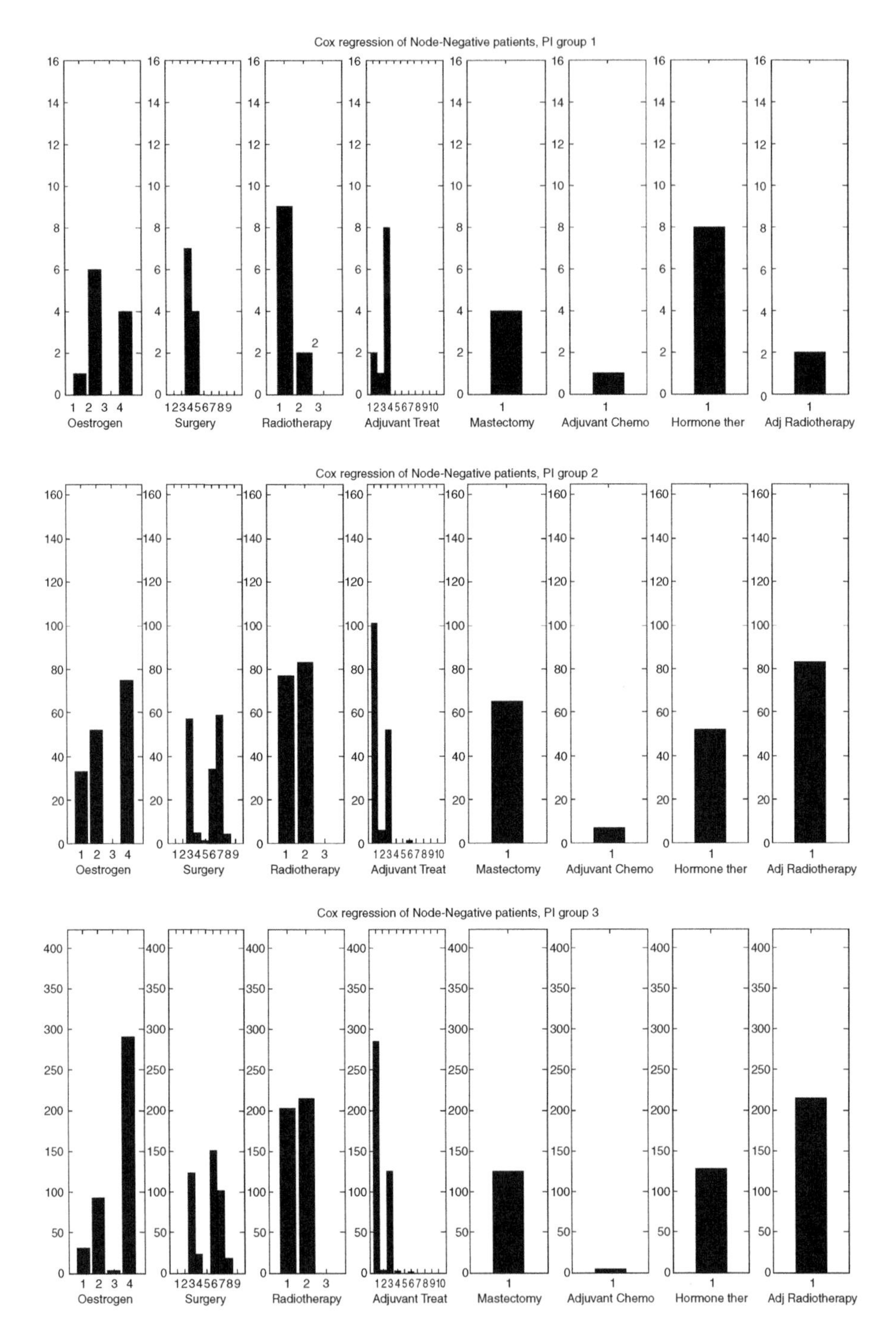

Fig. 7. Attribute profiles for oestrogen, surgery, radiotherapy, adjuvant treatment, mastectomy, adjuvant chemotherapy, hormone therapy and adjuvant radiotherapy for three risk groups identified in the node-negative patients by the proportional hazards model for the dataset collected between 1990 and 1993.

PI1 had infiltrating ductal carcinoma and NPI score equal to 5 which put them in the medium survival group of patients that may benefit from chemotherapy.

Overall there were 9 patients who died before the end of the study period of 5 years. It is worthy of further study to ascertain whether any of these patients might have benefited from adjuvant chemotherapy.

Finally, by inspecting the three risk groups it was observed that patients from within the same risk group and with similar oestrogen factor have received different therapies. This maybe because patients selected from the different choices of disease management or it maybe that these patients have significantly different characteristics of age and menopausal status. It is also possible that the prognostic tools available to the clinicians did not pick out these patients as having a different expected survival from the rest, hence requiring special care.

7.1. PLANN-ARD analysis for node-negative breast cancer prognosis

The variables used by PLANN-ARD for the node-negative patients from the dataset gathered between 1983 and 1989 were histology, pathological size and oestrogen.

In Fig. 8, the survivorship for two prognostic groups with 365 patients in the prognostic group PI1 and 250 patients in the prognostic group PI2 is shown.

There is a good similarity between the patients in the risk groups from Fig. 9 and the results obtained with Cox regression model and shown in Fig. 1.

For the dataset collected between 1990 and 1993 the Cox selected variables are histology, pathological size and number of nodes involved. Three risk groups were obtained with 11 patients in risk group PI1, 188 patients in risk group PI2 and 389 patients in risk group PI3. The survivorship for the three risk groups is shown in Fig. 10.

The attribute histogram for PI1, PI2 and PI3 groups from Fig. 10 are shown in Fig. 11. The characteristics of the attribute profiles obtained with PLANN-ARD resemble the ones shown in Fig. 9. A pathological pattern can be observed comparable with the results from the Cox regression: patients with histology attribute 1 (infiltrating ductal carcinoma), pathological size 2 and positive oestrogen factor (attribute 2) have lower 5-year survivorship than patients with positive or unknown oestrogen factor (attributes 2 and 4) but with histology attribute 2 (infiltrating lobular carcinoma) or histology attribute 3 (in situ and mixed/medullary/tubular micro invasive carcinoma) and pathological size 1.

7.2. Model selection with PLANN-ARD

The model selection is carried out by selecting the input variables with the lowest hyperparameters α_m following the training of PLANN-ARD with a set of input variables.

For the dataset collected between 1983 and 1989, PLANN-ARD was run with 11 variables from Table 1: age, menopausal status, side, tumour diameter, predominant site, histological grade, pathological size, number of nodes involved, number of nodes removed, nodes ratio and oestrogen factor. In Fig. 12, the hyperparameter values during the training of

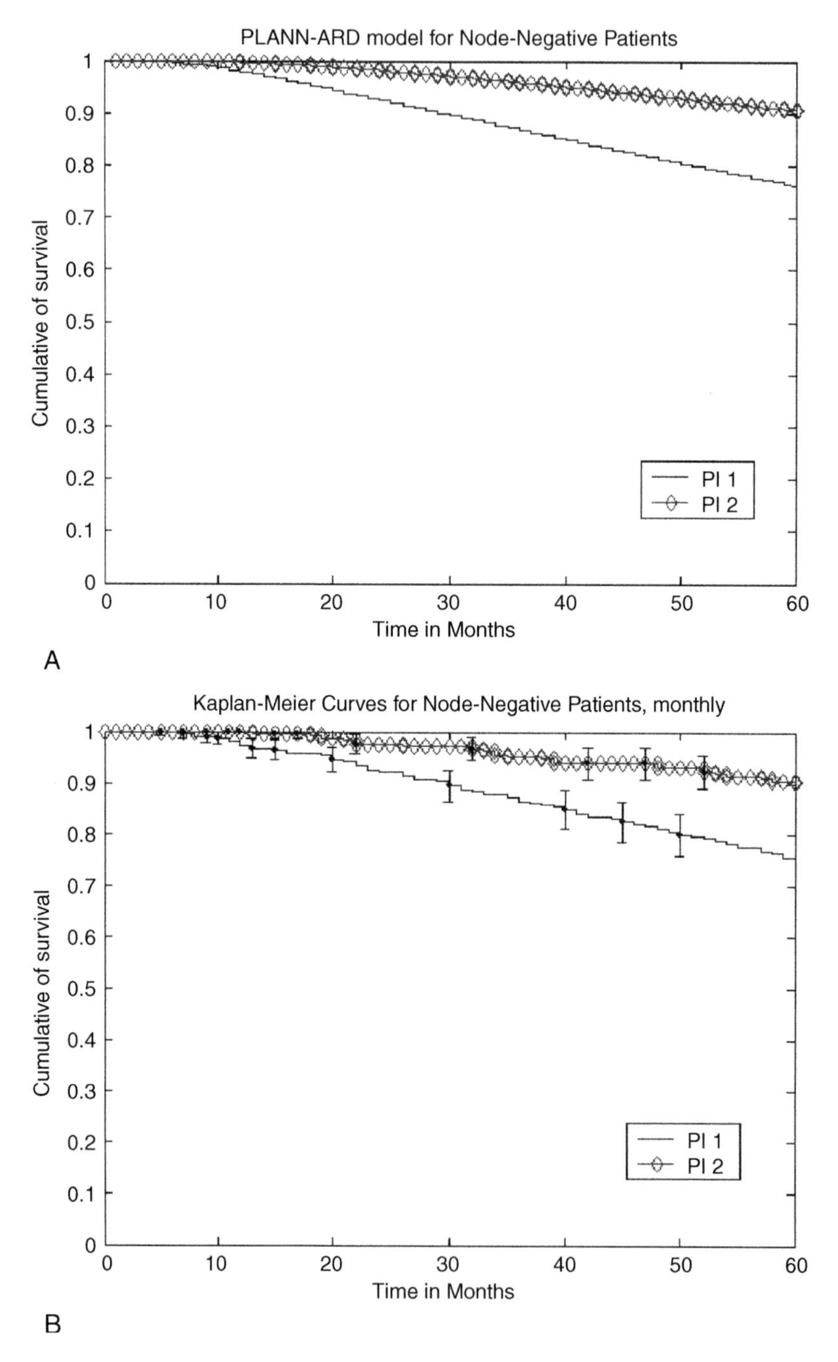

Fig. 8. (A) Partitioning of node-negative patients with log-rank test into two prognostic groups, with 365 patients in the prognostic group 1 and 250 patients in the prognostic group 2 and (B) the corresponding grouped Kaplan–Meier curves for the two risk groups.

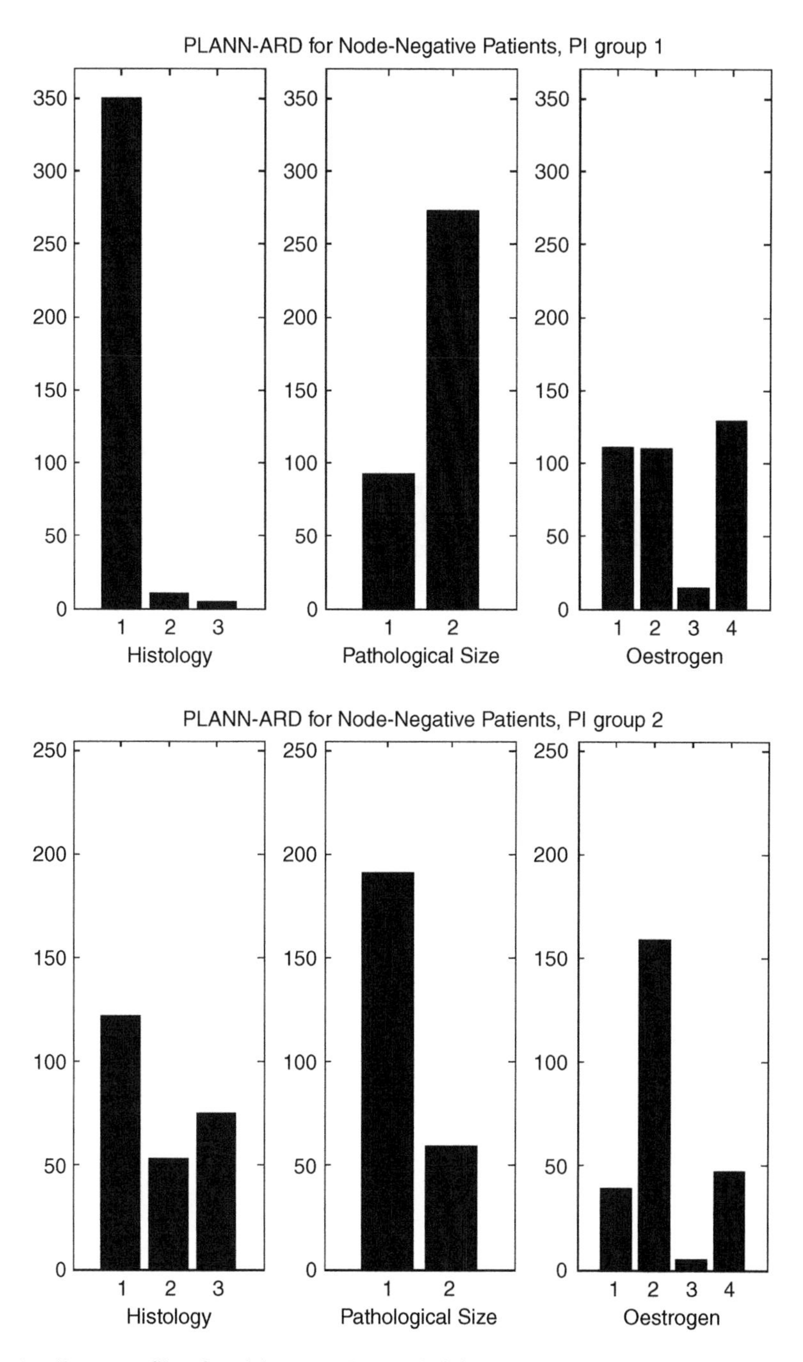

Fig. 9. Attribute profiles for risk group PI1 and risk group PI2 identified in node-negative patients by PLANN-ARD.

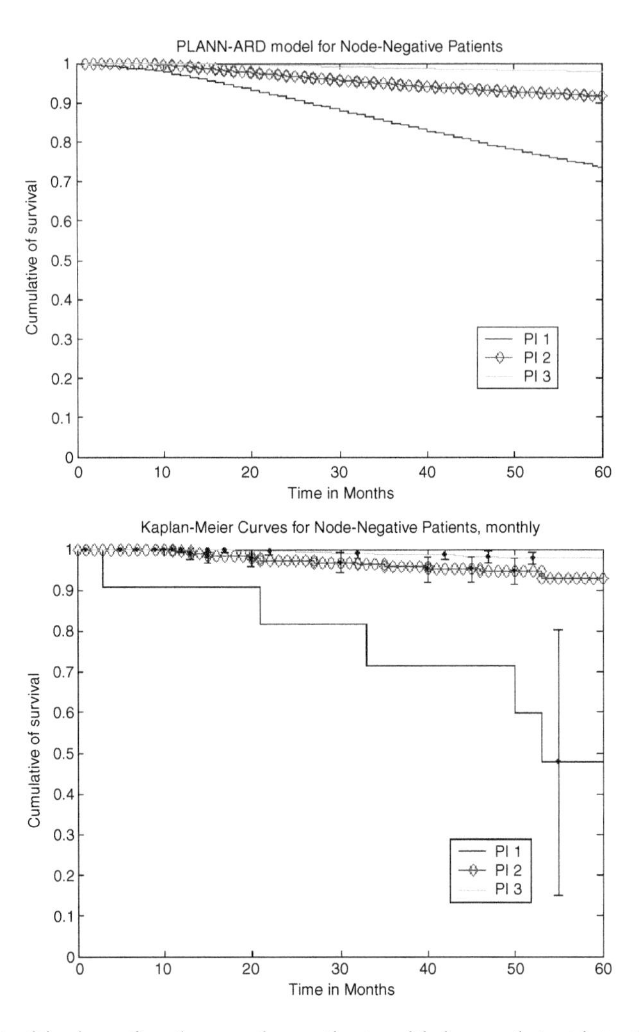

Fig. 10. (A) Partitioning of node-negative patients with log-rank test into three prognostic groups with 11 patients in risk group PI1, 188 patients in risk group PI2 and 389 patients in risk group PI3 and (B) the corresponding grouped Kaplan–Meier curves for the three risk groups.

PLANN-ARD with the 11 input variables from a year-long study are shown. The input variables with the smallest hyperparameters (α_m) are oestrogen factor, pathological size and histological grade. These three variables coincide with the variables from the stepwise model selection and the AIC for the same dataset. In Fig. 13A the survivorship obtained with PLANN-ARD is shown while in Fig. 13B the corresponding Kaplan–Meier curve

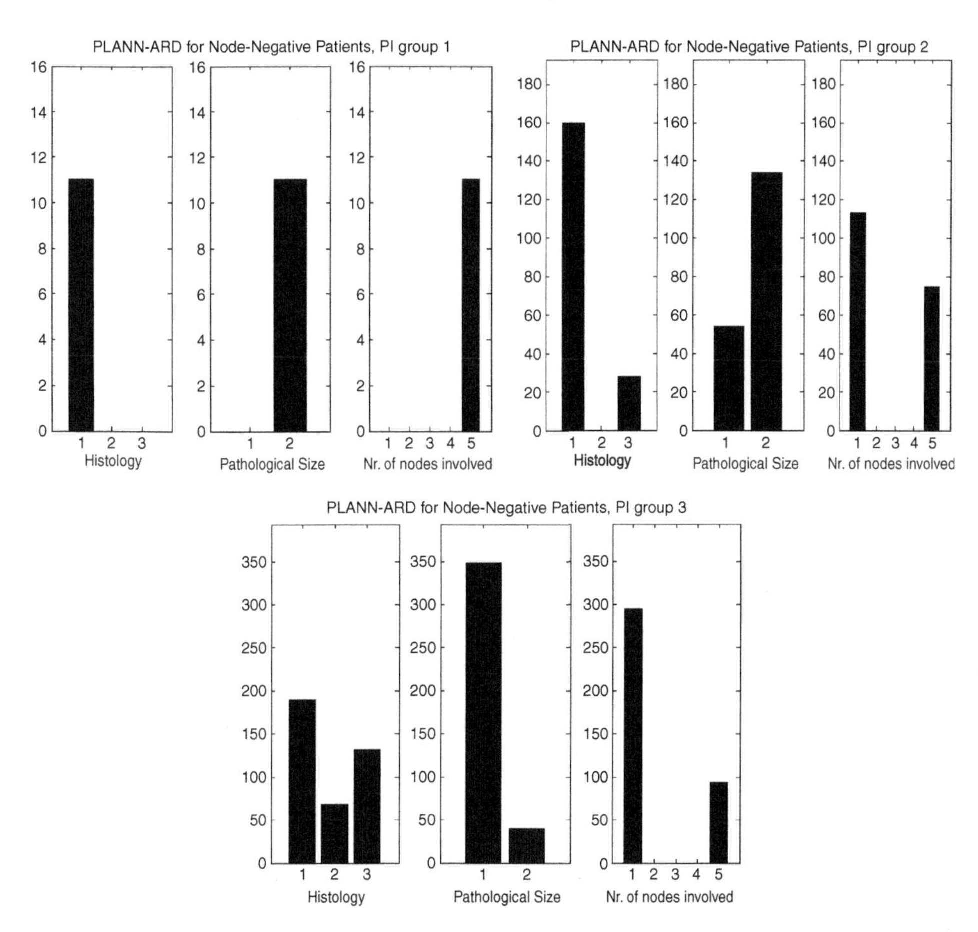

Fig. 11. Attribute profiles for risk group PI1, risk group PI2 and risk group PI3 identified in node-negative patients by PLANN-ARD.

is shown. The two curves show good similarity which proves the prognostic ability of PLANN-ARD.

The second dataset is used for training PLANN-ARD with similar input variables like the first dataset and also on a yearly study. The hyperparameter values are shown in Fig. 14. The model selection based on the hyperparameter values indicated the following input variables as variables with prognostic significance: pathological size, histological grade, oestrogen factor, menopausal status and number of nodes involved. The oestrogen factor and the menopausal status are variables which were not selected with the AIC during the Cox regression procedure. Figure 15A shows the survivorship obtained with PLANN-ARD while Fig. 15B shows the corresponding Kaplan–Meier curve. Following this, the PLANN-ARD model has been trained with the above-mentioned 5 selected variables and for a monthly study.

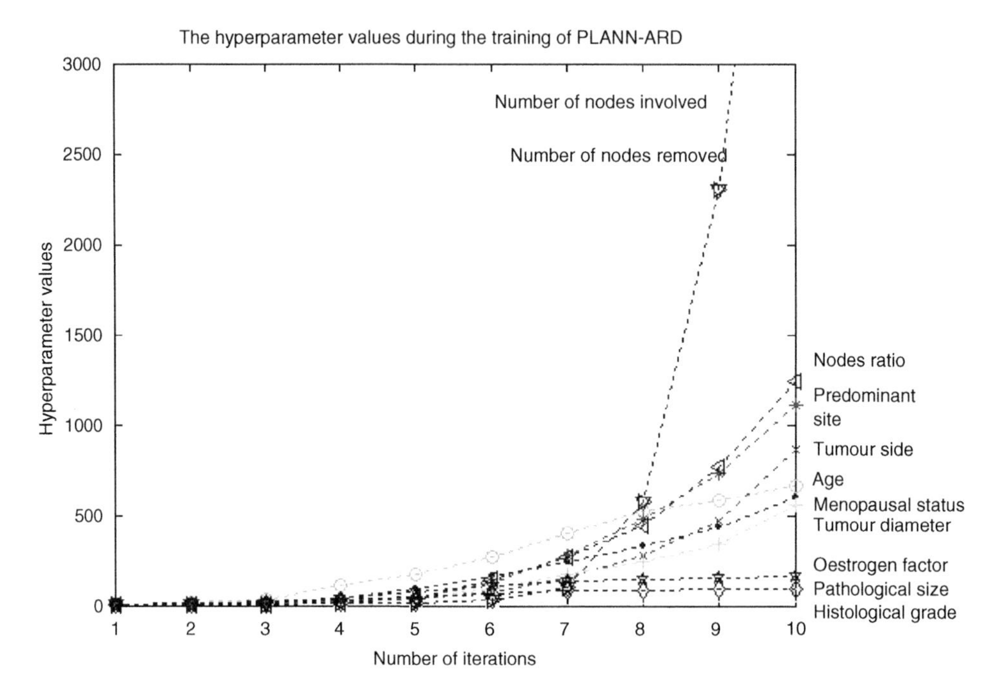

Fig. 12. The hyperparameter values during PLANN-ARD training.

With the five PLANN-ARD selected variables, three risk groups were obtained for the second dataset with the following patient distribution: 5 patients in risk group PI1, 226 patients in risk group PI2 and 357 patients in risk group PI3. The survivorship for the three risk groups is shown in Fig. 16A, while in Fig. 16B the corresponding Kaplan–Meier curves with confidence intervals are shown.

The attribute histogram for the three risk groups is shown in Fig. 17 and it displays a similar pathological pattern with the attribute histogram obtained with the Cox regression model and the PLANN-ARD model using the Cox-selected variables. In addition, the oestrogen factor has a well-differentiated pattern amongst the three risk groups.

The model selection performed with PLANN-ARD for this second dataset picked up three variables which are the same as the ones selected with the AIC: histology, pathological size and number of nodes involved. The inclusion of oestrogen factor by PLANN-ARD as a variable with prognostic importance seems to be justified by the attribute histograms shown in Fig. 17. Finally, from the five selected variables the hyperparameter value for the menopausal status was the highest which is the case of a variable with a less prognostic significance and it is sustained by the previous attribute histogram.

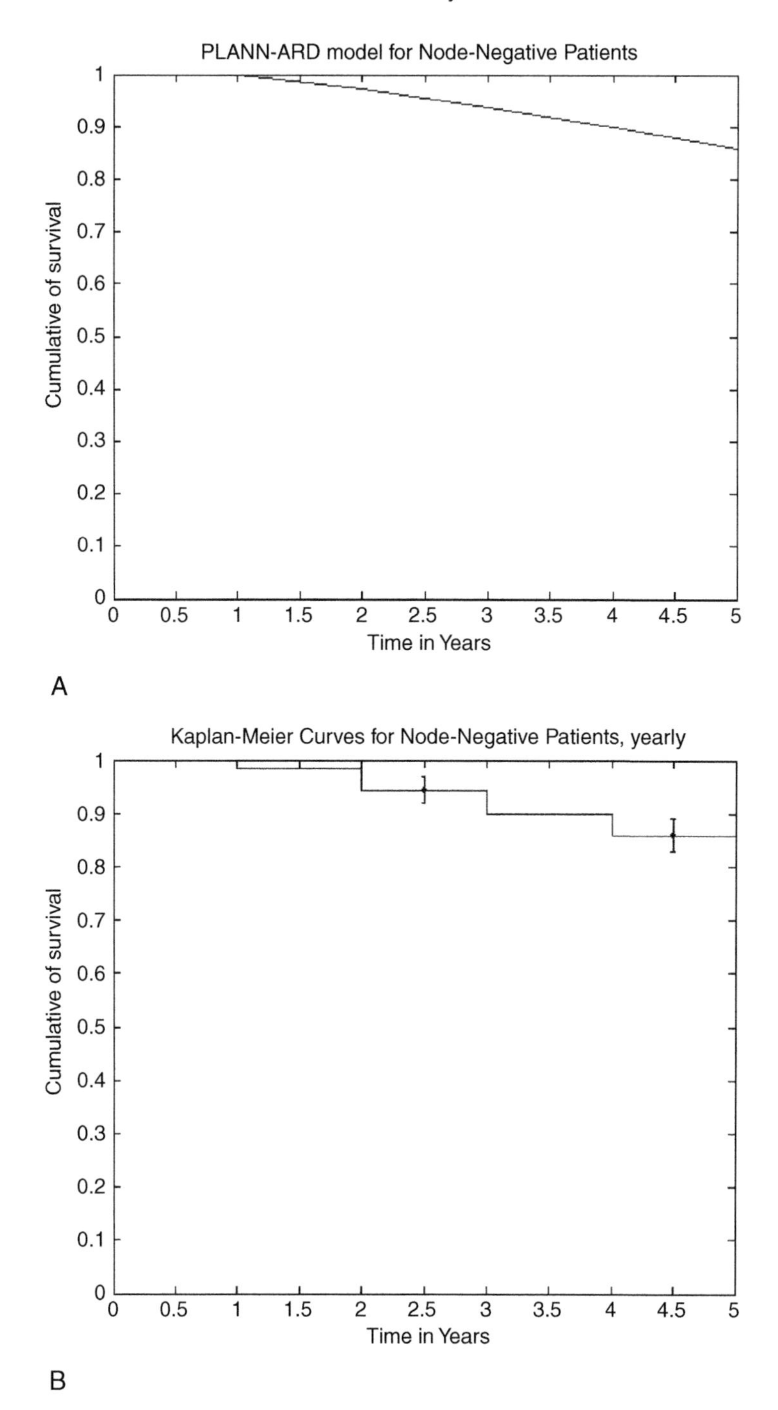

Fig. 13. (A) PLANN-ARD calculated survivorship for a dataset of 615 node-negative breast cancer patients and (B) the corresponding Kaplan–Meier curve.

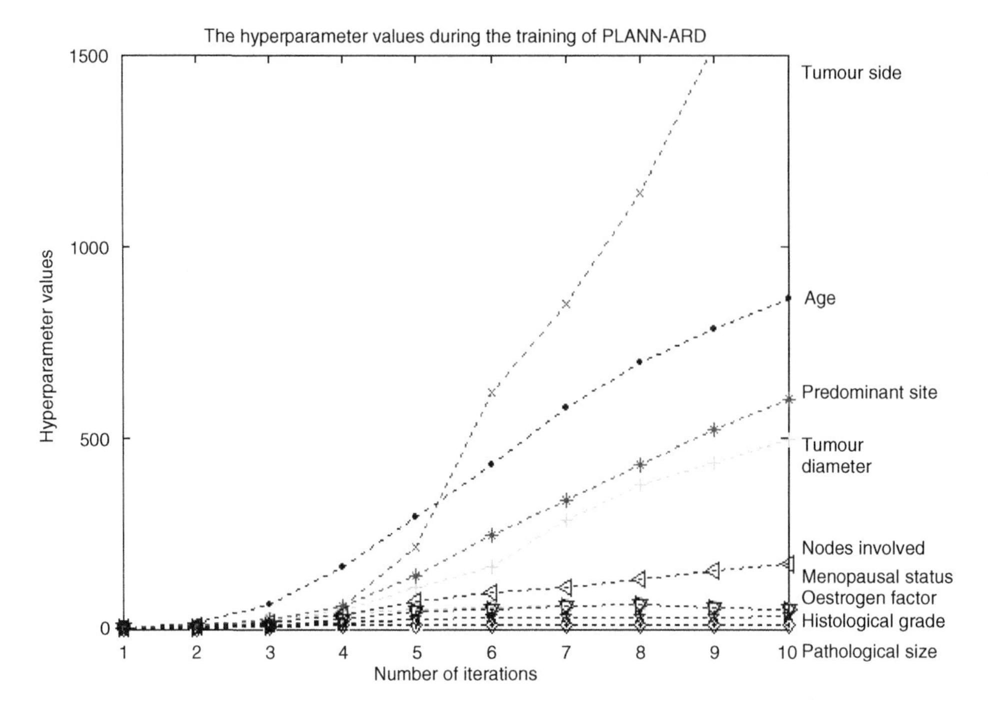

Fig. 14. The hyperparameter values during PLANN-ARD training.

8. CONCLUSIONS

A Bayesian framework with covariate-specific regularization has been used as an extension of a PLANN neural network for censored data to investigate the influence of different prognostic variables on node-negative breast cancer patients. The results of contrasting the PLANN-ARD with the clinically well-accepted proportional hazards model show that the two are consistent. Furthermore, the model selection carried out with PLANN-ARD indicated similar variables that have prognostic significance like the model selection performed with the Cox regression.

The regression models have been tested on datasets gathered at the same hospital but in different time intervals. It proved that the node-negative patients from the dataset gathered between 1990 and 1993 have higher survivorship than the patients collected between 1983 and 1989. This is because of the introduction of the Breast Screening Programmes since the beginning of 1990s in UK, which allowed the early detection of the disease. In accordance with this, by inspecting the attribute histograms of the two datasets, it is observed that a higher number of patients with increased pathological size and histological grade gathered before 1990s.

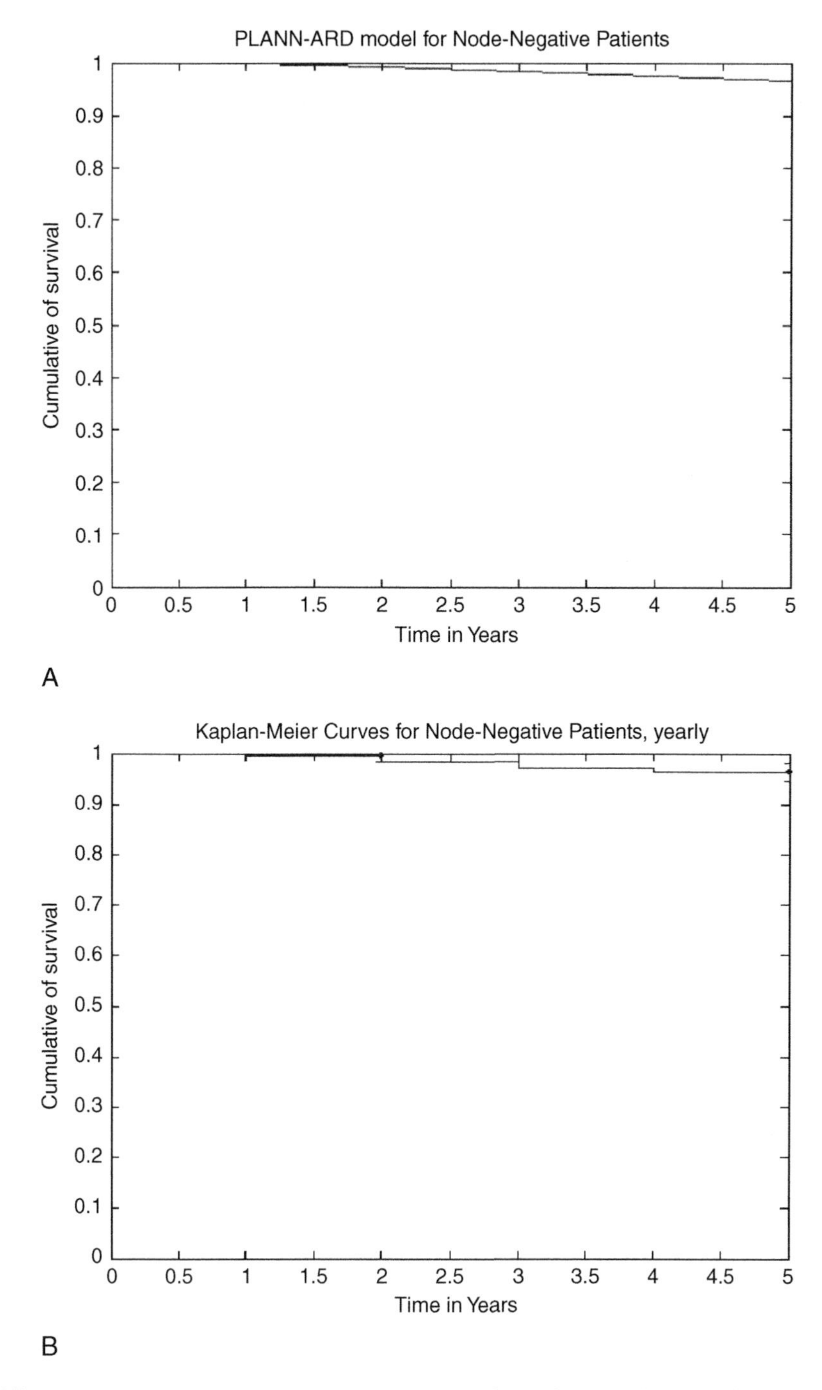

Fig. 15. (A) PLANN-ARD calculated survivorship for a dataset of 588 node-negative breast cancer patients and (B) the corresponding Kaplan–Meier curve.

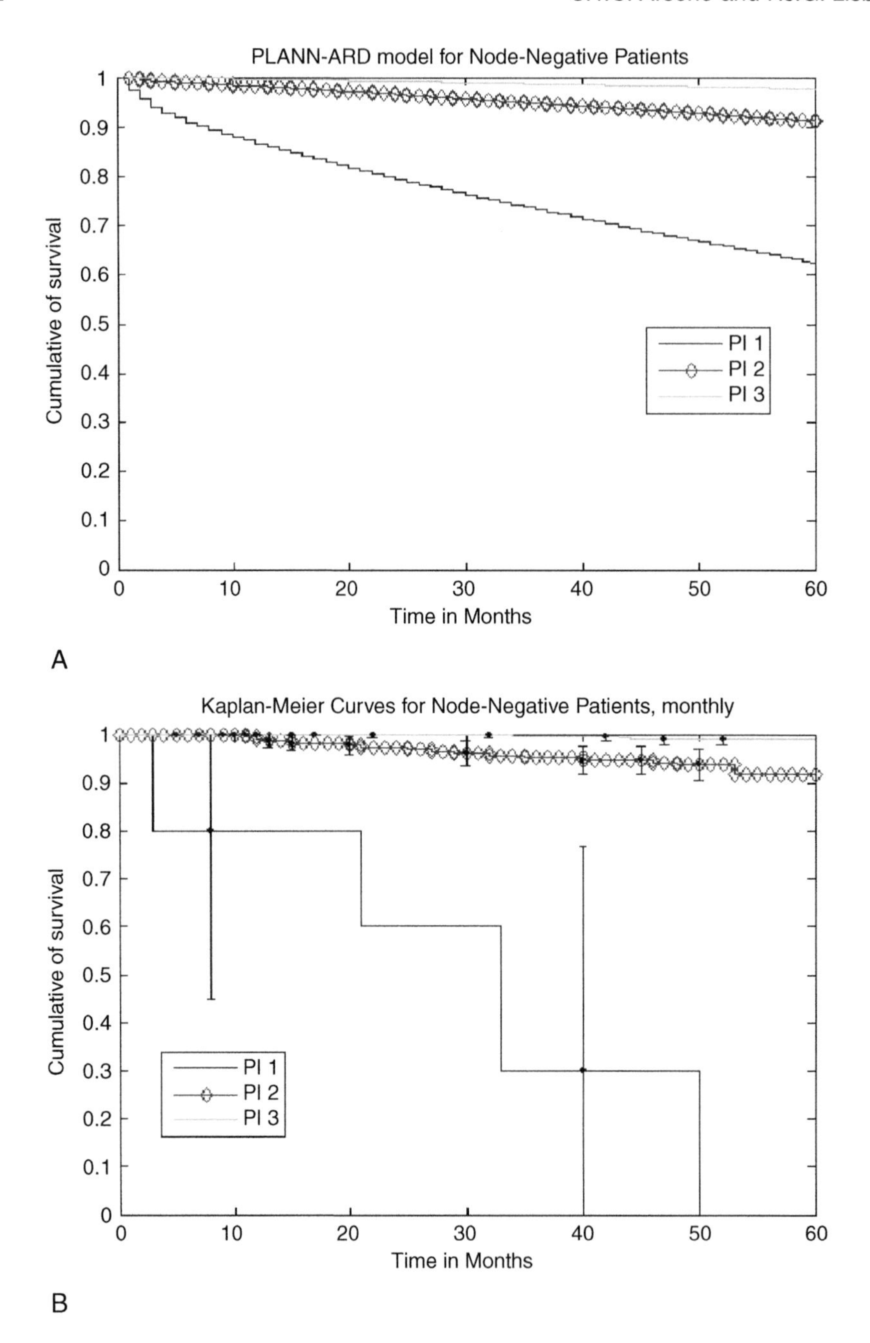

Fig. 16. (A) Partitioning of node-negative patients with log-rank test into three prognostic groups with 5 patients in risk group PI1, 226 patients in risk group PI2 and 357 patients in risk group PI3 and (B) the corresponding grouped Kaplan–Meier curves for the three risk groups.

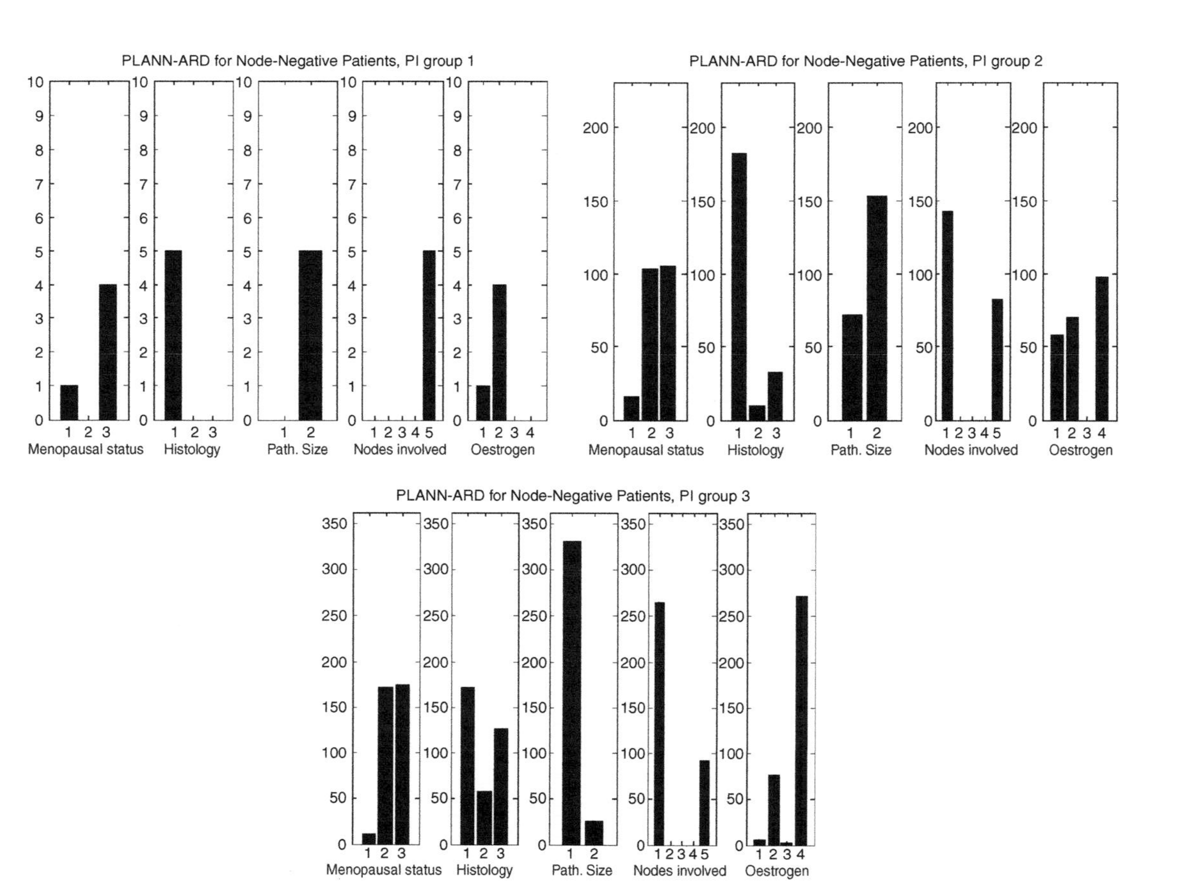

Fig. 17. Attribute profiles for risk group PI1, risk group PI2 and risk group PI3 identified in node-negative patients with PLANN-ARD-selected variable.

REFERENCES

Abner, A.L., J.L. Connolly, A. Recht, B. Bornstein, A. Nixon, S. Hetelekidis and B. Silver, 2000, The relation between the presence and extent of lobular carcinoma in situ and the risk of local recurrence for patients with infiltrating carcinoma of the breast treated with conservative surgery and radiation therapy. Cancer, 88(5), 1072–1079.

ACOR, 2004, Association of Cancer Online Resources (ACOR), www.ACOR.ORG.

Andersen, K.W., H.T. Mouridsen and Danish Breast Cancer Cooperative Group (DBCG), 1988, A description of the register of the nation-wide programme for primary breast cancer. Acta Oncol., 27, 627–643.

Arsene, C.T.C. and P.J.C. Lisboa, 2005, Node-negative breast cancer prognosis based on a Bayesian neural network approach with censored data, Second International Conference on Computational Intelligence in Medicine and Healthcare, CIMED'2005, pp. 147–202.

Aitkin, M., D. Anderson, B. Francis and J. Hindle, 1989, Statistical Modelling in GLM. Oxford University Press, New York.

Baxt, W.G., and H. White, 1995, Bootstrapping confidence intervals for clinical input variable effects in a network trained to identify the presence of acute myocardial infarction. Neural Comput., 7(3), 624–638.

Beahrs, O.H., D.E. Henson, R.V.P. Hutter and B.J. Kennedy, 1992, American Joint Committee on Cancer. Manual for Staging of Cancer, 4th ed. J.B. Lippincott, Philadelphia.

Biganzoli, E., P. Boracchi, L. Mariani and E. Marubini, 1998, Feed forward neural networks for the analysis of censored survival data: a partial logistic regression approach. Stat. Med., 17, 1169–1186.

Biganzoli, E., P. Boracchi, F. Ambrogi and E. Marubini, 2002, Artificial Neural Network Models for discrete cause specific hazards, 23rd Meeting of the International Society for Clinical Biostatistics, September 9–13, Dijon, France.

Biganzoli, E., P. Boracchi and E. Marubini, 2002, A general framework for neural network models on censored survival data. Neural Netw., 15, 209–218.

Bishop, C.M., 1995, Neural Networks for Pattern Recognition. Oxford University Press, New York.

Boracchi, P., E. Biganzoli and E. Marubini, 2001, Modelling cause specific hazards with radial basis functions artificial neural networks: an application to 2233 breast cancer patients. Stat. Med., 20, 3677–3694.

Boracchi, P., E. Biganzoli and E. Marubini, 2003, Joint modelling of cause-specific hazard functions with cubic splines: an application to a large series of breast cancer patients. Computat. Stat. Data Anal., 42, 243–262.

Bryce, T.J., M.W. Dewhirst, C.E. Floyd Jr., V. Hars and D.M. Brizel, 1998, Artificial neural network model of survival in patients treated with irradiation with and without concurrent chemotherapy for advanced carcinoma of the head and neck. Int. J. Radiat. Oncol. Biol. Phys., 41(2), 339–345.

Bugliosi, R., M. Tribalto, G. Avvisati, M. Boccardoro, C. de Martinis, R. Friera, F. Mandelli, A. Pileri and G. Papa, 1994, Classification of patients affected by multiple myeloma using neural network software. Eur. J. Haematol., 52(3), 182–183.

Burke, H.B., P.H. Goodman, D.B. Rosen, D.E. Henson, J.N. Weinstein, F.E. Harrell, J.R. Marks, D.P. Winchester and D.G. Bostwick, 1997, Artificial neural network improve the accuracy of cancer survival prediction. Cancer, 79, 857–862.

Camp, R.L., E.B. Rimm and D.L. Rimm, 2000, A high number of tumour free axillary lymph nodes from patients with lymph node negative breast carcinoma is associated with poor outcome. Cancer, 88, 108–113.

Campbell, M., R. Fitzpatrick, A. Haines, A.L. Kinmonth, P. Sandercock, D. Speigelhalter and P. Tryer, 2000, Framework for design and evaluation of complex interventions to improve health. BMJ, 321, 694–696.

Carter, C.L., C. Allen and D.E. Henson, 1989, Relation of tumour size, lymph node status, and survival in 24,740 breast cancer cases. Cancer, 63, 181–187.

Castiglione-Gertsch, M.M., 2002, Hormone receptor status determines benefit from hormonal therapy or chemotherapy for women with node-negative breast cancer, San Antonio Breast Cancer Symposium, Abstract #11.

Choong, P.L., C.J.S. deSilva, H.J.S. Dawkins and G.F. Sterrett, 1996, Entropy maximization networks: an application to breast cancer prognosis. IEEE Trans. Neural Netw., 7(3), 568–577.

Clark, G.M. and W.L. McGuire, 1991, Follow-up study of *HER/neu* amplification in primary breast cancer. Cancer Res., 51, 944–948.

Clark, G.M., L.G. Dressler, M.A. Owens, G. Pounds, T. Oldaker and W.L. McGuire 1989, Prediction of relapse or survival in patients with node-negative breast cancer by DNA flow cytometry. N. Engl. J. Med., 320, 627–633.

Cody, H.S., P.I. Borgen and L.K. Tan, 2004, Redefining prognosis in node-negative breast cancer: can sentinel lymph node biopsy raise the threshold for systemic adjuvant therapy? Ann. Surg. Oncol., 11, 227–230.

Collett, D., 1994, Modelling Survival Data in Medical Research. Chapman & Hall, London.

Collett, K., R. Skjaerven and B.O. Maehle, 1998, The prognostic contribution of oestrogen and progesterone receptor status to a modified version of the Nottingham Prognostic Index. Breast Cancer Res. Treat., 48, 1–9.

Coradini, D., P. Boracchi, M.G. Daidone, C. Pellizzaro, P. Miodini, M. Ammatuna, G. Tomasic and E. Biganzoli, 2001, Contribution of vascular endothelial growth factor to the Nottingham Prognostic Index in node negative breast cancer. Br. J. Cancer, 85, 795–802.

Cox, D.R., 1972, Regression models and life tables. J. Roy. Stat. Soc. Series B, 74, 187–220.

Dabiri, S., D. Huntsman, N. Makretsov, M. Cheang, B. Gilks, C. Badjik, K. Gelmon, S. Chia and M. Hayes, 2004, The presence of stromal mast cells identifies a subset of invasive breast with a favourable prognosis. Mod. Pathol., 17(6), 690–695.

Dales, J.P., S. Garcia, P. Bonnier, F. Duffaud, L. Andrac-Meyer, O. Ramuz, M.-N. Lavaut, C. Allasia and C. Charpin, 2003, CD105 expression is a marker of high metastatic risk and poor outcome in breast carcinomas correlations between immunohistochemical analysis and long-term follow-up in a series of 929 patients. Am. J. Clin. Pathol., 119, 374–380.

Dales, J.P., S. Garcia, S. Carpentier, L. Andrac, O. Ramuz, M.-N. Lavaut, C. Allasia, P. Bonnier and C. Charpin, 2004, Long-term prognostic significance of neoangiogenesis in breast carcinomas: comparison of Tie-2/Tek, CD105, and CD31 immunocytochemical expression. Hum. Pathol., 35(2), 176–183.

D'Eredita, G., C. Giardina, M. Martellota, T. Natale and F. Ferrarese, 2001, Prognostic factors in breast cancer: the predictive value of the Nottingham Prognostic Index in patients with a long-term follow-up that were treated in a single institution. Eur. J. Cancer, 37, 591–597.

de Placido, S., C. Carlomagno, F. Ciardiello, M. de Laurentiis, S. Pepe, A. Ruggiero, G. Tortora, L. Panico, A. D'Antonio, G. Pettinato, G. Petrella and A.R. Bianco, 1999, Measurement of neovascularization is an independent prognosticator of survival in node-negative breast cancer patients with long-term follow-up. Clin. Cancer Res., 5, 2854–2859.

Desch, C.E., B.E. Hillner, T.J. Smith and S.M. Retchin, 1993, Should the elderly receive chemotherapy for node negative breast cancer? A cost-effectiveness analysis examining total and active life-expectancy outcomes. J. Clin. Oncol., 11(4), 777–782.

Early Breast Cancer Trialists' Collaborative Group, 1998a, Tamoxifen for early breast cancer: an overview of the randomised trials. Lancet, 351(9114), 1451–1467.

Early Breast Cancer Trialists' Collaborative Group, 1998b, Polichemotherapy for early breast cancer: an overview of the randomized trials. Lancet, 352, 930–942.

Efficace, F., L. Biganzoli, M. Piccart, C. Coens, K. van Steen, T. Cufer, R.E. Coleman, H.A. Calvert, T. Gamucci, C. Twelves, P. Fargeot and A. Bottomley, 2004, Baseline health-related quality-of-life data as prognostic factors in a phase III multicentre study of women with metastatic breast cancer. Eur. J. Cancer, 40, 1021–1030.

Elandt-Johnson, R.C. and N.L. Johnson, 1980, Survival Models and Data Analysis. John Wiley & Sons, New York.

Eleuteri, A., R. Tagliaferri, L. Milano, S. de Placido and M. de Laurentiis, 2003, A novel neural network-based survival analysis model. Neural Networks, 16.

Ellenius, J., T. Groth and B. Lindahl, 1997, Neural network analysis of biochemical markers for early assessment of acute myocardial infarction. Stud. Health Technol. Inform., 43, 382–385.

Etchells, T.A. and P.J.G. Lisboa, 2003, On rule extraction from smooth decision surfaces, NNWSMED/CIMED, Proc. 5th International Conference, pp. 23–28.

Eubank, R.L., 1984, Approximate regression models and splines. Commun. Stat. A-Theor. 13, 433–484.

Farabegoli, F., M.A. Hermsen, C. Ceccarelli and D. Santini, 2004, Simultaneous chromosome 1q gain and 16q loss is associated with steroid receptor presence and low proliferation in breast carcinoma. Mod. Pathol., 17(4), 449–455.

Ferrero, J.M., A. Ramaioli, J.L. Formento, M. Francoual, M.C. Etienne, I. Peyrottes, F. Ettore, P. Leblanc-Talent, M. Namer and G. Milano, 2000, p53 determination alongside classical prognostic factors in node-negative breast cancer: an evaluation at more than 10-year follow-up. Ann. Oncol., 11(4).

Fisher, B., S. Anderson, E. Tan-Chiu, N. Wolmark, D.L. Wickerham, E.R. Fisher, N.V. Dimitrov, J.N. Atkins, N. Abramson, S. Merajver, E.H. Romond, C.G. Kardinal, H.R. Shibata, R.G. Margolese and W.B. Farrar, 2001a, Tamoxifen and chemotherapy for axillary node negative, estrogen receptor-negative breast cancer: findings from the National Surgical Breast and Bowel Project B-23. J. Clin. Oncol., 19(4), 931–942.

Fisher, B., J. Dignam, E. Tan-Chiu, S. Anderson, E. Fisher and N. Wolmark, 2001b, Prognosis and treatment of patients with breast tumors of #1 cm and negative axillary nodes. J. Nat. Cancer Inst., 93(2), 112–120.

Fisher, B., J.H. Jeong, J. Bryant, S. Anderson, J. Dignam and N. Wolmark, 2004, Treatment of lymph node-negative, estrogen receptor-positive breast cancer: long-term findings from National Surgical Adjuvant Breast and Bowel Project clinical trials. Lancet, 364, 858–868.

Galea, M.H., R.W. Blamey, C.E. Elston and I.O. Ellis, 1992, The Nottingham Prognostic Index in primary breast cancer. Breast Cancer Res. Treat., 22, 202–219.

Gasparini G., W.J. Gullik, P. Bevilacqua, J.R.C. Sainsbury, S. Meli, P. Boracchi, A. Testolin, G. La Malfa and F. Pozza, 1992, Human breast cancer: prognostic significance of the c-erbB2 oncoprotein compared with epidermal growth factor receptor, DNA ploidy and conventional pathologic features. J. Clin. Oncol., 10, 686–695.

Georgiadis, D., M. Kaps, M. Sielber, M. Hill, M. Konig, J. Berg, M. Kahl, P. Zunker, B. Diehl and E.B. Ringelstein, 1995, Variability of Doppler microembolic signal counts in patients with prosthetic cardiac valves. Stroke, 26(3), 439–443.

Glass, J.O. and W.E. Reddick, 1998, Hybrid artificial neural network segmentation and classification of dynamic contrast-enhanced MR imaging (DEMRI) of osteosarcoma. Magn. Reson. Imaging, 16(9), 1075–1083.

Goldhirsch, A., J.H. Glick, R.D. Gelber, A.S. Coates and H.J. Senn, 2001, International Consensus Panel on the Treatment of Primary Breast Cancer. Seventh International Conference on Adjuvant Therapy of Primary Breast Cancer. J. Clin. Oncol., 19, 3817–3827.

Goldstein, N.S., A. Mani, F. Vicini and J. Ingold, 1999, Prognostic features in patients with stage T1 breast carcinoma and a 0.5-cm or less lymph node metastasis. Significance of lymph node hilar tissue invasion. Am. J. Clin. Pathol., 111(1), 21–29.

Goodenday, L.S., K.J. Cios and I. Shin, 1997, Identifying coronary stenosis using an image-recognition neural network. IEEE Eng. Med. Bio. Mag., 16(5), 139–144.

Gore, S.M., S.J. Pocock and G.R. Kerr, 1984, Regression models and non-proportional hazards in the analysis of breast cancer survival. Appl. Statist., 33(2) 176–195.

Gray, R.J. 1996, Hazard rate regression using ordinary nonparametric regression smoother. J. Comput. Graph. Stat., 5, 190–207.

Greene, F.L., D.L. Page, I.D. Fleming, A. Fritz, C.M. Balch, D.G. Haller and M. Morrow, 2002, American Joint Committee on Cancer's Cancer Staging Manual, 6th ed. American Joint Committee on Cancer, US.

Hasebe, T., H. Tsuda, S. Hirohashi, Y. Shimosato, M. Iwai, S. Imoto and K. Mukai, 1996, Fibrotic focus in invasive ductal carcinoma: an indicator of high tumor aggressiveness. Jpn. J. Cancer Res., 87(4), 385–394.

Hasebe, T., S. Sasaki, S. Imoto and A. Ochiai, 2004, Histological characteristics of tumor in vessels and lymph nodes are significant predictors of progression of invasive ductal carcinoma of the breast: a prospective study. Hum. Pathol., 35, 298–308.

Hausen, S., D.A. Grabam, F.B. Sorensen, M. Bak, W. Vach and C. Rose, 2000, Vascular grading of angiogenesis: prognostic significance in breast cancer. Br. J. Cancer, 82, 339–386.

Haybittle, J.L., R.W. Blamey, C.W. Elston, J. Johnson, P.J. Doyle, F.C. Campbell, R.I. Nicholson and K. Griffiths, 1982, A Prognostic index in primary breast cancer. Br. J. Cancer, 45, 361–365.

Hilsenbeck, S.G., P.M. Ravdin and C.A. de Moor, 1998, Time-dependence of hazard ratios for prognostic factors in primary breast cancer. Breast Cancer Res. Treat., 52, 227–237.

Hosmer, D.W. and S. Lemeshow, 2000, Applied Logistic Regression, 2nd ed. John Wiley & Sons, New York.

Huang, J., P.H. Tan, J. Thiyagarajan and B.H. Bay, 2003, Prognostic significance of glutathione S-transferase-pi in invasive breast cancer. Mod. Pathol, 16(6), 558–565.

Huseby, R.A., H.E. Ownby, J. Frederick, S. Brooks, J. Russo and M.J. Brennan, 1988, Node-negative breast cancer treated by modified radical mastectomy without adjuvant therapies: variables associated with disease recurrence and survivorship. J. Clin. Oncol., 6.

Jacquemier, J., J.M. Kurtz, R. Amalric, H. Brandone, Y. Ayme and J.M. Spitalier, 1990, An assessment of extensive intraductal component as a risk factor for local recurrence after breast-conserving therapy. Br. J. Cancer, 61(6), 873–879.

Jagsi, R., R. Abi Raad, S. Goldberg, J. Michaelson and A. Taghian, 2003, Loco-regional recurrence rates and prognostic factors for failure in node-negative patients treated with mastectomy alone: implications for postmastectomy radiation, Proceedings from the 45th Annual Meeting of the American Society for Therapeutic Radiation and Oncology, Abstract #9.

Jarman, J. and P.J. Lisboa, 2004, A comparative study of NPI and PLANN-ARD by prognostic accuracy and treatment allocation for breast cancer patients, ENRICH Deliverables, http://www.cms.livjm.ac.uk/2nrich/deliverables2.asp

Jerez-Aragones, J.M., J.A. Gomez-Ruiz, G. Ramos-Jimenez, J. Munoz-Perez and E. Alba-Conejo, 2003, A combined neural network and decision trees model for prognosis of breast cancer relapse. Artif. Intell. Med., 27, 45–63.

Kalbfleisch, J.D. and R.L. Prentice, 1980, The Statistical Analysis of Failure Time Data. Wiley, New York.

Kaplan, S.A. and P. Meier, 1958, Nonparametric estimation from incomplete observations. J. Am. Stat. Assoc., 53, 457–481.

Klein, J.P. and M.L. Moeschberger, 1997, Survival Analysis. Techniques for Censored and Truncated Data. Springer, New York.

Klein, J.P., N. Keiding and C. Kamby 1989, Semiparametric Marshall–Olkin models applied to the occurrence of metastases at multiple sites after breast cancer. Biometrics, 45, 1073–1086.

Kleinbaum, D.G. 1997, Survival Analysis. Springer, New York.

Kooperberg, C. and D.B. Clarkson, 1997, Hazard regression with interval-censored data. Biometrics, 53, 1485–1494.

Kooperberg, C., C.J. Stone and Y.K. Truong, 1995, Hazard regression. J. Am. Stat. Assoc., 90(429), 78–94.

Kothari, R., H. Cualing and T. Balanchander, 1996, Neural network analysis of flow cytometry immunophenotype data. IEEE Biomed. Eng., 43(8), 803–810.

Larson, M.G., 1984, Covariate analysis of competing-risks data with log-linear models. Biometrics, 40, 459–468.

Lawless, J.F., 1982, Statistical Models and Methods for Lifetime Data. John Wiley & Sons, New York.

Lee, E.T., 1992, Statistical Methods for Survival Data Analysis. Wiley, New York.

Lindahl, D., J. Toft, B. Hesse, J. Palmer, S. Ali, A. Lundin and L. Edenbrandt, 2000, Scandinavian test of artificial neural network for classification of myocardial perfusion images. Clin. Physiol., 20(4), 253–261.

Lisboa, P.J.G., 2002, A review of evidence of health benefit from artificial neural networks in medical intervention. Neural Netw., 15, 11–39.

Lisboa, P.J.G., H. Wong, P. Harris and R. Swindell, 2003, A Bayesian neural network approach for modelling censored data with an application to prognosis after surgery for breast cancer. Artif. Intell. Med., 28, 1–25.

Lockwood, C.A., C. Ricciardelli, W.A. Raymond, R. Seshadri, K. McClaul and J.D. Horsfall, 1999, A simple index using video image analysis to predict disease outcome in primary breast cancer. Int. J. Cancer, 84, 203–211.

Lundin, J., M. Lundin, K. Holli, V. Kataja, L. Elomaa, L. Pylkkänen, T. Turpeeniemi-Hujanen and H. Joensuu, 2001, Omission of histologic grading from clinical decision making may result in overuse of adjuvant therapies in breast cancer: results from a nationwide study. J. Clin. Oncol., 19, 28–36.

Lundin, J., M. Lundin, J. Isola and H. Joensuu, 2003, A web-based system for individualised survival estimation in breast cancer. BMJ, 326(7379), 29.

Lundin, J., M. Lundin, J. Isola and H. Joensuu, 2004, Validation of a web-based prognostic system for breast cancer. Medinfo, 2004, 237–277.

Mangarisan, O.L., W.N. Street and W.H. Wolberg, 1995, Breast cancer diagnosis and prognosis via linear programming. Opera. Res., 43(4), 570–577.

Marcus, J.N., P. Watson, D.L. Page and H.T. Lynch, 1994, Pathology and heredity of breast cancer in younger women. J. Natl. Cancer Inst. Monogr, (16), 23–34.

Marubini, E. and M.G. Valsecchi, 1995, Analysing Survival Data from Clinical Trial and Observational Studies. Wiley, Chichester, pp. 331–361.

MacKay, D.J.C., 1992a, Bayesian interpolation. Neural Comput., 4, 415–447.

MacKay, D.J.C., 1992b, The evidence framework applied to classification networks. Neural Comput., 4(5), 720–736.

MacKay, D.J.C., 1995, Probable networks and plausible predictions – a review of practical Bayesian methods for supervised neural networks network-computation in neural systems. Network: Comput. Neural Syst., 6, 469–505.

McCullagh, P. and J.A. Nelder, 1989, Generalized linear models, 2nd ed. Chapman & Hall, London, UK.

Medri, L., O. Nanni, A. Volpi, E. Scarpi, A. Dubini, A. Riccobon, A. Becciolini, S. Bianchi and D. Amadori, 2000, Tumour microvessel density and prognosis in node-negative breast cancer. Int. J. Cancer, 20, 89(1).

Moore, A. and A. Hoang, 2002, A performance assessment of Bayesian networks as a predictor of breast cancer survival, Second International Workshop on Intelligent Systems Design and Application, Atlanta.

Nabney, I., 2001, NETLAB: Algorithms for Pattern Recognition. Springer, London.

Nakopoulou, L., S. Katsarou, I. Giannopoulou, P. Alexandru et al., 2002, Correlation of tissue inhibitor of metalloproteinase-2 with proliferative activity and patients' survival in breast cancer. Mod. Pathol., 15, 26–34.

National Institutes of Health Consensus Development Conference statement: adjuvant therapy for breast cancer, 2000, J. Natl. Cancer Inst. Monogr., 30, 5–15.

Neal, R.M., 1996, Bayesian Learning for Neural Networks. Springer, New York.

Neal, R.M. 2000, Slice Sampling. Technical Report No. 2005, Department of Statistics, University of Toronto.
Neal, R.M. 2001, Survival Analysis Using a Bayesian Neural Network. Joint Statistical Meetings Report, Atlanta.
NHS Breast Screening Programme, 2005, National Health Service Breast Screening Programme, London, UK, http://www.cancerscreening.nhs.uk/breastscreen.
Nicholas, S.A., P.E. Swanson, H. Linden, S.E. Hawes and T.J. Lawton, 2003, Androgen receptor expression in estrogen receptor-negative breast cancer immunohistochemical, clinical, and prognostic associations. Am. J. Clin. Pathol., 120, 725–731.
Noguchi, S., H. Koyama, J. Uchino, R. Abe, S. Miura, K. Sugimachi, K. Akazawa and O. Abe, 2005, Postoperative adjuvant therapy with tamoxifen, tegafur plus uracil, or both in women with node-negative breast cancer: a pooled analysis of six randomized controlled trials. J. Clin. Oncol., 23(10) 2172–2184.
O'Reilly, S.M., R.S. Camplejohn, D.M. Barnes, R.R. Millis, R.D. Rubens and M.A. Richards, 1990, Node-negative breast cancer: prognostic subgroups defined by tumor size and flow cytometry. J. Clin. Oncol., 8, 2040–2046.
Pantel, P., 1998, Breast cancer diagnosis and prognosis. Report. Department of Computer Science, The University of Manitoba, Canada.
Peto, R. and J. Peto, 1972, Asymptotically efficient rank invariant procedures. J. Roy. Stat. Soci. Series A., 135, 185–207.
Polak, M.J., S.H. Zhou, P.M. Rautaharju, W.W. Armstrong and B.R. Chaitan, 1997, Using automated analysis of the resting twelve-lead ECG to identify patients at risk if developing transient myocardial ischaemia – an application of an adaptive logic network. Physiol. Meas., 18(4), 317–325.
Quinlan, J.R. 1979, Discovering rules by induction from large collections of examples. In: D. Michie (Ed.), Expert systems in the Microelectronics Age. Edinburgh University Press, Edinburgh, pp. 168–201.
Quinlan, J.R. 1983, Learning efficient classification procedures. In: R.S. Michalski, J.G. Carbonell and T.M. Mitchell (Eds.), Machine Learning: An Artificial Intelligence approach. Tioga Press, Palo Alto, California.
Quinlan, J.R. 1986, Induction of decision trees. Mach. Learn., 1, 81–106.
Quinlan, J.R. 1993, C4.5: Programs for Machine Learning. Morgan Kaufmann Publishers, San Mateo, California.
Ramos-Jimenez, G., R. Moralez-Bueno and A. Villalba-Soria, 2000, CIDIM: control of induction by sample division method, Proceedings of IC-AI'2000, International Conference on Artificial Intelligence, Las Vegas, USA, CSREA Press, pp. 1083–1090.
Ravdin, P.M., A.S. Laura, J.D. Greg, M.B. Mercer, J. Hewlett, N. Gerson and H. Parker, 2001, Computer program to assist in making decisions about adjuvant therapy for women with early breast cancer. J. Clin. Oncol., 19(4), 980–991.
Reigitnig, P., F. Ploner, M. Marderbacher and S.F. Lax, 2004, Bilateral carcinomas of the breast with local recurrence: analysis of genetic relationship of the tumours. Mod. Pathol., 17(5), 597–602.
Ripley, B.D., 1996, Pattern Recognition and Neural Networks. Cambridge University Press, Cambridge.
Ripley, R.M., A.L. Harris and L. Tarassenko, 1998, Neural network models for breast cancer prognosis. Neur. Comput. Appl., 7, 367–375.
Ripley, B.D. and R.M. Ripley, 1998, Neural networks as statistical methods in survival analysis. In: R. Dybowski and V. Gant (Eds.), Artifical Neural Networks: Prospects for Medicine, Landes Biosciences Publishers.
Ross, J.S. and J.A. Fletcher, 1998, The HER-2/neu oncogene in breast cancer: prognostic factor, predictive factor and target for therapy. Oncologist, 3, 237–252.
Robert, C.P. 2001, The Bayesian Choice, 2nd ed. Springer, New York.
Ruiz-Gomez, J., G. Ramos-Jimenez and A. Villalva-Soria, 1999, Modelling based on rule induction learning. In: Computers and Computational Engineering in Control, WSES Press, Piraeus, Greece, pp. 158–163.
Saphner, T., D.C. Torney and R. Gray, 1996, Annual hazard rates of recurrence for breast cancer after primary therapy. J. Clin. Oncol., 14, 2738–2746.
Schmitz, K.J., F. Otterbach, R. Callies, B. Levkau, M. Holscher, O. Hoffmann, F. Grabellus, R. Kimmig, K.W. Schmid and H.A. Baba, 2004, Prognostic relevance of activated Akt kinase in node-negative breast cancer: a clinicopathological study of 99 cases. Mod. Pathol., 17(1), 15–21.
Selker, H.P., J.L. Griffith, S. Patil, W.J. Long and R.B. D'Agostino, 1995, A comparison of performance of mathematical predictive methods for medical diagnosis: identifying acute cardiac ischemia among emergency department patients. J. Investig. Med., 43(5), 468–476.
Seshadri, R., D.J. Horsfall, K. McCaul and A.S. Leong, 1997, A simple index to predict prognosis independent of axillary node information in breast cancer. Aust. N. J. Surg., 67.

Shim, J.Y., H.J. An, Y.H. Lee, S.K. Kim, K.P. Lee and K.S. Lee, 2003, Overexpression of cyclooxygenase-2 is associated with breast carcinoma and its poor prognostic factors. Mod. Pathol., 16(12), 1199–1204.

Si, Y., J. Gotman, A. Pasupathy, D. Flanagan, B. Rosenblatt and R. Gottesman, 1998, An expert system for EEG monitoring in the pediatric intensive care unit. Electroen. Clin. Neuro., 106(6), 488–500.

Sidoni, A., A. Bellezza, R. Cavaliere, M. Del Sordo, E. Scheibel and E. Bucciarelli, 2004, Prognostic indexes in breast cancer: comparison of the Nottingham and Adelaide indexes. The Breast, 13(1), 23–27.

Sigurdsson, H., B. Baldetorp, A. Borg, M. Dalberg, M. Ferno, D. Killander and H. Olsson, 1990, Indicators of prognosis in node-negative breast cancer. N. Engl. J. Med., 322, 1045–1053.

Smith, J.H., J. Graham and R.J. Taylor, 1996, The application of an artificial neural network to Doppler ultrasound waveforms for the classification of arterial disease. Int. J. Clin. Monit. Comput., 13(2), 85–91.

SPSS, 1999, SPSS Base 9.0/user's guide. SPSS Inc.

Stock, A., M.S. Rogers, A. Li and A.M. Chang, 1994, Use of the neural network for hypothesis generation in fetal surveillance. Baillieres. Clin. Ob. Gy., 8(3), 533–548.

Thor, A.D., D.H. Moore, S.M. Edgerton, E.S. Kawasaki, E. Reihaus, H.T. Lynch, J.N. Marcus, L. Schwartz, L.C. Chen and B.H. Mayall, 1992, Accumulation of p53 tumor suppressor gene protein: an independent marker of prognosis in breast cancers. J. Natl. Cancer Inst., 84, 845–855.

Toikkanen, S., H. Helin, J. Isola and H. Joensuu, 1992, Prognostic significance of HER-2 oncoprotein expression in breast cancer: a 30-years follow-up. J. Clin. Oncol., 10, 1044–1048.

van der Wal, B.C., R.M. Butzelaar, S. van der Meij and M.A. Boermeester, 2002, Axillary lymph node ratio and total number of removed lymph nodes: predictors of survival in stage I and II breast cancer. Eur. J. Surg. Oncol., 28(5), 481–490.

Veronesi, U., E. Marubini, M. Del Vecchio, A. Manzari, S. Andreola, M. Greco, A. Luini, M. Merson, R. Saccozzi, F. Rilke and B. Salvadori, 1995, Local recurrences and distant metastases after conservative breast cancer treatments: partly independent events. J. Nat. Cancer Inst., 87, 19–27.

Wait, S., P. Schaffer, B. Seradour, C. Guldenfels, B. Gairard, F. Morin and L. Piana, 2000, The cost of breast cancer screening in France. J. Radiol., 81(7), 799–806.

Weibull, A., 1951, A Statistical distribution function of wide applicability. J. Appl. Mech., 18, 293–297.

Wenger, C.R., S. Beardslee, M.A. Owens, G. Pounds, T. Oldaker, P. Vendely, M.R. Pandian, D. Harrington, G.M. Clark and W.L. McGuire, 1993, DNA ploidy, S-phase, and steroid receptors in more than 127,000 breast cancer patients. Breast Cancer Res. Treat., 28(1), 9–20.

Wiley, E.L., L.K. Diaz, S. Badve and M. Morrow, 2003, Effect of time interval on residual disease in breast cancer. Am. J. Surg. Pathol., 27(2), 194–202.

Wohlfahrt, J., P.K. Andersen and M. Melbye, 1999, Multivariate competing risks. Stat. Med., 18, 1023–1030.

Wolberg, W.H., W.N. Street and O.L. Mangasarian, 1993, Breast cytology diagnosis via digital image analysis. Anal. Quant. Cytol. Hist., 15(6), 396–404.

Wolberg, W.H., W.N. Street and O.L. Mangasarian, 1994, Machine learning techniques to diagnose breast cancer from image-processed nuclear features of fine needle aspirates. Cancer Lett., 77, 163–171.

Wong, H. 2001, A Bayesian neural network for censored survival data. Ph.D. Thesis, Liverpool John Moores University.

Zernikow, B., K. Holtmannspotter, E. Michel, F. Hornschuh, K. Groote and K.H. Hennecke, 1999, Predicting length-of-stay in pretermneonates. Eur. J. Pediatr., 158(1), 59–62.

Section 4

Application of Machine Learning Methods

Chapter 9

The Use of Artificial Neural Networks for the Diagnosis and Estimation of Prognosis in Cancer Patients

Alberto Mario Marchevsky

Department of Pathology, Cedars-Sinai Medical Center, 8700 Beverly Blvd, Los Angeles, CA 90048, USA
Email: Marchevsky@cshs.org

Abstract

Artificial neural networks (ANNs) are computational models that attempt to emulate the architecture of the human brain. Data is processed in discrete "elements" or "neurons" and transferred amongst these elements through "connections" that simulate neural synapses. Artificial neurons are usually organized in the following layers: input, hidden and output. The neurons in the input layer compute the data provided by the investigators; the elements in the single or multiple hidden layers allow for the development of multiple variations of the data; while the output layer calculates the "answer" estimated by the model. Various mathematical functions are applied to the data, resulting in several ANN models, such as backpropagation, probabilistic and others.

ANNs offer the advantage of being able to work with "uncertain" data and to benefit from the availability of numerous elements of information that may not appear on an intuitive basis to influence the solution of a particular problem. They are suitable models for the solution of classification and forecasting problems, as they calculate a value for individual members of a population.

ANNs have been applied in our laboratory and elsewhere to estimate the prognosis of cancer patients. For example, in a study of patients with non-small-cell carcinoma of the lung, probabilistic ANN models were able to accurately forecast, based on several clinico-pathologic features, whether individuals with the disease would be dead or alive at 5 years after diagnosis and initial treatment. In a recent study, ANNs could classify cell lines with small cell carcinoma and non-small-cell carcinoma of the lung, based on DNA hypermethylation data collected with molecular methods. ANNs and other multivariate classificatory and forecasting models can be influenced by data "overfit", resulting in estimations that are mostly due to chance. The results of various ANN models need to be validated with jackknife analysis and other methods.

Potential applications of ANNs for the diagnosis and estimation of prognosis in cancer patients are discussed, and the difficult problem of model accuracy validation is reviewed.

Keywords: Artificial neural networks, cancer prognosis, cancer diagnosis, multivariate statistical methods, neurons, neuronal architecture, backpropagation neural networks, probabilistic neural networks, data overfit, model validation.

Contents

Outcome Prediction in Cancer
Edited by A.F.G. Taktak and A.C. Fisher

© 2007 Elsevier B.V. All rights reserved

1. INTRODUCTION

Artificial neural networks (ANNs) are computational models that attempt to emulate the architecture and function of the human brain (Russell and Norvig, 1995). They offer the advantage of being able to work with "uncertain" data and are suitable for processing information that may not appear on an intuitive basis to influence the solution of a particular problem (Rolston, 1988). The specialized parallel processing architectures of ANNs have been used to solve problems related to language processing, character recognition, image data compression, pattern recognition and for the analysis of classification and forecasting problems (Eberhart et al., 1996). ANN models have been applied in our laboratory and elsewhere to the study of clinico-pathological, molecular and other laboratory data, in experimental efforts at classifying pathologic lesions and estimating the prognosis of individual cancer patients (Bellotti et al., 1997; Naguib and Sherbet, 1997; Marchevsky et al., 1998, 1999, 2004; Singson et al., 1999; Esteva et al., 2001; Naguib, 2001; Marchevsky and Wick, 2004).

This chapter will briefly review some of the basic concepts of ANN technology, describe various potential applications in clinical practice for the estimation of the prognosis of individual cancer patients and discuss the difficult problem of validating the accuracy of these computational models.

1.1. Brief history of artificial neural network technology

Since ancient Greek historic times, there has been a long-standing interest in understanding "intelligence" (Russell and Norvig, 1995). This quest was energized in the latter half of the twentieth century when the development of modern electronics and computers created new opportunities for the practical implementation of various theoretical mathematical concepts into software and hardware designed to solve practical problems (Rolston, 1988). In 1943, Warren McCulloch, a neurophysiologist, and Walter Pitts, a young mathematician, wrote an influential paper on artificial intelligence (AI), describing how neurons might work and modelling a simple artificial neural network with electrical circuits (Russell and Norvig, 1995). In 1949, Donald Hebb described several basic concepts about artificial neurons and their behaviour. Frank Rosenblatt, a neuro-biologist intrigued with the functioning of the eye of a fly, developed the Perceptron, the oldest neural network still in use today. The Perceptron was built in hardware and could classify a continuous-valued set of inputs into one of the two classes by computing a weighted sum of the inputs, subtracting a threshold, and giving out one of the two possible values as the result. In 1959, Bernard Widrow and Marcian Hoff of Stanford developed the ADALINE and MADALINE (Multiple ADAptive LINear Elements) ANN models. MADALINE provides an adaptive filter, which eliminates echoes on phone lines and was the first ANN to be applied to a real-world problem; it is still in commercial use today.

Unfortunately, these early successes led people to exaggerate the potential of ANNs, particularly in light of the limited electronics then available. Such optimism resulted in the formulation of unfulfilled, outrageous claims and in fears about the dangerous effects that "thinking machines" would have on humanity. The inevitable backlash to this excessive hype led to a marked decrease in the funding for AI and a long period of stunted growth that lasted through the early 1980s.

In 1982, two events caused a renewed interest in AI and ANN technology. First, John Hopfield presented an influential paper to the United States (US) National Academy of Sciences suggesting the need to create useful devices, rather than modelling brains with AI technology. Second, the US–Japan Joint Conference on Cooperative/Competitive Neural Networks was held in Kyoto, which resulted in the announcement by Japan of a "Fifth computer generation" effort. This announcement generated concerns that the US could be left behind and stimulated renewed funding for AI research. Today, multiple ANN models have been developed in software and in specialized, digital, analogue and/or optical "neuro-chips" for a wide variety of applications.

2. ARTIFICIAL NEURAL NETWORK ARCHITECTURE: BASIC CONCEPTS

ANNs are composed of processing elements or artificial neurons arranged in parallel layers (Rolston, 1988; Russell and Norvig, 1995; Eberhart et al., 1996). These layers comprise an input layer composed of neurons that receive numerical input collected by an investigator or a device. All numerical data are generally normalized to range from −1 to 1. The input layer is connected to one or more hidden layers, which create large numbers of numerical combinations of the data. An output layer then provides the solution or answer to a problem estimated by the ANN. The neurons of each layer are "connected" with certain "strength" to those of the next layer. The "connection" is a number ranging from −1 to +1; this "connection strength" is generated by the neurons of a particular layer and used as input by the neurons of the next layer. The artificial neurons of each layer "connect" with all the neurons of the next layer but not with each other. The neuronal connections form a numerical matrix that forms the "knowledge" of the ANN.

The "connection strengths" of an untrained ANN are initially given a default set of values (Rolston, 1988; Eberhart et al., 1996). The ANN is then trained by repeatedly exposing it to a training dataset. This process progressively changes the values of the various connection strengths, as described below. Once the ANN is fully trained, the matrix of connection strengths is fixed and the model can then be used to process unknown or "test" data.

2.1. Artificial neurons or processing elements

Artificial neurons or processing elements are the basic components of an ANN (Rolston, 1988; Eberhart et al., 1996). Artificial neurons can be built in hardware, as specialized "neuro-chips", or modeled in software. They transform the input numerical data, through the use of various mathematical functions, into numerical outputs. The output of each neuron is presented as "connection strength" to all the neurons of the next neuronal layer. The output of the neuron/neurons of the output layer is a number ranging from −1 to +1. Particular thresholds can be applied to these output numbers to represent numerically the "solution" to the problem being addressed by the ANN. For example, if an ANN is trying to estimate whether a patient will be dead or alive five years after the initial diagnosis of a disease, the investigator can programme the system to represent all values ≥ 0.5 to represent an "alive" output and all others to represent a "dead" output.

Artificial neurons have seven major components:

- Weighting factors;
- Learning function;
- Summation function;
- Transfer function;
- Scaling and limiting;
- Output function;
- Error function and back-propagated value.

2.1.1. Weighting factors

A neuron receives one or more numerical inputs and applies an adaptive coefficient of strength (i.e. "weighting factor") to each of them (Rolston, 1988; Eberhart et al., 1996). In this manner, the intensity of each input signal can be modified in response to various training sets through the use of learning rules. This operation enables the assignment of "relevance" to each input, impacting on the processing element's summation function. Weighting factors perform the same type of function as do the varying synaptic strengths of biological neurons. Some inputs are made more important than others so that they have a greater effect on the processing element as they combine to produce a neural response.

2.1.2. Learning function

The purpose of the learning function is to modify the input connection weights of the inputs during the training process (Rolston, 1988; Eberhart et al., 1996). This process of changing the weights of the input connections to achieve some desired result can also be called the adaptation function, as well as the learning mode.

2.1.3. Summation function

Artificial neurons compute the sum of all of the weighed inputs into a single number or vector, using a summation function (Rolston, 1988; Eberhart et al., 1996). This summation function can be more complex than just the simple input. The weighted sum of products and various algorithms for combining neural inputs have therefore been proposed for different ANN architectures and paradigms.

2.1.4. Transfer function

The result of the summation function is transformed into a working output through an algorithmic process known as the transfer function (Rolston, 1988; Eberhart et al., 1996). In the transfer function the summation total can be compared with some threshold, that is generally non-linear, to determine the neural output. If the sum is greater than the threshold value, the processing element generates a signal. If the sum of the input and weighted products is less than the threshold, no signal (or some inhibitory signal) is generated. Both types of response are significant.

2.1.5. Scaling and limiting

After processing the signal through the artificial neuron's transfer function, the value can be further modified by functions that scale and limit the output (Rolston, 1988; Eberhart et al., 1996). This scaling process simply multiplies the value by some scale factor and then adds an offset. Limiting is the mechanism which ensures that the scaled result does not exceed an upper or lower bound.

2.1.6. Output function (competition)

After processing the input data using the various functions described above, each artificial neuron generates one output signal that is transferred as "connection strength" to many other neurons, in a manner similar to biological neurons. Neurons are allowed to compete with each other using connection strengths that are either positive or negative numbers (Rolston, 1988; Eberhart et al., 1996).

2.1.7. Error function and back-propagated value

The difference between the current output and the desired output of an ANN is calculated during the training process (Rolston, 1988; Eberhart et al., 1996). The artificial neuron's error is then typically propagated into the learning function of other processing elements. These values are used by the ANN during the iterative training process.

2.2. Training or teaching artificial neural networks: training and testing datasets

ANNs are generally "taught" by exposing them to training datasets that include the corresponding desired output set (supervised training) (Rolston, 1988; Eberhart et al., 1996). They can also be trained in an unsupervised manner, using datasets that include no known desired output set (unsupervised training). In the latter situation, the ANNs are expected to develop their own classification or forecasting models, "unbiased" by human interaction.

In experimental studies, the data are usually randomly divided into two datasets: the training set, which includes the desired output information; and the testing set, which lacks the latter (Bellotti et al., 1997; Marchevsky et al., 1998, 1999, 2004; Singson et al., 1999;

Esteva et al., 2001). The characteristics of each trained ANN will depend to some extent on the characteristics of the individual cases or members of the "training set".

2.3. Supervised and unsupervised learning

The vast majority of artificial neural network solutions have been trained with supervision (Naguib, 2001). In this mode, the actual output of a neural network is compared to the desired output. Weights, which are usually randomly set to begin with, are then adjusted by the network so that the next iteration, or cycle, will produce a closer match between the desired and the actual output. The supervised learning method tries to minimize the current errors of all processing elements. This global error reduction is created over time by continuously modifying the input weights until acceptable network accuracy is reached.

Training sets need to be sufficiently large to contain all the required information if the network is to learn the features and relationships that are important. Not only do the sets have to be large but also the training sessions must include a wide variety of data.

Unsupervised learning is currently being used only for academic purposes and is limited to the use of ANN models known as self-organizing maps (Russell and Norvig, 1995). These ANNs look for regularities or trends in the input signals, and make adaptations using various mathematical functions.

2.4. Learning rates

Most learning functions have some provision for a constant called learning rate. This constant increases the connection strength values by some arbitrary number during training to allow the system to improve its performance during training (Rolston, 1988: Eberhart et al., 1996).

2.5. Learning rules

Many learning laws or rules have been proposed for a variety of ANN models. Most of these rules are some sort of variation of the best-known and oldest learning law, Hebb's Rule (Rolston, 1988: Eberhart et al., 1996). This rule indicates that if a neuron receives an input from another neuron, and if both are highly active (mathematically have the same sign), the weight between the neurons should be strengthened. Other learning rules, mostly derived from the Hebb's rule, include the Hopfield Law, Kohonen's Learning Law, Gradient Descent Rule, the Delta rule and others (Rolston, 1988). The Delta rule is the most commonly used learning law in current ANN software and is based on the simple idea of continuously modifying the strengths of the input connections to reduce the difference (the delta) between the desired output value and the actual output of a processing element. This rule changes the synaptic weights during training in the way that minimizes the mean squared error of the network.

2.6. Testing trained artificial neural network models

The accuracy of trained ANN models needs to be studied by the analysis of validation or "test" datasets that have data with desired output known to the investigator but not to the network (Rolston, 1988: Eberhart et al., 1996). ANNs that can analyze the test data with acceptable specificity have a good potential to yield valuable results. However, in any particular experiment, the fact that a trained ANN analyses correctly the test data offers no guarantee that the system will generalize to other datasets, as the characteristics of the trained ANN will depend on the variability of a particular training dataset that may not be representative of a much larger data sample.

2.7. Validation of artificial neural network models: cross-validation procedures

ANNs and multivariate statistical methods can yield apparently accurate results randomly. (Marchevsky and Wick, 2004; Marchevsky et al., 2004). The results of these analyses are frequently determined by the characteristics of the training dataset, where many of the variables may show auto-correlated values. Statisticians refer to this problem as data overfit or "shrinkage" (Looney, 2002). As a result of these problems, the characteristics of a trained ANN are strongly influenced by the data used for training and their output cannot be generalized with accuracy to the study of other datasets (Naguib, 2001).

Probably the best method to evaluate the accuracy of an ANN model is to test it with additional sets of data, which are different from those of the initial training and testing sets, using data collected from a variety of populations and under different conditions. As such data are not frequently available during development, various automatic jackknifed procedures have been proposed. In an iterative manner, a dataset is arbitrarily divided into training and testing sets using a proportion of cases for each set. For example, 80% of the cases may be used for training the ANN and the remaining 20% of the cases for testing the results. Several training and testing sets are organized using different cases. For example, the data from a particular patient may be used as a part of the training set in some of these "training–testing" combinations and as a part of the testing set in others (Marchevsky and Wick, 2004; Marchevsky et al., 2004). Jackknife procedures can also use all cases for training except for one case to be used as "one-out test" case. The results of these various ANNs trained and tested with similar but not identical data are compared to determine if their classification or prediction rates are comparable. If the majority of test cases are classified correctly by the various ANNs, then the results suggest that any of these ANNs could be applied in the future for the analysis of truly unknown data. The results of the various classifications obtained by different ANNs trained in this manner can be compared with Kappa statistics, designed to compare observations made by different observers. This method has been widely used for assessing intra-observer and inter-observer agreement for diagnoses provided by various observers. The kappa values allow for classification of agreements as: moderate (0.41–0.6), substantial (0.6–0.8) and almost perfect (0.81–1.00) (Marchevsky et al., 2004).

2.8. Artificial neural network model selection

Multiple ANN models have been developed for prediction, classification, data association, data conceptualization and data filtering (Naguib, 2001). It is beyond the scope of this chapter to describe these various models in detail. For example, backpropagation, delta bar delta, directed random search, higher order neural networks and self-organizing maps have been proposed for the analysis of problems related to prediction, where the input values are processed to predict an output such as stock prices, people at risk for a particular disease and others (Eberhart et al., 1996). ANN models, such as the learning vector quantization, counter-propagation models, probabilities neural network and others have been proposed for classification purposes, such as the determination of tumour cell type or the kind of airplane on a radar screen (Rolston, 1988). The probabilistic neural network provides a general solution to pattern classification problems by using Bayesian classifiers, developed in statistics (Russell and Norvig, 1995). Bayesian theory, developed in the 1950s, takes into account the relative likelihood of events and uses a priori information to improve prediction (Looney, 2002).

3. APPLICATION OF ARTIFICIAL NEURAL NETWORKS TO THE ESTIMATION OF THE PROGNOSIS OF INDIVIDUAL CANCER PATIENTS

The diagnosis of cancer is based on pathologic examination and classification of neoplasms into specific cell types (Marchevsky and Wick, 2004). The prognosis of a patient with a particular cancer type is usually determined using survival statistics by the combination of histopathologic, staging and other clinical or laboratory data. These forecasting models apply to large populations of patients having a particular diagnosis but do not estimate precisely the prognosis of an individual patient.

There is an increasing interest in the use of molecular data from human neoplasms for diagnostic and prognostic purposes (Narayanan et al., 2002). A prodigious amount of data regarding the molecular composition of a variety of neoplasms are being collected from tissue samples, but it is not yet clear how to analyze and interpret these data to yield diagnostic and prognostic information that will complement or replace the experience acquired over many years from the study of neoplasms with microscopy and other morphology-based methods. A recent review of the application of Evidence-Based Medicine and Decision to Pathology discussed the limitations of such general approaches to the prognostication of individual patients with cancer and other diseases (Marchevsky and Wick, 2004).

ANN models offer a potentially useful tool for the development of classification and prognostic models for patients with cancer, as they are well-suited to analyse multivariate data with somewhat "uncertain" characteristics and are designed to assign a classification or forecasting value to individual members of a population. Various studies in our laboratory and many others have applied backpropagation, probabilistic and other ANN models to the study of neoplasms (Becker, 1994; Attikiouzel and deSilva, 1995; Babaian and Zhang, 2001; Batuello et al., 2001; Abbass, 2002; Aoyama et al., 2002; Ball et al., 2002; Anagnostou et al., 2003).

A recent literature search using the terms "artificial neural network" and "cancer" yields a list of over 200 studies that have applied ANN technology for the diagnosis and prognosis of cancer patients (Binder et al., 1994; Burke, 1994; Droste et al., 1996; Burke et al., 1997; Buyse and Piedbois, 1997; Douglas and Moul, 1998; Fogel et al., 1998b; Biagiotti et al., 1999; Bostwick and Burke, 2001; Dreiseitl et al., 2001; Errejon et al., 2001; Djavan et al., 2002; Catto et al., 2003; Coppini et al., 2003; Danesi and Paolo, 2003; Bloom et al., 2004; Bollschweiler et al., 2004; Chen et al., 2004; Dua et al., 2004). Selected applications based on laboratory data and on imaging data are listed in Tables 1 and 2 (Becker, 1994; Naguib and Sherbet, 1997; Naguib et al., 1997, 1998; Biagiotti et al., 1999; Grumett and Snow, 2000; Murphy et al., 2000; Nakamura et al., 2000; Babaian and Zhang, 2001; Batuello et al., 2001; Han et al., 2001; Mattfeldt et al., 2001a,b; Montie and Wei, 2001; Abbass, 2002; Aoyama et al., 2002; Halkiotis and Mantas, 2002; Narayanan et al., 2002; Ng et al., 2002; Anagnostou et al., 2003; Fujikawa et al., 2003; Grey et al., 2003; Gamito and Crawford, 2004; Gulliford et al., 2004).

Table 1. Various experimental applications of artificial neural networks for the diagnosis and estimation of prognosis in cancer patients using laboratory data*

Clinical function	Application
Tumour grading	Bladder cancer
Diagnosis	Malignant lymphoma
	Lung cancer
	Malignant mesothelioma
	Liver dysplasia and cancer
	Ovarian dysplasia
Prediction of nodal spread and/or stage	Breast cancer
	Lung cancer
	Colon cancer
	Gastric cancer
	Prostate cancer
Prognosis	Breast cancer
	Lung cancer
	Neuroblastoma
	Prostate cancer
	Bladder cancer
	Ovarian cancer
	Colon cancer
	Head and neck cancer
Predict outcome of repeat prostate biopsies	

*This table is not intended to be all inclusive.

Table 2. Various experimental applications of artificial neural networks for the diagnosis and estimation of prognosis in cancer patients using imaging data*

Clinical Function	Application
Improve accuracy of staging of lung cancer patient using imaging methods	Analysis of solitary pulmonary nodules
	Analysis of magnetic resonance imaging for the diagnosis of breast cancer
	Detection of breast lesions with mammogram
	Detection of small lung nodules based on computed tomography
	Diagnosis of liver lesions based on ultrasound images
Analysis of multidisciplinary data	Prediction of prostate cancer stage based on magnetic resonance imaging, prostate specific antigen and Gleason score
	Prognosis of lung cancer patients based on genetic polymorphisms and clinical parameters

*This table is not intended to be all inclusive.

4. EXAMPLES OF ARTIFICIAL NEURAL NETWORK APPLICATIONS IN CANCER RESEARCH

4.1. Prediction of survival in patients with Stage I and II lung cancer

The prognosis of patients with Stage I and II non-small-cell lung cancer (NSCLC) can be estimated but cannot be definitively ascertained by the use of current clinicopathologic criteria and tumour marker studies. Our laboratory in collaboration with pathologists in Argentina studied sixty-seven patients with NSCLC, including 49 patients with Stage I NSCLC and 18 with Stage II disease (11 with squamous cell carcinomas, 35 with adenocarcinomas and 21 with large cell carcinomas), who were treated with lobectomy and followed for a minimum of 5 years (Bellotti et al., 1997). The tumours were studied with DNA flow cytometry and quantitative immunocytochemical studies for proliferation cell nuclear antigen, p53 protein, and MIB-1. The data were analysed with backpropagation neural networks, and statistical methods. The dependent variables were "free of disease" and "recurrence or dead from disease." Twenty neural network models were trained, using all cases but one, after 1883–2000 training cycles. All of the 20 models classified the test cases correctly.

A more recent study performed in collaboration with pathologists at the Baylor Medical College, Houston, Texas reported the use of a probabilistic ANN for the analysis of multiple prognostic factors (age, sex, cell type, stage, tumour grade, smoking history and immunoreactivity to *c-erbB-3*, *bcl-2*, *Glut1*, *Glut3*, *retinoblastoma* gene and *p53*

(Marchevsky et al., 1998). The ANN was trained to estimate the 5-year survival in 63 patients with Stage I or II NSCLC, treated solely by surgical excision. Several probabilistic ANNs with genetic algorithm models were developed using the prognostic features as input neurons and survival at 5 years (free of disease/dead of disease) as output neurons. The probabilistic ANN yielded excellent classification rates for dependent variable survival. The best model was trained with 52 cases and classified all 11 "unknown" test cases correctly.

Hsia et al. (2003) recently reported the use of ANNs to estimate the survival of 75 advanced lung cancer patients based on the analysis of data from genetic polymorphism of the *p21* and *p53* genes in conjunction with patients' general data. The predicted accuracy was 86.2%.

4.2. Lung cancer diagnosis using DNA hypermethylation data

A recent study from our laboratory reported the use of probabilistic ANNs for the classification of lung cancer cells, based on DNA hypermethylation data (Marchevsky et al., 2004). DNA methylation levels at 20 loci were measured in 41 SCLC and 44 NSCLC cell lines with the quantitative real-time PCR method MethyLight. The data were analysed with linear discriminant analysis (LDA) and ANNs to classify the cell lines into SCLC or NSCLC. Two significant LDA models correctly classified 84 and 82% of the cell lines, respectively. The data were sorted randomly by cell line into 10 different data sets, each with training and testing subsets composed of 80 and 20% of the cases. Ten different ANN models were trained and tested using these data sets, to cross-validate the results. Five of the ANN models used all 20 variables while five other ANN models used the same 5 variables selected by statistical analysis. The first five ANN models correctly classified 100% of the cell lines, while the latter five models correctly classified 87–100% of the cases. The classifications provided by the 10 different models were compared with kappa statistics, yielding kappa values ranging from 0.8 to 1.0, representing substantial to perfect concordance.

Hanai et al. (2003) in a recent study from Japan developed a prognostic model for 125 NSCLC patients with 17 potential input variables, including 9 clinico-pathological variables (age, sex, smoking index, tumour size, p factor, pT, pN, stage, histology) and 5 immunohistochemical variables (p27 percentage, p27 intensity, p53, cyclin D1, retinoblastoma (RB)), by using the parameter-increasing method (PIM). The ANN model correctly predicted the outcome in 104 of 125 patients (83%, judgment ratio (JR)) and accuracy for prediction of survival at 5 years was 87%.

Zhou et al. (2002) reported the use of ANNs to identify lung cancer cells in the images of specimens collected with needle biopsies and classify them first as either normal cells or cancer cells and thereafter as adenocarcinoma, squamous cell carcinoma, small cell carcinoma, large cell carcinoma or normal.

4.3. Prediction of nodal status in breast cancer and colon cancer patients

Axillary lymph node status is an important prognostic feature for patients with breast cancer, but the therapeutic value of axillary lymphadenectomy is controversial. We studied

279 patients with invasive breast carcinoma treated with modified radical mastectomy or with lumpectomy combined with axillary lymph node dissection in an attempt to develop predictive ANN models (Marchevsky et al., 1999). Prognostic factors evaluated were age, histologic type of invasive tumour, presence of associated ductal and/or lobular carcinoma in situ, lesion size, histologic and nuclear grades, DNA index, presence of multiploidy by flow cytometric analysis, and immunocytochemical expression of oestrogen and progesterone receptors, proliferating nuclear cell antigen, and *HER-2/neu* oncogene. Several probabilistic ANNs with genetic algorithms were developed using prognostic features as input neurons and lymph node status (positive or negative) as output neurons. The best ANN model was trained with 224 cases using 19 input neurons. It classified correctly 49 (89.0%) of 55 unknown cases (specificity, 97.2%; sensitivity, 80.0%; positive predictive value, 93.8%; negative predictive value, 87.5%). A study of colon cancer patients with similar methodology yielded comparable results (Singson et al., 1999).

Recently, Grey et al. (2003) developed ANN models that predict the nodal spread of breast cancer patients based on the analysis of *S100A2* and *nm23* gene expression and steroid receptor expression.

Other laboratories have also reported promising results using ANNs for the estimation of lymph node metastases in patients with gastric adenocarcinoma, and prostate cancer (Droste et al., 1996; Naguib et al., 1997, 1999; Batuello et al., 2001; Han et al., 2001; Seker et al., 2002; Bollschweiler et al., 2004).

4.4. Prediction of the clinical outcome of neuroblastoma patients

Wei et al. (2004), in a recent study at the National Cancer Institute (NCI), reported the use of ANNs and DNA microarrays to predict successfully the clinical outcome of patients diagnosed with neuroblastoma (NB). The ANNs identified a minimal set of 19 genes whose expression levels were closely associated with this clinical outcome. Gene expression analysis using cDNA microarrays containing over 25 000 genes was studied to create global gene expression profiles of 49 patients with primary NB and known clinical outcome. The patients were divided into either good (event-free survival for greater than three years) or poor (death due to disease) outcome groups. The ANNs could predict the clinical outcome from any individual gene profile with an accuracy of about 88%. As these gene profiles consisted of over 25 000 genes, the researchers tried to optimize the profiles and find the minimum number of genes (so-called "pruning process"), which could act as a predictor set. The ANNs identified 19 genes whose expression levels could accurately predict clinical outcome. When only looking at these 19 genes, prediction accuracy of ANNs increased to 95%.

5. CONCLUSIONS

It is beyond the scope of this chapter to review in detail the vast number of studies that have reported the use of ANNs for Cancer Diagnosis and Prognosis (Becker, 1994; Burke, 1994; Rogers et al., 1994; Deligdisch et al., 1995; Wu et al., 1995; Droste et al., 1996;

Bottaci et al., 1997; Douglas and Moul, 1998; Fogel et al., 1998a; Wei et al., 1998, 2004; Biagiotti et al., 1999; Ronco, 1999; Bigio et al., 2000; Grumett and Snow, 2000; Schwarzer et al., 2000; Babaian and Zhang, 2001; Batuello et al., 2001; Boracchi et al., 2001; Bostwick and Burke, 2001; Errejon et al., 2001; Sargent, 2001; Snow et al., 1999, 2001; Tourassi et al., 2001; Abbass, 2002; Aoyama et al., 2002; Ball et al., 2002; Djavan et al., 2002; Narayanan et al., 2002; Ochi et al., 2002; Seker et al., 2002; Selaru et al., 2002; Yang et al., 2002; Zhou et al., 2002; Anagnostou et al., 2003; Catto et al., 2003; Crawford, 2003; Danesi and Paolo, 2003; Fujikawa et al., 2003; Grey et al., 2003; O'Neill and Song, 2003; Porter and Crawford, 2003; Ringner and Peterson, 2003; Schumacher et al., 2003; Zlotta et al., 2003; Bloom et al., 2004; Bollschweiler et al., 2004; Dua et al., 2004; Gamito and Crawford, 2004; Szabo et al., 2004; Taktak et al., 2004).

These studies have generally validated the value of ANN technology as a classificatory and predictive tool for the analysis of a variety of data collected with pathological, image analysis, molecular studies, imaging and other modalities. However, most of these studies have been performed using relatively small data sets, multiple variables and a relatively small ratio of observations: numbers of variables, raising questions as to whether some of the optimistic results reported in the literature can be generalized to much larger populations of cancer patients. Further studies using data from hundreds or thousands of patients are needed in order to develop robust classificatory and predictive models based on ANN technology that could provide reliable prognostic and predictive information for the routine care of cancer patients. These studies are difficult to perform in one research institution and require the development of a research infrastructure that allows the collection of tissue, clinical data and other materials from many patients treated at multiple institutions (Marchevsky and Wick, 2004f). Such large studies will hopefully further the development of robust prognostic and predictive models for the treatment of cancer patients based on the use of ANN technology and multivariate statistical methods (Biganzoli et al., 2003).

REFERENCES

Abbass, H.A., 2002, An evolutionary artificial neural networks approach for breast cancer diagnosis. Artif. Intell. Med., 25(3), 265–281.

Anagnostou, T., M. Remzi, M. Lykourinas and B. Djavan, 2003, Artificial neural networks for decision-making in urologic oncology. Eur. Urol., 43(6), 596–603.

Aoyama, M., Q. Li, S. Katsuragawa, H. MacMahon and K. Doi, 2002, Automated computerized scheme for distinction between benign and malignant solitary pulmonary nodules on chest images. Med. Phys., 29(5), 701–708.

Attikiouzel, Y. and C.J. deSilva, 1995, Applications of neural networks in medicine. Australas. Phys. Eng. Sci. Med., 18(3), 158–164.

Babaian, R.J. and Z. Zhang, 2001, Computer-assisted diagnostics: application to prostate cancer. Mol. Urol., 5(4), 175–180.

Ball, G., S. Mian, F. Holding, R.O. Allibone, J. Lowe, S. Ali, G. Li, S. McCardle, I.O. Ellis, C. Creaser and R.C. Rees, 2002, An integrated approach utilizing artificial neural networks and SELDI mass spectrometry for the classification of human tumours and rapid identification of potential biomarkers. Bioinformatics, 18(3), 395–404.

Batuello, J.T., E.J. Gamito, E.D. Crawford, M. Han, A.W. Partin, D.G. McLeod and C. O'Donnell, 2001, Artificial neural network model for the assessment of lymph node spread in patients with clinically localized prostate cancer. Urology, 57(3), 481–485.

Becker, R.L., 1994, Computer-assisted image classification: use of neural networks in anatomic pathology. Cancer Lett., 77(2–3), 111–117.

Bellotti, M., B. Elsner, L.A. Paez De, H. Esteva and A.M. Marchevsky, 1997, Neural networks as a prognostic tool for patients with non-small-cell carcinoma of the lung. Mod. Pathol., 10(12), 1221–1227.

Biagiotti, R., C. Desii, E. Vanzi and G. Gacci, 1999, Predicting ovarian malignancy: application of artificial neural networks to transvaginal and color Doppler flow US. Radiology, 210(2), 399–403.

Biganzoli, E., P. Boracchi, D. Coradini, D.M., Grazia and E. Marubini, 2003, Prognosis in node-negative primary breast cancer: a neural network analysis of risk profiles using routinely assessed factors 2772. Ann. Oncol., 14(10), 1484–1493.

Bigio, I.J., S.G. Bown, G. Briggs, C. Kelley, S. Lakhani, D. Pickard, P.M. Ripley, I.G. Rose and C. Saunders, 2000, Diagnosis of breast cancer using elastic-scattering spectroscopy: preliminary clinical results. J. Biomed. Opt., 5(2), 221–228.

Binder, M., A. Steiner, M. Schwarz, S. Knollmayer, K. Wolff and H. Pehamberger, 1994, Application of an artificial neural network in epiluminescence microscopy pattern analysis of pigmented skin lesions: a pilot study. Br. J. Dermatol., 130(4), 460–465.

Bloom, G., I.V. Yang, D. Boulware, K.Y. Kwong, D. Coppola, S. Eschrich, J. Quackenbush and T.J. Yeatman, 2004, Multi-platform, multi-site, microarray-based human tumor classification. Am. J. Pathol., 164(1), 9–16.

Bollschweiler, E.H., S.P. Monig, K. Hensler, S.E. Baldus, K. Maruyama and A.H. Holscher, 2004, Artificial neural network for prediction of lymph node metastases in gastric cancer: a phase II diagnostic study. Ann. Surg. Oncol., 11(5), 506–511.

Boracchi, P., E. Biganzoli and E. Marubini, 2001, Modelling cause-specific hazards with radial basis function artificial neural networks: application to 2233 breast cancer patients. Stat. Med., 20(24), 3677–3694.

Bostwick, D.G. and H.B. Burke, 2001, Prediction of individual patient outcome in cancer: comparison of artificial neural networks and Kaplan-Meier methods. Cancer, 91(Suppl 8), 1643–1646.

Bottaci, L., P.J. Drew, J.E. Hartley, M.B. Hadfield, R. Farouk, P.W. Lee, I.M. Macintyre, G.S. Duthie and J.R. Monson, 1997, Artificial neural networks applied to outcome prediction for colorectal cancer patients in separate institutions. Lancet, 350(9076), 469–472.

Burke, H.B., 1994, Artificial neural networks for cancer research: outcome prediction. Semin. Surg. Oncol., 10(1), 73–79.

Burke, H.B., P.H. Goodman, D.B. Rosen, D.E. Henson, J.N. Weinstein, F.E. Harrell Jr., J.R. Marks, D.P. Winchester and D.G. Bostwick, 1997, Artificial neural networks improve the accuracy of cancer survival prediction. Cancer, 79(4), 857–862.

Buyse, M. and P. Piedbois, 1997, Artificial neural networks. Lancet, 350(9085), 1175–1176.

Catto, J.W., D.A. Linkens, M.F. Abbod, M. Chen, J.L. Burton, K.M. Feeley and F.C. Hamdy, 2003, Artificial intelligence in predicting bladder cancer outcome: a comparison of neuro-fuzzy modeling and artificial neural networks. Clin. Cancer Res., 9(11), 4172–4177.

Chen, Y.D., S. Zheng, J.K. Yu and X. Hu, 2004, Artificial neural networks analysis of surface-enhanced laser desorption/ionization mass spectra of serum protein pattern distinguishes colorectal cancer from healthy population. Clin. Cancer Res., 10(24), 8380–8385.

Coppini, G., S. Diciotti, M. Falchini, N. Villari and G. Valli, 2003, Neural networks for computer-aided diagnosis: detection of lung nodules in chest radiograms. IEEE Trans. Inf. Technol. Biomed., 7(4), 344–357.

Crawford, E.D., 2003, Use of algorithms as determinants for individual patient decision making: national comprehensive cancer network versus artificial neural networks. Urology, 62(6 Suppl 1), 13–19.

Danesi, R. and A.D. Paolo, 2003, Predicting survival with artificial neural networks. Clin. Colorectal Cancer, 2(4), 245.

Deligdisch, L., A.J. Einstein, D. Guera and J. Gil, 1995, Ovarian dysplasia in epithelial inclusion cysts. A morphometric approach using neural networks. Cancer, 76(6), 1027–1034.

Djavan, B., M. Remzi, A. Zlotta, C. Seitz, P. Snow and M. Marberger, 2002, Novel artificial neural network for early detection of prostate cancer. J. Clin. Oncol., 20(4), 921–929.

Douglas, T.H. and J.W. Moul, 1998, Applications of neural networks in urologic oncology. Semin. Urol. Oncol., 16(1), 35–39.

Dreiseitl, S., L. Ohno-Machado, H. Kittler, S. Vinterbo, H. Billhardt and M. Binder, 2001, A comparison of machine learning methods for the diagnosis of pigmented skin lesions. J. Biomed. Inform., 34(1), 28–36.

Droste, K., E. Bollschweiler, T. Waschulzik, T. Schutz, R. Engelbrecht, K. Maruyama and J.R. Siewert, 1996, Prediction of lymph node metastasis in gastric cancer patients with neural networks. Cancer Lett., 109(1–2), 141–148.

Dua, R., D.G. Beetner, W.V. Stoecker and D.C. Wunsch, 2004, Detection of basal cell carcinoma using electrical impedance and neural networks. IEEE Trans. Biomed. Eng., 51(1), 66–71.

Eberhart, R., P. Simpson and R. Dobbins, 1996, Computational Intelligence PC Tools. Academic Press, New York, NY.

Errejon, A., E.D. Crawford, J. Dayhoff, C. O'Donnell, A. Tewari, J. Finkelstein and E.J. Gamito, 2001, Use of artificial neural networks in prostate cancer. Mol. Urol., 5(4), 153–158.

Esteva, H., M. Bellotti and A.M. Marchevsky, 2001, Neural networks for the estimation of prognosis in lung cancer. In: R.N.G. Naguib (Ed.), Artificial Neural Networks in Cancer Diagnosis, Prognosis and Patient Management. CRC Press, Boca Raton, Florida, pp. 29–38.

Fogel, D.B., E.C. Wasson III, E.M. Boughton and V.W. Porto, 1998a, Evolving artificial neural networks for screening features from mammograms. Artif. Intell. Med., 14(3), 317–326.

Fogel, D.B., E.C. Wasson, E.M. Boughton, V.W. Porto and P.J. Angeline, 1998b, Linear and neural models for classifying breast masses. IEEE Trans. Med. Imaging., 17(3), 485–488.

Fujikawa, K., Y. Matsui, T. Kobayashi, K. Miura, H. Oka, S. Fukuzawa, M. Sasaki, H. Takeuchi and T. Okabe, 2003, Predicting disease outcome of non-invasive transitional cell carcinoma of the urinary bladder using an artificial neural network model: results of patient follow-up for 15 years or longer. Int. J. Urol., 10(3), 149–152.

Gamito, E.J. and E.D. Crawford, 2004, Artificial neural networks for predictive modeling in prostate cancer. Curr. Oncol. Rep., 6(3), 216–221.

Grey, S.R., S.S. Dlay, B.E. Leone, F. Cajone and G.V. Sherbet, 2003, Prediction of nodal spread of breast cancer by using artificial neural network-based analyses of S100A4, nm23 and steroid receptor expression. Clin. Exp. Metastasis, 20(6), 507–514.

Grumett, S.A. and P.B. Snow, 2000, Artificial neural networks: a new model for assessing prognostic factors. Ann. Oncol., 11(4), 383–384.

Gulliford, S.L., S. Webb, C.G. Rowbottom, D.W. Corne and D.P. Dearnaley, 2004, Use of artificial neural networks to predict biological outcomes for patients receiving radical radiotherapy of the prostate. Radiother. Oncol., 71(1), 3–12.

Halkiotis, S. and J. Mantas, 2002, Automatic detection of clustered microcalcifications in digital mammograms. Stud. Health Technol. Inform., 90, 24–29.

Han, M., P.B. Snow, J.M. Brandt and A.W. Partin, 2001, Evaluation of artificial neural networks for the prediction of pathologic stage in prostate carcinoma. Cancer, 91(Suppl 8), 1661–1666.

Hanai, T., Y. Yatabe, Y. Nakayama, T. Takahashi, H. Honda, T. Mitsudomi and T. Kobayashi, 2003, Prognostic models in patients with non-small-cell lung cancer using artificial neural networks in comparison with logistic regression. Cancer Sci., 94(5), 473–477.

Hsia, T.C., H.C. Chiang, D. Chiang, L.W. Hang, F.J. Tsai and W.C. Chen, 2003, Prediction of survival in surgical unresectable lung cancer by artificial neural networks including genetic polymorphisms and clinical parameters. J. Clin. Lab Anal., 17(6), 229–234.

Looney, S.W., 2002, Biostatistical Methods. Humana Press, Totawa, N.J.

Marchevsky, A.M. and M.R. Wick, 2004, Evidence-based medicine, medical decision analysis, and pathology. Hum. Pathol., 35(10), 1179–1188.

Marchevsky, A.M., S. Patel, K.J. Wiley, M.A. Stephenson, M. Gondo, R.W. Brown, E.S. Yi, W.F. Benedict, R.C. Anton and P.T. Cagle, 1998, Artificial neural networks and logistic regression as tools for prediction of survival in patients with stages I and II non-small-cell lung cancer. Mod. Pathol., 11(7), 618–625.

Marchevsky, A.M., S. Shah and S. Patel, 1999, Reasoning with uncertainty in pathology: artificial neural networks and logistic regression as tools for prediction of lymph node status in breast cancer patients. Mod. Pathol., 12(5), 505–513.

Marchevsky, A.M., J.A. Tsou and I.A. Laird-Offringa, 2004, Classification of individual lung cancer cell lines based on DNA methylation markers: use of linear discriminant analysis and artificial neural networks. J. Mol. Diagn., 6(1), 28–36.

Mattfeldt, T., H.A. Kestler, R. Hautmann and H.W. Gottfried, 2001a, Prediction of postoperative prostatic cancer stage on the basis of systematic biopsies using two types of artificial neural networks. Eur. Urol., 39(5), 530–536.

Mattfeldt, T., H. Wolter, R. Kemmerling, H.W. Gottfried and H.A. Kestler, 2001b, Cluster analysis of comparative genomic hybridization (CGH) data using self-organizing maps: application to prostate carcinomas. Anal. Cell Pathol., 23(1), 29–37.

Montie, J.E. and J.T. Wei, 2001, Artificial neural networks for prostate carcinoma risk assessment. An overview. Cancer, 91(Suppl 8), 1647–1652.

Murphy, G.P., P. Snow, S.J. Simmons, B.A. Tjoa, M.K. Rogers, J. Brandt, C.G. Healy, W.E. Bolton and D. Rodbold, 2000, Use of artificial neural networks in evaluating prognostic factors determining the response to dendritic cells pulsed with PSMA peptides in prostate cancer patients. Prostate, 42(1), 67–72.

Naguib, R.N.G., 2001, Artificial Neural Networks in Cancer Diagnosis, Prognosis, and Patient Management. CRC Press, Boca Raton, Florida, US.

Naguib, R.N. and G.V. Sherbet, 1997, Artificial neural networks in cancer research. Pathobiology, 65(3), 129–139.

Naguib, R.N., A.E. Adams, C.H. Horne, B. Angus, A.F. Smith, G.V. Sherbet and T.W. Lennard, 1997, Prediction of nodal metastasis and prognosis in breast cancer: a neural model. Anticancer Res., 17(4A), 2735–2741.

Naguib, R.N., M.C. Robinson, D.E. Neal and F.C. Hamdy, 1998, Neural network analysis of combined conventional and experimental prognostic markers in prostate cancer: a pilot study. Br. J. Cancer, 78(2), 246–250.

Naguib, R.N., H.A. Sakim, M.S. Lakshmi, V. Wadehra, T.W. Lennard, J. Bhatavdekar and G.V. Sherbet, 1999, DNA ploidy and cell cycle distribution of breast cancer aspirate cells measured by image cytometry and analyzed by artificial neural networks for their prognostic significance. IEEE Trans. Inf. Technol. Biomed., 3(1), 61–69.

Nakamura, K., H. Yoshida, R. Engelmann, H. MacMahon, S. Katsuragawa, T. Ishida, K. Ashizawa and K. Doi, 2000, Computerized analysis of the likelihood of malignancy in solitary pulmonary nodules with use of artificial neural networks. Radiology, 214(3), 823–830.

Narayanan, A., E.C. Keedwell and B. Olsson, 2002, Artificial intelligence techniques for bioinformatics. Appl. Bioinformatics, 1(4), 191–222.

Ng, E.Y., S.C. Fok, Y.C. Peh, F.C. Ng and L.S. Sim, 2002, Computerized detection of breast cancer with artificial intelligence and thermograms. J. Med. Eng Technol., 26(4), 152–157.

Ochi, T., K. Murase, T. Fujii, M. Kawamura and J. Ikezoe, 2002, Survival prediction using artificial neural networks in patients with uterine cervical cancer treated by radiation therapy alone. Int. J. Clin. Oncol., 7(5), 294–300.

O'Neill, M.C. and L. Song, 2003, Neural network analysis of lymphoma microarray data: prognosis and diagnosis near-perfect. BMC Bioinformatics, 4(1), 13.

Porter, C.R. and E.D. Crawford, 2003, Combining artificial neural networks and transrectal ultrasound in the diagnosis of prostate cancer. Oncology (Huntingt), 17(10), 1395–1399.

Ringner, M. and C. Peterson, 2003, Microarray-based cancer diagnosis with artificial neural networks. Biotechniques, 34(Suppl 3), 30–35.

Rogers, S.K., D.W. Ruck and M. Kabrisky, 1994, Artificial neural networks for early detection and diagnosis of cancer. Cancer Lett., 77(2–3), 79–83.

Rolston, D.W., 1988, Principles of Artificial Intelligence and Expert System Development. McGraw-Hill, New York, NY, USA.

Ronco, A.L., 1999, Use of artificial neural networks in modeling associations of discriminant factors: towards an intelligent selective breast cancer screening. Artif. Intell. Med., 16(3), 299–309.

Russell, S. and P. Norvig, 1995, Artificial Intelligence. A Modern Approach. Prentice Hall, Upple Saddle Valley, New Jersey.

Sargent, D.J., 2001, Comparison of artificial neural networks with other statistical approaches: results from medical data sets. Cancer, 91(Suppl 8), 1636–1642.

Schumacher, M., E. Graf and T. Gerds, 2003, How to assess prognostic models for survival data: a case study in oncology. Methods Inf. Med., 42(5), 564–571.

Schwarzer, G., W. Vach and M. Schumacher, 2000, On the misuses of artificial neural networks for prognostic and diagnostic classification in oncology. Stat. Med., 19(4), 541–561.

Seker, H., M.O. Odetayo, D. Petrovic, R.N. Naguib, C. Bartoli, L. Alasio, M.S. Lakshmi and G.V. Sherbet, 2002, Assessment of nodal involvement and survival analysis in breast cancer patients using image cytometric data: statistical, neural network and fuzzy approaches. Anticancer Res., 22(1A), 433–438.

Selaru, F.M., Y. Xu, J. Yin, T. Zou, T.C. Liu, Y. Mori, J.M. Abraham, F. Sato, S. Wang, C. Twigg, A. Olaru, V. Shustova, A. Leytin, P. Hytiroglou, D. Shibata, N. Harpaz and S.J. Meltzer, 2002, Artificial neural networks distinguish among subtypes of neoplastic colorectal lesions. Gastroenterology, 122(3), 606–613.

Singson, R.P., R. Alsabeh, S.A. Geller and A. Marchevsky, 1999, Estimation of tumor stage and lymph node status in patients with colorectal adenocarcinoma using probabilistic neural networks and logistic regression. Mod. Pathol., 12(5), 479–484.

Snow, P.B., D.M. Rodvold and J.M. Brandt, 1999, Artificial neural networks in clinical urology. Urology, 54(5), 787–790.

Snow, P.B., D.J. Kerr, J.M. Brandt and D.M. Rodvold, 2001, Neural network and regression predictions of 5-year survival after colon carcinoma treatment. Cancer, 91(Suppl 8), 1673–1678.

Szabo, B.K., M.K. Wiberg, B. Bone and P. Aspelin, 2004, Application of artificial neural networks to the analysis of dynamic MR imaging features of the breast. Eur. Radiol., 14(7), 1217–1225.

Taktak, A.F., A.C. Fisher and B.E. Damato, 2004, Modelling survival after treatment of intraocular melanoma using artificial neural networks and Bayes theorem. Phys. Med. Biol., 49(1), 87–98.

Tourassi, G.D., M.K. Markey, J.Y. Lo and C.E. Floyd Jr., 2001, A neural network approach to breast cancer diagnosis as a constraint satisfaction problem. Med. Phys., 28(5), 804–811.

Wei, J.S., B.T. Greer, F. Westermann, S.M. Steinberg, C.G. Son, Q.R. Chen, C.C. Whiteford, S. Bilke, A.L. Krasnoselsky, N. Cenacchi, D. Catchpoole, F. Berthold, M. Schwab and J. Khan, 2004, Prediction of clinical outcome using gene expression profiling and artificial neural networks for patients with neuroblastoma. Cancer Res., 64(19), 6883–6891.

Wei, J.T., Z. Zhang, S.D. Barnhill, K.R. Madyastha, H. Zhang and J.E. Oesterling, 1998, Understanding artificial neural networks and exploring their potential applications for the practicing urologist. Urology, 52(2), 161–172.

Wu, Y.C., K. Doi and M.L. Giger, 1995, Detection of lung nodules in digital chest radiographs using artificial neural networks: a pilot study. J. Digit Imaging, 8(2), 88–94.

Yang, J., G. Xu, H. Kong, Y. Zheng, T. Pang and Q. Yang, 2002, Artificial neural network classification based on high-performance liquid chromatography of urinary and serum nucleosides for the clinical diagnosis of cancer. J. Chromatogr. B. Analyt. Technol. Biomed. Life Sci., 780(1), 27–33.

Zhou, Z.H., Y. Jiang, Y.B. Yang and S.F. Chen, 2002, Lung cancer cell identification based on artificial neural network ensembles. Artif. Intell. Med., 24(1), 25–36.

Zlotta, A.R., M. Remzi, P.B. Snow, C.C. Schulman, M. Marberger and B. Djavan, 2003, An artificial neural network for prostate cancer staging when serum prostate specific antigen is 10 ng./ml. or less. J. Urol., 169(5), 1724–1728.

Chapter 10

Machine Learning Contribution to Solve Prognostic Medical Problems

Flavio Baronti, Alessio Micheli, Alessandro Passaro and Antonina Starita

Dipartimento di Informatica, University of Pisa, Pisa, Italy
Email: starita@di.unipi.it

Abstract

Exploring biomolecular and medical data is a challenging area where the need for data driven methodologies is constantly increasing. Machine Learning (ML) methods have the ability to learns from data, inferring from examples a general hypothesis that can approximate complex relationships in the data for descriptive or predictive aims.

The ML is particularly useful for poorly understood domains due to the lack of a clear theory where, however, there are collections of relevant real-world data, which can be affected by uncertain or noise, or characterized by complex relationships that standard approaches cannot properly face.

The achievement of successful results for problems in biochemical and medical domains may require the integration of different type of data (such as clinical, genetic, biochemical data), together with computational task (including descriptive or predictive purpose), model design, and learning methods.

This survey summarizes typical aspects of the ML approach to problems and tasks, and treats the characteristics of data sets, models, tools, and evaluation techniques, in the context of their application in medical data analysis and bioinformatics, with emphasis on emergent approaches and research perspectives.

Finally, we present and discuss some recent results, as a test application of a rule-based evolutionary classifier system to a concrete example of clinical and genetic data set, built up for studies on the susceptibility to cancer.

Acknowledgement

The work was sponsored by EC IST NoE BIOPATTERN, Contract No: 508803.

Keywords: Machine learning, data analysis, medical applications, clinical and genetic data, learning structured data, evolutionary classifier systems.

Contents

© 2007 Elsevier B.V. All rights reserved

1. INTRODUCTION

One of the emerging issues in medical research is data analysis. The widespread use of computers makes it easy to gather and manage large amounts of data from many different sources. A well-organized system can make available clinical, biological, genetic data, and all other information collected about patients. This data is often *complex*, meaning that it contains many elements related in non-obvious ways or characterized by explicit or implicit relationships and structures. Such integration is increasingly considered necessary in order to produce more accurate diagnoses. For instance, decoding of DNA gave rise to the promise of personalized medicine: knowledge of the genetic makeup is thought to allow for diagnoses and prescriptions tailored for the specific individual. The data analysis system is then required to accept all this data, possibly in the form which is closer to reality, which can mean not only a set of attribute-value pairs, but also sequences or other variable size structures.

In this chapter, we introduce the research area of Machine Learning (ML), with particular emphasis on its applications in medical problems. ML is concerned with inferring general hypotheses from experience, typically made available through a collection of "past" situations. The central objective is to learn a strategy from the past, with the concern to produce good results also for unseen situations. ML nowadays helps in the understanding of medical problems, particularly in such domains (like the genetic one) where the interactions between different factors have not been fully understood yet.

Traditionally, medical data analyses have been performed employing standard statistical methods, since clinicians can usually better understand them and are often already familiar with some of the statistical packages that are widely available. Despite their popularity, however, many statistical techniques are based on very simple models, which often fail to catch data complexity. In this regard, ML can provide quite useful tools, since its models are usually much more powerful and flexible and can actually tackle problems with complex data. The downside is that this greater flexibility generally comes at the cost of an increased variability and a lesser interpretability of results.

Section 2 gives a basic overview of the machine learning theory. Section 3 explains the general characteristics of medical data, and the typical goals of medical research. Section 4 gives an example of application of two machine learning approaches, evolutionary classifier systems and decision trees, to a medical problem, connecting clinical and genetic data. Section 5 summarizes emergent approaches and the results achieved by exploiting learning structured data methods for medicinal chemistry, and research directions for pharmacogenetics. Section 6 discusses the benefits of ML and draws conclusions.

2. MACHINE LEARNING

Here, we review some basic concepts and terms of Machine Learning (ML) theory, focusing on the approaches studied in the application part.

ML deals with the problem of inferring general functions from known data. ML methods are particularly useful for poorly understood domains, where the lack of a clear theory describing the underlying phenomena, or the presence of uncertain and noisy data, hampers the development of effective algorithms to solve specific problems. The techniques developed in the field of ML can be exploited for a variety of applications and they play a central role in other (related) disciplines also, such as "Knowledge Discovery in Databases", which deal with the overall cycle process of extracting unknown and useful information from the data.

For the sake of introduction, we find it useful to first describe the ML topics of our interest in terms of few key design choices concerning the data, the tasks, the models, and the learning algorithms:

- The *data* is the set of facts available for the problem at hand. Examples from the application domain are represented in a formalism that should be able to capture the structure of the analysed objects.
- The *task* defines the aim of the application. It implicitly defines the nature of the results, and thus how they can be used. The original problem is moved into the problem of learning some designed *target function*. The form of task is related to the type of feedback information available from the system that we are modelling. Tasks that we consider in the following can be, for example, roughly partitioned into predictive (classification and regression) or descriptive (cluster analysis, association analysis, summarization, etc.).
- The *model* is characterized by the type of *hypothesis*, i.e. the function fitting the data of interest, used to describe the solution for the task. The representation of such functions defines the *space of hypotheses*. In ML the hypothesis (model) is used to approximate the target function. In general, the hypothesis can be an expression in a given language that describes the relationships among the data.
- An *algorithm* is used to learn the best hypothesis according to the data, the task and the class of models considered.

The first design choice for a learning system is the collection and representation of the problems data. The set of represented data constitutes the training experience from which the system will learn. The type of information available can have a significant impact on the qualitative response of the learner. The instance of data entry for the system is a quantitative or structural description of an object referred as *pattern* (in ML terminology). The choice of the appropriate representation, considering both the selection of the representational types, and the selection of the set of distinguishing features that convey information, is a critical problem-oriented design step. The data that we consider can be of different types according to the representation formalism, as now described.

2.1. Single flat table

All the objects in the data set are represented by a matrix of data, where for each example, there is a fixed-size vector of object properties (measurements or *features*), according to an attribute-value language. The features can have real values (continuous attribute) or nominal values (discrete or categorical values).

Among vectorial patterns we can find, for instance, the pixel matrix of an image or the genetic expression profile obtained with microarray technology. The dataset analysed in Section 4 is an example of flat table.

2.2. Structured domain

The objects in the domain can be sequences (lists), hierarchical structures (e.g. trees), graphs, relational data, multi-table representations, and so on. In data mining, structured objects correspond to objects of different types (multiple relations in a relational database), for example, a database with more than one table. Note that labelled structures can represent both vector patterns and their relationships.

A large set of real-world data can be characterized by structured data, in particular for biological and medical domains. For instance, temporal events, signals, proteins, DNA and molecules are clear examples of data that can naturally be represented by sequences or graphs. In these cases, a structured representation is able to retain the meaning of the relationships among primitive elements conveyed by the original data.

The capability to deal with more complex source of data, including structured data, can be a key feature in ML to approach challenging tasks emerging from the integration of different fields, such as (for the purpose of this chapter) clinical, biochemical and genetic studies. This integration is actually the goal of the BIOPATTERN network of excellence, and the basic requirement to produce a *bioprofile*, that is the unification of a person's medical history with diagnosis and prediction of possible susceptibility to diseases.

In the ML area the tasks are mainly distinguished according to the type of information available as data. The task can be *supervised*, when information on the desired model response is given for each example (or sample), or *unsupervised* when this information is not available.

In the framework of supervised learning we distinguish the following terms, according to the two different computational tasks:

- *Classification*: means to approximate a discrete-valued function. The function maps a pattern into a M-dimensional decision space, where M is the number of categories or *classes* ($M \geq 2$). For $M > 2$ we speak of multi-class problems. A special case is given for binary classification, with $M = 2$, called also "concept learning" within the *pattern recognition* framework.
- *Regression*: means to approximate a real-valued target function. The function maps a pattern into a continuous space. The problem may be also viewed as "curve fitting" in multidimensional space.

In medicine, supervised learning is useful in many cases: we might want to decide whether or not a person has a certain disease, how high is his risk to develop oral cancer, or how long he will survive after a surgical intervention.

Now, we also consider an unsupervised task:

- *Clustering*: means to determine useful subsets of a unclassified set of data sample.

In medical domain, for instance, we might want to see if all the people who achieved complete remission form a homogeneous set, or if we can find some distinct sub-groups within them, which would point towards different remission causes.

To build a model able to capture the underlying relations among the data, according to the goal defined in the task, is the main aim of the machine learning methods. To specify a model, we need to delineate the class of functions that the learning machine can implement (hypothesis space).

The panorama of ML models is quite large. The classes of hypotheses that can be considered include: equations (e.g. logistic regression), classification and regression trees, predictive rules (e.g. evolutionary classifier systems), distance-based models, probabilistic models (Bayesian networks), neural net-works and kernel-based learning machines (e.g. SVM).

The *language* of the hypotheses can be more oriented towards logic (*symbolic* representation) or towards mathematics (*sub-symbolic* representation). A symbolic algorithm generates rules which relate the outcome to some characteristics of the input, performing comparisons and logical operations. An example of a symbolic hypothesis in human-readable form could be "If sex is male and either smoke is greater than 5 or exposure to pollutants is greater than 8, then the probability of getting oral cancer is 0.9". On the other side, sub-symbolic approaches deal only with numbers and mathematical functions; in the same setting, such an approach could instead derive the formula $p = 0.76 \times sex + 8.12 \times smoke + 3.15 \times poll$.

The symbolic approach has the strong advantage of being very close to human reasoning: this generally makes the results readily understandable by the researcher, which is very important in critical domains like medicine. On the other side, sub-symbolic models are generally more flexible; their mathematical nature can be exploited to explore cleverly the search space, and to demonstrate properties of the found solution.

Most of the known ML methods use a flat representation of data (fixed-size vectors of features in one table). However an attribute-value language is not able to capture in a natural way the complexity of a structured domain. ML models have been specifically investigated to handle structured data. The new and of increasing interest area of ML dealing with structured domains can be referred to as "relational data mining" or "structured domain learning". Inductive Logic Programming (Nienhuys-Cheng and de Wolf, 1997) has been proven successful for relational data mining tasks involving concept learning. Recurrent neural networks (Frasconi et al., 2001) have been applied to model sequences for several types of classification and regression tasks, while recursive neural networks (Frasconi et al., 2001) extend the input domain to more general hierarchical structures (see Section 5). More recently, kernel-based methods (Smola and Schölkopf, 2002) have been extended to process structured data (Gaertner, 2003 provides a good review on this topic).

Learning algorithms perform a (heuristic) search through the portion of the space of hypotheses which is valid for the given data. Each model listed above, that uses a parameterized space of hypotheses, has one (or more) corresponding learning algorithms allowing adaptation of the free parameters of the model to the task at hand. For example, we can mention multiple linear regression as a learning algorithm for equation models, or the covering algorithm as a learning algorithm for rule induction. Some other ML methods do not rely on the construction (and "learning") of a global hypothesis approximating the target function: for instance, in the class of distance-based methods, the *nearest neighbour* (and its variants, e.g. k-NN) and other more complex instance-based approaches, such as case-based reasoning.

Search algorithms can be grouped into broad sets which share similar basic ideas. The most simple search algorithm is *exhaustive search*. This involves simply trying every hypothesis in the hypothesis space, and choosing the best one. This method of course ensures optimality (and very often it is the only one so reliable); unfortunately, it is unfeasible for all the non-trivial cases, since the space is typically too big (or even infinite) to be completely explored in a reasonable amount of time.

At the other end of the spectrum lie the *Monte Carlo* methods: these algorithms choose a random subset of the space of hypotheses and explore only that. Choosing the size of the sample is a very easy method to limit the running time of search; of course, these methods generally do not offer guarantees on the quality of the solution found with respect to the true optimum.

In order to reduce the time necessary to find a solution, several *heuristic* methods have been developed. *Best first* search can be thought as a clever way to perform an exhaustive search. A start point is chosen (at random); then all of its *neighbours* (defined following a problem-dependent neighbourhood criterion) are ordered according to the "better than" relationship and recursively visited. With this strategy, the most promising paths are followed first, and then progressively worse-looking parts of the space are explored.

In order to cut down the complexity of this search, *beam search* explores only the best n solutions at each step. This however does not guarantee any more that the best solution will sooner or later be found; so often n is taken as 1, which is the case of *hill climbing*. In continuous domains (like in neural networks), this algorithm makes use of *gradient descent* techniques.

While at first glance this seems a much better solution than random or exhaustive search, it has some drawbacks. Often there is no clear definition of neighbouring solutions, or when there is one, the set could be too big or infinite to be explored exhaustively. The main drawback however is that this strategy is deceived by *local optima*, that is solutions which are best of their neighbourhood, but not the global optimum; in complex representations, this is a serious problem, also because there is no guarantee on the actual distance to the true optimum. These problems tend to be mitigated with other heuristic techniques, like *restarting* (performing hill climbing several times, each time with a different start point).

Finally, *evolutionary computation* is a relatively new search paradigm which promises to overcome these limitations, but at the price of introducing variability in the final solution (the algorithm makes probabilistic choices, resulting in executions with the same input and starting point not guaranteed to produce the same output). Regardless of the particular flavour of evolutionary algorithm, like genetic algorithms (GA) – which works on fixed-size solutions – or Genetic Programming – which works on variable-size solutions – the evolutionary keyword is of primary importance to understand how they work: in fact, much of the inspiration is taken from Darwin's evolution theory.

A genetic algorithm works not with a single hypothesis, but with a population of competing hypotheses (which in the GA jargon are called individuals). Like in nature, fitter individuals have greater choices to survive, and to propagate their genetic makeup to their children. Since every individual is a hypothesis, his "fitness" is related to how well the hypothesis explains the data. A genetic algorithm starts typically with random hypothesis;

some of them will casually have a better-than-average fitness, and will have greater chances to survive, and evolve towards even better solutions.

When an individual is selected for survival, he has two possibilities to carry his genetic makeup to the next generation: sexual and asexual reproduction. In the first case, the individual mates with another surviving one; two new individuals are created, constituted by a random recombination of the genetic makeup of the parents (crossover). In the second case, the individual is "cloned" to the next generation, but there is a small chance of a mutation happening during the process. It is important to note that the single individual cannot learn: learning comes from the adaptation of the whole population through generations.

The problem-solving power of genetic algorithms has been ascribed to their ability to escape local minima, thanks to the use of a population of hypotheses with varying degrees of fitness, and to the crossover method, which allows average fitness solutions to combine with each other, possibly resulting in a good advance in fitness. The latter issue in particular is related to the still quite debated *building blocks* hypothesis.

The GAs are employed as the search algorithm in the evolutionary classifier systems, described in Section 4.

Beyond the specific characteristics of the different models, there are some common concepts valid for every predictive machine learning model that we will use in the following discussion.

A ML model is supposed to be used in two different states (the two phases could be interleaved): the *learning phase* and the *prediction phase*. The learning phase corresponds to the building of the model. A hypothesis (a function h that fits the data of interest) is constructed on the basis of a set of known data, the *training data set*. The training data are the "experience" that the model tries to learn from. Therefore, this data set should be a representative sample of the real distribution of the problem at hand.

The prediction phase is the operative one. The model is used to compute an evaluation of the learned function over novel samples of data. The knowledge acquired in the learning phase should allow the model to predict with reasonable accuracy the correct response for previously unseen data. The estimation of this accuracy is the critical aspect of each ML application and the rational basis for the appropriate measures of the model performance. The *holdout* method is the most used approach for this estimation: a set of known data independent of the training set, called *test data set* is used to perform prediction. An appropriate measure of the performance over the test set can estimate the accuracy (or the generalization capacity) of the model. Different statistical techniques can be used to improve the estimation accuracy: e.g. *k-fold cross-validation*, *bootstrapping*, etc. (Bishop, 1995; Haykin, 1999). If the performance on the test set is used to choose between different models or different configurations of the current model (i.e. it is used to drive the building of the predictive model), another set of data called *validation set* is used to assess the final prediction accuracy of the system.

Committee and ensemble techniques can be used to improve the performance of single models (e.g. Bishop, 1995).

The formal framework which builds the theoretical foundations of ML is the statistical learning theory (Vapnik, 1995). In particular, it allows to formally study the conditions under which model performance on the real data distribution can be approximated by its performance on the sample used for training. In fact, while in practice the validity of this approximation is usually measured with the previously described validation techniques, a theoretical bound exists which is strictly related to a measure of model complexity, the Vapnik–Chervonenkis (VC) dimension of the hypotheses space, and to the amount of data used for training.

To further characterize the search of the best hypothesis h, it is possible to describe for each method the constraints imposed to the learner, referred as *inductive bias* (or simply *bias*). The representation of the hypotheses in a specific ML model defines the hypothesis space that the learner can explore to find h (*language bias*). The strategy adopted by the algorithm to search h over the hypothesis space is the *search bias*. Furthermore another decision concerns adding a strategy to control overfitting for the particular training data set (*overfitting-avoidance bias*). More formally, the inductive bias is the set of assumptions made by the learner in order to constrain the problem: such assumptions are necessary to extract regularities, since a learner without bias cannot extract any regularities from data, and reduces itself to a lookup-table system with loss of generalization properties (Mitchell, 1997).

As assured by the results of the statistical learning theory, there are benefits by limiting the complexity of the model. Practical approaches can be characterized by the bias that constrains the problem. The reduction of the hypothesis space, imposing language bias, can be well-motivated by a knowledge-driven process. If there is a priori knowledge on the expected solution, it is possible to effectively reduce the search space. For example, "regularization theory" is a framework where the search of hypothesis is subject to a smoothness constraint. The heuristics induced by the search bias are the basis to deal with the problem of a complete search on the hypothesis space, which is in general intractable.

On the other side, different ML methods (models and algorithms) correspond to different inductive bias. There is no universal "best" learning method. The lack of inherent superiority of any ML methods is formally expressed in the so-called "no free lunch theorem" by Wolpert and Macready (1997). Each method is more or less suitable according the specific task at hand. In particular, the language can be more or less appropriate to describe the relationships among the data of the application. Moreover, comparison parameters, such as predictive accuracy, speed (generating and using the model), robustness, scalability and interpretability can be considered to evaluate the quality of the method.

In Section 4, we focus on the class of hypothesis space and learning algorithms that characterize the evolutionary classifier system area. In fact, such algorithms will be used in a study on oral cancer development, involving clinical and genetic data.

3. CHARACTERISTICS OF MEDICAL APPLICATIONS

The characteristics of the data clearly depend on the problem being analysed. Medical data sets however have some recurring specificities, which are interesting to summarize in order to better understand the typical requirements of medical problems.

- Medical data are *heterogeneous*. Among the various recordings on each patient, there can be real values with different ranges, integer values, ordered or unordered classes. There can be images, variable-length strings; there could even be some non-standardizable natural language text (the physician's conclusions for a certain set of tests, for instance). It is almost impossible for a single technique to handle these kinds of data types.

- On the other hand, techniques which require only homogeneous data are of limited usefulness in medical data analysis.
- Medical databases are *incomplete*. Collection of data is generally a by-product of medical care, rather than an objective in itself; completeness is then not a requirement. There can be technical or economical reasons for which a value is not recorded; or even motivations pertaining the patient's health itself. Certain values for instance could require dangerous tests, which are performed only when considered strictly necessary.

A good methodology to manage medical data must then be tolerant to missing values.

- Medical data is inherently *noisy*. Not only can the recorded values be approximate or uncertain; even the classification can be imprecise or wrong. Noise tolerance is then a primary requirement for analysis.
- Medical problems can show *high dimensionality*. As we noted in the introduction, medicine is trying to consider complex interactions between many factors, in order to reduce prediction error. Moreover, some tests generate large quantity of data alone; think about computer tomography or microarray analysis.
- Medical data is often *unbalanced*. The class of people who have oral cancer for instance is certainly less numerous than the class of people who do not have it. Learning algorithms then should not suppose that the attributes have a balanced or normal distribution.
- Investigation results must be *interpretable*. Opaque methods, which cannot show in human-readable way the reasoning behind their answers, are unlikely to be accepted and used by physicians – even if they demonstrate a very good performance. Understandability of the model is probably more important than performance itself.

Managing medical data finally presents other issues (ethical and legal, for instance). Cios and Moore (2002) give an enlightening review on the topic.

3.1. Goals in medical data analysis

A prominent machine learning application in medicine is the prognostic process, where patient's information is gathered and interpreted to predict the future development of the patient's condition. Prognostic systems (see Lucas and Abu-Hanna, 1999 for a review) have to deal with high degrees of uncertainty and must exploit knowledge about the evolution of processes over time. Moreover, they are frequently used as tools to plan medical treatments.

The outcome predicted for a specific patient is generally influenced by the particular sequence of treatment actions to be performed, which in turn may depend on the information that is available about the patient before the treatment is started. Often the outcome is also influenced by progress of the underlying disease itself. The outcome of interest may be expressed by a single variable, e.g. when modelling life expectancy, but it may be more complex, when modelling not just the length of life but also various aspects pertaining to the quality of life. A subset of variables may then be used to express the outcome.

An application area for prognostic systems is treatment selection, which is the process of deciding upon the most appropriate treatment alternative for a specific patient. Reasoning about different treatments involves reasoning about the current situation of a patient and the effects to be expected from the treatments. The reasoning algorithms are therefore often embedded in a decision-support system that offers the necessary constructs from decision theory to select an optimal treatment given the predictions (Lucas et al., 1998; Andreassen et al., 1999).

Since the amount of biological and medical data that can be submitted to an automated system is steadily growing, methods able to discover functional interactions among data are of greatest interest. The kind of data to analyse can vary from clinical databases collected in research and health-care centres to genetic data, and can even be a mixture of the two. Moreover, since data are often collected over time, it is possible to analyse the temporal patterns to reveal how the variables interact as a function of time.

The discovery and study of genetic interactions is central to the understanding of molecular structure and function, cellular metabolism, development of cells and tissues, and response of organisms to their environments. If such interaction patterns can be measured for various kinds of tissues and the corresponding data can be interpreted, potential clinical benefits are obvious and novel tools for diagnostics, identification of candidate drug targets, and predictions of drug effectiveness for many diseases will emerge.

For example, finding interactions between genes based on experimentally obtained expression data in microarrays is currently a significant research topic. Microarray techniques, introduced by Schena et al. (1995), allow for the study of expression of thousands of genes simultaneously, so to be interpreted they obviously require knowledge discovery tools ranging from various clustering techniques to supervised learning methods.

4. APPLICATION

As we have seen above, medical data analysis presents many specific characteristics which a machine learning approach must take into account. In particular we focus on three of them: integration of heterogeneous data, support for incomplete data, and interpretability of results.

The need for integration of different kinds of data is one of growing importance in medical domains, mostly because genetic information is becoming more and more available. Studies combining genetic and clinical data can bring new and deeper insights on gene–effect relationships, disease susceptibilities, and gene interactions.

Although new techniques allow the acquisition of a vast amount of data, missing values are still very frequent in medical databases, so that data analysis methods which cannot deal with them often fail to exploit a lot of information. In fact, managing the missing values is not very easy: in many approaches only full rows can be used or the missing values must be filled, for example, with most common ones.

Finally, for a data analysis tool to be successful in medicine, it is crucial that its results are interpretable by physicians, rather than operate as a *black box*.

In order to fulfil these requirements, we chose XCS, a rule-based machine learning methodology which already reported interesting results in medical applications. In particular, it has the ability to provide meaningful insight of its classification process, instead of focusing exclusively on accuracy. In this regard, XCS showed many advantages over other well-established classification systems (for experimental comparison between XCS and other machine learning algorithms, see for instance Bagnall and Cawley, 2003). As seen in the works on Wisconsin Breast Cancer data by Wilson (2001b), and in the Holmes' study (2000) on epidemiologic surveillance data (using EpiCS, a similar classifier system), the use of explicit rules to match the input data allows an easy visualization of the criteria the system employs in each classification and a comparison with physicians' previous knowledge.

Moreover, XCS allows for a seamless management of missing values: an individual with missing data is matched only by those classifiers which do not rely on that value to make a prediction. The rationale underlying this choice is to avoid taking decisions based on data we do not have. Another possible approach is proposed by Holmes and Bilker (2002), where missing values are matched by every classifier, thus producing a kind of average value for that data.

Another key aspect which led us to choose XCS was the ease of integration of different kinds of data. In fact, whilst the original formulation of XCS is targeted to binary input, the shift to other data types, such as real or integer ones, has already been proven to be very easy (see respectively Wilson (2000, 2001b). In particular, we developed an XCS classifier system tailored to work with Boolean, integer, real, and gene-class value types.

Now, we provide a brief description of the XCS algorithms (full details can be found in Butz and Wilson, 2001). Then we will see its application on a dataset collected in a study on oral cancer susceptibility, where the main goal will be to obtain a small set of mixed clinical and genetic rules that could suggest to physicians which genes increase or reduce oral cancer risk, and the direction to follow for more focused genetic research.

Finally we show the results obtained on the same dataset with two other algorithms: logistic regression, a classical statistical tool, and decision trees, one of the most common methodologies in rule-based learning. The three algorithms are then evaluated with respect to descriptive power, predictive accuracy and actual usability of the results.

4.1. XCS

Learning classifier systems (LCS), first introduced by Holland (1976), exploit the ability of the genetic algorithm at their heart to search efficiently over complex search spaces. A learning classifier system represents its "genotypes" as production rules, providing a level of readability that is rarely found within sub-symbolic approaches without the need for additional post-processing. LCS combines reinforcement learning, evolutionary computing and other heuristics to produce adaptive systems. They maintain and evolve a population of classifiers (rules) through the genetic algorithm. These rules are used to match environmental inputs and choose subsequent actions. Environment's reward to the actions is then used to modify the classifiers in a reinforcement learning process. When used to classify, the set of rules provides a deterministic answer.

XCS is an evolution of learning classifier systems proposed by Wilson (1995, 1998) which demonstrated good performance in comparison to other machine learning techniques (results in Bagnall and Cawley, 2003). XCS introduces a measure of classifiers' fitness based on their accuracy, i.e. the reliability of their prediction of the expected payoff, and applies the GA only on the action set, the subset of classifiers which lead to the choice of the action. This gives the system a strong tendency to develop accurate and general rules to cover problem space and allow the system's "knowledge" to be clearly seen.

4.1.1. System description

The core component of XCS is a set of classifiers, that is condition-action-prediction rules, where the *condition* specifies a pattern over the input states provided by the environment, the *action* is the action proposed (e.g. a classification), and the *prediction* is the payoff expected by the system in response to the action. Additionally, each classifier has associated an estimate of the *error* made in payoff predictions, and a *fitness* value.

XCS implements a reinforcement learning process: at every step, the system is presented an individual from the data set and it examines its set of classifiers to select those matching the input situation. These classifiers form the *match set*. Then for each possible action, the system uses the fitness weighted average prediction of the corresponding classifiers to estimate environmental reward. At this point, the XCS can choose the best action looking for the highest predicted reward. However, during learning, the action is usually selected alternating the previous criterion with random choice, useful to better explore the problem space. The actual reward returned by the environment is then used to update the classifiers in the *action set*, i.e. the subset of the *match set* corresponding to the selected action. A genetic algorithm is also executed on this set to discover new interesting classifiers.

To reduce the number of rules developed, XCS implements various techniques, such as the use of macroclassifiers, the subsumption and the deletion mechanisms. In fact, the system uses a population of macroclassifiers, i.e. normal classifiers with a *numerosity* parameter, representing the number of their instances (microclassifiers). This helps in keeping track of the most useful rules and improves computational performance at no cost.

Subsumption is used to help generalization: when the GA creates a new classifier with a condition logically subsumed by his parent (i.e. matching a subset of the inputs matched by the parent's) it is not added to the population, but the parent's numerosity is incremented. A similar check is also occasionally done among all the classifiers in the current action set.

Finally the deletion mechanism keeps the number of microclassifiers under a fixed bound. The classifier to be removed is chosen with a roulette wheel selection biased towards low fitness individuals and assuring approximately equal number of classifiers in each action set.

As already stated, this process leads to the evolution of more and more general rules. For each classifier we can define a measure of generality following Wilson (2001b), ranging from 0 (most specific) to 1 (most general). A possible termination criterion is to stop evolution when the average generality value of the population gets stable.

4.1.2. Ruleset reduction

During learning XCS tends to evolve an accurate and complete mapping of condition-action-prediction rules matching the data. Consequently, in particular on a very sparse data set as in our study, the final number of rules is quite high. Similar problems, which break the knowledge visibility property, were experienced in other studies on "real" data sets, for instance by Wilson (2001a,b). These works suggest letting the system evolve many steps after reaching the maximum performance, and then to extract a small subset of rules which attain the same performance level. This is the function of the *Compact Ruleset Algorithm* (CRA), first proposed by Wilson (2001a).

4.2. Oral cancer – problem description

We applied XCS on the data collected in a study on the development of head and neck squamous cell carcinoma (HNSCC). Preliminary results of this application are presented in Baronti et al. (2004).

The data set we analysed was designed to explore the influence of genotype on the chance to develop HNSCC. It is already well-known that this kind of cancer is associated with smoking and alcohol-drinking habits, it is more common among males and its incidence increases with age. The individual risk however could be modified by genetic factors, such as polymorphisms of enzymes involved in the metabolism of tobacco carcinogens and in the DNA repair mechanisms. The patients were thus described with a combination of demographic and lifestyle data (sex, age, smoking and drinking habits) and genetic data (the polymorphisms of eleven genes believed to be relevant to this disease) along with a clinical value which stated if they had cancer or not when the database was compiled.

The genotype information provided by molecular testing regarded eleven genes involved with carcinogen-metabolizing (CCND1, NQO1, EPHX1, CYP2A6, CYP2D6, CYP2E1, NAT1, NAT2, GSTP1) and DNA repair systems (OGG1, XPD). Nine of these genes have two allelic variants; let us call them a_1 and a_2. Since the DNA contains two copies of each gene, there exist three possible combinations: a_1a_1, a_2a_2 (the homozygotes) and a_1a_2 (the heterozygote – order does not matter). The homozygotes where represented with values 0 and 2, while the heterozygote with 1. Due to dominance, the heterozygote is possibly equivalent to one of the homozygotes; however, for many of the considered genes this dominant effect is not known. So Class 1 can be either equivalent to Class 0 or to Class 2. The remaining two genes have 4 allelic variants, which result in 9 combinations; they were sorted by their activity level, and put on an integer scale from 0 to 8.

The full data consists of 355 records, with 124 positive elements (HNSCC patients) and 231 negative (controls). They were collected in different periods between 1997 and 2003; this has led to many missing data among the genotypic information of patients. Actually only 122 elements have complete genotypic description; the remaining 233 have missing values ranging from 1 to 9, with the average being 3.58. As an overall figure, of the $11 \times 355 = 3905$ genotype values, just 3070 are present: 21% of the genotype information is missing.

4.2.1. Adaptation to the problem

As we have seen above, the type of information contained in the data set varies from binary (i.e. sex), to continuous-valued (i.e. age, indicators of smoking and alcohol-drinking habits), and to a special class data for the genotype.

For the integer and real data types, possible XCS implementations already exist in the literature (Wilson, 2000, 2001b for instance). But for the genotypic values, we needed a slightly different treatment. Nine of the genes considered have two allelic variants, thus we need three classes (considering also the heterozygote) for the input values, but the classifiers have in fact to merge the heterozygote with either one of the homozygotes. So the values we used are the following: as input we have 00 for a_1a_1, 11 for a_1a_2, and 22 for a_2a_2; in classifiers 11 is not allowed, but we admit 01 (matching 00 and 11), 12 (matching 11 and 22) and ## (matching all values).

4.3. Results

We had two aims in testing the system: evaluating its ability to correctly classify unseen data after training and checking if it could find interesting rules. We applied a tenfold cross-validation and repeated the experiment ten times (each time with a different folding), in order to obtain results independent from the particular folding. Each experiment was allowed to run for 500 000 steps, as a few tests showed that the generality value reached stability by this point. Moreover, we employed a crossover rate of 0.80 and a mutation rate of 0.04, while the other parameters were chosen following Butz and Wilson (2001). The experiments were run with several population sizes, ranging from 6400 to 200 micro-classifiers. The final results are summarized in Table 1.

In the experiment with 6400 classifiers, the accuracy on the training set reached almost optimal value, while it decreased in the experiments with lower population sizes. However the accuracy on the test set was at least comparable and even showed a slightly increasing trend with smaller populations (see Fig. 1). This suggests that the high accuracy of the 6400 test is due to overfitting and lower population sizes are preferable. In particular, XCS performances appear stable for populations in the range from 200 to 600. The evolution of the system for a population of size 400 is plotted in Fig. 2.

Table 1. Summary of the ten 10-fold cross-validation experiments. Specificity and sensitivity are both relative to the test set

			Accuracy			
Max rules	CRA	Final rules	Training	Test	Specificity	Sensitivity
6400	Before	1659 ± 115	99 ± 1%	75 ± 2%	90 ± 2%	50 ± 5%
	After	47 ± 14	99 ± 1%	72 ± 3%	77 ± 2%	65 + 3%
800	Before	413 ± 25	93 ± 1%	77 ± 1%	87 + 2%	59 ± 3%
	After	49 ± 21	93 ± 1%	74 ± 2%	82 ± 1%	61 ± 5%
600	Before	333 ± 22	91 ± 2%	78 ± 2%	88 ± 2%	59 ± 3%
	After	34 + 11	91 + 2%	75 ± 2%	83 ± 3%	62 ± 3%
400	Before	236 ± 19	87 ± 2%	78 ± 2%	89 ± 3%	60 ± 2%
	After	16 ± 9	87 ± 2%	79 ± 1%	89 ± 2%	62 ± 3%
200	Before	119 ± 17	82 ± 4%	78 ± 2%	88 ± 5%	59 ± 5%
	After	9 ± 5	82 ± 4%	78 + 2%	90 ± 2%	56 ± 5%
See5		Not Applicable	79 ± 2%	69 ± 2%	76 ± 2%	57 ± 4%

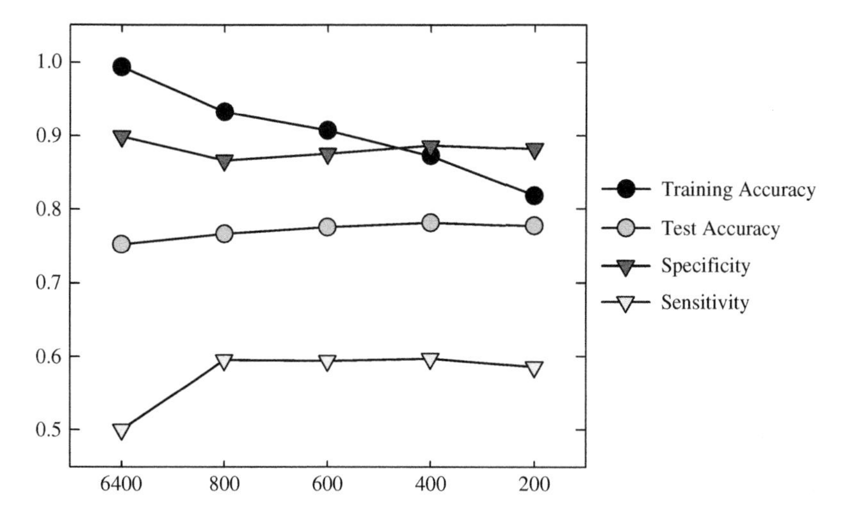

Fig. 1. XCS performances with varying population sizes.

The CRA successfully extracted a small subset of the original rules which maintained the maximum performance on the training set, while not getting worse significantly on the test set. Actually it could be more interesting to apply a pruning algorithm to the original population, designed to reduce the model complexity in order to achieve better generalization. Differently from CRA, such an algorithm should be allowed to lose some accuracy on the training set, in order to perform better on the test set.

Nevertheless the small sets of rules extracted made it feasible to manually look for possibly interesting rules. As an example we provide in Table 2, two of such rules in human readable form. The first rule is common knowledge rediscovered by the system. Instead the second one has been judged interesting by physicians: in fact a previous study by

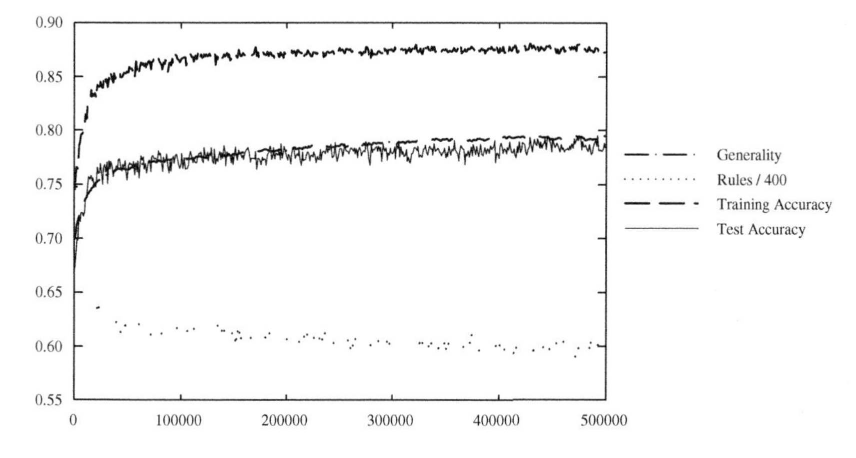

Fig. 2. Plot of average evolution in the experiments with a population of 400 microclassifiers.

Table 2. Examples of rules extracted by the system, with their correct/matched ratio

Rule	Ratio
IF $age \leq 40$ THEN $cancer = false$	(26/26)
IF $smoke \geq 12$ AND $EPHX1 \in \{11, 22\}$ AND $GSTP1 = 00$ THEN $cancer = true$	(38/40)

To-Figueras et al. (2001) already reported an increased lung cancer risk associated to GSTP1 in combination with EPHX1 polymorphisms, so it will be interesting to investigate on the role of these genes in relation to HNSCC risk.

4.4. Comparison with logistic regression

One of the most common data explanation methods in medicine is logistic regression (LR) (a detailed explanation of the method can be found in Hosmer and Lemeshow, 2000). The logistic regression method builds a probabilistic model of the outcome, obtained through a *logit* transformation of a linear combination of the input values.

The model is based on the following equation:

$$f(\mathbf{x}) = \frac{1}{1 + e^{\alpha + \beta \mathbf{x}}}, \tag{1}$$

where α is a scalar, β is a vector, and $\mathbf{x}$ is the input vector.

Skipping over the mathematical motivations, the usefulness of logistic regression is not only in building a model which can predict unseen data, but chiefly in the interpretation of the coefficients found (the βs in our equation). An important quantity relative to the input variables is the *odds ratio*; let us see for instance what this means for a single dichotomous input variable, $x_j \in \{0, 1\}$.

In this context, the odds ratio is simply calculated as e^{β_j}, and describes how much the outcome is more likely when the input condition is present ($x_j = 1$) with respect to when the input condition is not present ($x_j = 0$). This value is then clearly very important in deciding how much an input variable is influential on the final outcome. Similarly, for a real variable $x_j \in \Re$ the odds ratio $e^{c\beta j}$ quantify how much the outcome is more likely for an increase of c units of the variable.

Another advantage of LR models, aside from their strong mathematical and statistical foundations, is their simplicity of setup: there are no parameters to finetune like in most ML methods, and they are readily available in standard statistical analysis packages.

4.4.1. Logistic regression results

Applying logistic regression to the HNSCC dataset presents two main difficulties:

- The heterozygote should be considered equal to either one of the homozygotes. This relationship can either be ignored or manually enforced, since the logistic regression model cannot be instructed to automatically derive it.

- The dataset must be complete: no missing values are allowed. In order for this to happen, we removed from the dataset all the lines with at least one missing value. This however causes roughly two-thirds of the data to be thrown away. A better strategy is to identify some subsets of the attributes, and do the same procedure only on those subsets; having less attributes makes it more likely for an instance to be complete.

The first test was performed with all the attributes: after removing all the instances with missing data, only 120 were left. The only significant (Wald's test $z = 3.99$, $p = 10^{-4}$) variable found was *packyears*, with an odds ratio of 1.04 ± 0.01. These results were consistent even after manually deciding for each gene which homozygote the heterozygote it was equal to.

The next tests were performed splitting in two subsets the genes, and taking into account only one of the two groups; this means less columns, which in turn produces more full rows. The two tests could in fact use 141 and 302 instances respectively; however, the only strongly significant variable predicted was again *packyears*. On the second subset, containing only the *nat* and *cyp* genes, also *sex* was not rejected ($p = 0.003$).

The main drawback of logistic regression analysis on this dataset is probably not the need for complete data, but its limitation to consider only linear interactions between the risk factors. For instance, while the allelic variants of two genes do not singularly induce any increase in risk, it is possible that their combined effect does. LR cannot detect these non-linear associations, and thus is a limited tool to explore the possibly complex interactions between attributes.

4.5. Comparison with decision trees

The second comparison we show is to a different machine learning tool for classification and prediction: decision trees (Quinlan, 1986). Decision trees are a well-known machine learning method which comply with our requirements about interpretability, treatment of different data types, and robustness to missing data.

A decision tree is a classifier in the form of a tree structure, where each leaf node indicates the value of a target class and each internal node specifies a test to be carried out on a single attribute, with one branch and sub-tree for each possible outcome of the test. The classification of an instance is performed by starting at the root of the tree and moving through it until a leaf node is reached, which provides the classification of the instance.

Among the variety of algorithms for decision tree induction from data, probably the most known and used are ID3 and its enhanced version C4.5 (Quinlan, 1993). ID3 searches through the attributes of the training instances and extracts the attribute that best separates the given examples. The algorithm uses a greedy search, that is, it picks the best attribute and never looks back to reconsider earlier choices. The central focus of the decision tree growing algorithm is selecting which attribute to test at each node in the tree. The goal is to select the attribute that is most useful for classifying examples. A good quantitative measure of the worth of an attribute is a statistical property called information gain that measures how well a given attribute separates the training examples according to their target classification. This measure is used to select among the candidate attributes at each step while growing the tree.

4.5.1. Decision tree results

Decision tree induction on our dataset was performed using the See5 software by Rulequest Research (1994). After some testing, we found out that the default parameters (pruning CF = 25%, minimum case per branch = 4) worked well for this dataset; boosting was not employed, since it did not appear to improve performance. We applied a tenfold cross-validation and repeated it ten times, as in the experiments with XCS (that is, with 10 different foldings). In this case, results' variability is due only to the random folding in the cross-validation procedure, since the decision tree induction algorithm is deterministic.

The results are reported in Table 1, where the accuracy, sensitivity, and specificity obtained with See5 are compared with those obtained with XCS. Finally, the decision tree obtained with the execution of See5 on the entire dataset is reported in Table 3.

4.6. Results and discussion

The figures in Table 1 show a clear performance advantage of XCS over See5, both on training and test sets. This gives a quite good level of confidence on extracted rules, suggesting XCS managed to convey in them useful knowledge.

However, sets of rules obtained with XCS are slightly less readable and interpretable than decision trees. Moreover, XCS results show a quite high variability. In fact, classification accuracy does not change much between runs, but the actual rulesets appear quite different. Since interpretability is our main concern, this constitutes a remarkable problem: there is no evident way to get a single "final" set of rules. In this respect an appealing See5 characteristic is that it extracts a single decision tree from a given dataset.

An open question regards the fact that the reached performance value on test cannot be considered "high" in an absolute sense; however, given the particular nature of the input data, it is not completely clear how better this value could become. For instance, this data set is noisy not only on some input variables (smoke and alcohol habits), but also on the target: more than other diseases, cancer cannot be deterministically predicted. Regarding the first issue, it would be useful to perform some tests on the effects of noise in XCS.

Table 3. Decision tree obtained from the entire dataset, along with the correct/matched ratio for each branch

```
packyears <= 0.04875: false (135.9/158.9)
packyears > 0.04875:

:... age > 0.78: false (12/12)
    age <= 0.78:
    :... gstpl <= 0: true (63.3/102.1)
        gstpl > 0:
        :... nat2 <= 3: false (30/43.6)
             nat2 > 3: true (24.2/38.5)
```

Concerning the target variable, a possible direction is prediction of a risk factor instead of a raw class, as in Holmes (2000).

Another interesting aspect to investigate is the ruleset reduction algorithm: CRA is mainly focused on maintaining the training performance achieved, while a more pruning-like strategy could be beneficial for generalization. CRA should moreover include as a chief goal to regularize the algorithm output, in order to produce more stable results. The stability of results could also be achieved as a post-processing step; for instance, it could be possible to find similar rules recurring among different executions. This would require a measure of similarity between rules, and a clustering algorithm able to group them together.

5. LEARNING STRUCTURED DATA IN MEDICINAL CHEMISTRY AND PERSPECTIVES

As indicated in Section 1, structured data can play a relevant role in solving problems in complex domains. In fact, a central issue in modelling biochemical and medical domains is to provide the model with a proper and expressive representation of the real-world data. Structured data characterize many branches of natural sciences and prominent applications are emerging for the treatment of medical, biological and chemical structured data. For instance, biological and biochemical problems are characterized by quite complex domains where managing of relationships and structures, in the form of sequences, trees, and graphs, is important to achieve suitable modelling of the solutions. A specific interest in medicinal chemistry is to reduce costs and accelerate drug discovery cycles, including the studies on their potential genotoxicity, carcinogenicity, or other pharmaceutical toxicity, to anticipate adverse health effects, which provide a strong demand of high humanitarian and scientific value. To this aim, in parallel to the genetic and proteomic studies, an increasing attention is paid to studies on smaller organic molecules and their interactions with DNA and proteins.

One of the most elucidating examples of structured data in such fields is probably given by chemical structure formulas that determine primary structure of molecules, because of their natural graphical description. One of the principal goals in medicinal chemistry is to correlate the chemical structure of molecules with their properties, including their biological and pharmaceutical properties. The models developed for such analysis have been termed *Quantitative Structure–Property Relationship* (QSAR). Since molecules are naturally described via a varying size structured representation, general approaches to the processing of structured information are needed. In this area, the use of ML methods to deal with structured domain provides an opportunity to obtain a direct and adaptive relationship between molecular structures and their properties.

In the context of neural computing, recursive neural networks models have been exploited to tackle biological (proteins) and chemical (molecules) structured data (for example in Baldi et al., 1999 and Bianucci et al., 2003). In the following, we introduce some basic concepts of the *Recursive Neural Network* approach to show that Recursive Neural Network processing is a feasible way to do learning in structured domain and that it can provide new solutions for medicinal chemistry (the basic approach was introduced by Sperduti and Starita, 1997 and Frasconi et al., 1998; an extended survey of the approach appeared in

Frasconi et al., 2001; Micheli, 2003 provides for a unified presentation, recent developments and applications, and references for historical background).

The Recursive Neural Network (RNN) is a Neural Network model able to handle the complexity of variable-size structured data through a recursive encoding process. In particular, RNN can be exploited to work directly with hierarchical structured data that represent molecules. Such an approach offers an alternative to the traditional QSAR analysis, which is based on a flat representation of molecular compounds built through a case dependent extraction of numerical descriptors, guided by the knowledge of experts.

In the RNN approach, the encoding process mimics by construction the morphology of each input hierarchical structure. For each vertex of the structure, the model computes a numerical code using information both of the vertex label and of the code of the sub-graphs descending from the current vertex. At the end of the process, a code of the whole molecular structure is computed. Since the model is equipped with tunable free parameters, the encoding process can be adapted to the prediction task: the learning algorithm fits the parameters' values to the given set of input/output training examples.

From an external point of view, the model directly takes as input molecular structured representations and it simultaneously learns both how to numerically represent (encode) and to map chemical structures to their property/activity values. Through this adaptive encoding the model can compute structural descriptors that are specific for the data and computational problem at hand. In other words, the map of (chemical) similarities among molecules is automatically adapted by the model to the task, according to the property/activity target values. Note that the process can consider both the 2D graph topology and the atom types (or the chemical functionalities). Hence, a new perspective to the QSAR studies is offered by exploiting the richness of a structured molecular representation and avoiding the use of any fixed structure-coding (or similarity) scheme. For an overview of recent results on the application of RNN to QSPR/QSAR analysis, see Micheli et al., 2001, 2003 and Bianucci et al. (2003). It must be stressed that the proposed methodology, relying on the generality and flexibility of a structured representation, defines a unified approach that can be used to tackle different problems on different kinds of molecular data.

In particular, since universal approximation capabilities of the RNN have been proven (specifically in Hammer, 2000 for tree-structured domains), RNN can be considered a general tool useful especially to deal with new tasks where the relevance of the traditional molecular descriptors is unknown. More generally, the presented approach can be seen as a paradigmatic example of the studies aiming at extending machine learning techniques (considering either neural computing, kernel-based, probabilistic or symbolic approaches) to the treatment of various structured classes of data (see Micheli, 2003 and the references therein).

Our aim here is also to propose the new approach as a general methodology to tackle various structured problems in the area of medicinal chemistry and bioinformatics. The main potential developments concern hard tasks in toxicology and bioinformatics whenever it is natural to find useful structured representation of chemical/biological data.

The flexibility of the structured data learning approach can also be employed to integrate genetic, biological, clinical and chemical data, and to capture relevant information such as topological or functional description of the data that can characterize various tasks in medicinal chemistry and biology.

A further step to solve medical problems in complex domains can derive from the integrated analysis of genomic, clinical and chemical information. This includes the study of the integration of QSAR analysis with related disciplines such as genomics, proteomics, and the application of predictive ADME-Tox (adsorption, distribution, metabolism, elimination toxicity) for lead drugs.

In fact, the need for rapid and accurate prediction of pharmacokinetic properties, including individualized evaluation of drug effects, can be understood in the emergent situation characterized by the advancements in the sequencing of the human genome, in proteomics, in the anticipation of the identification of a vastly greater number of potential targets for drug discovery.

More specifically, *pharmacogenetics* studies aim at identifying the genetic basis of drug efficacy and adverse effects analysing the relationship between individual genotype and the response to drugs.

The integration of the analysis of genetic determinants of diseases into the drug discovery process may enable more effectively design and a more tailored treatment. Better and safer drugs can be developed and the selection of drugs and doses can be adapted to the genetic characteristics of the patient. *Individualized medicine* can be based on the analysis of pharmacogenetic information from clinical trials.

The introduction of a new relevant variable in the drug discovery and development process leads to a more complex design process, including both research, pre-clinical and clinical phases. Moreover, it should be taken into account, both the complexity of finding gene variations (polymorphisms) that affect drug response and the opportunity (and the need) to study multiple drug candidates tailored to different patients. All these factors stress the need of computational tools/machine learning techniques allowing a reliable and efficient evaluation of drug response on the basis of expressive representation of data from different sources. The availability of ML tools, able to deal with complex data domain, extends the possibility of treatment of such problems in the same computational frame.

6. CONCLUSIONS

In this chapter we presented a brief introduction to machine learning methodologies. In particular we focused our attention on the capability of ML approaches to face problems in poorly understood domains, to deal with uncertainty and noise, and to exploit relationships and structural information in the data.

These properties are extremely valuable in the applications on medical data analysis. In fact, the medical domain is characterized by the availability of vast amounts of data, collected by different sources and of different kinds, including clinical, biological, and genetic information about patients. ML approaches have the potential to exploit these complex data and to explore the relationships between them.

As an instance of ML methodology applied to a complex medical domain, we set up an XCS system to analyse heterogeneous data composed by mixed lifestyle, clinical, and genetic information, from a study on the risk of developing HNSCC. The long-term goal is to identify the genes actually involved in the susceptibility to oral cancer, and highlight possible interactions between them. XCS has confirmed its flexibility in adapting to different data types and seamless handling of missing values. The rules extracted from the first experiments suggest that the system can produce interesting results. Moreover, they are easily converted in human-readable form, and can be immediately evaluated by physicians.

Through the proposed methodology we intended to show that the ML-based modelling of complex systems can be effectively equipped with expressive representation of complex data in the form of structured representation.

In particular concerning biological and chemical problems, we discussed cases where predictions can be done directly from molecular structures, introducing potential benefits in the current QSPR/QSAR methodology.

Moreover, new methodologies of drug discovery are emerging from the techniques of managing and analysing biological, clinical and chemical data. The flexibility of the structured data learning approach can also be exploited to integrate genetic, biological, clinical and chemical data to introduce more general and flexible approaches into medicinal chemistry and biology for the individualized medicine needs.

REFERENCES

Andreassen, S., C. Riekehr, B. Kristensen, H. Schønheyder and L. Leibovici, 1999, Using probabilistic and decision-theoretic methods in treatment and prognosis modelling. Artif. Intell. Med., 15, 121–134.

Bagnall, A. and G. Cawley, 2003, Learning classifier systems for data mining: a comparison of XCS with other classifiers for the forest cover dataset, Proceedings of the IEEE/INNS International Joint Conference on Artificial Neural Networks (IJCNN-2003), Vol. 3, Portland, Oregon, USA, pp. 1802–1807.

Baldi, P., S. Brunak, P. Frasconi, G. Pollastri and G. Soda, 1999, Exploiting the past and the future in protein secondary structure prediction. Bioinformatics, 15(11), 937–946.

Baronti, F., V. Maggini, A. Micheli, A. Passaro, A.M. Rossi and A. Starita, 2004, A preliminary investigation on connecting genotype to oral cancer development through XCS, Proceedings of WIRN 2004, in press.

Bianucci, A., A. Micheli, A. Sperduti and A. Starita, 2003, A novel approach to QSPR/QSAR based on neural networks for structures. In: L. Sztandera and H. Cartwright (Eds.), Soft Computing Approaches in Chemistry. Springer-Verlag, Heidelberg, pp. 265–297.

Bishop, C.M., 1995, Neural Networks for Pattern Recognition. Oxford University Press Inc., Oxford.

Butz, M.V. and S.W. Wilson, 2001, An algorithmic description of XCS. In: P. L. Lanzi et al. (Eds.), IWLCS 2000, Vol. 1996 of LNAI. Springer-Verlag, Berlin, Germany, pp. 253–272.

Cios, K. J. and W.G. Moore, 2002, Uniqueness of medical data mining. Artif. Intell. Med., 26(1–2), 1–24.

Frasconi, P., M. Gori, A. Käuchler and A. Sperduti, 2001, Chapter 19, From sequences to data structures: theory and applications. In: J. Kolen and S. Kremer (Eds.), A Field Guide to Dynamical Recurrent Networks. IEEE Press Inc., New York, pp. 351–374.

Frasconi, P., M. Gori and A. Sperduti, 1998, A general framework for adaptive processing of data structures. IEEE Trans. Neural Netw., 9(5), 768–786.

Gaertner, T., 2003, A survey of kernels for structured data. Newsletter of the ACM Special Interest Group on Knowledge Discovery and Data Mining 5(1), 49–58.

Hammer, B., 2000, Learning with Recurrent Neural Networks, Vol. 254 of Springer Lecture Notes in Control and Information Sciences. Springer-Verlag, Berlin, Germany.

Haykin, S., 1999, Neural Networks, A Comprehensive Foundation, 2nd ed. Prentice Hall, Upper Saddle River, NJ, USA.

Holland, J.H., 1976, Adaptation. In: R. Rosen and F.M. Snell (Eds.), Progress in Theoretical Biology, 4. Plenum Press, New York.

Holmes, J.H., 2000, Learning classifier systems applied to knowledge discovery in clinical research databases. In: Lanzi et al. (Ed.), Learning Classifier Systems. From Foundations to Applications, Vol. 1813 of LNAI. Springer-Verlag, Berlin, Germany, pp. 243–261.

Holmes, J.H. and W.B. Bilker, 2002, The effect of missing data on learning classifier system learning rate and classification performance. In: Lanzi et al. (Ed.), IWLCS 2002. Vol. 2661 of LNAI. Springer-Verlag, Berlin, Germany, pp. 46–60.

Hosmer, D. and S. Lemeshow, 2000, Applied Logistic Regression, 2nd ed. Wiley, New York.

Lucas, P., H. Boot and B. Taal, 1998, Computer-based decision-support in the management of primary gastric non-hodgkin lymphoma. Meth. Inform. Med., 37, 206–219.

Lucas, P.J.F. and A. Abu-Hanna, 1999, Prognostic methods in medicine. Artif. Intell. Med., 15(2), 105–119.

Micheli, A., 2003, Recursive processing of structured domains in machine learning. Ph.D. Thesis, Department of Computer Science, University of Pisa, Pisa, Italy.

Micheli, A., A. Sperduti, A. Starita and A. Bianucci, 2001, Analysis of the internal representations developed by neural networks for structures applied to quantitative structure-activity relationship studies of benzodiazepines. J. Chem. Inf. Comput. Sci., 41(1), 202–218.

Mitchell, T.M., 1997, Machine Learning. McGraw-Hill, New York, USA.

Nienhuys-Cheng, S.-H. and R. de Wolf, 1997, Foundations of Inductive Logic Programming. Springer-Verlag, Berlin, lNAI 1228.

Quinlan, J.R., 1986, Induction of decision trees. Machine Learning, 1, 81–106.

Quinlan, J.R., 1993, C4.5: Programs for Machine Learning. Morgan Kaufmann Publishers Inc., San Francisco, CA, USA.

Rulequest Research, 1994, See5/C5.0. URL http://www.rulequest.com/.

Schena, M., D. Shalon, R. Davis and P. Brown, 1995, Quantitative monitoring of gene expression patterns with a complementary DNA microarray. Science, 270, 467–470.

Smola, A., B. Schölkopf, 2002, Learning with Kernels: Support Vector Machines, Regularization, Optimization and Beyond. MIT Press, Cambridge, MA, USA.

Sperduti, A. and A. Starita, 1997, Supervised neural networks for the classification of structures. IEEE Trans. Neural Netw., 8(3), 714–735.

To-Figueras, J., M. Gene, J. Gomez-Catalan, E. Pique, N. Borreg and J. Corbella, 2001, Lung cancer susceptibility in relation to combined polymorphisms of microsomal epoxide hydrolase and glutathione s-transferase p1. Cancer Lett., 173(2), 155–162.

Vapnik, V.N., 1995, The Nature of Statistical Learning Theory. Springer-Verlag, New York.

Wilson, S.W., 1995, Classifier fitness based on accuracy. Evol. Comput., 3(2).

Wilson, S.W., 1998, Generalization in the XCS classifier system. In: J.R. Koza et al. (Eds.), Genetic Programming 1998: Proceedings of the Third Annual Conference. Morgan Kaufmann, University of Wisconsin, USA, pp. 665–674.

Wilson, S.W., 2000. Get real! XCS with continuous-valued inputs. In: Lanzi et al. (Ed.), Learning Classifier Systems. From Foundations to Applications, Vol. 1813 of LNAI. Springer-Verlag, pp. 209–219.

Wilson, S.W., 2001a, Compact rulesets from XCSI. In: P.L. Lanzi et al. (Eds.), IWLCS 2001. Vol. 2321. Springer-Verlag, Berlin, pp. 197–210.

Wilson, S.W., 2001b, Mining oblique data with XCS. In: P.L. Lanzi, et al. (Eds.), IWLCS 2000. Vol. 1996 of LNAI. Springer-Verlag, Berlin, pp. 158–174.

Wolpert, D.H. and W.G. Macready, 1997, No free lunch theorems for optimization. Evol. Comput. 1(1), 67–82.

Chapter 11

Classification of Brain Tumours by Pattern Recognition of Magnetic Resonance Imaging and Spectroscopic Data

Andy Devos[1], Sabine van Huffel[1], Arjan W. Simonetti[1], Marinette van der Graaf[2], Arend Heerschap[2] and Lutgarde M.C. Buydens[3]

[1]*SCD-SISTA, Department of Electrical Engineering, Katholieke Universiteit Leuven, Kasteelpark Arenberg 10, 3001 Heverlee (Leuven), Belgium*
Email: andy.devos@hotmail.com, sabine.vanhuffel@esat.kuleuven.be, Arjan.Simonetti@philips.com
[2]*Department of Radiology, Radboud University Nijmegen Medical Centre, PO Box 9101, 6500 HB Nijmegen, The Netherlands*
Email: A.Heerschap@rad.umcn.nl, M.vanderGraaf@rad.umcn.nl
[3]*Laboratory for Analytical Chemistry, Radboud University Nijmegen, PO Box 9010, 6500 GL Nijmegen, The Netherlands*
Email: L.Buydens@science.ru.nl

Abstract

The medical diagnosis of brain tumours is one of the main applications of Magnetic Resonance (MR). Magnetic Resonance consists of two main branches: Imaging and Spectroscopy. Magnetic Resonance Imaging is the radiologic technique applied to produce high-quality images for diagnostic purposes. Magnetic Resonance Spectroscopy provides chemical information about metabolites present in the brain, such as their concentrations. Both Imaging and Spectroscopy can be exploited for the grading and typing of brain tumours, also called classification.

The present gold standard to diagnose an abnormal brain mass is the histopathological analysis of a biopsy. However, a biopsy is riskful for the patient and therefore it would be very benificial if a diagnostic tool based on non-invasive techniques such as MR would be used to aid or even avoid the current gold standard. Classification of brain tumours is very interdisciplinairy and involves many aspects of medicine, engineering and mathematics. The development of a medical decision support tool covers data collection, specific pre-processing, exploitation of the useful features for classification and testing of the classification. The domain-specific knowledge of neurologists and radiologists is invaluable to guarantee a diagnostic tool applicable in daily clinical practice.

This chapter provides an overview of the NMR methodology and its applications to brain tumour diagnosis. Spectral pre-processing issues such as normalization and baseline correction, which could have an influence on the accuracy of the classification, are discussed.

A wealth of methods exists for feature extraction and classification of MR data; principal component analysis and mixture modelling are covered as unsupervised techniques and linear discriminant analysis and support vector machines as supervised ones. The described methods were tested on MRI and MRS data of healthy as well as brain tumour tissue, acquired in the framework of the EU-funded INTERPRET project.

Results of the INTERPRET project illustrate that imaging and spectroscopic data are complementary for the accurate diagnosis of brain tumour tissue. The chapter arguments for a strong focus on the fusion of MR imaging and spectroscopic data and non-MR data, in the framework of further development and improvement of a medical decision support tool.

Outcome Prediction in Cancer
Edited by A.F.G. Taktak and A.C. Fisher
© 2007 Elsevier B.V. All rights reserved

Acknowledgements

The authors acknowledge Leentje Vanhamme, Lukas and Ron Wehrens for their contributions related to this chapter. This study was carried out at the ESAT laboratory and the Interdisciplinary Centre of Neural Networks (ICNN) of the Katholieke Universiteit Leuven, in the framework of the Belgian Programme on Interuniversity Poles of Attraction, initiated by the Belgian Federal Science Policy Office (IUAP Phase IV-02 and IUAP Phase V-22), the EU-funded projects BIOPATTERN (EU network of excellence; contract no. 508803), eTUMOUR (FP6 integrated project; contract no. 503094) and INTERPRET (IST-1999-10310), the Concerted Action Project MEFISTO and AMBIORICS of the Flemish Community, the FWO projects G.0407.02 and G.0269.02 and the IDO/99/03 and IDO/02/009 projects. AD research funded by a Ph.D grant of the Institute for the Promotion of Innovation through Science and Technology in Flanders (IWT-Vlaanderen).

Keywords: Brain tumours, classification, Magnetic Resonance Imaging (MRI), Magnetic Resonance Spectroscopy (MRS), Magnetic Resonance Spectroscopic Imaging (MRSI), Linear Discriminant Analysis (LDA), Least Squares Support Vector Machines (LS-SVM).

Contents

1. INTRODUCTION

Yearly, about 29 000 persons are diagnosed with a brain tumour in Europe (1998 estimates) (CaMon-project, 1998), a rate of 7 in every 100 000. Accurate diagnosis of these tumours is desirable. Prognosis largely depends on the tumour type and grade of malignancy; ranging from a median survival of 7–10 years for tumours of grade II, 2–5 years for grade III tumours and less than 1 year for grade IV tumours (Prados, 1991; Leibel et al., 1994; Aldape et al., 2003). Additionally, different tumour types respond differently to treatment, like radiotherapy or chemotherapy. Fast growing tumours are much more likely to emerge again after treatment than slow growing tumours, but high-grade tumours do respond better to radiotherapy and chemotherapy. Therefore, early detection and correct treatment based on accurate diagnosis are important to improve clinical outcome.

The present gold standard for diagnosis of an abnormal brain mass suspected of being a brain tumour is the histopathological analysis of a biopsy. A biopsy requires the use of a medical imaging technique to localize the tumour in order to retrieve the biopsy and to facilitate the diagnosis. A biopsy is not without risk of morbidity and mortality and can not be carried out in all instances (e.g. brain stem tumours, paediatric tumours). Additionally, there are inherent inaccuracies in the gold standard (Mittler et al., 1996), which can lead to misclassification or imprecision in establishing the final diagnosis. Therefore, it would be beneficial to the patient if the invasive biopsy is avoided and the diagnosis is made by means of non-invasive techniques.

Magnetic Resonance Imaging (MRI) is often used for clinical diagnosis of brain tumours due to its high spatial resolution and signal-to-noise ratio of the images. MRI is a non-invasive technique which does not involve any radiation risk for the patient. Using MRI, images of cross sections of the brain can be acquired with several contrasts, depending on the acquisition parameters. Images can also be acquired after intravenous administration of a contrast agent. Together, they provide the clinician with high-resolution images on which most tissue types and their morphology are clearly displayed. However, even with the precise morphologic information, it is not always able to distinguish between different tumour types or to indicate the spatial extent of the tumour.

More recently developed MRI techniques like diffusion- and perfusion-weighted MRI are other promising techniques for the characterization of brain tumours (Nelson and Cha, 2003; Rees, 2003). Diffusion-weighted MRI visualizes the tissue structure and is useful for assessing tumour cellularity, while perfusion-weighted MRI provides measurements that reflect changes in tumour vasculature and tumour grading.

Besides morphologic information available on images, additional valuable spectroscopic information can be provided by in vivo Magnetic Resonance Spectroscopy (MRS), which can be performed on the same MR scanner. MRS provides chemical information of metabolites present in living tissue and has the potential to facilitate the characterization of tissue, and in particular of human brain tumours (Mukherji, 1998; Smith and Stewart, 2002; Nelson, 2003). A relatively new spectroscopic technique, called Magnetic Resonance Spectroscopic Imaging (MRSI) or multivoxel MRS, is able to combine chemical and localized information, as it acquires a spectrum for each voxel or volume-element in a grid (Mukherji, 1998; Leclerc et al., 2002; Nelson et al., 2002; Nelson, 2003). This enables the construction of a spatial map of chemical information for each of the metabolites present in the tissue examined. The differentiation of abnormal brain tissues, including brain tumours, from normal brain forms a potentially major clinical application in which these MR techniques could have a large impact.

This chapter discusses the use of MRS(I) and the combination with conventional MRI for the automated characterisation of brain tumours. The development of a reliable and automated pattern recognition system requires the acquisition of a large amount of data. MR spectra are acquired at a high spectral dimension, which even strengthens the need of either a large database or a data reduction technique to restrict the number of features to a minimum. A pattern recognition system should be able to select or extract the biomedically relevant features and to exploit that information for diagnosis of brain tumours, in other words for the determination of the type and the grade of the tumour. This chapter explains the principle of NMR and its role for the characterization of brain tumours, as well as the different aspects of pattern recognition based on MR data. Further, the importance of a medical decision support system for clinical purposes is discussed which fuses data from several MR and non-MR techniques.

2. MAGNETIC RESONANCE

2.1. NMR versus other medical imaging techniques

Patients with symptoms of a brain tumour will be sent to a neuroscience unit for investigation, which involves a number of specialized tests to diagnose brain tumours. A neurological examination investigates the performance of all brain functions, like eye movement, sensory-motoric and muscular responses, reflexes, hearing, tactile and sensory sensation, movement, balance and coordination. Furthermore, medical imaging techniques can be applied to detect and localize a possible abnormal brain mass.

Computed Tomography (CT) uses X-ray radiation to construct detailed images of the brain from different angles. It can be performed with or without injecting a contrast agent. CT scans provide low levels of radiation, but can be regulated to provide the minimum amount of radiation exposure needed to produce the image.

Proton Emission Tomography (PET) and Single Photon Emission Computerized Tomography (SPECT) images are obtained by measuring local levels of injected contrast agents, such as glucose or methionine, that have been labelled with a radioactive tracer. SPECT is based on the principle of blood flow in the brain, which is directly related to brain activity. Areas of increased blood flow take up more radioactive tracer than areas of less blood flow. PET assesses changes in the function, circulation and metabolism of body organs and has emerged as a method of measuring body function and guiding disease treatment.

MRI applies a magnetic field to create high-resolution images of the brain and will be discussed further in the next sections. This technique has several advantages as it does not use X-rays or any other type of "ionizing" radiation. MRI in combination with MRSI is able to provide anatomical as well as chemical information.

2.2. The principle of NMR

Certain atomic nuclei, like ^{1}H (proton) and ^{31}P (phosphorus), possess an inherent angular momentum or spin. A magnetic property is associated with this spin and when these nuclei are subject to a static magnetic field B_0, their spin will be aligned with the magnetic field. Both ^{1}H and ^{31}P have a spin quantum number of 1/2, corresponding to two different spin or energy states and the energy difference between both states is proportional to the applied magnetic field

$$\Delta E = \gamma \hbar B_0, \quad \hbar = \frac{h}{2\pi}, \tag{1}$$

with γ the gyromagnetic ratio, characteristic of the isotope and h the Planck constant. To induce transitions between these energy states, an oscillating magnetic field is applied by a coil in a plane perpendicular to the static field B_0. This field has a frequency equal to the precession frequency of the nuclei

$$f_0 = \frac{\gamma B_0}{2\pi}. \tag{2}$$

The amount of energy absorbed by the nuclei (and emitted in a later stage) depends on the population difference between the two energy states. The population density of the nuclei in different energy states is determined by their Boltzmann distribution. In thermal equilibrium at absolute temperature T, the relative amounts n^- of the nuclei in the highest and n^+ of the nuclei in the lowest energy state are given by

$$n^- / n^+ = e^{(-\Delta E/kT)}, \tag{3}$$

where k is the Boltzmann constant. The ratio n^-/n^+ is very close to unity in normal circumstances, resulting in low absorption (and as a consequence emission) of energy. This explains the inherently low signal-to-noise ratio of the signal emitted when the spin system returns to equilibrium after excitation. This emitted signal is called a free induction decay (FID) signal, and corresponds to an exponentially decaying sinusoid in the time domain.

Nuclei of different atoms can be easily distinguished from one another since they have a different γ and consequently differ widely in resonance frequency. Nuclei of the same isotope which are not chemically equivalent are differentiable due to the effect of shielding. The amount of shielding, experienced by a nucleus, determines the effective magnetic field,

$$B_{\mathrm{eff}} = B_0(1-\sigma'), \tag{4}$$

where σ' is the shielding constant, a dimensionless unit that depends on the electrical environment of a nucleus. Therefore, nuclei in a different chemical environment emit signals with different frequencies. This phenomenon makes MRS a very attractive tool since it allows differentiation between molecular structures. Spin–spin (or J-) coupling, the interactions between neighbouring spins in the same molecule, induces a further differentiation in resonance frequencies.

2.3. Localization of the response

Due to the high concentration of proton spins in living beings, the use of proton NMR is very promising for biomedical research. However, till 1973 the signal measured corresponded to the global response of all spins around the coil. The main feature that was lacking to construct images of the distribution of water molecules was the identification of the spatial origin of the different signal components. Lauterbur solved this problem by introducing an additional small magnetic field, linearly varying as a function of the distance, while the spins are precessing around the magnetic field. Hence, this introduces a different strength of the magnetic field for each point inside the magnet.

The frequency of each spin is different and characteristic of its position in the magnet, which enabled the development of MRI and the introduction of the MR scanner in clinical radiological imaging. This technique produces high-resolution images without any danger of radiation or ionization.

The concept of the spatial localization also enabled the development of localized spectroscopy for biomedical purposes. MRS or single voxel spectroscopy produces one signal from a certain volume element, also called voxel (Fig. 1), while MRSI or multivoxel spectroscopy produces signals simultaneously from a two-dimensional grid of voxels. MRSI can facilitate the identification of heterogeneity of a tumourous region, since spatial

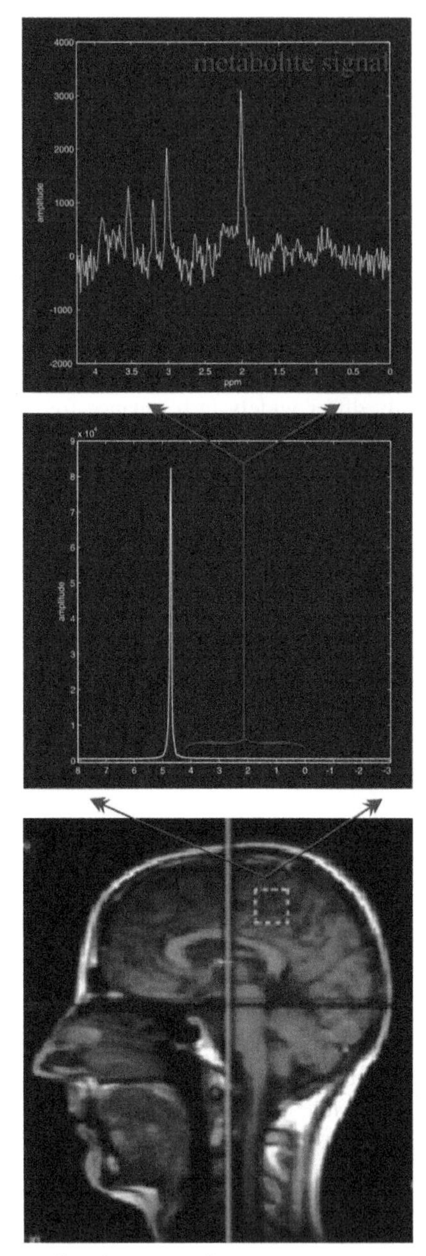

Fig. 1. Single voxel spectroscopy. Spatial localization techniques enable the selection of a small volume-element or voxel (bottom) to acquire a spectrum of the selected voxel (middle). The large peak corresponds to water, while the relevant resonance peaks (top) are more than 1000 times smaller and are situated at the right-hand side of the water peak.

variations of the tissue characteristics can be assessed at the metabolite level. For each of the voxels, the intensity of the biochemically relevant metabolites can be determined. This enables the development of metabolic imaging (Fig. 2), which constructs a spatial distribution or map of the intensity of any relevant metabolite over the selected brain region, while MRI only visualizes the spatial distribution of water. Therefore, MRSI has a large potential for clinical applications as it provides spectroscopic as well as spatial information of the brain tissue.

2.4. Characteristic information available in medical NMR

MRI has become one of the most important non-invasive aids in clinical diagnosis of brain tumours, because it enables the radiologist to assess the anatomical location, morphology and size of the tumour tissue with a relatively high spatial resolution. Normally, stacked images are recorded throughout the total volume of the brain in order to localize the tumour optimally. MR images with different contrasts are recorded, as the acquisition of only one type of image may not show the desired information. The contrast is obtained with specific acquisition parameters, resulting in T1-weighted, T2-weighted and proton density-weighted images, in which T1 and T2 are the two tissue-specific water relaxation time constants. These images are often followed by a T1-weighted image after intravenous administration of gadolinium-DTPA, to assess the blood–brain barrier viability. Next to this, also more modern MRI methods may be used, like diffusion-weighted imaging and functional MRI. During diffusion-weighted imaging, the water movement within the brain tissue is analysed at the molecular level. An abnormality can be detected and visualized on

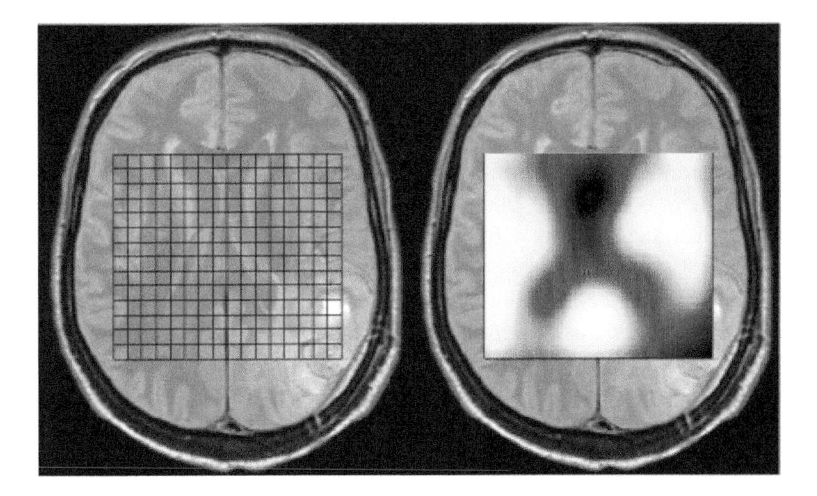

Fig. 2. MR enables the spectroscopic visualization of the whole brain. The left part shows an MR image (water content) of 256 × 256, while the right figure displays an MRS metabolite image (NAA) of 16 × 16.

diffusion-weighted images, since the normal water movement is restricted. With functional MRI it is possible to visualize which specific brain structure participates in a specific function, and is therefore important in the assessment of the function of the brain tissue surrounding a tumour.

MRS can be performed with several MR-sensitive nuclei. Next to the proton nucleus (^{1}H), other potentially useful nuclei for biomedical applications include ^{31}P, ^{19}F and ^{13}C. The use of ^{31}P MRS has been found important in the studies on energy metabolism, as the content of ATP, phosphocreatine (PCr) and inorganic phosphate during exercise can be followed (Gadian, 1995). It can also be used to calculate intracellular pH (Negendank, 1992), which is an important parameter in the study of tumours. Also, the signals of phosphomonoesters in tumours can be measured by ^{31}P MRS. These signals are found to be raised in tumours compared with normal tissue.

The metabolic information obtained by ^{1}H MRS has proven to be important in the investigation of brain tumours (Preul et al., 1996; Nelson et al., 1999). Several metabolite concentrations have found to be lowered or increased in tumours compared with normal tissue. This change in concentration can be used for specific tumour determination. The proton nucleus has a high MR sensitivity and its natural abundance is high. A large number of brain metabolites contain protons that generate signals at specific frequencies in the MR signal. The number of signals is so high that these actually crowd the MR spectrum and the overlap of signals is manifested. To influence the presence of signals from metabolites in the proton MR spectrum, acquisition protocols can be used that use different acquisition parameters. One of these parameters, the echo time (TE), has a direct influence on the signal of metabolites in the MR spectrum. After excitation of the proton spins, the signal decays by the T1- and T2- relaxation processes. These parameters, together with the concentration and the number of protons in the molecule, determine the height and shape of each resonance in the MR spectrum. The longer the TE, the more the signal has attenuated before acquisition. Hence, a short echo time spectrum (TE $\leq$ 50 ms) has larger peaks than a long echo time spectrum (TE $\geq$ 130 ms) (Fig. 3). A short echo time spectrum also contains more peaks, as resonances with a small T2 value (rapid T2 relaxation) or complex coupling pattern, like mI (myo-Inositol), Glu (glutamate) and Gln (glutamine) are less pronounced at longer echo times.

In several brain tumour studies (Smith and Stewart (2002) and references therein), differences in metabolic concentrations and their ratios between normal and cancerous tissue were reported, illustrated on Fig. 4 for short TE spectra: NAA (*N*-acetyl aspartate) and Cr (total creatine) levels are reduced, Cho (choline-containing compounds) is increased, and the ratios Cr: Cho and NAA: Cho are significantly reduced in all tumour types relative to control tissue (Christiansen et al., 1994; Manton et al., 1995). Differences in the levels of Asp (aspartate), Ala (alanine), mI (myo-inositol) and Glx (glutamine/glutamate) were found between normal cells and various tumour types. Differences in metabolite concentrations and ratios between different tumour types have also been reported (Kugel et al., 1990). For example, increasing Cho is correlated to the grade of malignancy. Lipids are found in areas of necrosis present in high-grade astrocytomas and metastases (Mukherji, 1998). The presence of this characteristic information motivates the use of MRS, as well as MRSI, for distinguishing several brain tumours according to their type and grade of malignancy.

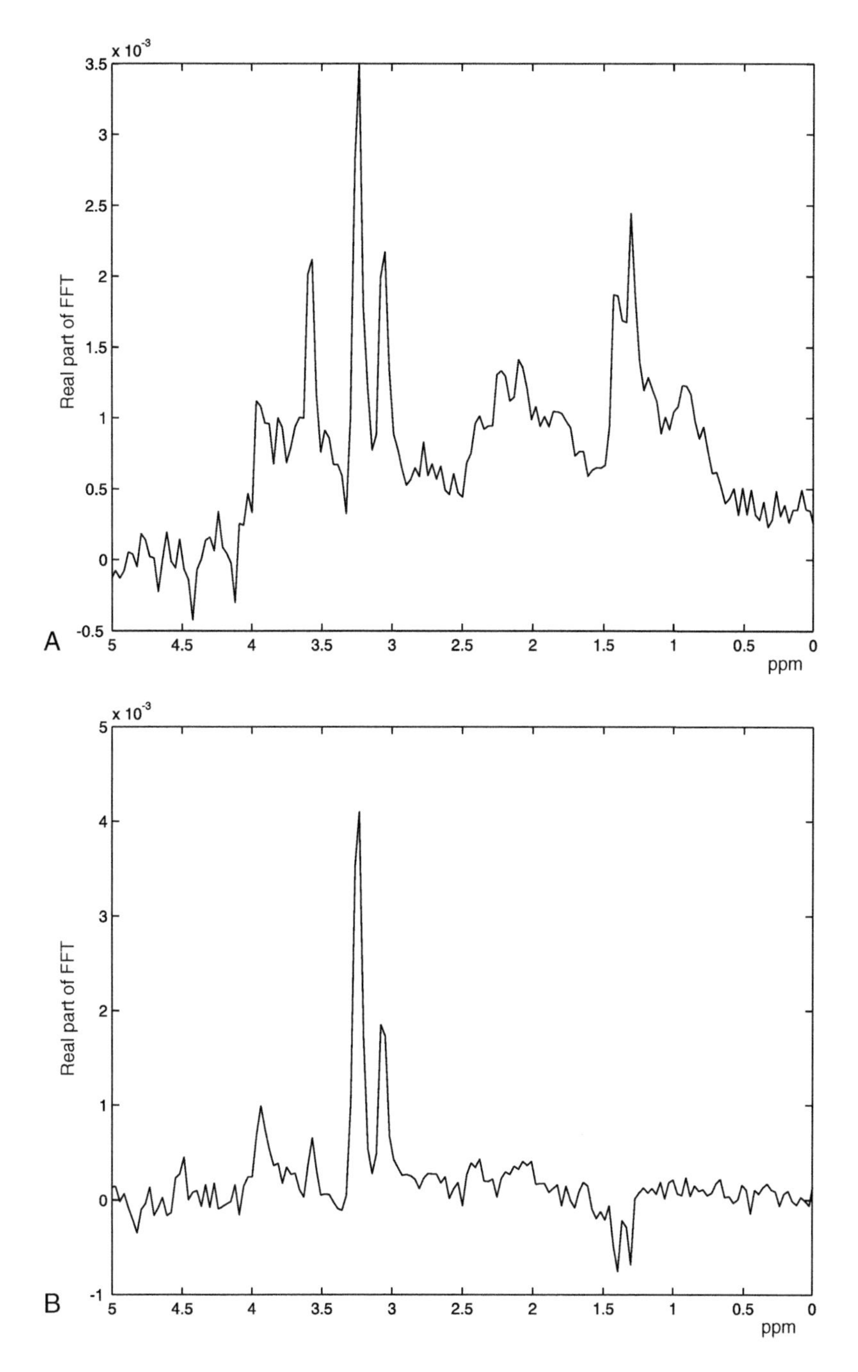

Fig. 3. Single voxel ^{1}H MR spectra at short (A) (TE = 20 ms) and long echo time (B) (TE =136 ms) of a patient with oligo-astrocytoma. Data are provided by UMCN (Nijmegen, The Netherlands), within the framework of INTERPRET (IST-1999-10310).

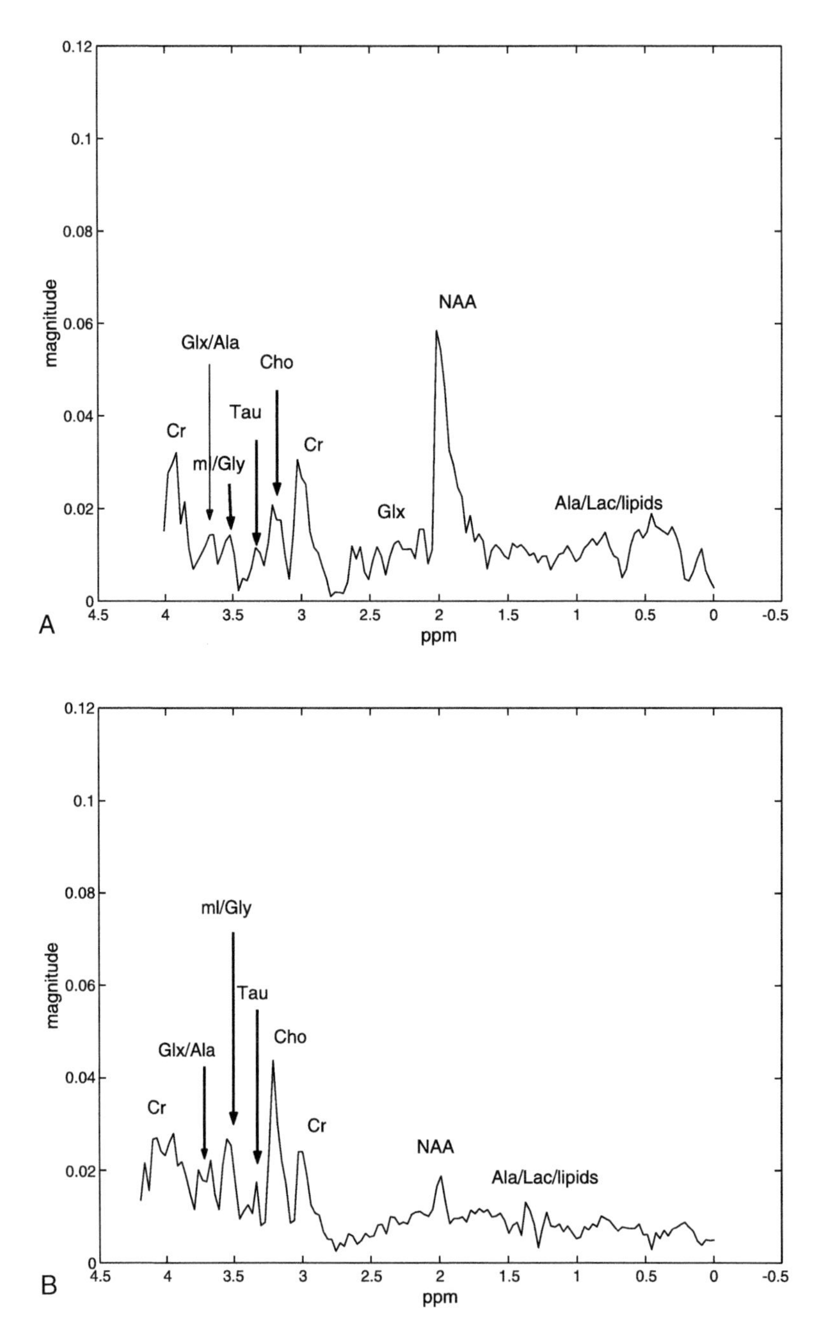

Fig. 4. Typical water normalized magnitude ^{1}H MR spectra (TE = 31 ms) of the normal tissue of a volunteer (A), an astrocytoma of grade II (B), a glioblastoma (C), a metastasis (D) (middle-right) and a meningioma (E). Data are provided by IDI (Barcelona, Spain), within the framework of INTERPRET (IST-1999-10310).

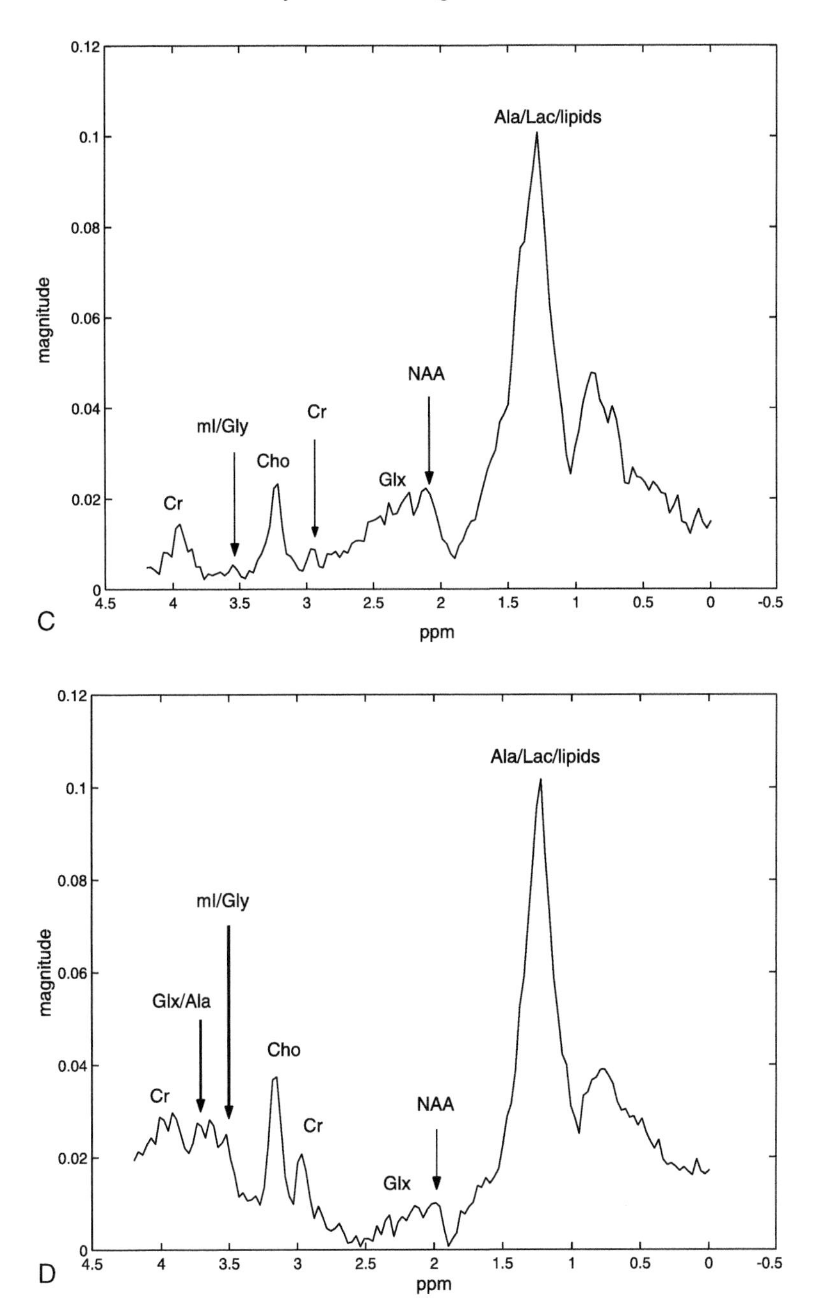
0.12
0.1
0.08
0.06
0.04
0.02
0
magnitude
Ala/Lac/lipids
NAA
Cr
mI/Gly
Cho
Glx
Cr
4.5
4
3.5
3
2.5
2
1.5
1
0.5
0
-0.5
C
ppm
0.12
0.1
0.08
0.06
0.04
0.02
0
magnitude
Ala/Lac/lipids
mI/Gly
Glx/Ala
Cho
Cr
Cr
NAA
Glx
4.5
4
3.5
3
2.5
2
1.5
1
0.5
0
-0.5
D
ppm

Fig. 4. cont'd

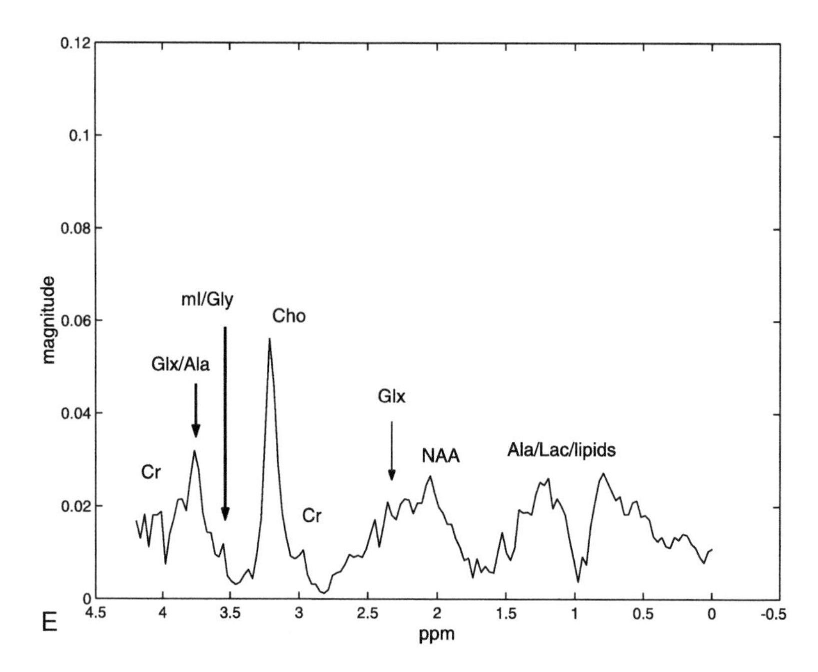

Fig. 4. cont'd

3. PATTERN RECOGNITION

Pattern recognition may be suited for several purposes. By extracting characteristic information, the data may be significantly reduced in size and noise. It may also serve as a basis for a more comprehensive visualization of the multidimensional data and it can be used for statistical interpretation. Last, pattern recognition can be applied for classification, which assigns a sample to a certain group.

The development of a pattern recognition system involves the following steps, as illustrated in Fig. 5: (1) data acquisition and collection, (2) pre-processing, (3) construction and testing of the classifier and (4) measuring the performance.

Each of these steps is discussed in the next paragraphs.

3.1. Data acquisition and collection

The results of pattern recognition are very much dependent on the quality of the data. It is of utmost importance to develop a detailed acquisition protocol in advance in order to obtain reproducible high-quality data. Depending on the purposes of the study, single or multivoxel data, at short or long echo time spectra should be acquired. If, in the area of MR,

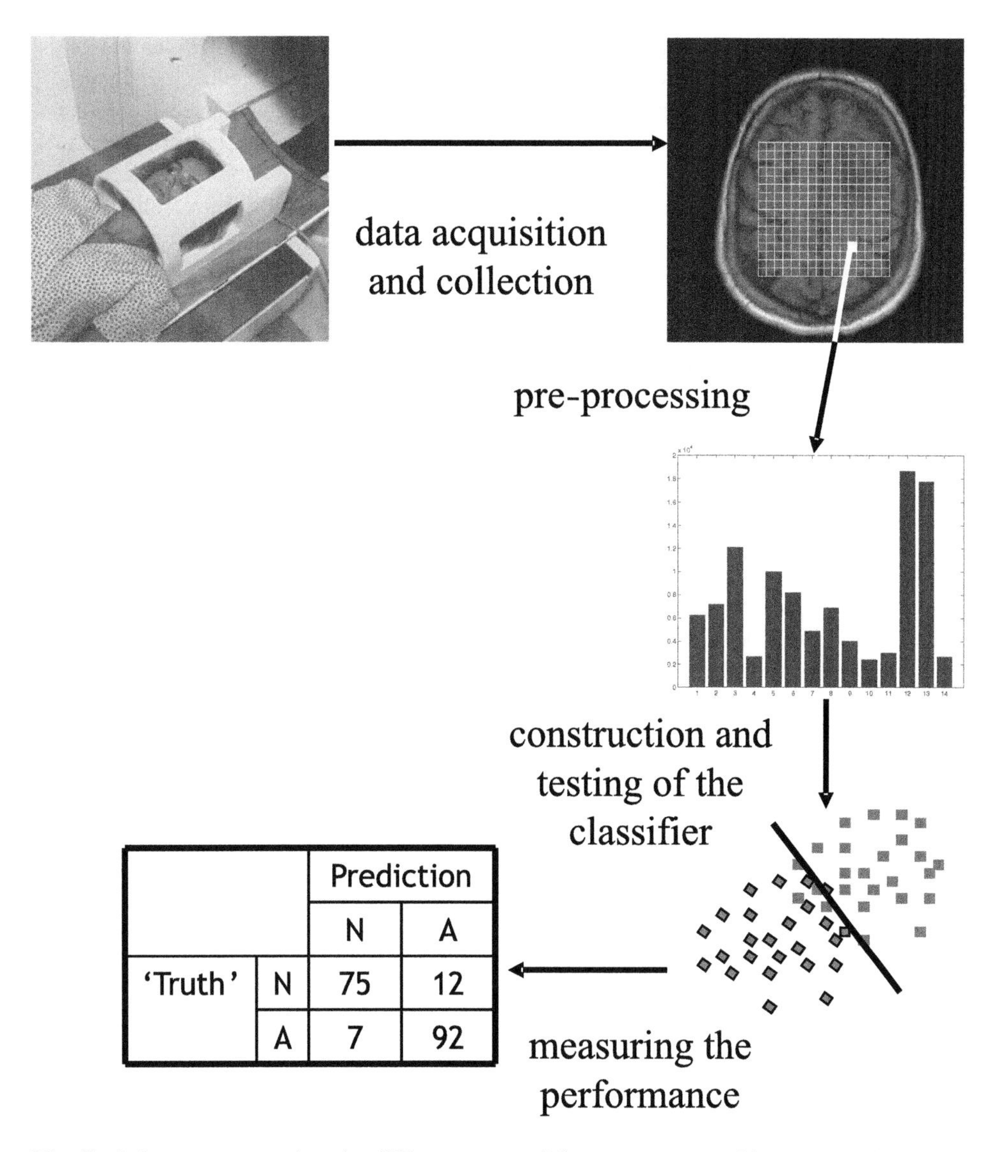

		Prediction	
		N	A
'Truth'	N	75	12
	A	7	92

Fig. 5. Scheme representing the different steps of the pattern recognition process based on MR data. First, using an MR scanner (top-left) a large database of high-quality signals is acquired; here a T1-weighted image of a patient with grade III oligodendroglioma is displayed (top-right). Second, the MR signals and other medical data are pre-processed in order to enhance the biomedically relevant information; here, several MR intensities (middle-right) are shown from one selected voxel on the grid. Based on these features a classifier (bottom-right) can be optimally constructed and tested. The classification result is evaluated using a particular performance measure; here using a contingency table.

a research purpose is to investigate the combined use of spectral and clinical features, it is advisable to collect as many samples as possible that include these features.

Issues in spectral quality and quality control are in general underestimated. There is no worldwide consensus or detailed criteria for quality control of MR spectra. Kreis (2004) discusses several topics in quality assessment, including the reproducibility of spectra, the signal-to-noise ratio and the suppression of several artefacts. A multicentre collaboration was carried out for quality control assessment; Bovée et al. (1995) focused on the protocols for quality assessment, Leach et al. (1995) discussed how an appropriate phantom can be developed, while Keevil et al. (1995) investigated the multicentre trial of several test cases and the validation of the quality assessment. For the EU-funded INTERPRET project (IST-1999-10310), all partners reached a consensus (van der Graaf, 2001) about the acquisition protocol for MRS and MRSI measurements. This facilitated the combined use of data acquired at different centres and using MR scanners from different manufacturers.

3.2. Pre-processing of NMR signals

The aim of the pre-processing step is to remove irrelevant information, while enhancing the key features in order to simplify the pattern recognition task. A few of the pre-processing steps are noise and artefact filtering, and normalization. Phase correction, line broadening and baseline removal are pre-processing steps specifically for the field of MRS. Also, feature extraction and selection can be regarded as a kind of pre-processing, that find a small amount of features with as much valuable information as possible. Typically, feature extraction is performed by the so-called unsupervised techniques (see Section 3.3), as clustering and PCA techniques.

3.2.1. Spectral pre-processing

MRS signals are affected by the presence of artefacts, instrumental errors, noise and other unwanted components. The spectral quality can be considerably improved by appropriate manipulation of the data prior to Fourier transformation. The signal-to-noise ratio can be enhanced by apodisation which multiplies the time domain signal by a decaying exponential function, which broadens the resonance peaks in the frequency domain.

In case a water unsuppressed signal is available together with the water suppressed signal, the method of Klose (1990) can be carried out. This corrects for eddy currents (caused by instrumental imperfections) by dividing the water suppressed signal by the phase term of the water unsuppressed signal. As a result of this operation the signal is more or less phase corrected and aligned.

The proton MRS signal is composed of many resonances including several unwanted components, like the dominant residual water peak, artefacts and noise. Filtering the MRS signal to eliminate the unwanted features is advised prior to further processing. Residual water removal can be performed by a subspace-based modelling approach (Barkhuysen et al., 1987; Laudadio et al., 2002) or by filtering (Kuroda et al., 1989; Sundin et al., 1999). Vanhamme et al. (2000) compared several methods for residual water removal.

In the following sections, a few pre-processing aspects are discussed in detail.

Normalization of Spectra. A normalization procedure should be applied that tries to compensate for signal intensity differences between spectra due to effects independent of the type of tumour tissue. Two main normalization approaches can be applied to MRS signals; normalization with respect to a particular mathematical norm and normalization by division by an intensity of a particular molecule.

- Mathematical normalization: if the spectrum is considered as a vector, then the L1-norm is defined as the sum of the elements in that vector, which is corresponding to the integral of the spectrum. Each spectral value is then divided by the L1-norm of the spectrum, in order to obtain an L1-normalized spectrum. The spectral vector can also be divided by its L2-norm, which is defined as the square root of the sum of the squares of the elements in that vector (Tate et al., 1996, 1998, 2003; Usenius et al., 1996; Devos et al., 2004a; Lukas et al., 2004). After division, the spectrum has unity norm with respect to the L2-norm.
- Normalization by an intensity of a molecule: a common normalization approach in NMR quantification is normalization with respect to the amplitude of creatine (Cr) (Preul et al., 1996), which is assumed to reach constant values over the complete brain region in normal tissue as well as in many pathologies. Nevertheless, Li et al. (2003) found that this normalization method increases variability. An alternative method divides the spectrum by the intensity of water, estimated from a spectrum without water suppression (Usenius et al., 1996; Devos et al., 2004a,b). This requires an additional measurement of a corresponding water unsuppressed signal, acquired with the same acquisition parameters and originating from the same voxel. The intensity of the water peak can be estimated, for example, by taking the highest value in the time domain signal, by peak integration in the frequency domain (Meyer et al., 1988), by modelling the water unsuppressed signal using Hankel Singular Value Decomposition (HSVD) (Barkhuysen et al., 1987) or Hankel Lanczos Singular Value Decomposition using PROPACK (HLSVD-PRO) (Laudadio et al., 2002). A more accurate and robust approach computes a Voigt model (Marshall et al., 1997) for the water unsuppressed signal based on a nonlinear least squares estimation (Devos et al., 2004a).

Magnitude Versus Real Spectra. An MRS signal is typically represented by its real and imaginary parts, and the process of "phasing" is required to correctly produce the real part of the spectrum for classification. Although automated phasing techniques exist, they are less suitable for in vivo data with large background signals. An alternative to using phased spectra is to calculate the magnitude spectrum (Lukas et al., 2004), which makes the signal phase independent. However, magnitude calculation yields a significant broadening of the peaks and results in a larger overlap of the individual peaks (Hoch and Stern, 1996).

Baseline Correction. Short echo time ^{1}H MRS signals are characterized by the presence of an unknown broad baseline underlying the sharper resonances of the metabolites of interest, that hinders the assessment of the intensity (i.e. quantification) of low-weight metabolites. In order to correct the signal for the baseline, most approaches first obtain an approximation of the baseline and then subtract that approximation from the original signal. A few of these methods are mentioned below:

- Measurement of the baseline and subtraction from the original FID (Behar et al., 1994; Bartha et al., 1999). This assumes that the baseline has a similar pattern independent of the pathology, which is in general not the case.

- Parametric and nonparametric approaches that model the macromolecular baseline (Provencher, 1993; Hofmann et al., 1999, 2002; Soher et al., 2001; Lemmerling et al., 2002; Seeger et al., 2003). Most of these techniques are integrated as part of a quantification approach to estimate the MRS parameters. Baseline modelling can be done, for example, by wavelets (Young et al., 1998; Soher et al., 2001), polynomial or spline functions (Provencher, 1993; Lemmerling et al., 2002). This requires the selection of several spectral points to define the fitted baseline, a process which is heavily user-dependent.
- Multiplication of the FID by an exponentially decaying function. The baseline is fitted as a product of the original FID and an exponentially decreasing apodization function (Campbell et al., 1973; Simonetti et al., 2003; Devos et al., 2004a), which requires only the decay as a parameter to be selected. As the baseline consists of broad fast decaying components, their main contribution is in the first part of the FID. After multiplication with a decaying function, the resulting function will mainly contain the broad baseline components.
- Truncation of the initial points in the FID (Ratiney et al., 2004). By removing the initial part of the FID, the baseline components are separated from the metabolite contributions.

3.2.2. Feature selection and extraction applied to brain tumour diagnosis using NMR

Based on MR data, several features can be used for brain tumour diagnosis. Pattern recognition can be based on the complete spectrum or on selected or extracted features. Typically, the goal of feature selection and feature extraction is to retain the most characteristic information and hence to perform dimensionality reduction. Feature extraction can be carried out by, for example, PCA or ICA (Huang et al., 2003). However, also biomedically relevant features can be exploited, obtained by quantification.

It is well known that characteristic resonance peaks correspond to important brain metabolites (Murphy et al., 1993; Mukherji, 1998; Leclerc et al., 2002; Majós et al., 2002; Smith and Stewart, 2002; Howe et al., 2003). It seems reasonable then, that these peaks might be used as discriminatory features to distinguish tumour types, in particular for those regions of the ^{1}H spectrum which are clearly different between spectra of different tumour types. Thus, as an alternative to using complete spectra, selected frequency regions or parameter estimates obtained by quantification can be used which are assumed to contain most of the information. Hence, the redundancy generated by spectral noise and artefacts in the spectrum is reduced. Selected frequency regions are taken as intervals around the resonance frequencies (Govindaraju et al., 2000) of several characteristic metabolites, amplitude estimates can be obtained by peak integration around the selected resonances or by a more accurate model-based approach (Provencher, 1993; Vanhamme et al., 1997; Lemmerling et al., 2002). For an overview of time domain quantification approaches, we refer to Vanhamme et al. (2001).

At long echo time (e.g. Lukas et al., 2004; Szabo de Edelenyi et al., 2000), the metabolite peaks of interest are L2 (lipids at ≈ 0.90 ppm); L1 (lipids at ≈ 1.25 ppm); Lac ($^3CH_3$ group at central frequency 1.31 ppm); Ala ($^1CH_3$ group at central frequency 1.47 ppm); NAA (*N*-acetyl aspartate, $^2CH_3$ group 2.01 ppm); Cr (total creatine, $N(CH_3)$ group at 3.03 ppm and $^2CH_2$ group at 3.91 ppm); Cho (choline-containing compounds, $N(CH_3)_3$ group at 3.18 ppm); Gly (glycine, $^2CH_2$ group at 3.54 ppm). At short echo time (e.g. Devos et al.

(2004a, 2005); Simonetti et al. (2004)), an extended set of metabolite peaks can be selected, because several additional metabolites (e.g. Glx, mI, Tau) are more visible in short echo time spectra. This additional set covers metabolite peaks of, for example, Glx ($^3CH_2$, $^4CH_2$ group; at several resonances between 2.03 and 2.45 ppm; ^2CH groups at 3.75 ppm); mI (^5CH, ^1CH, ^3CH, ^4CH and ^6CH groups at 3.26, 3.52 and 3.61 ppm); Tau (taurine, $^2CH_2$ and $^1CH_2$ group at 3.24 and 3.42 ppm); Ala (^2CH group at 3.77 ppm).

Furthermore, also amplitude ratios can be provided as input features to discriminate brain tumours. Opstad et al. (2004) calculated the lipid peak area (LPA) ratio as the ratio of the amplitude of the peaks around 1.25 ppm over that of the peaks around 0.90 ppm (in high-grade tumours mainly containing lipids), resulting in a good classification of glioblastomas and metastases.

Tate et al. (1998, 2003) proposed another approach based on correlation analysis to select the most important features. The method searches for the resonance frequencies with the highest correlation coefficient between their intensity values (in the frequency domain) and their class labels. Related resonance frequencies are avoided by selecting a threshold on the intercorrelation coefficient between their intensities. The feature selection is performed for a binary classification problem, but multiclass classification can also be performed using a common set of features. Although this approach is statistically based, the results could be largely affected by the possible misalignment of spectra.

3.3. The construction and testing of a classifier

In pattern recognition a distinction is made between unsupervised and supervised techniques, based on their approach to the learning process. Unsupervised techniques try to group samples based on their similarities with each other, without knowing the exact grouping. The similarity measure can be based on the distance of the samples in the multidimensional feature space constructed by the observed data features. Clustering techniques (Duda et al., 2001), Self-Organizing Maps (SOMs) (Kohonen, 2001), Principal Component Analysis (PCA) (Duda et al., 2001) are a few common unsupervised techniques.

Supervised techniques explicitly exploit the concept of training and test phase. The learning or training process is guided by a virtual "teacher" providing the target values for each of the training samples. Training is performed to construct a classifier that separates the training data in the feature space in an optimal manner according to some criterion. The resulting classifier is then tested on a test set of unseen data and evaluating the test results with respect to the correct test targets. Typically two-third of the samples are randomly selected as training set and the remainder as independent test set. *k*-nearest neighbours (Duda et al., 2001) and artificial neural networks (Bishop, 1995) are a few of the most well-known supervised techniques.

Although it is desirable to build a classifier with the highest performance, one should avoid overfitting. In such a case the classifier almost perfectly fits the training data, but cannot generalize on an independent test set. This leads to a low performance upon the insertion of new samples. A common setup to avoid overfitting is by introducing a validation set which is used to evaluate the classification performance during training (Fig. 6). In this scheme the total number of data is divided into a training set, a validation set and a

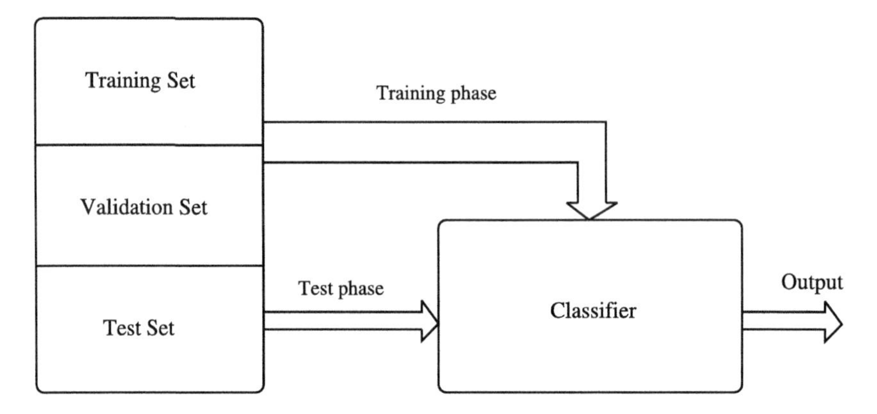

Fig. 6. The data set is divided into training, validation and test sets. The validation set is used in the training process to obtain a good generalization, e.g. to avoid overfitting. The test set is used to measure the performance of the classifier on the independent/unseen data.

test set. The classifier is trained with the training set, while the validation set is used to decide when to stop training (i.e. when a minimal error on this validation set is reached). The test data are only used after the training by means of which an independent classification performance can be measured.

3.4. Performance measures

3.4.1. Correct classification rate

There are many statistical methods for evaluating and estimating the performance of a classifier. Some of the best-known methods are leave-one-out, *N*-fold cross-validation and bootstrapping methods (Bishop, 1995; Duda et al., 2001). The goal should be to obtain as honestly as possible an estimation about the classification accuracy of the system. The correct classification rate shows the proportion of correct classifications to the total number of classification tests. However this test depends on the assessment setup.

Leave-one-out cross-validation (LOOCV) can be used as a method to estimate the classifier performance in an unbiased manner. Here, leaving only one case out of the total data set, the classifier is trained and then the classifier is tested using the left out data point. This procedure is repeated until each data point has been left out once. The classification performance is calculated by taking the average of the number of correct classifications.

One should also realize that in real-life cases, such as in clinical medicine there is virtually no perfect test. All tests will have an error rate and on occasion will either fail to identify an abnormality, or identify an abnormality which is not present. It is common to describe this error rate by the terms true and false positive and true and false negative as follows:

True Positive (TP): the test result is positive in the presence of the clinical abnormality.

Table 1. Contingency table commonly used in clinical medicine to assess the classifier performance in correctly predicting the clinical abnormality to the true diagnosis

	Predicted group	
Actual group	Normal	Abnormal
Normal	TN	FP
Abnormal	FN	TP

True Negative (TN): the test result is negative in the absence of the clinical abnormality.
False Positive (FP): the test result is positive in the absence of the clinical abnormality.
False Negative (FN): the test result is negative in the presence of the clinical abnormality.
A tabular format, known as contingency table is illustrated in Table 1. Table 2 defines various terms used to describe the clinical efficiency of a test based on the terms above.

3.4.2. Receiver operating characteristic

Receiver Operating Characteristic (ROC) curve analysis (Swets, 1979; Obuchowski, 2003) is an objective and highly effective technique for assessing the performance in binary classification or diagnostic test. A data sample is assigned to one of the two groups or classes (e.g. normal or abnormal) depending on the output value of the pattern recognition system relative to a certain threshold. The adequacy of the diagnostic test is often judged on the basis of its sensitivity (the proportion of abnormal subjects correctly identified) and its specificity (the proportion of normal subjects correctly classified).

Table 2. The definition of various terms used to describe the clinical efficiency of a test

Sensitivity	TP/(TP + FN)
Specificity	TN/(FP + TN)
Predictive value (positive)	TP/(FP + TP)
Predictive value (negative)	TN/(FN + TN)
Relative risk	$\dfrac{TP/(FP + TP)}{FN/(FN + TN)}$
Likelihood ratio	$\dfrac{TP/(TP + FP)}{FP/(TN + FP)}$ or $\dfrac{\text{Sensitivity}}{1 - \text{Specificity}}$
Odds	Probability/(1 − probability)
Accuracy	(TP + TN)/total

The ROC curve is a graphical presentation of sensitivity versus 1−specificity (or false positive rate) as the threshold is varying. Each point on the graph is generated by using a different cut-off point (Obuchowski, 2003). The area under the ROC curve (AUC) gives then a global measure of the clinical efficiency over a range of test cut-off points on the ROC curve. For example, as shown in Fig. 7 a test with an AUC of 1.0 is perfectly accurate as the sensitivity is 1.0 when the specificity is 1.0 (perfect test). In contrast, a test with an AUC of 0.0 is perfectly inaccurate. The line segment from (0,0) to (1,1) has an area of 0.5 and is called the chance diagonal (Fig. 7). Tests with an AUC value larger than 0.5 have at least some discrimination ability. The closer the AUC reaches 1.0, the better the diagnostic test. The AUC can also be interpreted as the average value of sensitivity for all possible values of specificity (Obuchowski, 2003). Hence, the AUC is independent of the cut-off points used or the prevalence of disease and is therefore a good summary measure of test accuracy.

ROC analysis and the AUC calculation can be used to choose the best of a host of different candidate diagnostic measures or to establish a trade-off between the number of false positives and false negatives.

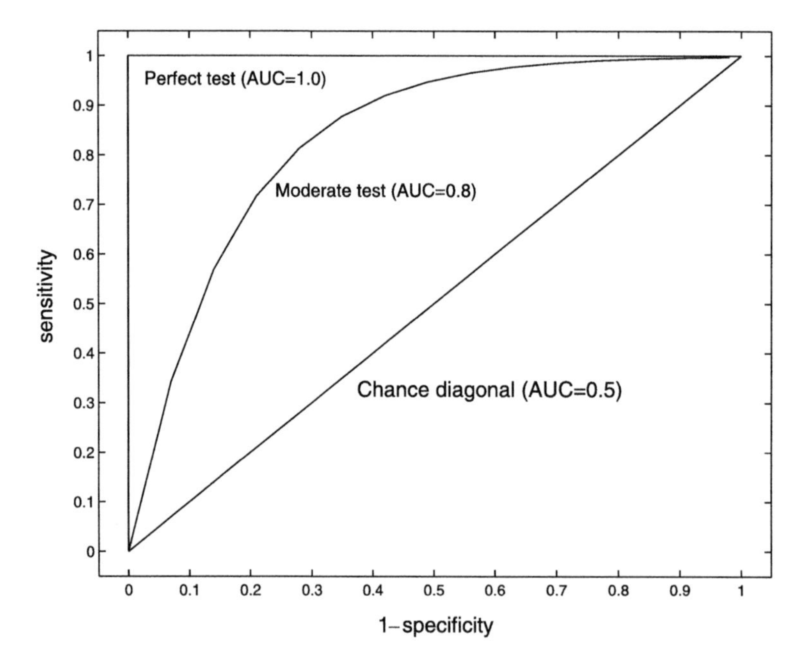

Fig. 7. ROC curve for different cases. Area under ROC curve (AUC) serves as a well-established index of diagnostic accuracy. ROC following diagonal line results in AUC = 0.5 (chance diagonal), whereas the maximum value of 1.0 corresponds to perfect assignment (unity sensitivity for all values of specificity).

3.4.3. Statistical analysis

This section describes the statistical comparison of the areas under the ROC curves derived from the same set of patients by taking into account the correlation between the areas that is induced by the paired nature of the data. In Devos et al. (2004a, 2005) and Lukas et al. (2004) this is used to compare the performance of different classifiers which are applied on M runs of randomized splitting of the data set into a training and test set.

Consider two classifiers C_1 and C_2 that handle the same input data; e.g. C_1 is Classifier 1 and C_2 is Classifier 2 applied to separate input into class 1 or 2. Let the AUC of each classifier C_I, $I = 1, 2$ be $A_{i,l}$ with standard error $SE_{i,l}$, $i = 1, 2$; $l = 1,\dots, M$, with M the number of stratified randomizations ($M = 100$). The pooled statistics are then given by A_i and SE_i ($i = 1, 2$), where n_l is the amount of samples for the stratified randomization $l = 1,\dots, M$ (Montgomery and Runger, 1994; Rice, 1995):

$$\overline{A_i} = \frac{1}{M}\sum_{l=1}^{M} A_{i,l} \quad (5)$$

$$SE_i = \sqrt{\frac{1}{N-M}\sum_{l=1}^{M}(n_l - 1)SE_{i,l}^2} \quad (6)$$

$$= \sqrt{\frac{1}{M}\sum_{l=1}^{M} SE_{i,l}^2} \quad (7)$$

Equation (7) is only satisfied if the test set contains an equal amount of samples for each stratified randomization, i.e. $\forall l n_l = n, N = \sum_{l=1}^{M} n_l$

A general approach to statistically test whether the areas under two ROC curves derived from the same samples differ significantly from each other is then given by the critical ratio z, defined as (Hanley and McNeil, 1983):

$$z = \frac{\overline{A_1} - \overline{A_2}}{\sqrt{SE_1^2 + SE_2^2 - 2rSE_1SE_2}}$$

in which r is a quantity representing the correlation introduced between the two areas by studying the same samples. The z value can be calculated using Eq. (5)–(7) based on the pooled statistics $\overline{A}_i$, SE_i, $i = 1, 2$ from M runs. If the resulting z value satisfies $z \geq 1.96$, then $\overline{A}_1$ and $\overline{A}_2$ are statistically different. The cut-off value 1.96 is taken as the quantity for which, under the hypothesis of equal AUCs ($\overline{A}_1 = \overline{A}_2$), $z \geq 1.96$ occurs with a probability of $\alpha = 0.05$ assuming a normal distribution.

This ROC analysis can be performed for binary classification. Although ROC analysis has been extended to multiclass classification (Srinivasan, 1999), the result is generally non-intuitive and computationally expensive. This motivates the use of the correct classification rate as performance measure for multiclass classification.

4. PATTERN RECOGNITION TECHNIQUES

4.1. Unsupervised techniques

In the research area of in vivo NMR signals, data can be generated at a relatively high dimension with respect to the amount of data, involving high complexity. The aim of unsupervised techniques is to reduce the complexity and retain the most valuable information. We will discuss Principal Component Analysis (PCA) and mixture modelling.

4.1.1. Principal component analysis

Linear Principal Component Analysis (PCA) is one of the most common statistical methods to reduce high-dimensional data. It consists of a transformation of the original variables into a new set of uncorrelated variables, called principal components (PCs). These new variables are linear combinations of the original ones, ranked based on the variance they retain. If the original variables are highly correlated, then the first few PCs will account for most of the variation and the remaining PCs can be discarded with slight loss of information. The more the PCs are used the better the reconstructed data fits the original noisy data.

Basically, PCA maps data into an orthogonal space, where the axes of this new coordinate system lie along the direction of maximum variance of the original data. By this transformation, it allows the mapping of vectors $\mathrm{x} \in \mathbb{R}^{\mathrm{n}}$ into a lower dimensional vectors $\mathrm{z} \in \mathbb{R}^{\mathrm{m}}$ with $m < n$. The covariance matrix can be estimated by

$$\hat{\mathrm{S}} = \frac{1}{N-1}\sum_{k=1}^{N}(\mathrm{x}_k - \mu)(\mathrm{x}_k - \mu)^{\mathrm{T}}, \tag{8}$$

where $\mu = \frac{1}{N}\sum_{k=1}^{N} x_k$ and computes the eigenvalue decomposition:

$$\hat{\mathrm{S}}u_i = \lambda_i u_i. \tag{9}$$

Taking the m largest eigenvalues and their corresponding eigenvectors, the score or transformed variables can be calculated using:

$$z_i = u_i^{\mathrm{T}}(\mathrm{x} - \mu), i = 1, \ldots, m. \tag{10}$$

PCA is expected to eliminate a significant number of dimensions by partitioning the feature space into subspaces of signal and noise. This assumes that most of the variance in the data can be explained by the retained components and small contributions by the noise. In this case, taking the first PCs which cover a certain amount of variance, e.g. 85%, will significantly reduce the dimension while keeping most information and filtering out noise.

4.1.2. Mixture modelling

Mixture modelling is an approach to clustering where the data are described as mixtures of distributions, usually multivariate normal distributions (Fraley and Raftery, 1998;

McLachlan and Peel, 2000). Each Gaussian can be considered as one cluster, or a cluster with a non-normal shape can be described by two or more Gaussians. Several advantages to model-based clustering over other, more common forms of clustering can be identified:

- The clustering has a statistical basis, which allows for inference. It is, for example, possible to derive uncertainty estimates for individual classifications, as well as for the clustering as a whole.
- Several criteria can be used to assess the optimal number of clusters, a direct consequence of the statistical model used to describe the data. This is a large advantage compared to, e.g. hierarchical clustering methods, where a cut-off value must be chosen by the user. In most cases, no clear criteria exist for such a choice.
- The clustering method can be selected according to the same criteria used for the choice of the number of clusters. As is the case in hierarchical clustering, several closely related clustering methods exist, and the one that fits the data best can be distinguished in an objective way.
- Noisy objects can be explicitly incorporated in the clustering procedure; these objects are then treated as one separate, widely spread cluster polluting the neat grouping of the other objects. In the current application, this feature is not used.
- Visualisation of the cluster shapes is possible in the space of the original variables. In some cases, this allows for an easier interpretation of the results; e.g. in the current application, neurologists can use domain knowledge to label the different clusters.

Describing a multivariate data set by a mixture of normal distributions is analogous to curve fitting in one dimension, where peaks in, e.g. a chromatogram can (ideally) be described by one or several gauss functions. The sum of these Gaussians should fit the original spectrum as close as possible. In mixture modelling, it is the density of the points in multivariate space that should be described by the mixture of normal distributions. This is visualized in Fig. 8.

The parameters of these Gaussians, means, covariance matrices and proportions, must be estimated from the data. If the class of each object is known, maximum likelihood can be used to obtain these parameters. The density at point x_i of a multivariate normal distribution, characterized by the mean μ and covariance matrix Σ is given by:

$$\phi(x_i \mid \mu, \Sigma) = (2\pi)^{-p/2} \, |\Sigma|^{-1/2} \, e^{-\frac{1}{2}(x_i-\mu)'\Sigma^{-1}(x_i-\mu)}. \tag{11}$$

The likelihood $L(\theta|x)$ that all objects are coming from a specific distribution, characterized by $\theta = (\mu, \Sigma)$, is the product of the densities:

$$L(\theta \mid x) = \prod_{i=1}^{n} \phi(x_i \mid \theta). \tag{12}$$

The estimates for the distribution describing the data optimally are those that maximize the likelihood $L(\theta|x)$. Many methods can be used for this. Often, the log-likelihood $l(\theta|x) = \log L(\theta|x)$ is maximized instead of the likelihood. In the case of mixture modelling, objects

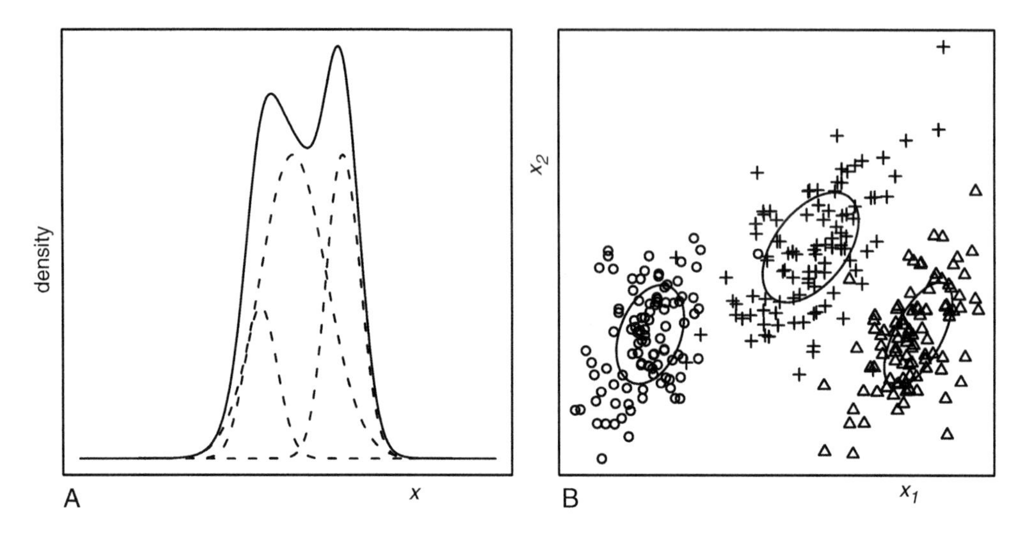

Fig. 8. The analogy between curve fitting and mixture modelling; in A, a curve (e.g. a chromatogram) is modelled by the sum of several Gaussians. In B, the density of points in two-dimensional space is modelled by a mixture of Gaussians (indicated by ellipses).

may belong to one of several distributions, or clusters:

$$\phi_k(\mathrm{x}_i \mid \mu_k, \Sigma_k) = (2\pi)^{-p/2} \mid \Sigma_k \mid^{-1/2} \mathrm{e}^{-\frac{1}{2}(\mathrm{x}_i-\mu_k)'\Sigma_k^{-1}(x_i-\mu_k)}, \tag{13}$$

where ϕ_k is the density of the data from cluster k, and μ_k and Σ_k are the mean vector and covariance matrix, respectively, of cluster k. In the case of G clusters, the likelihood is given by

$$L(\tau, \mu, \Sigma \mid \mathrm{x}) = \prod_{i=1}^{n} \sum_{k=1}^{G} \tau_k \phi_k(\mathrm{x}_i \mid \mu_k, \Sigma_k), \tag{14}$$

where τ_k is the fraction of objects in cluster k.

The problem now is that the classes of the objects x_i are unknown. The Expectation–Maximisation (EM) algorithm by Dempster et al. (1997), and McLachlan and Krishnan (1997) iteratively solves this problem. The first step in the EM algorithm for mixture models is the calculation of $\mathbf{z}_{ik}$, the conditional probability that object i belongs to class k, given an initial guess for the parameters $\theta(= \tau, \mu, \Sigma)$:

$$z_{ik} = \phi_k(\mathrm{x}_i \mid \theta_k) / \sum_{j=1}^{K} \phi_j(\mathrm{x}_i \mid \theta_j) \tag{15}$$

This is done for all objects and all classes. This is the expectation step; the second step is the maximisation step, in which the parameters θ for the mixture model are estimated.

The z_{ik} are used in this estimation and therefore these parameters (graphically expressed as the ellipses in Fig. 8) may differ from the initial estimates. The E- and M-steps alternate until convergence. Eventually, objects can be classified to the cluster with the highest z_{ik} value for that object: $\max_k (z_{ik})$.

Usually, one do not start the EM algorithm with initial values for θ, but with an initial partitioning and the M-step. Since the choice for an initial partitioning can influence the eventual classification significantly (McLachlan and Peel, 2000), most applications start from a number of different starting points and use the one leading to the best clustering, or use another clustering method to obtain the initial classification.

4.2. Supervised techniques

The supervised approach uses a "training set" to build a statistical classifier which classifies the samples in an optimal manner and is tested on an independent "test set". There exist several types of supervised techniques that can be applied to MR data. For an overview of supervised techniques like partial least squares, neural networks and *k*-nearest neighbour analysis we refer to (Duda et al., 2001; Lindon et al., 2001). This section mainly focuses on one classical and one kernel-based technique, respectively Linear Discriminant Analysis (LDA) and Least-Squares Support Vector Machines (LS-SVM).

4.2.1. Linear discriminant analysis

Linear Discriminant Analysis (LDA) originally was designed by Fisher (1936) for taxonomic classification, but has been widely applied for several classification purposes. Suppose L represents the linear transformation that maps the original n-dimensional space onto an m-dimensional feature subspace where normally $m \ll n$. The new feature vectors $z_k \in \mathbb{R}^m$ are defined by $z_k = L^T x$, $k = 1,\ldots, N$.

LDA searches for those vectors in the underlying space that best discriminate among classes (rather than those that best describe the data). More formally, given a number of independent features relative to which the data is described, LDA creates a linear combination of these which yields the largest mean differences between the desired classes.

For all samples of the classes, we define two measures (Martinez and Kak, 2001). The first one is called *within-class* scatter matrix, as given by

$$S_w = \sum_{j=1}^{n_C} \sum_{k=1}^{N_j} (x_k^j - \mu_j)(x_k^j - \mu_j)^T, \tag{16}$$

where x_k^j is the kth sample of class j, μ_j is the mean of class j, n_C is the number of classes and N_j is the number of samples in class j.

The second measure is called *between-class* scatter matrix

$$S_b = \sum_{j=1}^{n_C} (\mu_j - \mu)(\mu_j - \mu)^T, \tag{17}$$

where μ represents the mean of all classes.

The goal is to maximize the between-class measure while minimizing the within-class measure. A common way to do this is by maximizing the ratio $\det(S_b)/\det(S_w)$. It has been proven (Fisher, 1936) that if S_w is a non-singular matrix then this ratio is maximized when the column vectors of the projection matrix, L, are the eigenvectors of $S_w^{-1}S_b$. However, it should be noted that there are at most $n_C - 1$ nonzero generalized eigenvectors and, so, an upper bound on m is $n_C - 1$. We also require at least $n + n_C$ samples to guarantee that S_w does not become singular. Problems arise when dealing with high-dimensional data. The main difficulty in this case lies in the fact that the within-class scatter matrix is almost always singular, therefore the standard algorithm cannot be used. Another disadvantage is the high computational complexity of solving $S_w^{-1}S_b$ when working with the high-dimensional input space. To solve this (Swets and Weng, 1996; Belhumeur et al., 1997) propose the use of an intermediate space.

Often, PCA is performed to reduce the dimensionality of the data, followed by applying LDA to this data in the lower dimensional space. This method was shown efficient by empirical testing but had no theoretical background upon which it was proven correct (Fidler and Leonardis, 2003).

4.2.2. Support vector machines

Quite often, different classes do not have equally distributed data points and their distributions are also overlapping among classes, which causes the problem to be linearly non-separable. Two kernel-based classifiers SVM and LS-SVM are assessed. SVM and LS-SVM with linear kernel can be regarded as regularized linear classifiers, while LS-SVM with RBF kernel is regarded as a regularized nonlinear classifier.

A Support Vector Machine (SVM) (Vapnik, 1995, 1998) is a universal learning machine, which has become more established and performs well in many classification problems. The principles of SVM are as follows:

(1) Consider the training samples:

$$\{x_k, y_k\}_{k=1}^{N}, \quad x_k \in \mathbb{R}^n, \quad y_k \in \{-1, +1\}$$

The classifier in the primal space is defined by:

$$y(x) = sign[\mathrm{w}^{\mathrm{T}}\varphi(\mathrm{x}) + b],$$

$k = 1, \ldots, N$, in which w is a weighting function.

(2) The SVM performs a nonlinear mapping φ of the input vectors $\mathrm{x}_k \in \mathbb{R}^n$ from the input space into a high-dimensional feature space. Some kernel functions can be used for this mapping, e.g. linear, polynomial, RBF kernels.

(3) In the feature space, an optimal linear decision rule is constructed by calculating a separating hyperplane which has the largest margin:

$$\min_{\mathrm{w},e_k} J(\mathrm{w},e_k) = \tfrac{1}{2}\mathrm{w}^{\mathrm{T}}\mathrm{w} + C\sum_{k=1}^{N} e_k$$
$$\text{s.t. } y_k[\mathrm{w}^T\varphi(x)+b] \geq 1-e_k,$$
$$e_k \geq 0, \qquad k=1,\ldots N$$

in which C is a regularization constant.

(4) This hyperplane is the solution of the following quadratic programming (QP) problem:

$$\max_{\alpha} J(\alpha) = \sum_{k=1}^{N}\alpha_k - \frac{1}{2}\sum_{k=1}^{N}\sum_{l=1}^{N}\alpha_k\alpha_l y_k y_l K(x_k, x_l)$$

satisfying the constraints $\Sigma_{k=1}^{N}\alpha_k y_k = 0$ and $0 \leq \alpha_k \leq C$ for $k = 1,\ldots, N$, where $\{x_k \in \mathbb{R}^n | k = 1,\ldots, N\}$ is the training sample set, and $\{y_k \in \{1, +1\} | k = 1,\ldots, N\}$ the corresponding class labels. $K(x, x_k)$ is a symmetric kernel function in the input space which satisfies Mercer's theorem: $K(x, x_k) = \varphi(\mathrm{x})^{\mathrm{T}}\varphi(x_k)$.

(5) Those input vectors $x^k \in \mathbb{R}^n$ with corresponding nonzero α_k are called support vectors. They are located in the boundary margin and contribute to the construction of the separating hyperplane.

(6) Classification in the input space is calculated by mapping the separating hyperplane back into the input space (SV = set of support vectors):

$$y(x) = \mathrm{sign}\left[\sum_{x_k \in SV}\alpha_k y_k K(x, x_k) + b\right]$$

Recently, a least squared version called least squares support vector machines (LS-SVM) has been proposed (Suykens and Vandewalle, 1999; Suykens et al., 2002), incorporating equality instead of inequality constraints as in the SVM case. This simplifies the computation of the solution, namely by solving a set of linear equations. The modifications are:

(1) The constrained optimization problem in the primal space is reformulated as

$$\min_{\mathrm{w},b,e} J(\mathrm{w},b,e) = \tfrac{1}{2}\mathrm{w}^{\mathrm{T}}\mathrm{w} + \gamma\tfrac{1}{2}\sum_{k=1}^{N} e_k^2$$
$$\text{s.t. } y_k[\mathrm{w}^{\mathrm{T}}\varphi(x_k)+b] = 1-e_k, \quad k=1,\ldots,N$$
$$\text{The conditions for optimality are } y_k[\mathrm{w}^{\mathrm{T}}\varphi(x_k)+b]-1+e_k = 0,$$
$$\alpha_k = \gamma e_k, \sum_{k=1}^{N}\alpha_k y_k = 0, \quad \text{and} \quad \mathrm{w} = \sum_{k=1}^{N}\alpha_k y_k \varphi(x_k), \quad k=1,\ldots,N.$$

(2) Here, nonzero support values α_k are spread over all data points. Each α_k value is proportional to the error of the corresponding data point. No sparseness property arises as in the standard SVM case. But, interestingly, in the LS-SVM case one can relate a high support value to a high contribution of the data point on the decision line.

(3) Elimination of w and e from the previous equations gives

$$\left[\begin{array}{c|c} 0 & Y^{\mathrm{T}} \\ \hline Y & \Omega+\gamma^{-1}I \end{array}\right]\left[\begin{array}{c} b \\ \hline \alpha \end{array}\right]=\left[\begin{array}{c} 0 \\ \hline 1_v \end{array}\right] \tag{18}$$

with $Y = [y_1 \cdots y_N]^{\mathrm{T}}$, $1_v = [1 \cdots 1]^{\mathrm{T}}$, $e = [e_1 \cdots e_N]^{\mathrm{T}}$, $\alpha = [\alpha_1 \cdots \alpha_N]^{\mathrm{T}}$, $(\Omega)_{kl} = y_k y_l K(x_k, x_l)$. This set of linear equations is easier to solve rather than the QP problem as in the standard SVM.

5. TOWARDS A MEDICAL DECISION SUPPORT SYSTEM USING MR DATA

In the diagnosis, therapy prediction and assessment of brain tumours, imaging techniques play a critical role. Currently, the most commonly used techniques for diagnosing brain tumours are CT, MRI and PET. Several specialized modalities that can be performed with the above imaging techniques are under development. In case of MR for example, conventional MRI has been extended with fMRI, diffusion- and perfusion-weighted MRI and MRSI. However, the application of different MR approaches results in scattered information within a large amount of data, from which it may be difficult to derive a final diagnosis. For the clinician, it becomes especially difficult to interpret non-anatomical data, e.g. from MRSI, and extract the relevant information for determining the pathology. Normally, this type of data requires extensive processing before the tumour-specific information can be visualized. This is not only time consuming, but also requires high expertise. Furthermore, it is difficult for a clinician to extract correlations between data from different MR approaches, while these correlations have been proven to exist and helpful for a reliable diagnosis.

As explained in Sections 3 and 4, statistics and pattern recognition are very suited to deal with the processing, data reduction, data fusion and classification of MR data. Progress has been reported in automated pattern recognition for brain tumour diagnosis based on MRI or MRS data separately or the fusion of data from both MRI and MRSI. As the computer-aided diagnosis has made much progress in the past decades, one can imagine that computers will play a very large role in the clinical decision-making process of the future. Since computers are especially powerful in automatically combining, comparing and correlating data, it is only a matter of time until all available clinical information will be collectively used for the assessment of the patients' diagnosis. A tool that enables the decision-making can be called a computer-guided decision support system. It is foreseen that such systems will not only be developed for brain tumour diagnosis, but also they will be of great importance for many diseases. This could be especially true when MR techniques are combined with methods in the field of genomics or proteomics (micro array analysis) since the amount of data generated by these latter methods is huge.

The first steps in the development of a decision support system for brain tumour diagnosis have already been set by the INTERPRET consortium. This EU-funded research project has developed a large database of brain tumour patients and developed specific processing techniques for automated brain tumour classification. The project proposed to fuse data from MRI as well as MRSI. Szabo de Edelenyi et al. (2000) combined the information of one type of MR image with metabolic maps (see Section 2.3) obtained from MRSI to construct a classification map of the human brain, called a nosologic image. This image could be interpreted by the clinician like an original MR image and thus showing the spectral profiles was avoided.

A more advanced way to present information to the clinician was developed by Simonetti (2004). The proposed support system is driven by pattern recognition and provides the clinician with all kind of information displayed in a user interface. More specifically, the method uses data from MR images with four different contrast and MRSI data. First, through pre-processing and data reduction, tumour discriminating features are extracted from the data. These features are used to cluster the data (Fig. 9), in order to segment the brain without any prior knowledge (Fig. 9B). In the example, results for a 3, 4, 5 and 6 segment solution are presented, since it is until now difficult to estimate the optimal

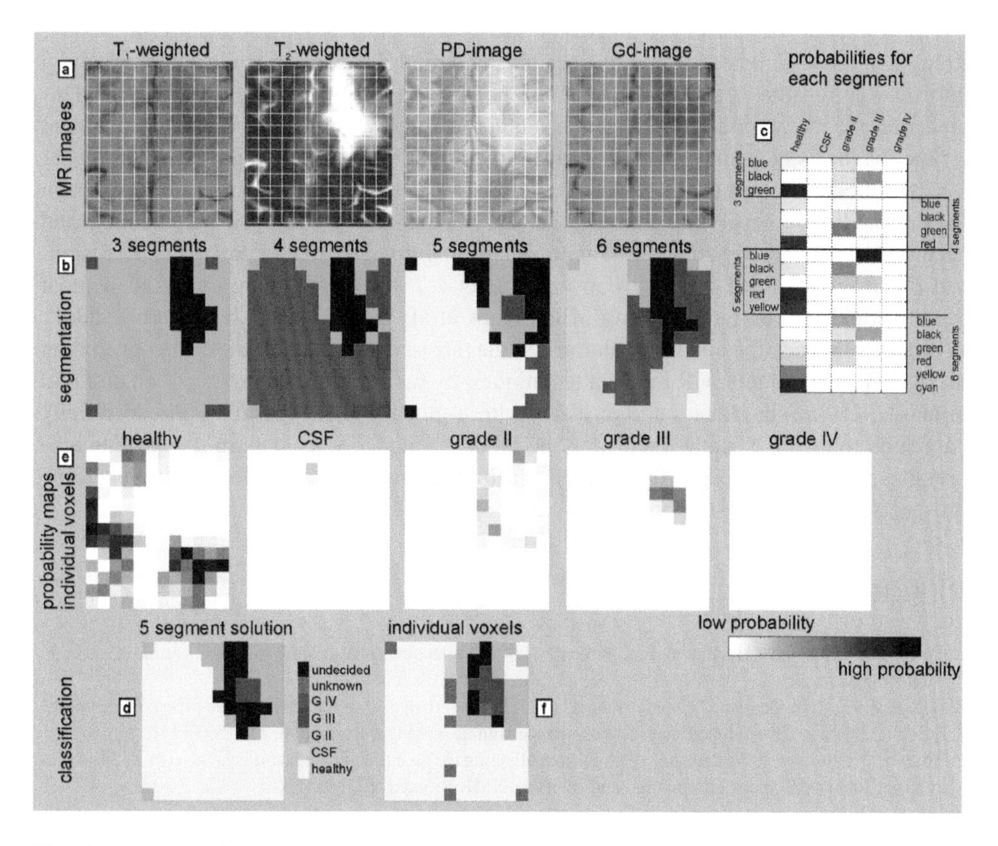

Fig. 9. Results of a medical support system for a patient with grade III glial tumour. See text for the explanation of the figures.

number of segments. The segmentation provides objective information about the heterogeneity of the tissue and can be compared with the MR images (Fig. 9A). The clinician can then select the number of segments such that, according to the medical expertise, the segmentation corresponds best with the morphological information. Additionally, the clinician can take into account the probability of each segment for a specific class membership (Fig. 9C). This not only helps in deciding the number of segments, but also gives an insight into whether a segment is appointed to a class with a high certainty. This kind of information may facilitate the acceptance of computed diagnosis, since it informs about the reliability of the classification results. After the selection of the number of segments, each cluster centroid (giving information about the type of tissue in the segment) is classified to reveal its class membership. It is also possible to classify each voxel separately, to obtain mutual information (Fig. 9D and 9F). It may well be that the classification of segments reveals the global (and reliable) tumour type of the patient, while the classification of separate voxels gives more insight into the heterogeneity and local differences in tumour grade. The probability maps are also shown (Fig. 9E) for the separate voxel classification. Since such a support system is very flexible, it could be of more help to the clinician than several independent pattern recognition methods.

The results of a few INTERPRET studies (Devos et al., 2005; Simonetti et al., 2004) strengthen the statement that imaging features and metabolic data provide complementary information for the accurate discrimination between several brain tissue types. This motivates the integration of MRSI into a standard clinical examination which is performed for the diagnosis of brain tumours. For example, in an MRI classification study (Ye et al., 2002) of brain gliomas also several other diagnostic factors were found to be important for the prediction of tumour grading like age, oedema, blood supply, calcification and haemorrhage. Characteristic brain tumour features were identified in data from perfusion- and diffusion-weighted imaging (Covarrubias et al., 2004), including an assessment of these methods in combination with MRSI (Law et al., 2002, 2003; Chiang et al., 2004). In order to enhance the quality of automated diagnosis, a fusion of all these data–including the aforementioned non-MR medical techniques–by means of pattern recognition could in principle lead to classification algorithms with a much higher sensitivity and specificity compared to methods using data from one modality alone. Since pattern recognition also provides handles to present fused data in a highly interpretable and objective way, the prospects of a decision support system based upon pattern recognition is high.

REFERENCES

Aldape, K., M. Okcu, M. Bondsy and M. Wrensch, 2003, Molecular epidemiology of glioblastoma. Cancer J., 9(2), 99–106.

Barkhuysen, H., R. de Beer and D. van Ormondt, 1987, Improved algorithm for non-iterative time-domain model fitting to exponentially damped magnetic resonance signals. J. Magn. Reson., 73, 553–557.

Bartha, R., D. Drost and P. Williamson, 1999, Factors affecting the quantification of short echo in-vivo ^{1}H MR spectra: prior knowledge, peak elimination, and filtering. NMR Biomed. 12, 205–216.

Behar, K., D. Rothman, D. Spencer and O. Petroff, 1994, Analysis of macromolecule resonances in ^{1}H NMR spectra of human brain. Magn. Reson. Med., 32, 294–302.

Belhumeur, P., J. Hespanha and D. Kriegman, 1997, Eigenfaces vs. fisherface: recognition using class specific linear projection. IEEE Trans. Pattern Anal. Mach. Intell., 19(7), 711–720.

Bishop, C., 1995, Neural Networks for Pattern Recognition. Oxford University Press, Oxford.

Bovée, W., S. Keevil, M. Leach and F. Podo, 1995, Quality assessment in in-vivo NMR spectroscopy: Ii. a protocol for quality assessment. EEC concerted research project. Magn. Reson. Imag., 13(1), 123–129.

CaMon-project, 1998, Comprehensive cancer monitoring programme in Europe. URL: http://www-dep.iarc.fr/hmp/camon.htm

Campbell, I., C. Dobson, R. Williams and A. Xavier, 1973, Resolution enhancement of protein pmr spectra using the difference between a broadened and a normal spectrum. J. Magn. Reson., 11, 172–181.

Chiang, I., Y. Kuo, C. Lu, K. Yeung, W. Lin, F. Sheu and G. Liu, 2004. Distinction between high-grade gliomas and solitary metastases using peritumoral 3-T magnetic resonance spectroscopy, diffusion, and perfusion imagings. Neuroradiology, 46(8), 619–627.

Christiansen, P., P. Toft, P. Gideon, G. Danielsen, P. Ring and O. Henriksen, 1994, MR-visible water content in human brain: a proton MRS study. Magn. Reson. Imag., 12(8), 1237–1244.

Covarrubias, D., B. Rosen and M. Lev, 2004, Dynamic magnetic resonance perfusion imaging of brain tumors. The Oncologist, 9, 528–537.

Dempster, A., N. Laird and D. Rubin, 1997, Maximum likelihood from incomplete data via the em algorithm. J. Royal Stat. Soc. B, 39(1), 1–38.

Devos, A., L. Lukas, J. Suykens, L. Vanhamme, A. Tate, F. Howe, C. Majós, A. Moreno-Torres, M. van der Graaf, C. Arús and S.Van Huffel, 2004a, Classification of brain tumours using short echo time ^{1}H MR spectra. J. Magn. Reson., 170(1), 164–175.

Devos, A., A. Simonetti, M. Van der Graaf, L. Lukas, J. Suykens, L. Vanhamme, L. Buydens, A. Heerschap and S. van Huffel, 2004b, The use of multivariate MR imaging intensities versus metabolic data from MR spectroscopic imaging for brain tumour classification. J. Magn. Reson., 173(2), 218–228.

Duda, R., P. Hart and D. Stork, 2001, Pattern Classification, 2nd ed. John Wiley & Sons, New York.

Fidler, S. and A. Leonardis, 2003, Robust LDA classification by subsampling. Proc. of IEEE Workshop on Statistical Analysis in Computer Vision, Madison, Wisconcin, USA, p. CDROM. URL: http://www.cse.lehigh.edu/~rjm2/SACV

Fisher, R., 1936, The use of multiple measurements in taxonomic problems. Annals of Eugenics, 7, 179–188.

Fraley, C. and A. Raftery, 1998, How many clusters? Which clustering method? Answers via model-based cluster analysis. Computer J., 41, 578–588.

Gadian, D., 1995, NMR and its applications to living systems, 2nd ed. Oxford Science publishers, Oxford.

Govindaraju, V., K. Young and A. Maudsley, 2000, Proton NMR chemical shifts and coupling constants for brain metabolites. NMR Biomed, 13, 129–153.

Hanley, J. and B. McNeil, 1983, A method of comparing the areas under receiver operating characteristic curves derived from the same cases. Radiology, 148, 839–843.

Hoch, J. and A. Stern, 1996, NMR Data Processing. John Wiley & Sons, New York.

Hofmann, L., J. Slotboom, C. Boesch and R. Kreis, 1999, Model fitting of ^{1}HMR spectra of the human brain: incorporation of short-T1 components and evaluation of parametrized vs. non-parametrized models. Proceedings of the 7th Scientific Meeting & Exhibition (ISMRM99), Philadelphia, USA, p. 586.

Hofmann, L., J. Slotboom, B. Jung, P. Maloca, C. Boesch and R. Kreis, 2002, Quantitative ^{1}H-magnetic resonance spectroscopy of human brain: influence of composition and parameterization of the basis set in linear combination model-fitting. Magn. Reson. Med., 48, 440–453.

Howe, F., S. Barton, S. Cudlip, M. Stubbs, D. Saunders, M. Murphy, P. Wilkins, K. Opstad, V. Doyle, M. McLean, B. Bell and J. Griffiths, 2003, Metabolic profiles of human brain tumours using quantitative in vivo ^{1}H magnetic resonance spectroscopy. Magn. Reson. Med., 49, 223–232.

Huang, Y., P. Lisboa and W. El-Deredy, 2003, Tumour grading from magnetic resonance spectroscopy: a comparison of feature extraction with variable selection. Stat. Med., 22, 147–164.

Keevil, S., B. Barbiroli, D. Collins, E. Danielsen, J. Hennig, O. Henriksen, M. Leach, R. Longo, M. Lowry, C. Moore, E. Moser, C. Segebarth, W. Bovée and F. Podo, 1995, Quality assessment in in-vivo NMR spectroscopy: IV. A multicentre trial of test objects and protocols for performance assessment in clinical NMR spectroscopy. Magn. Reson. Imag., 13(1), 139–157.

Klose, U., 1990, In-vivo proton spectroscopy in presence of eddy currents. Magn. Reson. Med., 14, 26–30.

Kohonen, T., 2001. Self-Organizing Maps, 3rd ed. Springer Series in Information Sciences Vol. 30., Springer, New York.

Kreis, R., 2004, Issues of spectral quality in clinical ^{1}H-magnetic resonance spectroscopy and a gallery of artefacts. NMR Biomed., 17, 361–381.

Kugel, H., W. Heindel, R.-I. Ernestus, J. Bunke, R. du Mesmil and G. Friedmann, 1990, Human brain tumors: spectral patterns detected with localized H-1 MR spectroscopy. Radiology, 183(3), 701–709.

Kuroda, Y., A. Wada, T. Yamazaki and K. Nagayama, 1989, Postacquistion data processing method for suppression of the solvent signal. J. Magn. Reson., 84, 604–610.

Laudadio, T., N. Mastronardi, L. Vanhamme, P. Van Hecke and S. Van Huffel, 2002, Improved lanczos algorithms for blackbox MRS data quantitation. J. Magn. Reson., 157, 292–297.

Law, M., S. Cha, E. Knopp, G. Johnson, J. Arnett and A. Litt, 2002, Highgrade gliomas and solitary metastases: differentiation by using perfusion and proton spectroscopic MR imaging. Radiology, 222, 715–721.

Law, M., S. Yang, H. Wang, J. Babb, G. Johnson, S. Cha, E. Knopp and D. Zagzag, 2003, Glioma grading: Sensitivity, specificity and predictive values of perfusion MR imaging and proton MR spectroscopic imaging compared with conventional MR imaging. AJNR Am. J. Neuroradiol., 24, 1989–1998.

Leach, M., D. Collins, S. Keevil, I. Rowland, M. Smith, O. Henriksen, W. Bovée and F. Podo, 1995, Quality assessment in in-vivo NMR spectroscopy: III. Clinical test objects: design, construction, and solutions. Magn. Reson. Imag., 13(1), 131–137.

Leclerc, X., T. Huisman and A. Sorensen, 2002, The potential of proton magnetic resonance spectroscopy (^{1}H-MRS) in the diagnosis and management of patients with brain tumours. Curr. Opini. Oncol., 14, 292–298.

Leibel, S., C. Scott and J. Loeffler, 1994, Contemporary approaches to the treatment of malignant gliomas with radiation therapy. Semin. Oncol., 21, 198–219.

Lemmerling, P., L. Vanhamme, H. in't Zandt, S. Van Huffel and P. Van Hecke, 2002, Time-domain quantification of short-echo-time proton MRS. MAGMA, 15, 178–179.

Li, B., H. Wang and O. Gonen, 2003, Metabolite ratios to assumed stable creatine level may confound quantification of proton brain MR spectroscopy. Magn. Reson. Imag., 21, 923–928.

Lindon, J., E. Holmes and J. Nicholson, 2001, Pattern recognition methods and applications in biomedical magnetic resonance. Prog. Nucl. Magn. Reson. Spectrosc., 39, 1–40.

Lukas, L., A. Devos, J. Suykens, L. Vanhamme, F. Howe, C. Majós, A. Moreno-Torres, M. van der Graaf, A. Tate, C. Arús and S.Van Huffel, 2004, Brain tumour classification based on long echo proton MRS signals. Artif. Intell. Med., 31(1), 73–89.

Majós, C., J. Alonso, C. Aguilera, M. Serrallonga, J. Acebes, C. Arús and J. Gili, 2002, Adult primitive neuroectodermal tumor: Proton MR spectroscopic findings with possible application for differential diagnosis. Radiology, 225, 556–566.

Manton, D., M. Lowry, S. Blackband and A. Horsman, 1995, Determination of proton metabolite concentrations and relaxation parameters in normal human brain and intracranial tumours. NMR Biomed., 8, 104–112.

Marshall, I., J. Higinbotham, S. Bruce and A. Freise, 1997, Use of Voigt lineshape for quantification of in-vivo ^{1}H spectra. Magn. Reson. Med., 37, 651–657.

Martinez, A. and A. Kak, 2001, PCA versus LDA. IEEE Trans. Pattern Anal. Mach. Intell., 23(2), 228–233.

McLachlan, G. and T. Krishnan, 1997, The EM Algorithm and Extensions. John Wiley & Sons, New York.

McLachlan, G. and D. Peel, 2000, Finite Mixture Models. John Wiley & Sons, New York.

Meyer, R., M. Fisher, S. Nelson and T. Brown, 1988, Evaluation of manual methods for integration of in vivo phosphorus NMR spectra. NMR Biomed., 1(3), 131–135.

Mittler, M., B. Walters and E. Stopa, 1996, Observer reliability in histological grading of astrocytomas stereotactic biopsies. J. Neurosurg., 85, 1091–1094.

Montgomery, D. and G. Runger, 1994, Applied Statistics and Probability for Engineers. John Wiley & Sons, New York.

Mukherji, S. (Ed.), 1998, Clinical Applications of Magnetic Resonance Spectroscopy. Wiley-Liss, New York.

Murphy, M., A. Loosemore, A. Clifton, F. Howe, A. Tate, S. Cudlip, P. Wilkins, J. Griffiths and B. Bell, 1993, The contribution of proton magnetic resonance spectroscopy (^{1}HMRS) to clinical brain tumour diagnosis. Magn. Reson. Med., 30, 518–519.

Negendank, W., 1992, Studies of human tumours by MRS: a review. NMR Biomed., 5, 302–324.

Nelson, S., 2003, Multivoxel magnetic resonance spectroscopy of brain tumours. Molecular cancer therapeutics, 2(2), 497–507.

Nelson, S. and S. Cha, 2003, Imaging glioblastoma multiforme. Cancer J., 9(2), 134–145.

Nelson, S., D. Vigneron and W. Dillon, 1999, Serial evaluation of patients with brain tumours using volume MRI and 3D ^{1}H MRSI. NMR Biomed, 12, 123–138.

Nelson, S., E. Graves, A. Pirzkall, X. Li, A. Chan, D. Vigneron and T. McKnight, 2002, In vivo molecular imaging for planning radiation therapy of gliomas: an application of ^{1}H MRSI. J. Magn. Reson. Imag., 16, 464–476.

Obuchowski, N., 2003, Receiver operating characteristic curves and their use in radiology. Radiology, 229, 3–8.

Opstad, K., M. Murphy, P. Wilkins, B. Anthony Bell, J. Griffiths, B. Bell and F. Howe, 2004, Differentiation of metastases from high-grade gliomas using short echo time ^{1}H spectroscopy. J. Magn. Reson. Imag., 20, 187–192.

Prados, M., 1991, Treatment strategies for patients with recurrent brain tumours. Semin. Radiat. Oncol., 1, 62–68.

Preul, M., Z. Caramanos, D. Collins, J. Villemure, R. Leblanc, A. Olivier, R. Pokrupa and D. Arnold, 1996, Accurate, non-invasive diagnosis of human brain tumours by using magnetic resonance spectroscopy. Nat. Med., 2(3), 323–325.

Provencher, S., 1993, Estimation of metabolite concentrations from localized in-vivo proton NMR spectra. Magn. Res. Med., 30, 672–679.

Ratiney, H., Y. Coenradie, S. Cavassila, D. van Ormondt and D. Graveron-Demilly, 2004, Time-domain quantitation of ^{1}H short echo-time signals: background accommodation. MAGMA, 16, 284–296.

Rees, J., 2003, Advances in magnetic resonance imaging of brain tumours. Current Opinion in Neurology, 16, 643–650.

Rice, J., 1995, Mathematical Statistic and Data Analysis, 2nd Ed., Duxbury Press, Wadsworth Publishing Company, Belmont, California.

Seeger, U., U. Klose, I. Mader, W. Grodd and T. Nägele, 2003, Parametrized evaluation of macromolecules and lipids in proton MR spectroscopy of brain diseases. Magn. Res. Med., 49, 19–28.

Simonetti, A., 2004, Investigation of brain tumour classification and its reliability using chemometrics on MR spectroscopy and MR imaging data. Ph.D. Thesis, Catholic University, Nijmegen.

Simonetti, A., W. Melssen, M. van der Graaf, G. Postma, A. Heerschap and L. Buydens, 2003, A new chemometric approach for brain tumour classification using magnetic resonance imaging and spectroscopy. Anal. Chem. 75(20), 5352–5361.

Simonetti, A., W. Melssen, F. Szabo de Edelenyi, J. van Asten, A. Heerschap and L. Buydens, 2004, Combination of feature-reduced MR spectroscopic and MR imaging data for improved brain tumour classification. NMR Biomed., 17, 1–10.

Smith, I. and L. Stewart, 2002, Magnetic resonance spectroscopy in medicine: clinical impact. Prog. Nucl. Magn. Reson. Spectrosc., 40, 1–34.

Soher, B., K. Young and A. Maudsley, 2001, Representation of strong baseline contribution in ^{1}H MR spectra. Magn. Res. Med., 45, 966–972.

Srinivasan, A., 1999, Note on the Location of Optimal Classifiers in n-dimensional ROC Space. Tech. Rep. Technical Report PRG-TR-2-99, Oxford University Computing Laboratory, Oxford, England.

Sundin, T., L. Vanhamme, P. van Hecke, I. Dologlou and S. Van Huffel, 1999, Accurate quantification of ^{1}H spectra: from finite impulse response filter design for solvent suppression to parameter estimation. J. Magn. Reson., 139, 189–204.

Suykens, J. and J. Vandewalle, 1999, Least squares support vector machine classifiers. Neur. Proc. Lett., 9(3), 293–300.

Suykens, J., T. van Gestel, J. de Brabanter, B. de Moor and J. Vandewalle, 2002, Least Squares Support Vector Machines. World Scientific Publishing Co., Singapore.

Swets, D. and J. Weng, 1996, Using discriminant eigenfeatures for image retrieval. IEEE Trans. Pattern Anal. Mach. Intell., 18(8), 831–836.

Swets, J., 1979, ROC analysis applied to the evaluation of medical imaging techniques. Invest. Radiol., 14(2), 109–121.

Szabo de Edelenyi, F., C. Rubin, F. Estéve, S. Grand, M. Décorps, V. Lefournier, J. Le Bas and C. Rémy, 2000, A new approach for analyzing proton magnetic resonance spectroscopic images of brain tumours: nosologic images. Nat. Med., 6, 1287–1289.

Tate, A., S. Crabb, J. Griffiths, S. Howells, R. Mazucco, L. Rodrigues and D. Watson, 1996, Lipid metabolite peaks in pattern recognition analysis of tumour in vivo MR spectra. Anticancer Res., 16, 1575–1580.

Tate, A., J. Griffiths, I. Martinez-Pérez, A. Moreno, I. Barba, M.C. Nas, D. Watson, J. Alonso, F. Bartumeus, F. Isamat, I. Ferrer, F. Villa, E. Ferrer, A. Capdevila and C. Arús, 1998, Towards a method for automated classification of ^{1}H MRS spectra from brain tumours. NMR Biomed. 11, 177–191.

Tate, A., C. Majós, A. Moreno, F. Howe, J. Griffiths and C. Arús, 2003, Automated classification of short echo time in in-vivo ^{1}H brain tumour spectra: a multicenter study. Magn. Reson. Med., 49, 29–36.

Usenius, J., S. Tuohimetsa, P. Vainio, M. Ala-Korpela, Y. Hiltunen and R. Kauppinen, 1996, Automated classification of human brain tumours by neural network analysis using in vivo ^{1}H magnetic resonance spectroscopic metabolite phenotypes. Neuroreport, 7(10), 1597–1600.

van der Graaf, M., 2001, Deliverable number 4. d2.2: Data protocols (MRS). EU-IST-1999-10310. URL: http://carbon.uab.es/INTERPRET/mrs data/mrs data.html

Vanhamme, L., T. Sundin, P. Van Hecke and S. Van Huffel, 2001, MR spectroscopy quantitation: a review of time-domain methods. NMR Biomed., 14, 233–246.

Vanhamme, L., T. Sundin, P. Van Hecke, S. Van Huffel and R. Pintelon, 2000, Frequency-selective quantification of biomedical magnetic resonance spectroscopy data. J. Magn. Reson., 143(1), 1–16.

Vanhamme, L., A. van den Boogaart and S. Van Huffel, 1997, Improved method for accurate and efficient quantification of MRS data with use of prior knowledge. J. Magn. Reson., 129, 35–43.

Vapnik, V., 1995, The Nature of Statistical Learning Theory. Springer, New York.

Vapnik, V., 1998, Statistical Learning Theory. John Wiley & Sons, New York.

Ye, C., J. Yang, D. Geng, Y. Zhou and N. Chen, 2002, Fuzzy rules to predict degree of malignancy. Med. Biol. Eng. Comput., 40, 145–152.

Young, K., B. Soher and A. Maudsley, 1998, Automated spectral analysis II: application of wavelet shrinkage for characterization of non-parameterized signals. Magn. Reson. Med., 40, 816–821.

Chapter 12

Towards Automatic Risk Analysis for Hereditary Non-Polyposis Colorectal Cancer Based on Pedigree Data

Münevver Köküer[1], Raouf N.G. Naguib[1], Peter Jančovič[2], H. Banfield Younghusband[3] and Roger Green[3]

[1]*Biomedical Computing Research Group (BIOCORE), School of Mathematical and Information Sciences, Coventry University, Coventry, UK*
[2]*Electronic, Electrical & Computer Engineering, University of Birmingham, Birmingham, UK*
[3]*Faculty of Medicine, Memorial University of Newfoundland, St. John's, Newfoundland, Canada*
Email: r.naguib@ieee.org

Abstract

Hereditary non-polyposis colorectal cancer (HNPCC) is one of the most common autosomal dominant diseases in the developed countries. Here, we report on a system to identify the risk of a family having HNPCC based on its history. This is important since population-wide genetic screening for HNPCC is not currently considered feasible due to its complexity and expense. If the risk of a family having HNPCC can be identified/assessed, then only the high-risk fraction of the population would undergo intensive screening. We compare artificial neural networks and statistical approaches for assessing the risk of a family having HNPCC and discuss the experimental results obtained by these two approaches.

Keywords: HNPCC, cancer risk assessment, pedigree analysis, artificial neural networks, Kohonen's self-organizing maps, principal component analysis.

Contents

1. INTRODUCTION

Colorectal cancer (CRC) is one of the most common malignancies in developed countries and represents a significant public-health issue. The United States and the United Kingdom

© 2007 Elsevier B.V. All rights reserved

are two of the high-incidence countries, with about 148 300 new cases and 56 600 deaths (Jemal et al., 2002) in the United States and 30 941 new cases and 17 000 deaths in the United Kingdom (CancerData, 2000) per year. In Canada, 18 100 new cases and 8200 deaths were estimated in 2003 (CancerStat, 2003).

It remains the second leading cause of cancer-related deaths in Western countries despite advances in screening, diagnosis and treatment which have contributed to a slight but steady decline in CRC mortality rates over the last 30 years. Many cases have a poor prognosis due to their disease being detected at a late stage when it is difficult to treat it effectively. The severity of CRC is indicated by a 5-year relative survival rate of around 50% following diagnosis of colon cancer (Rabeneck et al., 2005), although cases detected at an early stage have a better overall survival.

While genetic factors (e.g. family history and mutations in mismatch repair genes) are established as the strongest risk factors for CRC, these cannot account for the majority of CRC cases. About 20–30% of all colon cancer cases have a significant inherited component and 3–5% of cases occur in genetically defined high-risk colon cancer family syndromes (Mecklin, 1987; Rodriguez et al., 1997; Aaltonen et al., 1998).

Hereditary non-polyposis colorectal cancer (HNPCC), also known as Lynch syndrome, is the most common autosomal dominant disease characterized by the development of colon cancers at an early age (early-onset CRC) and the occurrence of various other cancers at other anatomic sites. Until recently, the genetic basis of most HNPCC cases was unknown. To assist the clinical diagnosis of HNPCC and to promote consistency among researchers, the Amsterdam Criteria (AC) for high-risk families was established (Vasen et al., 1991):

- At least three family members in two or more successive generations must have CRC, one of whom is a first-degree relative of the other two;
- Cancer must be diagnosed before the age of 50 in at least one family member; and
- Familial adenomatous polyposis must be ruled out.

Colorectal tumours in patients with HNPCC are characterized by a high frequency of DNA replication errors (Aaltonen et al., 1994). While such errors of replication are usually corrected in normal cells by specialised DNA repair systems, these errors remain uncorrected in HNPCC tumours resulting in the accumulation of mutations within the tumour. The specific pathway affected is termed the mismatch repair (MMR) system and depends on the coordinated action of proteins coded by MMR genes. As a result, inherited mutations in MMR genes predispose to HNPCC.

Commercial genetic testing is available for two MMR genes (hMSH2 and hMLH1) but population-wide genetic screening for HNPCC is not currently considered feasible because of its complexity and expense (Statement, 1996). If the risk of a family having HNPCC can be assessed, then only that fraction of the population that is at high risk needs to undergo intensive clinical screening.

2. DESCRIPTION OF THE PEDIGREE DATABASE

The cohort studied consists of members of 313 pedigrees. A pedigree refers to an extended family containing one or more groups of related individuals (i.e. at least two generations are involved) (Elston and Stewart, 1971). Our pedigree data consists of approximately 6800 individuals covering four or more generations. Pedigrees are constructed using the *Cyrillic 3* software (Cyrillic, 1999). This software uses a graphical user interface to manipulate pedigree data maintained in an underlying Microsoft Access database.

Figure 1 shows an example of a pedigree. The square symbol denotes male, a circle female and a diamond, an unknown sex. The diagonal slash on the symbol indicates a deceased member. A proband (initial recognised case of CRC in a family) is indicated by an arrow. Affected and non-affected members are shown as solid and open symbols, respectively. The black shading indicates CRC, checkerboard other HNPCC-related cancer (i.e. endometrial, gastric, small bowel, gastroesophageal, liver, pancreas, biliary duct, ovarian, kidney, ureter, brain) and diagonal shading indicates any cancer not related to HNPCC. Two shadings indicate a member affected by two types of cancer.

The 313 pedigrees represent the families of a consecutive series of all colon cancer patients diagnosed within the Canadian province of Newfoundland and Labrador during the years 1999–2001. These patients and their families are being followed as part of a study of the genetic basis of colon cancer funded by the Canadian Institutes of Health Research. Information on family history, age of onset of clinical manifestation, type of cancer, and cause of death was collected from family members and confirmed by hospital records (where possible) and death certificates. Whenever possible, living family members were interviewed and counselled by a genetic counsellor. The present study was approved by the Human Investigation Committee of the Faculty of Medicine, Memorial University of Newfoundland, Canada, and written consent was obtained from all probands.

In the pedigree database, 636 patients were diagnosed with CRC as depicted in Table 1. The mean age at diagnosis was 62 years. Ten of the 313 families met the Amsterdam Criteria (AC). HNPCC-related cancer was diagnosed in 365 individuals at the mean age of 60. They were scattered in 176 families, five of whom met the AC for HNPCC. As can be seen in Table 1, multiple colorectal cancers afflicting one single patient were diagnosed in four families at a mean age of 46. One of these four families met the AC. Amongst 2 3 families for whom a single patient was diagnosed with concomitant HNPCC-related cancers, there were effectively 27 patients with a mean age of 65 and only one of these families met the AC.

Moreover, in 87 families, there were at least 3 family members affected by CRC and only in 33 of those families, these members were first-degree relatives affected by CRC. In 103 families, CRC was diagnosed in all affected patients below the age of 50 years. In 156 families, two or more generations were affected by CRC.

Table 2 indicates the number of families and their percentages in our pedigree database who meet the clinical diagnosis criteria used by the genetic counsellor as shown in Table 3, Section 3. HR1, HR2 and HR3 are the three conditions used to define the Amsterdam Criteria. To designate a family as high-risk of HNPCC, all three conditions must be met. Ten families met these criteria. The IMR1 and IMR2 risk conditions were the intermediate-risk conditions observed most frequently, with percentages of 43.45 and 10.54%, respectively. No families met IMR7 or IMR8.

A total of 161 out of 313 families (51.4%) met neither the AC nor any of the intermediate risk criteria and were therefore designated as low risk.

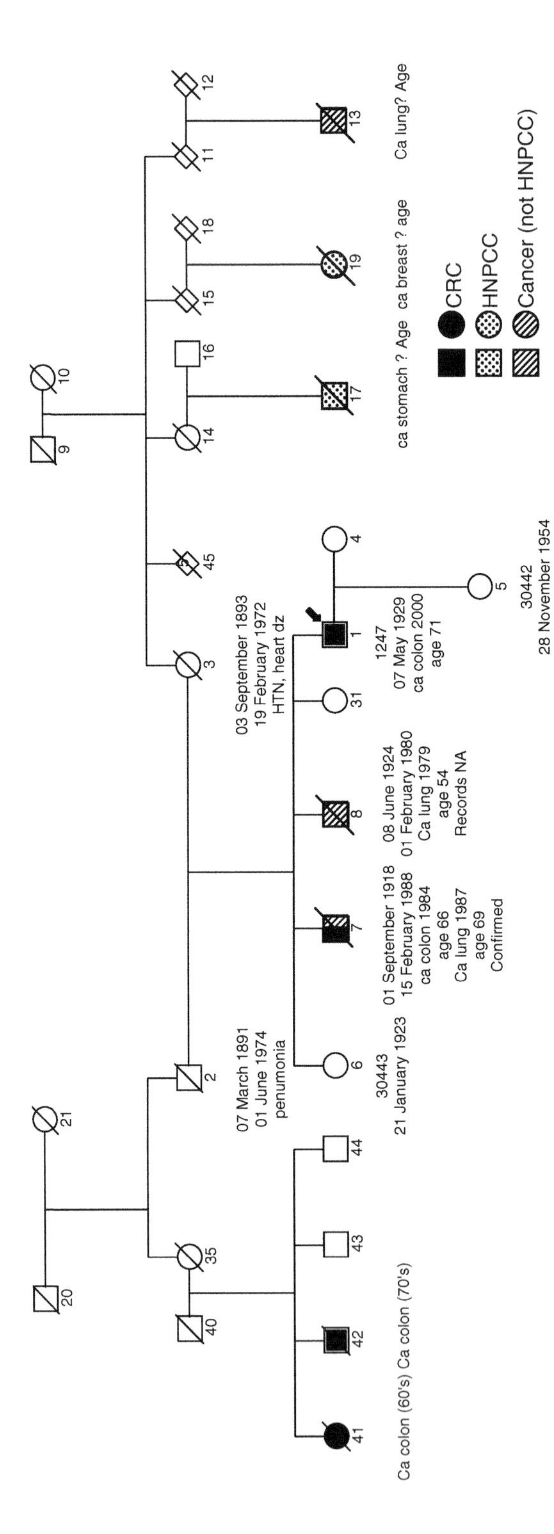

Fig. 1. An example of a family pedigree from the Cyrillic 3 software (Cyrillic, 1999).

Table 1. Descriptive data of families in the pedigree database

Cancer site	Number of patients	Mean age at diagnosis	Number of families	
			AC met	AC not met
Colorectal cancer (CRC)	636	62	10	303
Any HNPCC-related cancer	365	60	5	171
Multiple CRC in a single patient	4	46	1	3
Concomitant HNPCC-related cancer in a single patient	27	65	1	22

3. HNPCC RISK ASSESSMENT

The HNPCC risk assessment is currently performed by a genetic counsellor who makes the decision based on the criteria depicted in Table 3. HR1, HR2 and HR3 comprise the AC and a family who meets all three conditions is considered as having a high-risk for HNPCC. A family with any of the eight intermediate-risk (IMR) conditions is considered as having an intermediate-risk of an HNPCC. Any family that does not meet any of the high- or intermediate-risk conditions is considered as being of low-risk. A schematic diagram of how the counsellor identifies the risk of a family is shown in Fig. 2. However, the complexity of patient-related data (pedigree) could easily be misinterpreted or overlooked even by the specialist, and may result in a wrong assessment.

First, in order to be able to verify our results, we employed a rule-based system using the same criteria used by the counsellor (see Table 3 and Fig. 2) and refer to it as actual, or true. We found that in about 6% of the cases, the counsellor's decision was incorrect.

Table 2. Number and percentage of families in the database who meet the clinical risk criteria used by genetic counsellor (see Table 3)

Diagnostic criteria	Number of families	% families
HR1	33	10.54
HR2	84	26.84
HR3	71	22.68
High risk	10	3.19
IMR1	136	43.45
IMR2	33	10.54
IMR3	8	2.56
IMR4	3	0.96
IMR5	5	1.6
IMR6	5	1.6
Intermediate risk	142	45.36
Low risk	161	51.43

Table 3. Designation of families into different risk categories based on the counsellor diagnostic criteria

Risk category	Clinical diagnostic criteria used by genetic counsellor	
High	A family who meets all three HRs (Vasen et al., 1991)	
	HR1	at least 3 family members with CRC,
	HR2	two consecutive generations represented
	HR3	at least 1 subject <50 years at diagnosis
Intermediate	A family who meets any of the 8 IMRs (Cotterchio et al., 2005)	
	IMR1	proband + 2 relatives with any of the HNPCC associated cancers and 2 of the 3 are first-degree relatives
	IMR2	any family member with one of the above cancer < 35 years
	IMR3	proband <50 and relative with colon <50 (first- or second-degree relatives only)
	IMR4	proband <35 years
	IMR5	proband with multiple primary CRC reported via Family History Questionnarie (FHQ)
	IMR6	proband with other primary HNPCC associated cancer reported via FHQ
	IMR7	meets at least 1 pathologic criterion for intermediate risk
	IMR8	Ashkenazi Jewish
Low	A family who meets none of the above HRs and IMRs	

Next, in order to assess the risk of a family having HNPCC, we developed two Artificial Neural Networks (ANNs), a Multi-Layer Feed-Forward Neural Network (MLFFNN) and Kohonen's Self-Organizing Maps (SOM), to classify families into high-, intermediate- and low-risk categories on the basis of their pedigree data. We selected SOM (i.e. an unsupervised network) to determine how the network organises itself based on the underlying structure in the data without any structure being imposed. We then studied the accuracy with which these ANNs can predict the risk class of a family. We compared the results with those obtained from traditional statistical approaches; in this case, logistic regression (LR) and principal component analysis (PCA) with the *k*-nearest neighbour rule (*k*NN). The following section provides a brief introduction to the feature representation and classification methods used. The results obtained based on both ANNs and statistical approaches are presented and discussed in Section 4.

3.1. Feature representation and training-testing procedure

The pedigree data for each family is represented as a D-dimensional feature vector $\mathbf{x} = (x_1, x_2, \ldots, x_D)$ where each element corresponds to one of the following criteria: three

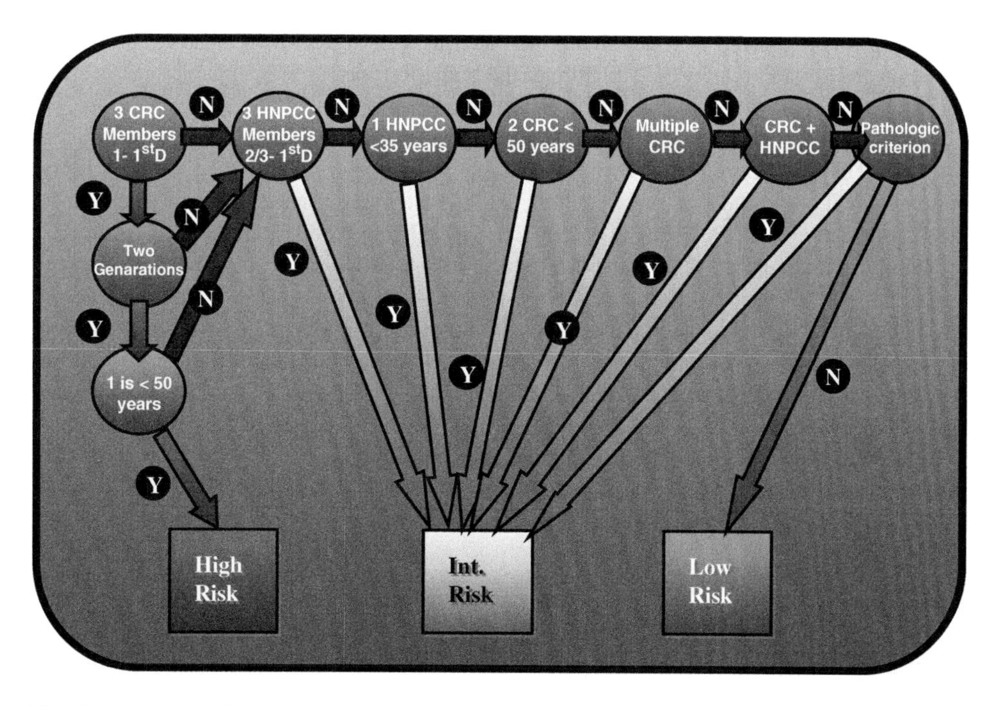

Fig. 2. An illustrative example of how a counsellor identifies the risk of a family (counsellor's criteria).

HRs (HR1–HR3) and six IMRs (IMR1–IMR6) criteria given in Table 3, and ratio of colorectal cancer and HNPCC-related cancers in the family (each obtained by dividing the number of affected individuals by the total number of persons in the family). Elements of the feature vector are binary variables except for two ratios which are continuous.

Since our data set (i.e. number of pedigrees) is small, we cannot afford to use an independent test set for assessing the performance of the systems developed. To overcome this difficulty, we employed the leave-one-out method. One input feature vector (pedigree) is left out from the training data and each system is trained/modelled using all the remaining training data. After training of the system is completed, the unseen input feature vector is presented to the trained/modelled system and analysed in a single cycle. In the case of SOM and PCA, a k-nearest neighbour (kNN) rule with $k = 3$ is used to decide the risk class of the testing family pedigree. This training-testing leave-one-out procedure is repeated for each pedigree in the database.

3.2. Artificial neural network analysis

The use of artificial neural networks (ANNs) in cancer research has increased substantially over the past years. ANNs are parallel, distributed information processing structures consisting of processing elements interconnected together (Hecht-Nielsen, 1990). These elements are modelled after the structure of the brain, thus perform in a manner that is analogous to most elementary functions of the biological neurons.

ANNs offer an alternative method of interpreting and recognising complex patterns in data sets. Their ability to model complex nonlinear relationships explains their popularity in the medical community as most medical data is inherently nonlinear in character (Baxt, 1995; Burke et al., 1997; Guthie and Monson, 1997; Naguib and Sherbet, 1997, 2001).

The operation of an ANN essentially consists of two phases: training and testing. Depending on whether or not the desired response of the network is provided, ANNs can be divided into supervised and unsupervised networks. In a supervised training environment, the network is "thought" to give the desired response by presenting it, the input data with the actual output. In an unsupervised training environment, the network gives response without exposing it to the desired output. Learning, instead, "emerges" from the data.

Here we employed both supervised and unsupervised ANNs: Multi Layer Feed-Forward Neural Network (MLFFNN) as a supervised ANN and Kohonen's Self-Organizing Maps (SOM) as an unsupervised ANN.

3.2.1. Classification based on multi-layer feed-forward neural networks

In multi-layer neural networks, neurons are organized into an input layer, one or more hidden layers and an output layer. Data is presented through the input layer. No processing is performed in these input neurons. Hidden layer(s) is/are the layer(s) where processing takes place: they provide the learning nonlinearity required for the solution of complex problems. The output layer produces the response of the network to a given input data. The network topology is constrained to be feed-forward; there are no recurrent or backward connections as shown in Fig. 3.

We use a standard back-propagation algorithm to train the MLFFNN. Back-propagation uses supervised learning and provides a way to train networks with any number of hidden neurons arranged in any number of layers (Bishop, 1995). Training continues iteratively: at each iteration all the input data and desired outputs are presented as they all contribute towards the estimation of the error gradient. Then the error is back-propagated to the previous layers of the network to adjust the weights and bias to reduce the overall error (see Fig. 3).

Let us denote the output values of neurons in a hidden layer by $h_1, h_2, \ldots, h_N$, where N is the number of neurons in that hidden layer, and the value of the kth output neuron by y_k. Then the mathematical representation of the MLFFNN would be:

$$h_n = f(w_{n1}^h x_1 + w_{n2}^h x_2 + \cdots + w_{nD}^h x_D) \quad (1)$$

$$y_k = g(w_{k1}^y h_1 + w_{k2}^y h_2 + \cdots + w_{kN}^y h_N), \quad (2)$$

where f and g are nonlinear transfer functions and w^h and w^y are the weights to the hidden and output neurons, respectively.

The number of neurons in the input layer corresponds to the number of elements in the feature vector described in Section 3.1. The number of neurons in the hidden layer is

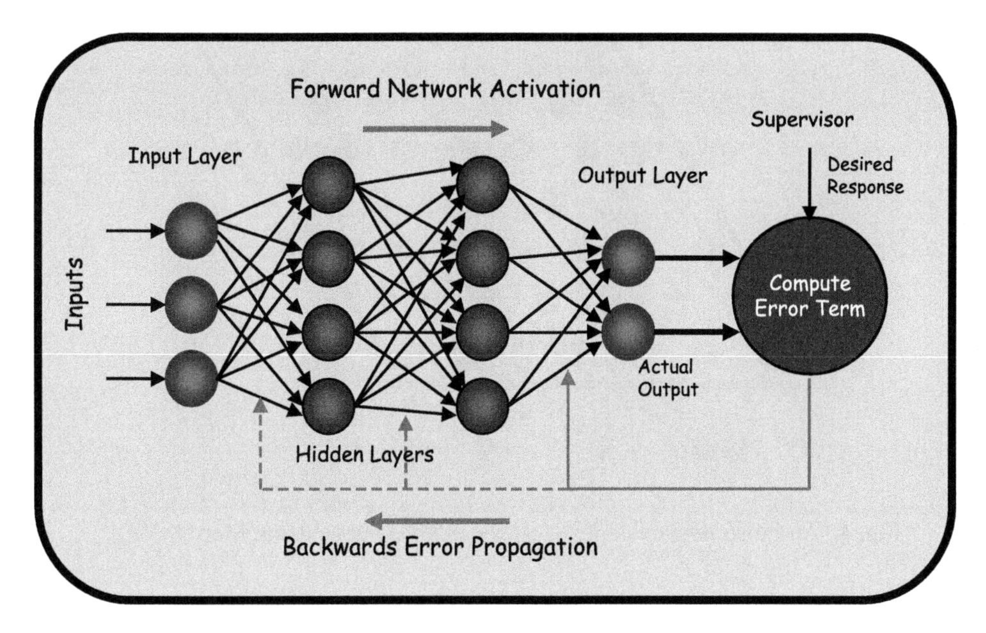

Fig. 3. An illustrative example of a Multi-Layer Feed-Forward Neural Network (MLFFNN).

selected as half of the input neurons, as suggested by Livingstone et al. (1997), i.e. six in this case. A hyperbolic tangent sigmoid transfer function is used at each of these hidden layer neurons. Three neurons with the logistic activation function are used in the output layer.

The neural network was created with the Neural Network Toolbox (V4.0.1) in Matlab™. Various back-propagation algorithms to train the network were used and similar performance was observed. The presented results were obtained by using the resilient back-propagation algorithm (Riedmiller and Braun, 1993) as it showed fast convergence. The learning rate was set to 0.01 and training was stopped when the minimum gradient (set to 1e-6) was reached.

3.2.2. Classification based on Kohonen's self-organizing maps

Kohonen's Self-Organizing Map (SOM) is one of the major unsupervised learning methods in the ANN family (Kohonen, 2001). The SOM algorithm creates mappings which transform high-dimensional data space into low-dimensional space in such a way that the topological relations of the input patterns are preserved.

SOM takes a set of input data and maps it onto neurons of a (usually) two-dimensional grid, see Fig. 4. Each neuron in the 2D grid is assigned a weight vector $\mathbf{w} = (w_{j1}, w_{j2}, \ldots, w_{jD})$ with the same dimensionality as that of the input vector, where $j = (1, 2, \ldots, L)$ and L is the total number of neurons in the network. The weights represent the associated memory.

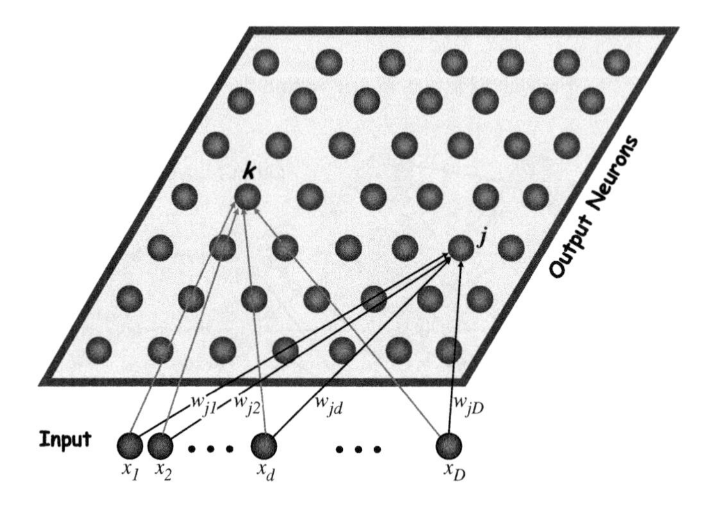

Fig. 4. An illustrative example of Kohonen's Self-Organizing Map (SOM).

The computational algorithm of SOM consists of two basic procedures, finding a winning neuron and adjusting weights of the winning neuron, as well as its neighbouring neurons.

During the training process, the weights of the winning neuron and neurons in a pre-defined neighbourhood are adjusted towards the input vector based on Eq. (3):

$$w_{jd}^{t+1} = w_{jd}^{t} + \eta h(j,k)\,(x_d - w_{jd}^{t}), \quad \text{for } 1 \le d \le D, \tag{3}$$

where η is the learning rate parameter and $h(j, k)$ is the neighbourhood function which has a value 1 at the winning neuron k, and decreases as the distance between j and k increases. At the start of the training process, the radius of the neighbourhood is fairly large, but it is made to shrink during the training. This guarantees that the global order is obtained at the beginning, whereas towards the end, as the radius gets smaller, stable convergence of the map will be achieved. The learning rate parameter η also decreases during training to help the map converge.

The SOM configuration used in this study is implemented in JAVA (Campbell et al., 2001) using a 2D output map with 400 neurons (20 × 20), a rectangular topology and Euclidean distance calculation for the network weights.

3.3. Statistical analysis

In order to evaluate ANNs the data are also analysed using conventional statistics. The methods used are logistic regression (LR) and principal components analysis (PCA). Both LR and PCA are implemented in a Matlab™ environment.

3.3.1. Classification Based on Logistic Regression

Logistic regression is part of a category of statistical models called "generalized linear models" and many of its applications can be found in the medical field. An assessment of clinical findings in HNPCC is given in Wijnen et al. (1998).

The logistic regression is a method for classifying a given input vector $x = (x_1, x_2, \ldots, x_D)$ into one of two classes. It is based on a model that the logarithm of the odds of belonging to one class is a linear function of the feature vector elements used for classification, i.e.

$$ln(p/1-p) = \alpha + \beta_1 x_1 + \beta_2 x_2 + \cdots + \beta_D x_D, \quad (4)$$

where p is the probability of belonging to one class, $p/(1-p)$ is the odds ratio, and α and $\beta_1, \beta_2, \ldots \beta_D$ are regression coefficients that are to be estimated based on the data. The most widely used method to estimate these coefficients is the maximum likelihood.

Due to the above-mentioned characteristics of the LR, HNPCC pedigree data are analysed separately for each of the risk classes (high, intermediate and low), in turn, to predict the probability of belonging to that class; i.e. in each risk class, the other two are combined together.

3.3.2. Classification based on principal component analysis

In order to compare the ANNs (i.e. MLFFNN and SOM) modelling to conventional statistical methods, this time, we employed the principal component analysis (PCA) for feature extraction and k-nearest neighbour (kNN) rule for classification. The PCA is widely used for various data classification problems (Lavine, 2003; Köküer et al., 2003). PCA projects high-dimensional data onto a lower-dimensional space (called the principal component space) by using the projection that best represents the data in a least-squares sense (Duda et al., 2000). The principal components are arranged such that the amount of variance of the data reflected by each principal component is non-increasing. Often, only the first few principal components are necessary to represent the information contained within the data.

The first step in the PCA is, based on the feature vectors of the entire training data set, to compute the PCA transformation matrix. Let us denote the covariance matrix calculated from the entire training feature set by **S**. The PCA decomposes the covariance matrix **S** into $\mathbf{S} = \mathbf{ULU}'$ where **L** is a diagonal $d \times d$ matrix containing the eigen values sorted in a non-increasing order of magnitude, and **U** is a $d \times d$ matrix containing corresponding eigen vectors. The PCA transformation matrix **W** is then formed by the eigen vectors corresponding to the first $\boldsymbol{M}$ highest eigen values. The value of $\boldsymbol{M}$ is usually low and can be decided upon empirically based on the amount of variance reflected by the eigen values.

The PCA then transforms each training feature vector **x** into the space defined by the $\boldsymbol{M}$ principal components, resulting in a new feature vector **y**,

$$\mathbf{y} = \mathbf{W}'(\mathbf{x} - \bar{\mathbf{x}}), \quad (5)$$

where $\bar{\mathbf{x}}$ is the mean vector of the training data. This feature vector **y** determines the location of the pedigree in the principal plane.

In the testing phase, an unknown input feature vector **x** is transformed into the PCA space by using Eq. (5) and then kNN classification rule is used to decide its class.

4. RESULTS AND DISCUSSION

We studied the accuracy with which ANNs (both supervised and unsupervised) can predict the risk class of a family having HNPCC. Then we compared the results with those obtained from traditional statistical approaches (LR and PCA). Evaluations were performed in terms of confusion matrices and then in terms of sensitivity, specificity and accuracy for each risk class that are defined as,

$$\text{Sensitivity} = \frac{\text{TP}}{\text{TP} + \text{FN}}$$

$$\text{Specificity} = \frac{\text{TN}}{\text{TN} + \text{FP}}$$

$$\text{Accuracy} = \frac{\text{TP} + \text{TN}}{\text{TP} + \text{TN} + \text{FP} + \text{FN}},$$

where TP is true positive (i.e. the correct prediction of an actual positive event), TN is true negative and FP and FN are the false positive and negative, respectively. The sensitivity measures the system's ability to correctly identify the presence of a disease whereas specificity indicates how precisely the system finds just the positive events. Note that there are three classes; thus, to define the sensitivity, specificity and accuracy for each class, the other two classes are combined together in turn.

Initially, in order to visualize the clustering of the risk classes formed by the SOM and PCA, the network is trained/modelled considering all 313 family pedigrees and the resultant SOM map and PCA plot are depicted in Fig. 5 (A and B) respectively. Each family is sign-coded based on the true risk class: the circle sign shows high-, plus intermediate-, and diamond low-risk, respectively. Note that the location of each family in

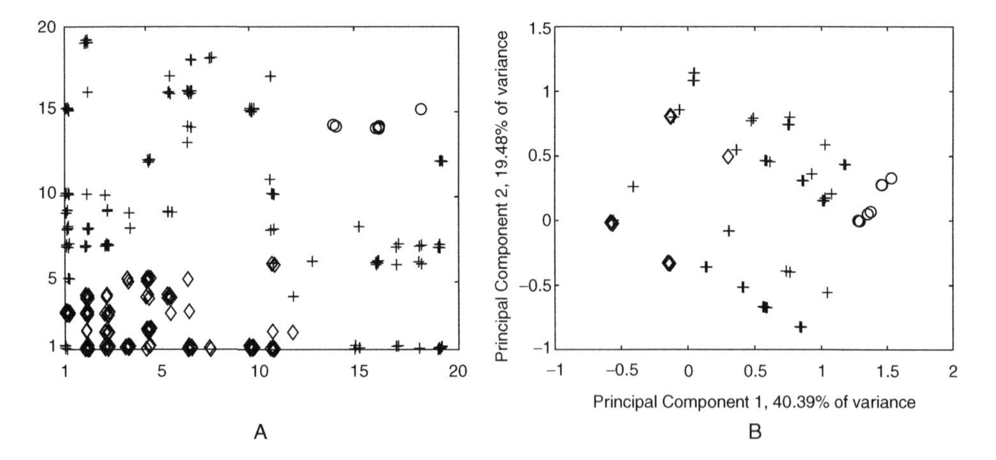

Fig. 5. The location of the families based on the pedigree data (A) by SOM and (B) PCA system. The circle, plus, and diamond signs indicate high-, intermediate- and low-risk cases, respectively.

the SOM has been randomized around the actual SOM neuron in order to provide better visualization. As can be seen from Fig. 5A, the risk classes are well clustered on the map.

It can be seen from Fig. 5B, where the PCA-space defined by the first two principal components, that the data corresponding to high risk class are well separated. In Fig. 6, we see that principal component (PC) 1 accounts for over 40% of the variance, PC 2 over 19%, and cumulatively with principal components 3, 4, 5 and 6 account for over 95%. Therefore, based on the feature set used, we can conclude that six latent variables account for most of the information content in our data set. However, using more than the first two principal components did not improve the classification performance in our experimental evaluation.

The results given hereafter are obtained with the leave-one-out procedure: after training of the system is completed with 312 pedigrees, the left-out pedigree is presented to the trained/modelled system and analysed in a single cycle in order to simulate prospective usage of the developed system in a real-world health care system. This procedure is repeated for each pedigree in the database.

The obtained classification results by using this procedure in the form of confusion matrices are shown in Table 4 (a–c) for MLFFNN, SOM and PCA, respectively, while the classification data for LR in high-, intermediate- and low-risk cases are depicted in Table 5. The sensitivity, specificity and accuracy results are displayed in Fig. 7.

As can be seen from Table 4 (a), all the intermediate and low-risk families are correctly identified by the MLFFNN. However, two out of ten cases in the high-risk families were misclassified. In the case of SOM (Table 4 (b)), two cases in the high risk families were also misclassified. The misclassification in the high-risk cases for both MLFFNN and SOM may be due to the insufficient number of example families in this class to train the network. The PCA-based system performed very well in classifying the high-risk

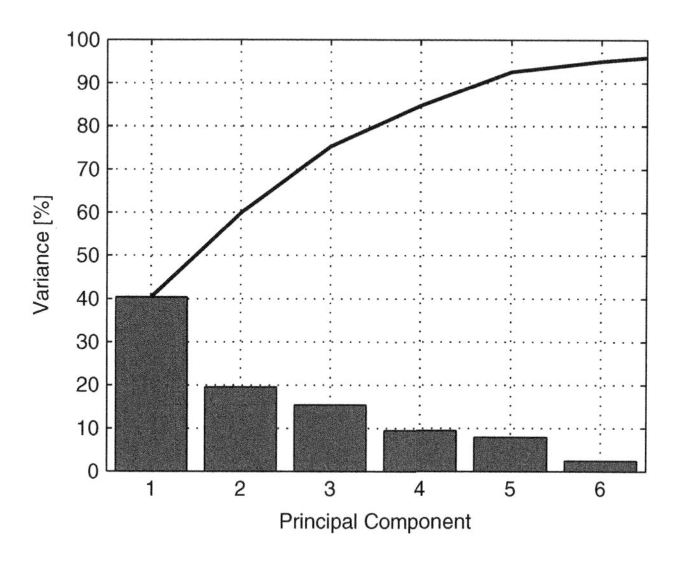

Fig. 6. A plot of the percentage variability of PCA: six latent variables account for most of the information content in the data set.

Table 4. Classification results of HNPCC risk based on the pedigree data obtained by the (a) MLFFNN, (b) SOM and (c) PCA systems

Actual risk	Estimated risk class		
class	High	Intermediate	Low
High	8	2	0
Inter	0	142	0
Low	0	0	161

(a)

Actual risk	Estimated risk class		
Class	High	Intermediate	Low
High	8	2	0
Inter	0	139	3
Low	0	1	160

(b)

Actual risk	Estimted risk class		
class	High	Intermediate	Low
High	10	0	0
Inter	0	137	5
Low	0	2	159

(c)

families (see Table 4 (c)); however, its performances in classifying the intermediate- and low-risk cases were poorer than those of MLFFNN and SOM.

Due to the nature of the LR, HNPCC risk analysis was performed separately for each of the risk classes in turn. In each risk class, the other two are aggregated together. The resultant confusion matrices for high, intermediate-, and low-risk are shown in Table 5 (a–c). For the high-risk case, 7 out of 10 cases were misclassified. In the intermediate- and low-risk classes, 12 out of 142 and 1 out of 161 were misclassified, respectively. It is evident that LR's predictive accuracy in finding the correct risk class is less accurate than any of the other systems illustrated in Table 4 (a–c). These results show that ANN models typically outperform the LR model and are consistent with other ANN research (e.g. (Leon, 1994; Naguib and Sherbet, 2001)).

Further differentiations in terms of the sensitivity, specificity and accuracy are as follows: The sensitivities of classification by MLFFNN and SOM were equal but less than that of the PCA for the high-risk class, and greater for the intermediate- and low-risk classes (see Fig. 7). As can be seen from Fig. 7A the PCA has the highest sensitivity for the high-risk class. High sensitivity in the high-risk class is desirable in order not to leave out any family that is potentially at high-risk from the genetic screening test. The LR's sensitivity was the poorest for the high- and intermediate-risk classes.

The specificities of classification by the MLFFNN, SOM and PCA were equal (100%) for the high-risk classes and the MLFFNN and SOM were greater than those of the LR and PCA for the low-risk case. High specificity will reduce the number of patients who unnecessarily undergo the genetic screening test and consequently reduce the screening costs.

The accuracies of the MLFFNN in the detection of the intermediate- and low-risk cases were greater than those of the SOM, LR and PCA (see Fig. 7B and C); though, for the high-risk class, the PCA gave the highest accuracy (Fig. 7A). However, the accuracy of the PCA for the low-risk class was the lowest amongst the others. In the high- and intermediate-risk classes, the accuracy of the LR was the lowest.

The above results show that LR is not able to operate as an accurate predictor of the HNPCC risk compared to ANNs. The PCA-based system performed very well in classifying the high-risk families, however the overall performance of the MLFFNN in predicting the risk classes (99%) was higher than that of the PCA (97%). We believe that ANNs, with sufficient exemplar families, offer not only better modelling of complex relationships but also better generalization.

The research is still in progress and our pedigree database is being enlarged day-by-day. We anticipate that greater understanding of the complex relationship between the disease and the family history can be gained by having a database with a larger number of pedigrees and extracting features that are more salient to the underlying structure of the pedigree of each family. Future research will concentrate around the selection of those features and incorporate other hereditary and pathological information when they become available.

5. SUMMARY

We have developed a classification system to assess the risk of a family having HNPCC, purely on the basis of pedigree data. This is currently performed by a genetic counsellor who makes the decision based on some pre-defined criteria.

Table 5. Classification results of HNPCC (a) high-risk, (b) intermediate-risk and (c) low-risk obtained by the LR system based on the pedigree data

Actual risk	Estimated risk class	
class	High	Intermediate+low
High	3	7
Intermediate + low	10	293

(a)

Actual risk	Estimated risk class	
class	Intermediate	High+low
Intermediate	130	12
High+low	7	164

(b)

Actual risk	Estimted risk class	
class	Low	High+intermediate
Low	160	1
High+intermediate	5	147

(c)

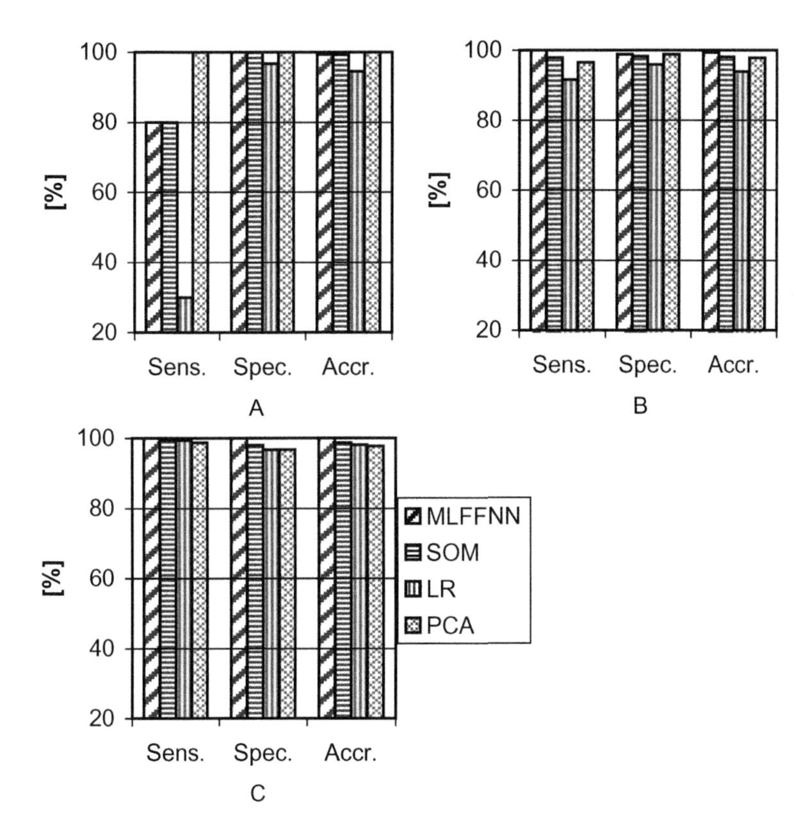

Fig. 7. Results of the comparison between the four different methods: MLFFNN, SOM, LR and PCA. Sensitivity, specificity and accuracy of risk classification are presented for the (A) high-, (B) intermediate- and (C) low-risk cases by MLFFNN, SOM, LR and PCA.

However, the complexity of patient-related data (pedigree) could easily be misinterpreted or overlooked even by the specialist, and may result in a wrong assessment. The proposed automated system can eliminate human errors associated with human fatigue and habits.

The automatic risk assessment system developed was based on ANNs (i.e. MLFFNN and SOM) and was compared with those based on statistical methods (i.e. LR and PCA). All were analysed and comparisons between them were presented.

Overall, the MLFFNN outperformed the SOM, LR and PCA in terms of the number of cases correctly classified. Two out of 313 cases were misclassified by the MLFFNN as opposed to 6, 7 and 20 by SOM, PCA and LR, respectively. However, the sensitivity of the MLFFNN system in the detection of the high-risk cases was less than that of the PCA. Higher sensitivity in the high-risk cases (i.e. to identify every high-risk family or potentially high-risk family) is desirable in order not to leave out any family that is potentially at high-risk from the genetic screening test.

Only in the PCA-based system were all the high-risk families correctly classified; hence it has the highest sensitivity for the high-risk cases. Since sensitivity in these cases measures the system's ability to correctly identify the presence of a disease, the output of the PCA-based system may be construed as performing better (though not reaching statistical significance with a 95% confidence interval). Nevertheless, the 2 out of 10 misclassified cases in MLFFNN and SOM may be due to the insufficient number of exemplars of high-risk families in our dataset to train the network.

Future analysis will have to be based, not only on Amsterdam or rule-based criteria, but will also have to take into consideration genetic mutations and other hereditary and pathological factors when they become available. It is the uncertainty behind the causes of cancer incidence, in general, and HNPCC, in particular, that makes the analysis more prone to modelling through an AI approach rather than a rule-based approach. We believe that having a database with a larger number of pedigrees, extracting features that are more salient to the underlying structure of the pedigree of each family and incorporating other hereditary and pathological information would reveal a better understanding of the relationship between the disease and family history. This is the next task that we shall pursue.

REFERENCES

Aaltonen, L.A., P. Peltomaki, J.P. Mecklin, H. Javinen, J.R. Jass, J.S. Green, H.T. Lynch, P. Watson, G. Tallqvist, M. Juhola, P. Sistonen, K.W. Kinzler, B. Vogelstein and A. de la Chapelle, 1994, Replication errors in benign and malignant tumours from hereditary non-polyposis colorectal cancer patients. Cancer Res., 54, 1645–1648.

Aaltonen, L.A., R. Salovaara, P. Kristo, F. Canzian, A. Hemminki, P. Peltomaki, R. B. Chadwick, H. Kaariainen, M. Eskelinen, H. Jarvinen, J. P. Mecklin and A. de la Chapelle, 1998, An incidence of hereditary non-polyposis colerectal cancer and the feasibility of molecular screening for the disease. N. Engl. J. Med., 338, 1481–1487.

Baxt., W.G., 1995, Application of artificial neural networks to clinical medicine. The Lancet, 346, 1135–1138,

Bishop, C.M., 1995, Neural Networks for Pattern Recognition. Oxford, UK: Oxford University Press.

Burke, H.B., P.H. Goodman, D.B. Rosen, D.E. Henson, J.N. Weinstein, F.E. Harrell, J.R. Marks, D.P. Winchester and D.G. Bostwick, 1997, Artificial neural networks improve the accuracy of cancer survival prediction. Cancer, 79, 857–862.

Campbell, J.G., F. Murtagh and M. Köküer, 2001, DataLab-J: a signal and image processing laboratory for teaching and research. IEEE Trans. Education, 44(4), 329–335.

CancerData, 2000, United Kingdom Cancer Registry Data. Her Majesty's Stationary Office, UK.

CancerStat, 2003, Canadian Cancer Statistics. National Cancer Institute of Canada, Toronto, Canada.

Cotterchio, M., M. Manno, N. Klar, J. McLaughlin and S. Gallinger, 2005, Colorectal screening is associated with reduced colorectal cancer risk: a case-control study within the population-based Ontario familial colorectal cancer registry. CCC, 16, 865–875.

Cyrillic, 1999, Cyrillic 3. Cherwell Scientific, Oxford, UK.

Duda, R.O., P.E. Hart and D.G. Stork, 2000, Pattern Classification, 2nd ed. Hoboken, NJ, USA: John Wiley and Sons Inc.

Elston, R.C and J. Stewart, 1971, A general model for the genetic analysis of pedigree data. Hum. Hered., 21, 523–542.

Guthie, G.S and J.R.T. Monson, 1997, Artificial neural networks applied to outcome prediction for colorectal cancer patients in separate institutions. The Lancet, 350, 469–472.

Hecht-Nielsen, R., 1990, Neurocomputing, Reading, MA, USA: Addison-Wesley.

Jemal, A.A., Thomas, T. Murray and M. Thun, 2002, Cancer statistics. CA Cancer J. Clin., 52, 23–47.

Kohonen, T., 2001, Self Organizing Maps, 3rd ed. Secaucus, NJ, USA: Springer-Verlag.

Köküer, M., F. Murtagh, N.D. McMillan, S. Riedel, B. O'Rourke, K. Beverly, A.T. Augusti and J. Mason, 2003, A wavelet, Fourier and PCA data analysis pipeline: application to distinguishing mixtures of liquids. J. Chem. Inf. Comput. Sci., 43, 587–594.

Lavine, B.K., 2003, Clustering and classification of analytical data. Encyclopaedia of Analytical Chemistry: Instrumentation and Applications, Chichester, West Sussex, UK: John Wiley and Sons Ltd, pp. 9689–9710.

Leon, M.A., 1994, Binary response forecasting: comparison between neural networks and logistic regression analysis. World Congress Neural Networks, 244–247.

Livingstone, D.J., D.T. Manallack and I.V. Tetko, 1997, Data modelling with neural networks: advantages and limitations. J. Comp. Aid. Mol. Design., 11, 135–142.

Mecklin, J.P. 1987, Frequency of hereditary colorectal carcinoma. Gastroenterology, 93, 1021–1025.

Naguib, R.N.G and G.V. Sherbet, 1997, Artificial neural networks in cancer research. Pathobiology, 65, 129–139.

Naguib, R.N.G and G.V. Sherbet. 2001, Artificial neural networks in cancer diagnosis, prognosis, and patient management. Boca Raton, Florida, USA: CRC Press.

Rabeneck, L., J.A. Davila, M. Thompson and H.B. El-Serag, 2005, Surgical volume and long-term survival following surgery for colorectal cancer in the Veterans Affairs Health-Care System. Am. J. Gastroenterol., 100(1), 250.

Riedmiller, M. and H. Braun, 1993, A direct adaptive method for faster backpropagation learning: The RPROP algorithm. Proceedings of the IEEE International Conference on Neural Networks.

Rodriguez, B., C.R. Boland, S.R. Hamilton, D.E. Henson, J.R. Jass, P.M. Khan et al., 1997, A national cancer institute workshop on hereditary nonpolyposis colerectal cancer syndrome: meeting highlights and Bedhesda guidelines. J. Natl. Cancer Inst., 89, 1758–1762.

Statement, 1996, Statement of the American Society of Clinical Oncology: genetic testing for cancer susceptibility, adopted on February 20, 1996. J. Clin. Oncol., 14, 1730–1736.

Vasen, H.F.A., J.P. Mecklin, P.M. Khan and H.T. Lynch, 1991, The International Collaborative Group on Hereditary Non-Polyposis Colerectal Cancer (ICGHNPCCC). Dis. Colon. Rectum., 34, 424–425.

Wijnen, J.T., H.F.A. Vasen, P.M. Khan, A.H. Zwinderman, H.V.D. Klift, A. Mulder, C. Tops, P. Moller and R. Fodde, 1998, Clinical findings with implications for genetic testing in families with clustering of colerectal cancer. N. Engl. J. Med. 339(8), 511–518.

Chapter 13

The Impact of Microarray Technology in Brain Cancer

M. Kounelakis[1], M. Zervakis[1] and X. Kotsiakis[2]

[1]*Department of Electronic and Computer Engineering, Technical University of Crete, Chania 73100, Greece*
Email: mkoune@danai.systems.tuc.gr
Email: michalis@danai.systems.tuc.gr
[2]*Department of Neurosurgery, General Hospital of Chania, Chania, Crete, Greece*
Email: xenofon7@otenet.gr

Abstract

The analysis of global gene expression patterns (expression profiling) produced from the microarray technology (cDNAs and tissue microarrays), has made important contributions to our understanding of the regulation of biological systems and gene function. Recently, it is becoming increasingly significant for the diagnosis, prognosis and treatment of brain cancer.

Conventional methods used for brain tumour diagnosis utilize modalities (CT, MRI, PET, EEG, Biopsy and Lumbar Puncture) that provide medical information. The genomic analysis used to supplement such medical information is expected to provide appropriate tools for early diagnosis and effective therapy of cancer. Microarray-based clustering and classification methods have been used to reclassify the brain tumours already known by the World Health Organization (WHO) and/or discover new sub-types. Unsupervised and supervised classification methods that have been tested on different brain tumour types using gene expression data as input, have shown promising efficiency. This fact offers great potential to the clinicians that are now able to develop new methods of treatment based on gene therapy instead of applying the traditional ones (surgery, radiation, chemotherapy etc.).

This chapter attempts to reveal the important role of genomics in brain cancer. Several genomic-based methods for brain cancer analysis are reviewed and compared to traditional ones with an emphasis to DNA microarray technology that was recently introduced. Finally, feature genomic-based developments that will assist the diagnosis, prognosis and treatment of brain cancer are presented.

Acknowledgement

This work was supported in part by the EC IST project BIOPATTERN, Contract No: 508803.

Contents

© 2007 Elsevier B.V. All rights reserved

1. INTRODUCTION

DNA microarray technology offers today the opportunity to analyse brain cancer in depth through the examination of its gene expression profile. Recent studies have shown that this technology facilitates the discovery of hidden information related to brain cancer genesis and also leads to a new era in genomic-based medicine.

Brain tumours (DeAngelis, 2001; Levin et al., 2001) can be classified into two groups primary and secondary or metastatic. Tumours that begin in brain tissue (Fig. 1) are known as primary brain tumours. Primary brain tumours are classified by the type of tissue in which they begin. The most common brain tumours are gliomas, which begin in the glial (supportive) tissue. There are several types of gliomas:

- *Astrocytomas* arise from small, star-shaped cells called astrocytes. They may grow anywhere in the brain or spinal cord. In adults, astrocytomas most often arise in the cerebrum. In children, they occur in the brain stem, the cerebrum, and the cerebellum.

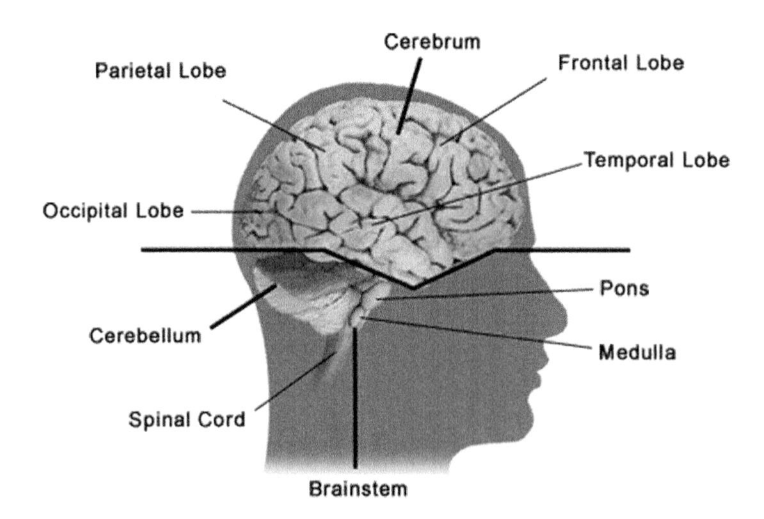

Fig. 1. Human brain parts.

A grade III astrocytoma is sometimes called anaplastic astrocytoma. A grade IV astrocytoma is usually called glioblastoma multiforme.

- *Brain stem gliomas* occur in the lowest, stem-like part of the brain. The brain stem controls many vital functions. Tumours in this area generally cannot be removed. Most brain stem gliomas are high-grade astrocytomas.
- *Ependymomas* usually develop in the lining of the ventricles. They may also occur in the spinal cord. Although these tumours can develop at any age, they are most common in childhood and adolescence.
- *Oligodendrogliomas* arise in the cells that produce myelin, the fatty covering that protects nerves. These tumours usually arise in the cerebrum. They grow slowly and usually do not spread into surrounding brain tissue. Oligodendrogliomas are rare. They occur most often in middle-aged adults but have also been found in people of all ages.

There exist other types of brain tumours that do not begin in the glial tissue. Some of the most common ones are described below:

- *Medulloblastomas* were once thought to develop from glial cells. However, recent research suggests that these tumours develop from primitive (developing) nerve cells that normally do not remain in the body after birth. For this reason, medulloblastomas are sometimes called primitive neuroectodermal tumours (PNET). Most medulloblastomas arise in the cerebellum; however, they may occur in other areas as well. These tumours occur most often in children and are more common in boys than in girls.
- *Meningiomas* grow from the meninges. They are usually benign. Because these tumours grow very slowly, the brain may be able to adjust to their presence; meningiomas often grow quite large before they cause symptoms. They occur most often in women between 30 and 50 years of age.
- *Schwannomas* are benign tumours that begin in Schwann cells, which produce the myelin that protects the acoustic nerve – the hearing nerve. Acoustic neuromas are a type of schwannoma. They occur mainly in adults. These tumours affect women twice as often as men.
- *Craniopharyngiomas* develop in the region of the pituitary gland near the hypothalamus. They are usually benign; however, they are sometimes considered malignant because they can press on or damage the hypothalamus and affect vital functions. These tumours occur most often in children and adolescents.
- *Germ cell tumours* arise from primitive (developing) sex cells, or germ cells. The most frequent type of germ cell tumour in the brain is the germinoma.
- *Pineal region tumours* occur in or around the pineal gland, a tiny organ near the centre of the brain. The tumour can be growing slowly (pineocytoma) or rapidly (pineoblastoma). The pineal region is very difficult to reach, and these tumours often cannot be removed.

Secondary brain tumours are tumours caused by cancer that originates in another part of the body. Cancer that spreads to the brain is the same disease and has the same name as the original (primary) cancer. Brain metastases outnumber primary neoplasm by at least 10 to 1, and they occur in 20–40% of cancer patients. The most common primary cancers metastasizing to the brain are lung cancer (50%), breast cancer (15–20%), unknown primary cancer (10–15%), melanoma (10%), and colon cancer (5%). Eighty percent of brain metastases occur in the cerebral hemispheres, 15% occur in the cerebellum, and 5% occur in the brain stem. Metastases to the brain are multiple in more than 70% of cases, but solitary metastases also occur. Brain involvement can occur with cancers of the nasopharyngeal region by direct extension along the cranial nerves or through the foramina at the base of the skull. Dural metastases may constitute up to 9% of total CNS metastases.

The diagnosis of brain metastases in cancer patients is based on patient history, neurological examination, and diagnostic procedures. Computed tomography scans with contrast or MRIs with gadolinium are quite sensitive in diagnosing the presence of metastases. Positron emission tomography scanning and spectroscopic evaluation are new strategies for diagnosing cerebral metastases and for differentiating the metastases from other intracranial lesions.

Brain cancer can be regarded as a genetic disease (Bodey et al., 2004) occurring as a result of the progressive accumulation of genetic aberrations. The aetiology of brain cancer is a complex interplay of numerous acquired genetic abnormalities, including amplifications of oncogenes, deletion of tumour suppressor genes, gene rearrangements, and loss or gain of functional mutations. Although a number of oncogenes and tumour suppressor genes have already been discovered using traditional techniques of molecular biology, recent insight into the *genetic expression profile* of cancer suggests that hundreds to thousands of important cancer-related genes remain yet to be discovered.

Numerous approaches have been used in recent years to identify cancer-specific and cancer-associated genes. These techniques include various microarray-based approaches that allow for global, systematic, and high throughput comparisons of the gene expression differences between normal and cancerous tissues. In the field of cancer research, the most commonly used microarray techniques for the molecular profiling of human tumours have been *cDNA* and *oligonucleotide microarrays*. Most of the unsupervised and supervised classification methods using gene expression profiles have been applied to primary brain tumour types.

It is widely believed that thousands of genes and their products (i.e. RNA and proteins) reside in a given living organism and function in a complicated and orchestrated way that creates the mystery of life. However, traditional methods in molecular biology generally work on a "one gene in one experiment" basis, which means that the output is very limited and the "whole picture" of gene function is hard to obtain.

In the past several years, a new technology called DNA microarray (Yang and Speed, 2002) (Fig. 2 (A and B)) has attracted tremendous interest among biologists. This technology promises to monitor the whole genome on a single chip so that researchers can have a better picture of the interactions among thousands of genes simultaneously.

Terminologies that have been used in the literature to describe this technology are included, but not limited to: biochip, DNA chip, DNA microarray, gene array, gene chip and genome chip. Microarray provides a medium for matching known and unknown DNA samples based on base-pairing rules (A–T and G–C) and automating the process of identifying the unknowns. An array experiment can make use of common assay systems, such as microplates or standard blotting membranes, and can be created by hand or make use of robotics to deposit the sample. In general, arrays are described as *macroarrays* or *microarrays*, the difference being the size of the sample spots. Macroarrays contain sample spot sizes of about 300 μm or larger and can be easily imaged by existing gel and blot scanners. The sample spot sizes in microarray are typically less than 200 μm in diameter and these arrays usually contain thousands of spots.

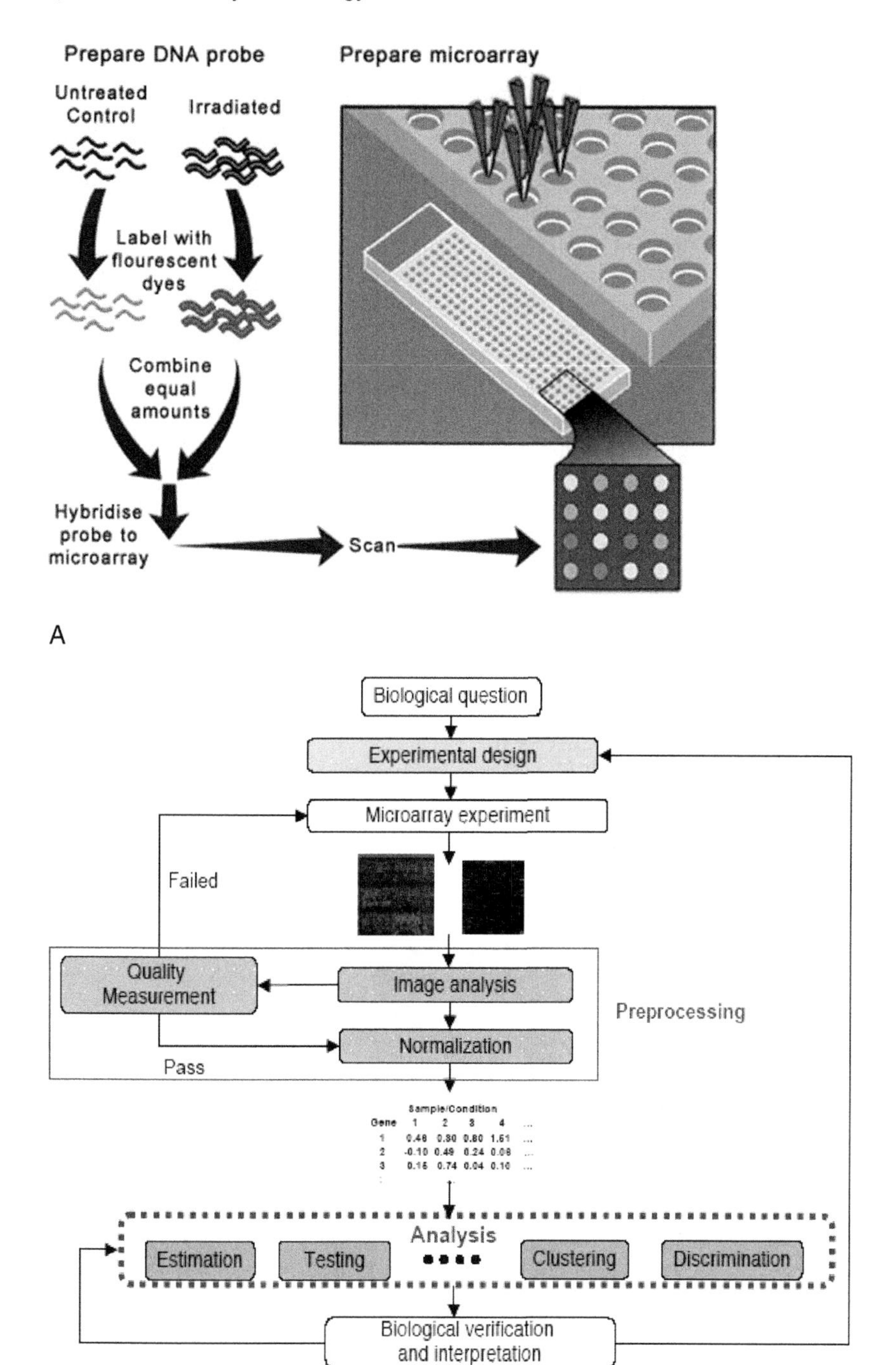

Fig. 2. Microarray experimental procedure.

Microarrays require specialized robotics and imaging equipment that generally are not commercially available as a complete system. DNA microarrays or DNA chips are fabricated by high-speed robotics, generally on glass but sometimes on nylon substrates, for which probes with known identity are used to determine complementary binding, thus allowing massively parallel *gene expression* and gene discovery studies. An experiment with a single DNA chip can provide researchers information on thousands of genes simultaneously – a dramatic increase in output.

The main reasons for using microarray technology to analyse the expression profiles of brain tumours can be summarized below:

- Identify differentially expressed genes in two or more situations/samples;
- Discover groups of genes that are co-regulated (clustering);
- Identify which genes form "interesting" groups and examine their function;
- Discriminate between two or more groups/types/situations and predict the class of a new sample (classification); and
- Examine how the genes and/or their groups function.

Due to the mass information delivered in microarrays, the target question and the experimental procedure must be carefully designed. A rigorous setup of such a microarray

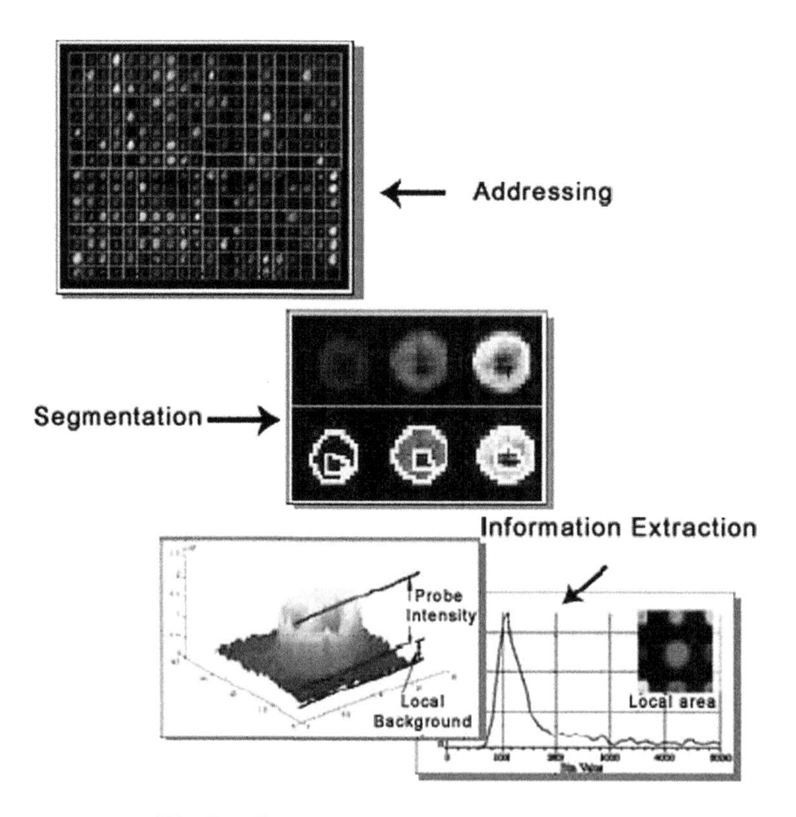

Fig. 3. Microarray image analysis procedure.

experiment is presented in Fig. 3. It is expected, however, that if science can provide answers to the issues above, genomic analysis will significantly aid the diagnosis, prognosis and treatment of cancer.

Preprocessing microarray (Chuaqui et al., 2002; Carter et al., 2005) data is a crucial task for preserving the maximum possible quality of relevant data to be analysed. Acquiring reliable data leads to a more accurate and robust approach for subsequent cluster/classification procedures. Preprocessing microarray data includes several sub-tasks that must be accomplished in order to proceed with analysis. These tasks include image analysis and normalization feature selection. They are explained in more detail later in Section 2.

Image analysis is based on the fact that the resulting images from the microarray experiment have to be processed to eliminate those factors that influence the quality of each spot-gene (noise, background intensity, etc) on the slide. For this reason, a sequential procedure takes place that is described through three phases: *addressing, segmentation* and *information extraction*.

Normalization (Quackenbush, 2002; Bolstad et al., 2003) manages to minimize, or even eliminate, systematic variations due to experimental features of microarray experiments that are present in most large microarray datasets. Many different experimental features can cause biases including different sources of RNA, different production lots of microarrays or different microarray platforms. These systematic biases are manifested as differences in gene expression patterns when one set of microarrays is directly compared with a second set of microarrays. When using "supervised" statistical analyses, systematic biases demonstrate themselves as a subset of genes that tend to be more highly expressed in one set of microarrays versus another and a concomitant subset of genes that are lower in expression in one set versus the other. These biases can typically be identified because they perfectly correlate with non-biological properties like where the samples were isolated and processed (source bias), or what print batch of microarrays the samples were tested on (batch effect bias). As can be expected, these systematic biases compromise the integrity of the data, and are especially troublesome in experiments in which many samples are assayed over a long time period, as these studies typically get assayed on many different print batches of microarrays.

Gene selection (Troyanskaya et al., 2002; Wang et al., 2005) methods are very important in microarray data analysis too. It is well understood that a massive number of gene expression values is produced from a microarray experiment. In order to proceed with the main analysis of these data, useless gene expression values must be filtered out in order to reduce the computational time and the complexity of the overall dataset. Filter and wrapper methods have been introduced to facilitate this feature (gene) reduction procedure.

Following the preprocessing stage, unsupervised and supervised learning usually takes place in order to identify different classes of genes that facilitate several other observations, such as classifying new data, understanding the behavior of genes of same and/or different class etc. In unsupervised learning (cluster analysis), the classes are unknown a priori and the goal is to discover these classes from the data whereas in supervised learning (classification analysis), the classes are predefined and the goal is to understand the basis for the classification from a set of labeled objects (learning) and build a predictor (classifier) for future unlabeled observations.

The main disadvantage of supervised methods is that they are limited to *hypothesis testing*. If one has some prior knowledge, which can lead to a hypothesis, supervised methods will help to accept or reject it. They will *not reveal* the unexpected and *never lead* to new hypotheses, or to new partitions of the data. For example, if the tumours break into two unanticipated classes on the basis of their expression profiles, a supervised method will not be able to discover this. Another shortcoming is the possibility of misclassification of some samples. A supervised method will not discover, in general, samples that were incorrectly labeled and used in, say, the training set. The alternative is to use unsupervised methods of analysis. These aim at exploratory analysis of the data, introducing as little external knowledge or bias as possible, and "*let the data speak*." Therefore the examination of the structure of the data on the basis of correlations and similarities is what really matters. A more detailed presentation of the clustering and classification algorithms used for the analysis of the brain tumour gene expression data follows in Sections 3 and 4.

2. PREPROCESSING MICROARRAY DATA

A very important issue when examining microarray data is the preprocessing procedure. The experimental outcome must be carefully assessed in order to proceed to clustering and classification and obtain correct results. Detailed microarray image analysis and normalization is essential to confirm the quality of the measurements.

The first issue to consider is the quality of the data. RNA samples, cell viability, array quality, etc. must all be checked before carrying out the experiment. Erroneous data can always be identified if a sufficient number of repeat experiments are performed. The same logic can be extended to "post-experimental" factors, such as image analysis and normalization methods. Certain techniques could therefore yield better results than others, depending on array type, dye types, etc.

Other hands-on methods, although more laborious, could serve to *verify* whether the observed expression levels on the array have really occurred. Such methods include:

- PCR (Polymerase Chain Reaction),
- Reverse Transcription (RT) PCR (Polymerase Chain Reaction),
- Northern Blot and Western Blot analyses,
- SAGE (Serial Analysis of Gene Expression),
- Dot Blot analysis,
- RNase Protection Assay, and
- FISH.

However, repeating this for all genes is not only extremely intensive but it also defeats the purpose of a high-throughput system! It would therefore be more appropriate to restrict these techniques to the small number of genes that are of interest or whose expression levels are in question.

2.1. Image analysis of microarray data

The processing of scanned images usually involves three tasks.

(1) *Addressing* or *gridding* which is the process of assigning coordinates to each of the spots,

(2) *Segmentation*, which allows the classification of the pixels either as foreground or as background. Methods for segmentation contain:

- fixed circle segmentation;
- adaptive circle segmentation;
- adaptive shape segmentation; and
- histogram segmentation.

(3) *Information* (or *intensity*) *extraction*, which implies calculating, for each spot on the array, red and green foreground fluorescence intensities, background intensities and, in some cases, quality measures like:

- variability measures in pixel values within each spot mask;
- spot size;
- circularity measures; and
- relative signal to background intensity.

Background adjustment is necessary because measured intensities include a contribution due to the non-specific hybridization of the target to other elements in the slides (chemicals, etc). The most commonly used procedure to remove this background effect is subtracting the fluorescence intensity measured around the spots.

Nevertheless, the use of mean or median around the spot tends to produce noisy measures. Some software packages use morphological opening, which is a way of calculating an average of the background along windows that can be subtracted from the signal. This method performs better than the subtraction of a constant average, which can cause negative intensity values.

2.2. Normalization of microarray data

In practice, every repeat experiment will give rise to a certain amount of variation. These changes are termed *systematic* and *random variations* and together make up the experimental error inherent in the procedure. A statistical method must be applied to minimize these variations, which in turn allows comparison of the expression levels between multiple microarray experiments. Normalization procedures rely on the fact that gene expression data can follow a normal distribution and therefore the entire distribution can be transformed about the population mean and median without affecting the standard deviation (i.e. the variation of the data).

2.2.1. cDNA microarray normalization

For spotted arrays, the array itself is already hybridized with two types of mRNA or cDNA, each of which has been labeled with a different fluorescent dye. Most often these are Cy3 (Red = R) and Cy5 (Green = G). In order to show the equations involved in normalization techniques, the letters R and G are used instead of Cy3 and Cy5.

The main purpose of making comparisons is to calculate the expression ratio of the genes that participate in a microarray experiment. If G is the reference and R the experimental sample then:

$$T_i = \frac{R_i}{G_i} \text{ or log ratio} = \log_2 \frac{R_i}{G_i}, \tag{1}$$

where T_i is the normalization ratio of gene i of the array. Two types of normalization are applied to spotted arrays; *across-slide* and *within-slide* normalization.

2.2.2. Across-slide normalization

There are several types of normalization that may be used in this case:

- mean or median normalization;
- scaling normalization; and
- rank distribution normalization.

In *mean* or *median normalization* all data (genes) is adjusted to have the same mean or median value. This is usually achieved by multiplying all data with a *normalization factor*, which is given by:

$$N_{\text{total}} = \frac{\sum_{i=1}^{N_{\text{array}}} R_i}{\sum_{i=1}^{N_{\text{array}}} G_i}, \tag{2}$$

where N_{total} is the normalization factor, R and G the two channels, i is each gene of the array and N_{array} is the total number of genes on the array.

In *scaling normalization*, the process is more or less the same as the simple mean/median normalization procedures, except the *distributions* about the median for each array are made to be equivalent.

$$T'_i = \frac{(T_i - \text{median}_a)}{\text{mad}_a}, \quad \text{where mad}_a = \text{median}_a \left| T_i - \text{median}_a \right| \tag{3}$$

is the *median absolute deviation* of the array.

In *rank normalization*, the distribution of every array becomes identical. Each gene in every array is sorted such that the individual intensities (for 1-channel) or ratios (for 2-channel) are arranged in descending order. The highest rank (No. 1) will therefore be assigned to the gene with the highest numerical value.

2.2.3. *Within-slide normalization*

The point to within-slide normalization is to make the resulting ratio (denoted T_i') for each gene (i) independent of spot intensity and location on the array. The same techniques considered thus far can be applied to a single array too. However, there are more methods worth mentioning at this point; one in particular is Lowess (Loess) normalization (Fig. 4).

A Loess curve is first drawn on the RI (ratio–intensity) plot. The curve is calculated by a regression process. The regression process essentially calculates the *dependence of the ratio on the intensity* and puts it in a mathematical context. It is possible then to calculate this dependence for *each* gene (i) by observing its distance from the curve.

2.2.4. *Oligonucleotide microarray normalization*

There are two normalization procedures, which operate on the average difference values and therefore allow one to compare two or more arrays; global normalization and global scaling.

In the global normalization, the average intensity (i.e. the mean of all the average difference values excluding the lowest and highest 2%) of an experimental array is transformed to be numerically equivalent to the average intensity of the baseline (reference) array. This is achieved with the use of a normalization factor (Eq. (4)).

In the global scaling procedure, the average intensities of all arrays that are going to be compared are multiplied by normalization factors (NFs) so that all average intensities are made to be numerically equivalent to a preset amount (termed target intensity). In the research literature, the target intensity is most often 200 (Eq. (5)).

$$\mathrm{NF} = \frac{a_{\text{baseline}}}{a_{\text{experimental}}} \tag{4}$$

$$\mathrm{NF} = \frac{200}{\text{array}_x} \tag{5}$$

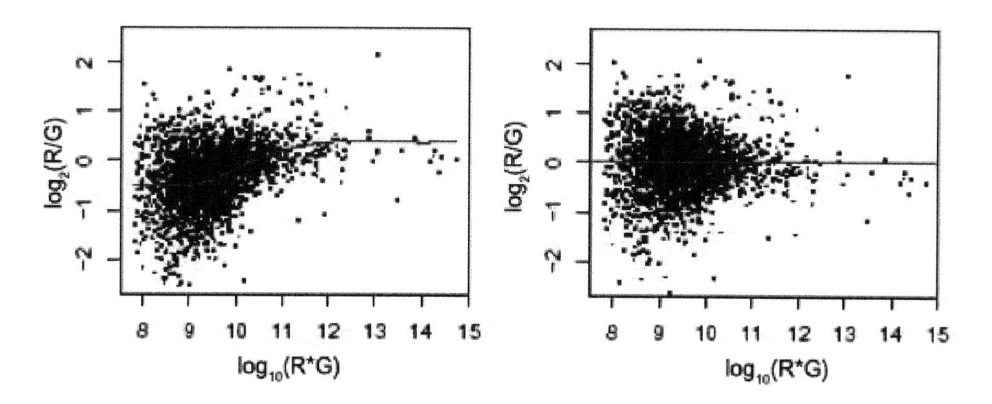

Fig. 4. Loess normalization procedure (log ratio).

2.3. Gene selection techniques

Preprocessing microarray data is a key issue before proceeding with data mining techniques (clustering and classification). Due to the fact that a set of microarray experiments, generating gene expression profiles, frequently contains a considerable number of genes that do not really contribute to the biological process that is being studied, *gene selection techniques* are necessary to overcome the problems of getting genes that have seemingly random and meaningless profiles or profiles containing many missing values.

Gene selection therefore is essential for robust data mining analysis. Another main benefit is also the dimensionality reduction that is obtained after the application of these techniques, which in turn assists the clustering-classification algorithms to produce more accurate results. Two general approaches are used for gene selection: filter methods and wrapper methods.

In filter methods, features are scored individually (e.g. using statistical methods). These are applied before clustering-classification. In wrapper methods, a classification algorithm uses an internal process to eliminate redundant features. The essential difference between these approaches is that a wrapper method makes use of the algorithm that will be used to build the final classifier, while a filter method does not. Thus, given a classifier C and given a set of features F, a wrapper method searches in the space of subsets of F, and compares the performance of the trained classifier C on each tested subset. A filter method on the other hand, does not make use of C, but rather attempts to find predictive subsets of the features by making use of simple statistics computed from the empirical distribution.

The most known filter methods are:

2.3.1. PCA (Principal Component Analysis) and ICA (Independent Component Analysis)

PCA finds the directions of maximal variation in the microarray data and uses the direction of the largest variation as factor one, the direction of the second largest variation as factor two, and so on. In addition, PCA assumes that all factors are orthogonal. In contrast, ICA computes the components by assuming that the "causes" that shape the data are statistically independent. ICA finds the coordinate system that makes the information given by each IC component maximally statistically independent of the information given by the other components.

2.3.2. Fisher discriminant criterion

In this method, high dimensional data (genes) is projected onto a line and discrimination is obtained in one-dimensional space. The projection maximizes the distance between the means of the two classes while minimizing the variance within each class.

2.3.3. PPR (Projection Pursuit Regression)

Projection pursuit is a procedure for searching high-dimensional data for interesting low-dimensional projections via the optimization of a criterion function called the projection pursuit index.

2.3.4. TNoM (Threshold Number of Misclassification)

Threshold number of misclassification, or TNoM score, is a simple threshold-based method that uses a given expression level, for a given gene, to predict the cluster label of a given test sample.

2.3.5. EM (Expectation Maximization)

The EM method is a parameter estimation method which falls into the general framework of maximum-likelihood estimation, and is applied in cases, like microarrays, where part of the data can be considered incomplete or "hidden".

2.3.6. SVMs (Support Vector Machines) and NNets (Neural Networks)

SVM and NNets are relatively new supervised learning algorithms commonly applied in microarray analysis. They have been previously used successfully in a number of applications. A more detailed analysis of these two algorithms is presented in the fourth sub-section.

2.3.7. RFE (Recursive Feature Elimination)

This is the most important wrapper method applied in microarray data for gene selection. This method works with Support Vector Machines (SVMs). The method recursively removes features (genes) based upon the absolute magnitude of the hyperplane elements. Given microarray data with n genes per sample, the SVM outputs the normal to the hyperplane, **w**, which is a vector with n components, each corresponding to the expression of a particular gene.

2.3.8. UAF (Univariate Association Filtering)

In this method, an ordering of all predictors according to their strength (i.e. its association with the target) is performed. Then a selection of the first K predictors is made and feeds them to the classifier of choice. Various measures of association may be used here, like correlation measures.

Several other wrapper methods also used for gene selection are the: ARD (Automatic Relevance Determination) and the Backward/Forward Wrapping providing reliable results.

3. CLUSTERING OF MICROARRAY DATA OF BRAIN CANCER

Reliable and precise clustering (Moreau et al., 2002; Shannon et al., 2003) of brain tumours is essential for successful diagnosis and treatment of brain cancer and the discovery of new subtypes. Current methods for unsupervised classification of brain tumour malignancies rely on a variety of morphological, clinical, and molecular variables. In spite of recent progress, there are still uncertainties in diagnosis.

3.1. Clustering microarray data (unsupervised learning)

Microarrays may be used to characterize the molecular variations among brain tumours by monitoring gene expression profiles on a genomic scale. This may lead to a more reliable characterization and classification of tumours.

Before presenting the clustering techniques applied today on microarray data of brain tumours, it is necessary to give some theoretical and mathematical background of gene expression data produced by a microarray.

The *gene expression data* (also called gene expression profile, or gene expression signature or level) is mathematically represented by the following table (Fig. 5), where the gene expression profiles of each one of the G genes are positioned in rows and the samples (tumour types) or observations n (different experiments) are positioned in columns. Therefore X_{gi} is the gene expression level of gene g $(g=1\ldots G)$ in sample or observation i $(i=1\ldots n)$. $X_i = (X_{i1}, X_{i2}, \ldots, X_{iG})$ is the gene expression profile and the (feature) vector for sample i, while Y_i is the tumour class or response for sample i.

The main task in clustering is to identify similar genes on the basis of their gene expression levels and group them together (row clustering). Even more, clustering could be applied to identify similar samples (column clustering) (Fig. 6).

3.1.1. *Common clustering techniques*

Several clustering algorithms have been recently applied to microarray data. The most important ones are described below.

Hierarchical Clustering. This is the most common clustering approach for gene expression data and can be considered as the *de facto* standard (Fig. 7). It exists in two modes; one-way and two-way clustering. Hierarchical clustering (Eisen et al., 1998) has the advantage that the results can be properly visualized. Two approaches have been considered extensively:

- a top-down approach (divisive clustering) and
- a bottom-up approach (agglomerative clustering)

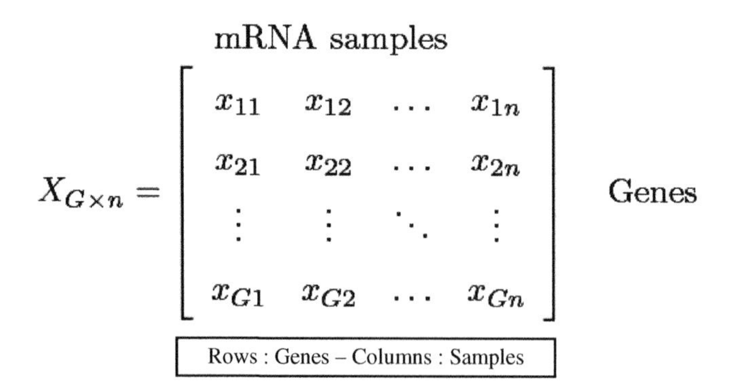

Fig. 5. Gene expression matrix.

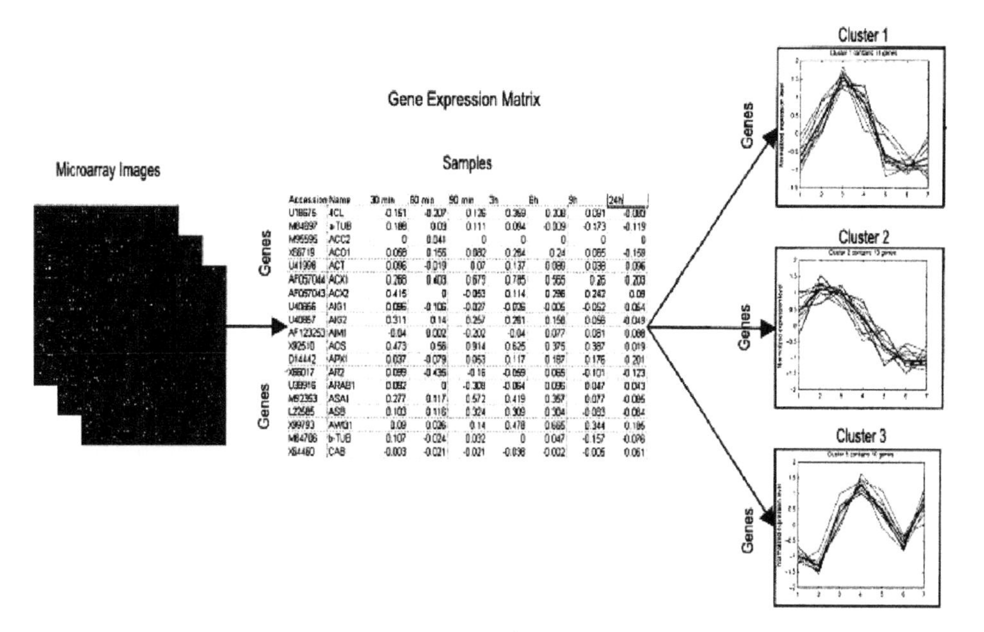

Fig. 6. Clustering microarray data procedure.

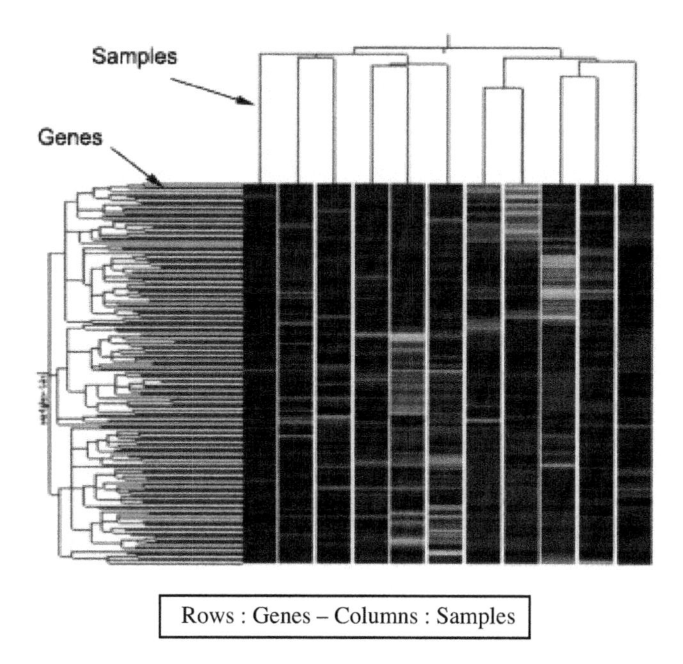

Fig. 7. Hierarchical clustering output image.

The latter is the most commonly used. The algorithm of hierarchical clustering proceeds as follows:

Algorithm:

- Assign all the gene expression profiles to initial clusters.
- The distance between every couple of clusters is calculated according to a certain distance measure (this results in a pairwise distance matrix).
- Iteratively (and starting from all singletons as clusters), the two closest clusters are merged, and the distance matrix is updated to take this cluster merging into account.
- This process gives rise to a tree structure where the height of the branches is proportional to the pairwise distance between the clusters. Merging stops if only one cluster is left.
- Finally, clusters are formed by cutting the tree at a certain level or height.

A major drawback is that the memory complexity is quadratic in the number of gene expression profiles, which can be a problem when considering large datasets.

***K*-means Clustering.** *K*-means clustering (Herwig et al., 1999) results in a partitioning of the data (every gene expression profile belongs to exactly one cluster) using a predefined number of partitions or clusters (Fig. 8). This is a top-down approach and is used for both one-way and two-way clustering. The algorithm is described below:

Algorithm:

- Divide up all the gene expression profiles among initial clusters.
- Iteratively, the centre (which is nothing more than the average expression vector) of each cluster is calculated, followed by a reassignment of the gene expression vectors to the cluster with the closest cluster centre.
- Convergence is reached when the cluster centres remain stationary.

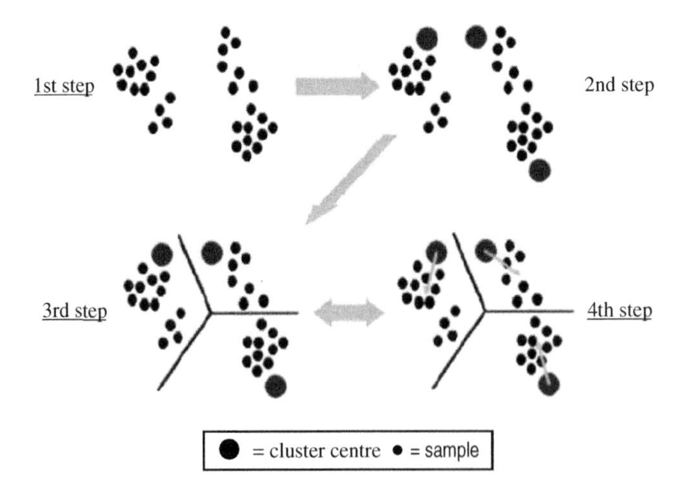

Fig. 8. *K*-means clustering.

A main disadvantage of this algorithm is that the user predefines the number of clusters (K), which might not be equal to the true clusters.

Self-Organizing Maps (SOMs). In SOMs (Tamayo et al., 1999), the user has to predefine a topology or geometry of nodes (e.g. a two-dimensional grid, one node for each cluster), which again is not straightforward. The algorithm of SOM is presented below:

Algorithm:

- The nodes are mapped onto the gene expression space (X_1, X_2) initially at random and iteratively adjusted.
- In each iteration a gene expression profile is randomly picked, and the node that maps closest to it is selected.
- This selected node (in gene expression space) is then moved (Fig. 9) into the direction of the selected expression profile. The other nodes are also moved into the direction of the selected expression profile but to an extent proportional to the distance from the selected node in the initial two-dimensional node topology.

The algorithm works well with large datasets and appropriates neural network implementation.

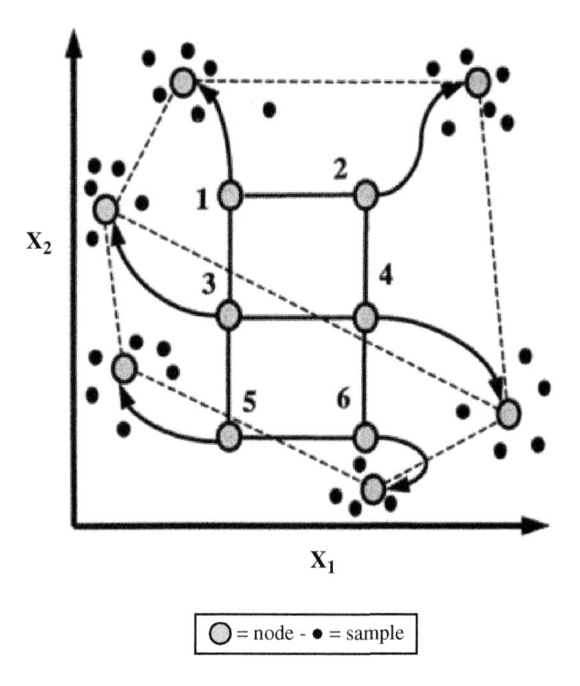

Fig. 9. Self-organizing maps.

Singular Value Decomposition (or Principal Component Analysis). Considering K tumour samples (or observations) as points in an n-dimensional space (i.e. the space of n genes), the aim is to reduce the dimension of the space while retaining as much of the variation of the data as possible. Principal component analysis (Alter et al., 2000) identifies the direction in this space with maximal variance (of the observations projected onto it). This gives the first principal component (PC). The $(i + 1\text{st})$ PC is the direction with maximal variance among those orthogonal to the first i PCs. The data projected onto the first PC may then be visualized in scatter plots.

A PCA analysis (Fig. 10) of DNA microarray data considers the genes, or the test cases as variables, or both. When genes are variables, the analysis creates a set of "*principal gene components*" that indicate the features of genes that best explain the experimental responses they produce. When experiments are the variables, the analysis creates a set of "*principal experiment components*" that indicate the features of the experimental conditions that best explain the gene behaviors they elicit. When both experiments and genes are analysed together, there is a combination of these affects, the utility of which remains to be explored.

The approach is efficient for comparisons of the expression of different genes across different samples.

Block Clustering. Block Clustering (Tibshirani et al., 2001) is a two-way clustering technique. It simultaneously clusters both genes and samples.

Algorithm:

- Begin with the entire matrix in one block.
- At each stage find the best row and column split.
- Split continued until a large number of blocks are obtained.
- Some blocks are recombined until the optimal number of blocks is obtained.

Gene Shaving Clustering. The goal of this Gene Shaving Clustering (Hastie et al., 2000) is to find several small, possibly overlapping blocks of genes, with small variance within blocks.

Algorithm:

- Start with the whole gene expression matrix **Y**.
- Find the first principal component of the genes.
- For each gene, compute the absolute value of its correlation with the first principal component.
- Remove the 10% of the genes having the smallest absolute correlation (and return to second step).

The algorithm produces a set of nested gene groups (cluster). Gene Shaving is a subset clustering approach.

Although it is possible to obtain biologically meaningful results with these algorithms, some of their characteristics often complicate their use for clustering expression data. They require, for example, the predefinition of one or more user-defined parameters that are hard to estimate by a biologist (e.g. the predefinition of the number of clusters in K-means and SOM, which is almost impossible to predict in advance). Moreover, changing parameter settings often has a strong impact on the final result. These methods therefore need extensive parameter fine-tuning, which means that a comparison of the results with different parameter settings is almost always necessary, with the additional difficulty that comparing the quality of the different clustering results is hard.

Another problem is that first-generation clustering algorithms often force every data point into a cluster. In general, a considerable number of genes included in the microarray experiment do not contribute to the biological process studied, and these genes will therefore lack co-expression with other genes (they will have seemingly constant or even random expression profiles). Including these genes in one of the clusters will "contaminate" their content (these genes represent noise) and make these clusters less suitable for further analysis.

Finally, the computational and memory complexity of some of these algorithms often limit the number of expression profiles that can be analysed at once. Considering the nature of our datasets (number of expression profiles often running up into the tens of thousands), this constraint is often restrictive.

Other clustering algorithms have also been developed that present satisfactory efficiency like CAST (Cluster Affinity Search Technique) and CLICK (Cluster Identification via Connectivity Kernels), SOTA (Self-Organizing Tree Algorithm). Furthermore, clustering of gene expression data of brain cancer often employs combination of several algorithms, although it is true that *today's clustering algorithms* are based more on Block Clustering and Gene Shaving techniques.

3.2. Cluster validity measures

It is evident that clustering approaches of gene expression data may produce different results, due to the fact that the choice of preprocessing, algorithm, and distance/correlation measures differs in each method. This raises the question of validating the relevance of the cluster results; in other words, the efficiency of each clustering method.

Validation (Dunn, 1974; Hubert and Schultz, 1976; Davies and Bouldin, 1979; Rousseeuw, 1987; Viks, et al., 2003) of an algorithm and its results can be either *statistical* or *biological*. Statistical cluster validation can be done by assessing cluster coherence, examining the predictive power of the clusters, or by testing the robustness of a cluster result against the addition of noise. Alternatively, the relevance of a cluster result can be assessed by a biological validation. It is extremely difficult to select the best cluster output, since "*the biologically best*" solution will be known only if the biological system studied is completely characterized. Although some biological systems have been described extensively, no such completely characterized benchmark system is now available.

Some of the most acceptable statistical and biological clustering validation measures are presented below.

3.2.1. Statistical measures

Cluster Coherence. In this method, the cluster is considered reliable if the within-cluster (intra-cluster) distance is small (i.e. all genes in cluster are tightly co-expressed) and the cluster has an average profile well delineated from the remainder dataset (inter-cluster distance is maximum).

Such measures are:

- Sum of squares of K-means;
- Silhouette coefficients (or index);
- Fisher's index;
- Dunn's validity index;
- Davies-Bouldin index; and
- Hubert's Γ Statistic.

These measures can be used as stand alone statistics to compare cluster results.

Figure of Merit (FOM) In this method, the clustering algorithm is applied to all experimental observations or samples (the data variables) except for one left-out condition. If the algorithm performs well, it is expected that all genes from the left-out condition or sample, have highly correlated values. Therefore, the FOM is computed for a clustering result by summing, for the left-out condition, the squares of the deviations of each gene relative to the mean of the genes in its cluster *for this condition or sample*. In this perspective, FOM measures the within-cluster similarity of the expression values of the removed experiment and therefore reflects the predictive power of the clustering. It is expected that removing one experiment from the data should not interfere with the cluster output if the output is robust.

Cluster Sensitivity Gene expression levels reflect the superposition of real biological signals and experimental errors. A way to assign confidence to a cluster membership of a gene consists in creating new *in silico* replicas of the microarray data by adding to the original data a small amount of artificial noise (similar to the experimental noise in the data) and clustering the data of those replicas. If the biological signal is stronger than the experimental noise in the measurements of a particular gene, adding small artificial variations (in the range of the experimental noise) to the expression profile of this gene will not drastically influence its overall profile and therefore will not affect its cluster membership. In this case, the cluster membership of that particular gene is robust with respect to sensitivity analysis, and a reliable confidence can be assigned to the clustering result of that gene. However, for genes with low signal-to-noise ratios, the outcome of the clustering result will be more sensitive to adding artificial noise. Therefore the key issue here is to choose the noise level to be applied for further sensitivity analysis. This is usually done through a Bootstrap analysis (bootstrapping is adding residual noise to data).

3.2.2. Biological measures

One way to biologically validate the results of clustering algorithms is to compare the gene clusters with existing functional classification schemes. In such schemes, genes are allocated to one or more functional categories (classes) representing their biochemical properties, biological roles, and so on. Finding clusters that have been significantly enriched for genes with similar function is a proof that a specific clustering technique produces biologically relevant results.

Apart from the validity measures mentioned, combined clustering techniques are also used to validate the clustering results. This method sometimes provides better clustering output which matches better with the real redefined classes (prior knowledge).

3.3. Recent work

Significant research has been accomplished over the last five years, where important observations were derived from the application of known clustering methods on gene expression profiles of different tumours. The most recent ones are shown below:

- Hierarchical Clustering applied to Diffuse large B-cell lymphoma (DLBCL), the most common subtype of non-Hodgkin's lymphoma and clinically heterogeneous, to discover distinct types (Alizadeh et al., 2000).
- Hierarchical Clustering applied to gene expression profiles of three temporal lobe brain tissues (normal) and four primary glioblastoma multiforme (GBM) tissues using oligonucleotide microarrays (Market et al., 2001).
- Hierarchical Clustering applied to astrocytomas to identify genes with distinct expression patterns in high-grade and low-grade gliomas (Rickman et al., 2001).
- Hierarchical Clustering and Self-Organizing Maps (SOMs) applied to seven (7) brain tumours to discriminate them based on their previously assigned WHO grade and discover possible interrelations (Watson et al., 2001).
- Hierarchical Clustering and SOM applied to 314 brain tumours and 98 normals to detect gene expression profiles differences that will assist for a better diagnosis (Ramaswamy et al., 2001).
- Hierarchical Clustering applied to diffuse large B-cell lymphoma (DLBCL), the most common lymphoid malignancy in adults, to identify different patterns of genes (Shipp et al., 2002).
- Different clustering techniques (Hierarchical, SOM, ...) applied to cDNA microarray data of brain tumours (oligodendroglioma, medulloblastoma and ependynoma) to derive differences on gene basis (Jiang et al., 2002).
- Hierarchical Clustering applied to high-density microarray data of varying WHO grade meningiomas to assess their cancer-related gene expression profiles (Watson et al., 2002).
- Hierarchical Clustering applied to four types of glioma: (a) oligodendroglioma; (b) anaplastic oligodendroglioma; (c) anaplastic astrocytoma; and (d) glioblastoma multiforme to define combined gene sets (Kim et al., 2002).
- Principal Component Analysis (or SVD) applied to lymphoma data (Alizadeh et al., 2000) to obtain links between patterns in the genes and patterns in the samples (tissues) (Misra et al., 2002).
- Hard *K*-means Clustering (C-means) and other clustering techniques (Hierarchical, SOM) applied to microarray data of brain tumour (10 medulloblastoma, 10 malignant

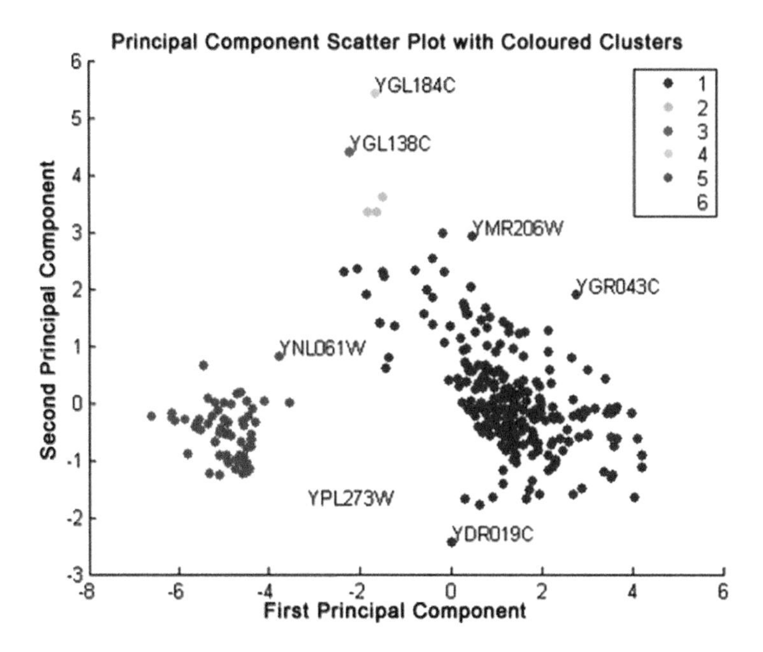

Fig. 10. Principal components analysis.

gliomas, 10 atypical teratoid/rhabdoid tumours (Rhab), 8 primitive neuroectodermal (PNET) and 4 normal cerebella tumours (Ncer)) to discover similar patterns of gene expressions (Wang et al., 2003).

- Hierarchical Clustering applied to diffuse astrocytoma of World Health Organization (WHO) grade II, which has an inherent tendency to spontaneously progress to anaplastic astrocytoma (WHO grade III) and/or glioblastoma (WHO grade IV). Gene expression profiles are also compared (van de Boom et al., 2003).
- Hierarchical Clustering and Principal Component Analysis (PCA or SVD) applied to malignant high-grade astrocytoma and benign low-grade astrocytoma to find progression factors of the tumour (Khatua et al., 2003).
- *K*-means Clustering applied to Affymetrix high-density oligonucleotide arrays to identify the global gene expression signatures associated with gliomas of different types and grades (glioblastomas, lower grade astrocytomas and oligodendrogliomas) The results defined molecular subsets of gliomas, which may be potentially used for patient stratification, and suggest potential targets for treatment (Shai et al., 2003).
- Block clustering applied to cDNA microarray data of 53 patient biopsies, comprising low-grade astrocytoma, secondary glioblastoma (respective recurrent high-grade tumours), and newly diagnosed primary glioblastoma. It is demonstrated that human gliomas can be differentiated according to their gene expression (Godard et al., 2003).
- Hierarchical Clustering applied to several brain tumours microarray datasets (Pomeroy et al., 2002: embryonic tumours, Ramaswamy et al., 2001: primary tumours,

Shipp et al., 2002: lymphoma, Alizadeh et al., 2000: lymphoma, MacDonald et al., 2001: medulloblastoma, Khatua et al., 2003: astrocytoma, and Rickman et al., 2001: gliomas), to define possible co expression of genes (Lee et al., 2004).

4. CLASSIFICATION OF MICROARRAY DATA OF BRAIN CANCER

As mentioned above, in supervised classification, the main goal is to understand the basis of the classification rule from a set of labeled objects (learning set) and build a predictor (classifier) for future unlabeled observations (test set) (Fig. 11).

Here, the classes are predefined and associated with each sample/observation is a *class label* or *response* Y_i and a set of G genes that form the feature vector X_i. Classifying a sample/observation into one of the K classes on the basis of an observed measurement X reduces to predict Y from this X.

A classifier or predictor for K tumour classes partitions the space X of gene expression profiles into K disjoint and exhaustive subsets, $A_1, \ldots, A_K$, such that for a sample with expression profile $X = (X_1, \ldots, X_G) \in Ak$ the predicted class is K. Classifiers are built from past experience, i.e. from observations which are known to belong to certain classes. Such observations comprise the learning (training) set (L)

$$L = \{(X_1, Y_1), \ldots, (X_n, Y_n)\} \tag{6}$$

4.1. Common classification techniques

There are several classification techniques that have been applied to microarray data of brain tumour. The most important ones are presented below.

4.1.1. Decision trees or classification trees

Decision tree algorithms (Murthy et al., 1994) (Fig. 12) form a class of popular pattern recognition algorithms, whose basic principle is to *divide and conquer*. Each decision node

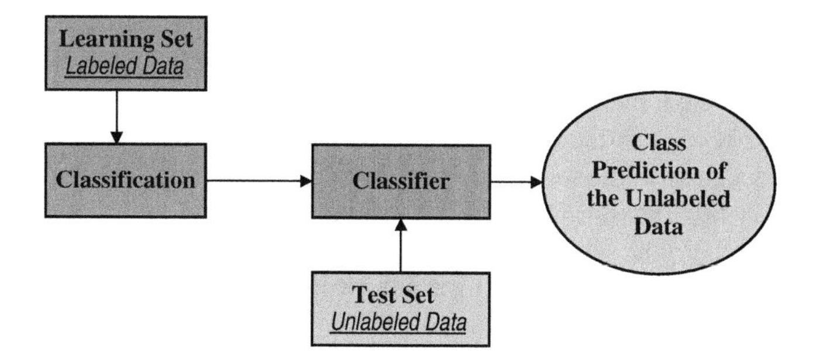

Fig. 11. Classification process.

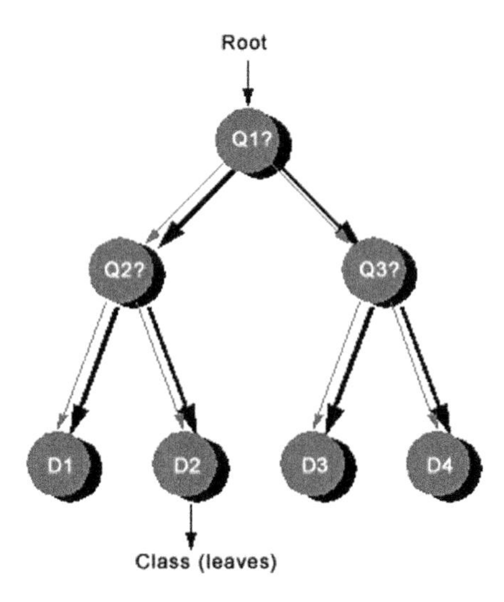

Fig. 12. Decision tree classifier structure.

in a tree divides a dataset into two parts. The partition only happens when it needs to. When a partition is needed, it means that there are two classes of patterns in the dataset. This means that the dataset is not pure or the *purity* is not satisfied. In practice, *impurity* measures, such as entropy, are often used. The most commonly used decision tree algorithms are CART (Breiman et al., 1984) and ID3, C4.5, C5 (Quinlan, 1993).

Algorithm:

- Each variable (observed measurement X) is selected through maximizing its capability to separate the given data. To measure this capability, impurity is used.
- If a variable can separate two classes perfectly, the impurity measure will be zero. For a variable with the impurity measure as zero, the genes whose experimental measurement values are less than an optimally determined threshold belong to one class while the genes whose experimental measurement values are greater than the threshold belong to the other class.
- The variable with the lowest impurity measure will be selected first as the root node in a decision tree. For instance, if experimental measurement α has a lower impurity measure than experimental measurement β, α will be selected as a decision node before β.
- After α tree has been constructed, a decision will be made in a progressive way. The root will pass the decision to the left sub-tree if the specified experimental measurement of a novel gene is less than an optimally determined threshold associated with the root node, otherwise the right sub-tree.
- Regarding the top node as a root in a sub-tree, the above process continues until approaching a leaf with a class label attached.
- When approaching a leaf, the *novel gene* will then be classified as a member of the class associated with the leaf.

Decision or Classification trees are also used for gene selection while other classifiers like FLDA (Fisher's Linear Discriminant Analysis), ANNs (Artificial Neural Networks) etc. require preliminary analysis. Decision trees do not perform well in small data sets.

4.1.2. K-nearest neighbours

Nearest neighbour (Duda et al., 2001) methods are based on a measure of distance between observations/samples such as the Euclidean distance or one minus the correlation between two gene expression profiles (Fig. 13).

Algorithm:

- Find the k observations in the learning set that are closest to X.
- Predict the class of X by majority vote i.e. choose the class that is most common among those k observations.

The size of k has to be predetermined manually. The usual values are 3, 5, and 9.

4.1.3. Artificial neural networks (ANNs)

The first generation of ANNs (Dayhoff and DeLeo, 2001), the so-called perceptrons, was simple linear logistic regression tools. More elaborate ANNs in the form of a multilayer perceptron form another machine learning approach that has proven to be powerful when classifying tumour array-based expression data (Fig. 14).

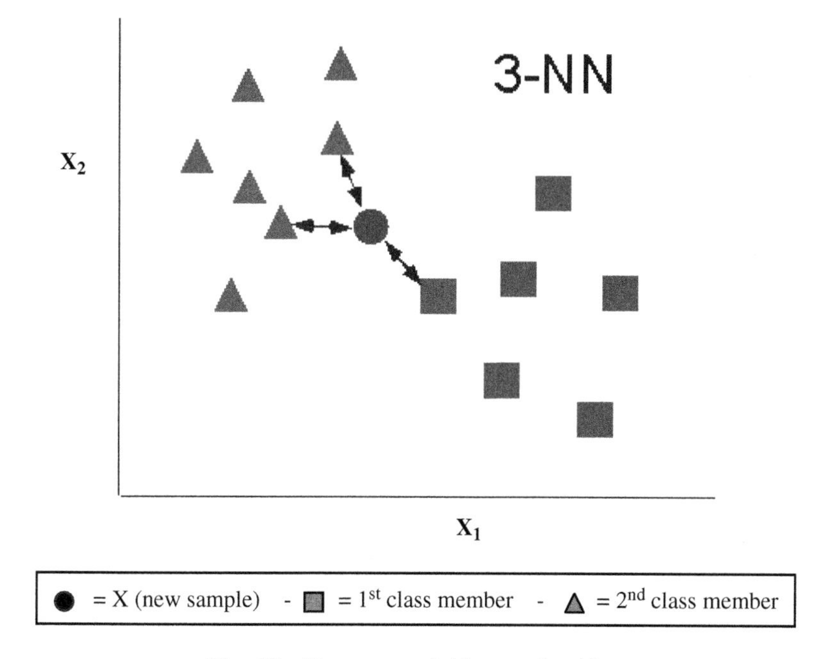

Fig. 13. *K*-nearest neighbours classifier.

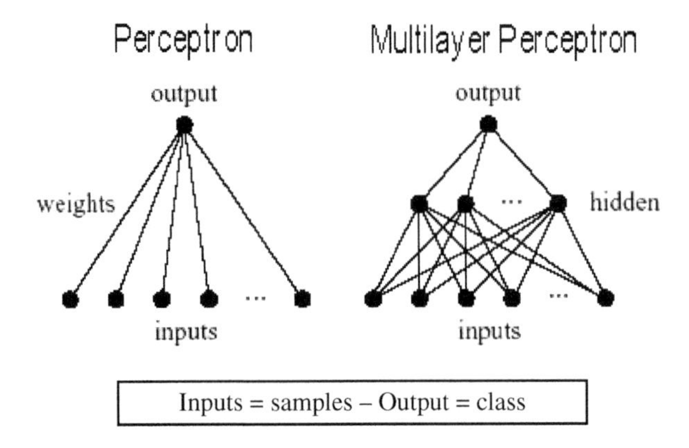

Fig. 14. Single layer and multilayer perceptrons.

A multilayered perceptron consists of a set of layers of perceptrons, modeled on the structure and behavior of neurons in the human brain. The input data, in this case the gene expression data, is fed into the so-called input layer and triggers a response in the following so-called hidden layer(s). The response in the hidden layer(s) in turn triggers a response in the output layer. In the case of classification, each perceptron in the output layer typically represents a class. When the gene expression pattern of a sample is fed into the ANN, ideally only the output perceptron representing the class that the sample belongs should respond.

For calibration, samples belonging to the classes of interest are presented to the ANNs, which are trained to recognize them in a supervised fashion by a process of error minimization. Since the number of perceptrons in the input layer depends on the dimension of the input data, a large number of perceptrons is needed for high dimensional data.

Furthermore, the more perceptrons used in the ANN, the more training samples are needed to calibrate all the perceptrons in such a way that the classifier has good predictive power. In the case of array data, where the number of samples is much less than the number of measured genes, this leads to a large risk of over fitting.

There are two parts to the solution of this problem. First, the dimension of the data can be reduced, either by using a dimensional reduction algorithm such as PCA or by selecting a smaller set of genes as input to the classifier in a supervised way by using a discriminatory score like *t*-test, S/N statistics etc. Second, the learning process can be carefully monitored using a cross-validation scheme (description below) to avoid over training. In this form, neural networks are efficient for high-dimensionality problems.

4.1.4. Support Vector Machines

Support Vector Machines (SVMs) (Vapnik, 1998) are a family of learning algorithms, which is currently considered as one of the most efficient methods in many real world applications.

The theory behind SVMs was developed in the 1960s and 1970s by Vapnik and Chervonenkis, but the first practical implementation of SVM was only published in the early 1990s. Since then the method gained more and more attention among the machine learning community thanks to its ability to outperform most other learning algorithms (including neural networks on decision trees) in many applications.

Recently, SVMs have been applied to biological problems (Guyon et al., 1999) including gene expression data analysis or protein classification, particularly because of the high dimensionality of the data.

SVM is a binary classification method and is mostly used for two class discrimination problems. In other words, the 2 classes are associated with +1, −1 labels, Y_i {+1, −1}.

Therefore,

$$x_i \cdot w + b \geq +1$$
$$x_i \cdot w + b \leq -1, \tag{7}$$

where x_i is the sample i, w is the normal to the hyperplane, and b the bias. Y_i can be either +1 or −1, as mentioned above.

The SVM classifier is based on the principle of finding the maximum margin hyperplane that best distinguishes the two classes (e.g. tumourous versus normal). The classifier is trained using only the *support vector*s (i.e. the samples that lay on the two hyperplanes parallel to the optimal one) (Fig. 15).

This method works remarkably well due to its ability to map a non-separable dataset onto a separable one using a "Kernel" function (linear, polynomial, radial basis and sigmoid). In this way classification becomes easy.

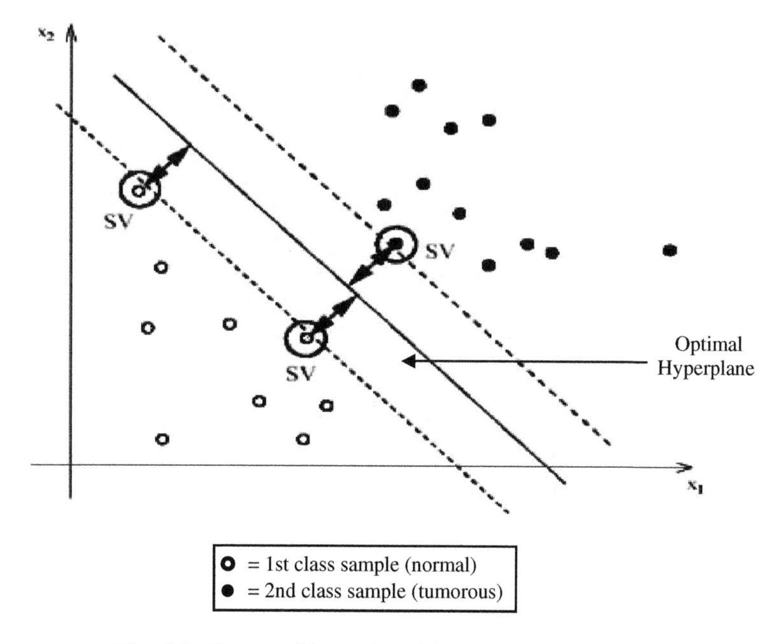

Fig. 15. Support Vector Machines (SVMs) classifier.

Algorithm:

- Select the gene expression data matrix;
- Select the Kernel function to use;
- Execute the training algorithm using QP (Quadratic programming) solver to obtain the λ_i values (Lagrange multipliers); and
- Unseen data can be classified using the λ_i values and the support vectors (sv).

SVMs achieve good performance due to dimensionality reduction employed. Furthermore, an SVM can be regarded as a type of Neural Networks.

4.1.5. Bayesian networks

Bayesian Networks (Friedman et al., 1997) represent statistical relationships among various variables and are useful in analyzing gene expression patterns and examining statistical properties of dependence and conditional independence in the data. The nodes in the Bayesian network correspond to each gene and the values of the nodes represent the gene expression level. There are several Bayesian methods for classification like: Naïve Bayes, Bayesian Belief Networks, and Expectation Maximization. Here, a brief description of the Naïve Bayes method is given, which is the most commonly applied method for gene expression data classification.

Naïve Bayesian Classifier assumes independence among features. The assumption seems unrealistic. For example, if we take expression data for a given sample/observation as the input features, there is no reason to say they are independent. Interestingly however, this method is competitive with state-of-the-art classifiers such as Decision trees (C4.5, C5.0) This classifier learns from training data the conditional probability of each sample X given the class label Y. Classification is then done by applying Bayes rule to compute the probability of Y given the particular instance (sample) of $X_1, \ldots, X_n$ (where n = number of genes) and then predicting the class with the highest posterior. i.e. **Posterior probability of X_i belonging to class Yi = Prior probability of Y_i * likelihood of X_i given Y_i.**

4.1.6. Fisher Linear Discriminant Analysis (FLDA)

Discriminant analysis can be distinguished into two categories: *linear or quadratic* (*called LDA* and *QDA*, respectively). Fisher's Linear Discriminant Analysis (Fig. 16) belongs to the *linear* case. This method is often applied for classification of gene expression data (Golub et al., 1999).

Algorithm:

- Find linear combination of the gene expression profiles $X = X_1, \ldots, X_G$ with large ratios of between-groups to within-groups sums of squares (discriminant variables); and
- Assign the new sample X to that class whose mean vector is closest to X in terms of the discriminant variables.

The method performs well, but may be unstable in high-dimensionality problems.

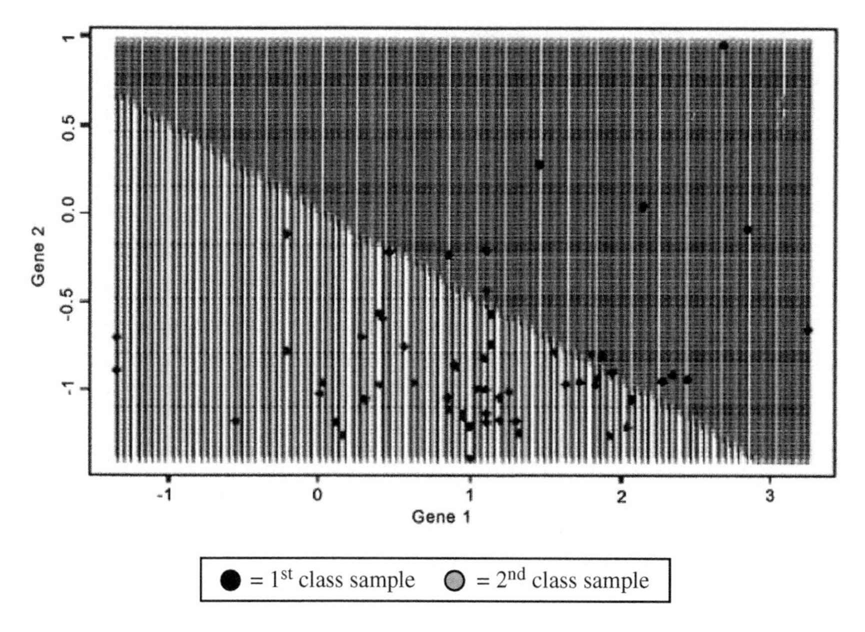

Fig. 16. Fisher's Linear Discriminant Analysis.

4.1.7. Voted classification

Methods for voting classification algorithms, such as Bagging and Boosting, have been shown to be very successful in improving the accuracy of certain classifiers for artificial and real-world datasets.

Recently, they have been applied to microarray data (Dudoit et al., 2002) to enhance the decision tree algorithm efficiency.

Voting algorithm takes a classifier and a training set as input and trains the classifier multiple times on different versions of the training set. The generated classifiers are then combined to create a final classifier that is used to classify the test data. Voting algorithms can be divided into two types: those that adaptively change the distribution of the training set based on the performance of previous classifiers (Boosting) and those that do not (Bagging).

Boosting (mainly AdaBoost) Algorithm:

- Train a classifier on the training set;
- The trained classifier is assigned a voting weight based on its accuracy;
- Calculate the classification result for each sample of the training set, based on the weighted voting of all trained classifiers; and
- Modify the probability of each sample appearing in the training set based on the classification correctness.

Bagging (Bootstrap Aggregating) Algorithm:

- Randomly select *T* samples from the original learning (training) set;
- Train the classifiers on these samples;
- Apply these classifiers to the test samples; and
- Choose the classifier with best accuracy on the selected samples, i.e. the one who takes the most votes.

4.1.8. Genetic Algorithms

The Genetic Algorithm (GA) (Karzynski et al., 2003) works by creating many random "solutions" to the problem at hand. Being random, these starting "solutions" are not very good: schedules overlap and itineraries do not traverse every necessary location.

All of these solutions are coded the only way computers know: as a series of zeroes and ones. The evolution-like process consists in considering these 0s and 1s as genetic "chromosomes" that, like their real-life, biological equivalents, will be made to "mate" by hybridization, also throwing in the occasional spontaneous mutation. The "offspring" generated will include some solutions that *are better than the original*, purely random ones. The best offspring are added to the population while inferior ones are eliminated. By repeating this process among the better elements, repeated improvements will occur in the population, survive and generate their own offspring.

GAs may represent another useful tool in the classification of biological phenotypes based on gene expression data. Several papers have described the use of GAs for binary class prediction problems. However, despite their suitability for addressing problems involving large solution spaces, the potential for using GAs in multiple-class prediction settings has to date remained unexplored. GAs are also used for gene selection problems and with a combination of a neural network, provide great accuracy in classification matters.

4.2. Classification performance estimation

There are several methods to measure the performance (Ambroise and McLachlan, 2002; Aliferis et al., 2003) of the classifiers described above. These methods reflect the efficiency and robustness of classifiers. A brief analysis is given below.

4.2.1. Resubstitution estimation

The error rate on the learning set is calculated. The limitation of this method is that, it can be severely biased downward.

4.2.2. Test set estimation

In the absence of a genuine test set, cases in the learning set *L* may be repeatedly randomly divided into two sets, *L*1 and *L*2; the classifier is built using *L*1 and the error rate is computed for *L*2. The limitation of this method is that, it reduces effective sample size;

there are no widely accepted guidelines for choosing the relative size of these artificial learning sets and test sets.

4.2.3. V-Fold Cross-Validation (CV) Estimation

Cases in the learning set L are randomly divided into V subsets Lv, $v = 1, \ldots, V$, of as nearly equal size as possible. Classifiers, at each iteration are trained on $L-Lv$ learning sets, leaving one of the Lv subsets out from the initial L set to be used as test set. The error rates are computed for test subset Lv, and averaged over v. Bias–variance trade-off: small V typically gives a larger bias, but a smaller variance and mean squared error.

4.2.4. Leave-One-Out Cross-Validation (LOOCV)

This is a special case of cross validation mentioned. Training of the classifier is done by leaving one sample out of the learning set at each step, and uses this sample for test. In general, this method has low bias but high variance estimates of classification error. For stable (low variance) classifiers such as k-nearest neighbour, LOOCV provides good estimates of generalization error rates.

4.2.5. Out-of-bag estimation

Drawing a random sample of size n from the empirical distribution, a bootstrap sample of size n covers approximately 2/3 of the observations of the learning sample. The observations, which are not in the bootstrap sample, are called out-of-bag sample and may be used for estimating the misclassification error or for improved class probability estimates.

The performance evaluation measures used in the methods applied to measure the performance of the classifier are:

4.2.6. Error rate

The predictive accuracy (A_{cc}) of the classifier measures the proportion of correctly classified instances:

$$A_{cc} = \frac{\mathrm{TP} + \mathrm{TN}}{\mathrm{TP} + \mathrm{TN} + \mathrm{FP} + \mathrm{FN}} \tag{8}$$

where true positives (TP) denote the correct classifications of positive examples; true negatives (TN) are the correct classifications of negative examples; false positives (FP) represent the incorrect classification of negative examples into the positive class; and false negatives (FN) are the positive examples incorrectly classified into the negative class.

4.2.7. ROC

A ROC curve (Fig. 17) displays the relationship between the proportion of true positive and false positive classifications resulting from each possible decision threshold value in a two-class classification task. The area under the curve is a measure of test accuracy, and when applied to a gene expression profile, it provides an estimate of the probability that a

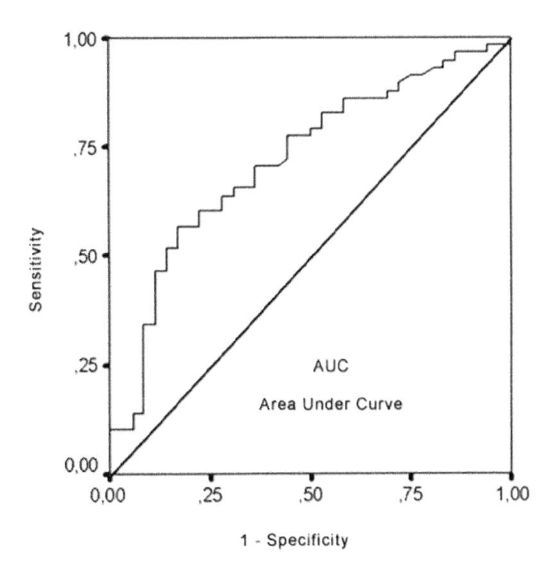

Fig. 17. ROC curve.

gene is up or down-regulated in a given group, e.g. patients with cancer versus healthy controls.

$$S_n = \frac{TP}{TP + FN} \tag{9}$$

$$S_p = \frac{TN}{TN + FP}, \tag{10}$$

where TP is the sensitivity, TN is the specificity, FP is the 1 − specificity and FN is the 1 − sensitivity. Under the null hypothesis of no difference in expression, its value is close to 0.5, i.e. probability of a correct classification equal to 50% for groups of equal size, and the ROC curve overlaps the rising diagonal (chance line). On the contrary, when the distance between groups increases, the area under the ROC curve is higher and the curve tends to approach the left-hand corner, corresponding to the highest theoretical value of accuracy (probability of a correct classification = 100%).

4.2.8. Confusion matrix

A confusion matrix contains information about actual and predicted classifications done by a classification system. Each column shows the real classes (already known) and each row presents the predicted ones. Performance of classifiers is commonly evaluated using the data in the matrix.

Table 1. Confusion matrix – presents actual and predicted classifications done by a classification system

		Confusion matrix			
		Real classes			
		AS	EP	MD	OL
Classification	AS	5			
	EP	1	7	1	
	MD			7	1
	OL				1
	Sum	6	7	8	2
	Sensitivity	0.83	1	0.88	0
	Specificity	0.98	0.96	0.98	1

Table 1 presents 6 cases of astrocytomas (AS), 7 cases of ependynomas (EP), 8 cases of medulloblastomas (MD) and 2 cases of oligodendrogliomas (OL). The predicted classes (rows) as compared to the actual ones (columns), determine the classifier's efficiency and the sensitivity-specificity values.

4.3. Recent work

Recent studies involving the application of microarrays in the classification of cancer have proved the effectiveness of this new technology. Gene expression profiles provide detailed analysis of cancer malignancies and assist the discovery of new types of cancer. Some of the most important findings are presented below:

- SVM algorithm applied to 314 brain tumours and 98 normals to detect gene expression profiles differences that will assist for a better diagnosis. The expression levels of 16 063 genes and expressed sequence tags are used to evaluate the accuracy of a multi-class classifier based on a SVM algorithm (Ramaswamy et al., 2001).
- Genetic Algorithms and *K*-nearest neighbour classifiers applied to Alizadeh et al. (2000) dataset to identify genes that can jointly discriminate between classes of samples (Li et al., 2001).
- Fisher's Linear Discriminant Analysis, Nearest Neighbours, Decision trees and Boosting – Bagging algorithms applied to Alizadeh et al. (2000) dataset to compare their results and their efficiency (Dudoit et al., 2002).
- *K*-nearest neighbours classifier applied among others (Average Difference and Δ values) to compare the results of classification of lymphoma and medulloblastoma data sets (Antipova et al., 2002).
- Three supervised machine-learning techniques applied to Pomeroy et al. (2002) dataset (Central Nervous System Embryonal Tumour Outcome) to assess the results of

cancer classification. These classifiers were: Decision tree (C4.5), Boosting, and Bagging (Pomeroy et al., 2002).
- *K*-nearest neighbour classifier applied to patients' data included 60 children with medulloblastomas, 10 young adults with malignant gliomas (WHO grades III and IV), 5 children with AT/RTs, 5 with renal/extrarenal rhabdoid tumours, and 8 children with supratentorial PNETs (Nutt et al., 2003).
- Supervised classification techniques applied to Shipp MA microarray dataset (lymphoma) to identify differences in the gene expression profiles (Shipp et al., 2002).
- Microarray analysis is used in (Tan and Gilbert, 2003) to determine the expression of 12 000 genes in a set of 50 gliomas, 28 glioblastomas and 22 anaplastic oligodendrogliomas. Supervised learning approaches were used to build a two-class prediction model based on a subset of 14 glioblastomas and 7 anaplastic oligodendrogliomas with classic histology. A 20-feature *k*-nearest neighbour model correctly classified 18 of the 21 classic cases in leave-one-out cross-validation when compared with pathological diagnoses.
- Multi-layer perceptron, *k*-nearest neighbour, SVM and structure adaptive self-organizing map have been used for classification of different lymphoma dataset (Alizadeh et al.). Combination of the classifiers has been done to achieve better classification results (Alizadeh et al., 2000).
- Supervised classification methods applied to brain cancer dataset (low-grade astrocytoma, secondary glioblastoma and newly diagnosed primary glioblastoma) to identify similar gene expression levels of the samples (Cho and Won, 2003).

5. CLINICAL VERSUS GENETIC ANALYSIS OF BRAIN CANCER

5.1. Diagnosis, prognosis and treatment of brain cancer

As mentioned in Section 1, brain cancer is distinguished into two different categories: *primary* and *secondary* or *metastatic*. At the time being, research is mainly focused on primary brain tumours and more specifically on *gliomas* (Astrcytomas, brain stem gliomas, ependynomas and oligodendrogliomas), which are mostly encountered (50% of all primary brain tumours) and have the worst prognosis. Several approaches (Barkovich 1992; Abdullah and Mathews, 1999; Delbeke 1999; Hustinx and Alavi, 1999; Devos et al., 2005) for diagnostic, prognostic and treatment purposes have been already generated and widely applied providing valuable information to the clinicians. The low-resolution data derived from these approaches assist the clinicians in deciding the therapy path that they have to follow to treat brain cancer.

But is this enough? Do they possess all the information needed to choose the best treatment way? What is missing? The high-resolution data, which can be derived using genetics, will confirm and test the accuracy of the conventional/traditional methods applied so far, but even more will provide a new way of dealing with brain cancer.

Before analyzing the emerging role of genetics and the application of the DNA microarray technology on brain cancer, it is appropriate to present research efforts that have been accomplished for diagnosis, prognosis and treatment purposes.

5.1.1. Diagnosis

Diagnosis plays a key role in understanding the type and the characteristics of brain tumour. False diagnosis can often lead to a false prognosis and treatment path. Current diagnostic approaches offer the ability to observe the morphology, size and stage of the tumour and decide the therapy that has to be followed. The most recent diagnostic approaches are presented in the following with a brief analysis and discussion.

A neurological examination is usually the first test given when a patient complains of symptoms that suggest a brain tumour. The examination includes checking eye movements, hearing, sensation, muscle movement, sense of smell, and balance and coordination. The clinician will also test mental state and memory.

A variety of imaging techniques have been introduced and applied today. The most important ones are:

- *X-rays* of the skull were once standard diagnostic tools but are now performed only when more advanced procedures are not available;
- *Magnetic Resonance Imaging* (*MRI*) is the gold standard for diagnosing a brain tumour. It does not use radiation and provides pictures from various angles that can enable doctors to construct a three-dimensional image of the tumour.
- A variant called *magnetic resonance spectroscopy* (*MRS*) provides metabolite information which enables a clinician to acquire information about the grading and type of brain tumour.
- *Computed Tomography* (*CT*) uses a sophisticated X-ray machine and a computer to create a detailed picture of the body's tissues and structures. It is not as accurate as an MRI and does not detect about half of low-grade gliomas.
- *Positron Emission Tomography* (*PET*) provides a picture of the brain's activity rather than its structure by tracking substances that have been labeled with a radioactive tracer. PET is not routinely used for diagnosis, but it may complement MRI to help determine tumour grade after a diagnosis.

Lumbar puncture (or spinal tap) is employed to obtain a sample of spinal fluid, which is examined for the presence of tumour cells. A CT scan or MRI should generally be performed before a lumbar procedure thus ensuring safe procedure.

Biopsy is a surgical procedure in which a small sample of tissue is taken from the suspected tumour and examined under a microscope for malignancy. The results of the biopsy also provide information on the cancer cell type.

5.1.2. Prognosis

The "prognosis" of brain cancer usually refers to the likely outcome of brain cancer. The prognosis of brain cancer may include the duration of brain cancer, chances of complications of brain cancer, probable outcomes, prospects for recovery, recovery period for brain cancer, survival rates, death rates, and other outcome possibilities in the overall prognosis of brain cancer. Naturally, such forecast issues are by their nature, unpredictable. The survival rates in people with brain tumours depend on many different variables. The most important are shown below:

- Whether the tumour is malignant or benign;
- Cancer cell type and location (location affects whether the tumour can be removed surgically or not);

- Tumour grade (this is the tendency to spread and the growth rate);
- Patient's age (the outlook is poorer in the very youngest and very oldest patients, although younger patients who survive two years after diagnosis have a much better outlook than older patients);
- Patient's ability to function; and
- Duration of symptoms.

Latest researches have revealed additional prognosis estimation methods. The most important ones are presented below:

Elevated levels of certain cancer-associated molecules may be correlated with poor or positive prognosis in patients with specific types of brain cancer cells. Such markers include genetically mutated p53 and PTEN proteins and elevated levels of epidermal growth factor receptor (EGFR) (Bodey et al., 2004; Hilton and Melling, 2004).

Analyses that identify genetic types may soon help clinicians determine if patients with specific brain tumour cells respond better to one treatment than another. For example, specific genetic profiles of oligodendrogliomas have been associated with predictable responses to certain agents called nitrosourea alkylating agents (especially carmustine).

5.1.3. Treatment

The approach for treating brain tumours is to reduce the tumour as much as possible using surgery, radiation treatment (radiotherapy), chemotherapy and investigative procedures

The intensity, combination, and sequence of these treatments depend on the glioma subtype, its size and location, and patient age, health status, and medical history.

Recent advances in surgical and radiation treatments have significantly extended average survival times compared to those of standard therapy. Investigative treatments, such as with monoclonal antibodies and gene therapies also show promise for a great future.

The standard procedure is called craniotomy: The neurosurgeon removes a piece of skull bone to expose the area of brain over the tumour. The tumour is located and then removed. The surgeon has various surgical options for breaking down and removing the tumour. They include:

- Standard surgical procedures;
- Laser microsurgery (which produces great heat and vaporizes tumour cells); and
- Ultrasonic aspiration (which uses ultrasound to break the glioma tumour into small pieces, which are then suctioned out).

Relatively benign, grade-I gliomas may be treated only by surgery. Some controversy exists over whether surgery for low-grade astrocytomas improves survival, although insufficient research has been conducted to prove its benefits or lack thereof these gliomas. Most malignant tumours require additional treatments, including repeated surgery. Additional procedures to enhance brain surgery have been developed in order to allow maximum removal of the cancerous tissue without affecting the healthy brain parts (cells). Some of them are: *stereotaxy*, *cortical localization*, *image-guided surgery*, and *magnetic-tipped catheters*.

Radiotherapy plays a central role in the treatment of most brain tumours, whether benign or malignant. There are different phases where radiotherapy could be applied.

- *Radiotherapy after surgery*. Even when it appears that the entire tumour has been surgically removed, microscopic cancer cells often remain in the surrounding brain tissue.
- *Radiotherapy when surgery is not appropriate*. Radiotherapy may be used instead of surgery for inaccessible tumours or for tumours that have properties that are particularly responsive to radiotherapy.
- *Radiotherapy and chemotherapy*. Combining chemotherapy with radiotherapy is beneficial in some patients with high-grade tumours.
- *Stereotactic Radiosurgery*. It has been developed to allow highly targeted radiation to be delivered directly to the small tumours while avoiding healthy brain tissue. The term radiosurgery is used because the destruction is so precise that it acts almost like a surgical knife. Some studies are finding that stereotactic radiosurgery improves survival, even in patients with the highly aggressive glioblastoma multiforme brain cancer. The procedure is being tested to boost standard radiotherapy.

Chemotherapy involves the use of toxic drugs to kill cancer cells. They may be given orally, intravenously, or administered directly into the central nervous system. Chemotherapy is not an effective initial treatment for low-grade brain tumours, mostly because standard drugs cannot pass through the blood–brain barrier. Recently, however, researchers have identified certain genetic arrangements in specific brain tumours that make them sensitive to the effects of chemotherapy. Some of the drugs used in Chemotherapy are: *Carmustine* (also called BCNU) and *PCV*. Each of these drugs is also used separately and in other combinations. Examples include the following: *Procarbazine*, *Carboplatin*, *Temozolomide* and other chemotherapy agents.

Several other promising treatment paths have been introduced. Some of them are: Immunotherapy, Gene Therapy, Angiogenesis Inhibitors, Transplantation Procedures and High-Dose Chemotherapy, and Photodynamic Therapy.

5.2. Genetic analysis of brain cancer

The revolution of Genomics and Proteomics (Zhang et al., 1997; Gray and Collins, 2000; Sallinen et al., 2005), over the last few decades has offered the opportunity to clinicians, biologists and engineers to cooperate in order to investigate their involvement in brain cancer pathogenesis and behavior. The outcome of many experiments and research efforts has proved that specific genes clearly contribute to cancer formation and growth.

However, significant questions are still to be answered before evaluating the full benefits of genomics.

- Is there only one or a group of markers that assist the growth of brain cancer and its development?
- Are there any specific codes of behavior under which they function that might change under the influence of environmental, nutritional or other factors? Which are these factors?
- Are there any means to observe and record their function and bring it back to normal whenever necessary?
- Are there any gene markers that verify cancer outcome (aggressiveness, growth, etc.)?

- Are there any ways to regulate the function of a gene or a group of them in order to control cancer or even eliminate it?

Genomics (Ramaswamy and Golub, 2002; Wadlow and Ramaswamy, 2005), due to their great importance have already influenced the conventional ways for diagnosis, prognosis and treatment of brain cancer. Clinicians now think of genomics as the new era in medicine. Many of them believe that most of the traditional methods for diagnosis, prognosis and therapy will be augmented, or even substituted by genomic-based approaches in the near future. Others, the more skeptics, believe that genomics will be the main "weapon" in dealing with brain cancer, but an improvement of the conventional methods will also offer great support.

Recently, many new bio-technologies have been introduced to assist the biologists and clinicians in their research. The most promising though are the *DNA Microarrays* that managed to generate a new way of studying genes and their changes using their gene expression ratios that show the degree of change of their functional behavior. Simple numbers now describe these changes that can be measured under different disease stages and / or different patients.

5.2.1. The role of genomics in diagnosis-prognosis of brain cancer

It is now widely acceptable that brain cancer is the result of genetic abnormalities (Yoon et al., 2001; Nayak et al., 2004) that affect the function of genes and that may happen due to different reasons (environmental, nutritional etc.). Genes determine the form, function, and growth patterns of cells. Those that accelerate or suppress growth are often involved in cancer. For example, many cancers have an abnormality in a gene that is responsible for stimulating cellular growth and / or the gene that normally prevents cancer is not working properly. Both of these genetic abnormalities can result in uncontrolled and excessive cellular growth, the hallmark of cancer. Some of the most common abnormalities detected in brain cancer are the following:

- *Translocations* – the changing places of a gene from one chromosome with a gene on another chromosome;
- *Deletions* – a gene or sequence of nucleotides is missing in the DNA; and
- *Polymorphisms* – variations in nucleotide sequence.

Tumour genesis involves an interplay between at least two classes of genes: *oncogenes* and *tumour suppressor* genes. Oncogenes are abnormally activated versions of cellular genes that promote cell proliferation and growth. Activated oncogenes thereby result in an exaggerated impulse for a cell to grow and divide. Tumour suppressor genes, on the other hand, are normal genes that act to inhibit tumour cell proliferation and growth. The inactivation of these genes results in tumour formation or progression. The most common scenario for inactivation of both copies of a tumour suppressor gene is mutation of one allelic copy, followed by loss of all or part of the chromosome bearing the second allele. Consequently, the identification of consistent regions of chromosomal loss in specific tumour types suggests a tumour suppressor gene in that chromosomal region. These basic themes of oncogene activation and tumour suppressor gene inactivation underlie the current molecular understanding of human tumour formation.

Recent laboratory tests and research studies have managed to identify genetic differentiations in primary brain tumours caused by gene mutations (activations, inactivations, translocations, deletions, etc.). The results of these tests determined the genes and the growth factors involved in the tumour genesis of astrocytomas, ependynomas, stem gliomas and oligodendrogliomas. An analysis of the most important gene factors of brain cancer found already is presented in the following.

Diffuse Astrocytic Tumours. The p53 gene, a tumour suppressor gene located on chromosome 17p13.1, has an integral role in a number of cellular processes, including cell cycle arrest, response to DNA damage, apoptosis, angiogenesis and differentiation; as a result, p53 has been dubbed the "guardian of the genome". The p53 gene is involved in the early stages of astrocytoma tumour genesis. For instance, p53 mutations and allelic loss of chromosome 17p are observed in approximately one-third of all three grades of adult astrocytomas, suggesting that inactivation of p53 is important in the formation of the grade II tumours. Moreover, high grade astrocytomas with homogeneous p53 mutations evolve clonally from subpopulations of similarly mutated cells present in initially low-grade tumours. Such mutation studies are complemented by functional studies that have recapitulated the role of the p53 inactivation in the early stages of astrocytoma formation.

A number of genetic abnormalities have been associated with anaplastic astrocytoma, and recent studies have suggested that most of these abnormalities converge on one critical cell-cycle regulatory complex which includes the p16, cyclin-dependent kinase 4 (cdk4), cyclin D1 and retinoblastoma (Rb) proteins. Individual components in this pathway are altered in up to 50% of anaplastic astrocytomas and in the majority of GBM.

Chromosome 9p loss occurs in approximately 50% of anaplastic astrocytomas and GBMs, with 9p deletions occurring primarily in the region of the CDKN2/p16 (or MTS1) gene, which encodes the p16 protein. The frequency of 9p loss increases not only at the transition from astrocytoma to anaplastic astrocytoma, but also at the transition from anaplastic astrocytoma to GBM, implying that the 9p tumour suppressor plays a role in different stages of astrocytoma progression.

Loss of chromosome 13q occurs in one-third to one-half of high-grade astrocytomas, suggesting the presence of a progression-associated astrocytoma tumour suppressor gene on that chromosome. The 13q14 region containing the RB (retinoblastoma) gene is preferentially targeted by these losses and inactivating mutations of the RB gene occur in primary astrocytomas. Overall, analysis of chromosome 13q loss, RB gene mutations and Rb protein expression suggests that the RB gene is inactivated in about 20% of anaplastic astrocytomas and 35% of GBM. Interestingly, RB and CDKN2/p16 alterations in primary gliomas are inversely correlated, rarely occurring together in the same tumour.

Allelic losses on 19q have been observed in up to 40% of anaplastic astrocytomas and GBMs, indicating a progression-associated glial tumour suppressor gene on chromosome 19q. This tumour suppressor gene may be unique to glial tumours and is involved in all three major types of diffuse cerebral gliomas (astrocytomas, oligodendrogliomas, and oligoastrocytomas).

Chromosome 10 loss is a frequent finding in GBM, occurring in 60–95% of GBMs but only rarely in anaplastic astrocytomas. Attempts to identify this tumour suppressor gene by deletion mapping, however, have been hampered by the observation that, in most cases, the entire chromosome is lost.

Platelet derived growth factor (PDGF) is over expressed, together with its receptors, in both low- and high-grade astrocytic tumours. However, the mechanism for this is unclear as the PDGFa gene is amplified in only 16% of glioblastomas.

Epidermal growth factor receptor (EGFR) is over expressed in about 40% of adult primary glioblastomas, with amplification of the gene in the form of extra-chromosomal double-minutes. This is often associated with gene rearrangement, which is strongly associated with chromosome 10 loss. EGFR amplification is not a feature of secondary glioblastomas and is uncommon in childhood malignant astrocytic tumours. Although glioblastomas that over-express EGFR may respond less well to radiotherapy, most studies have found that demonstration of EGFR expression does not add any useful prognostic information. Though, with the development of therapeutic antibodies targeted at the EGFR, tumour expression of EGFR may become clinically important.

A number of other growth factors, including vascular endothelial growth factor (VEGF) may be over expressed in diffuse astrocytic tumours. This has been correlated with an adverse prognosis in low-grade diffuse astrocytic tumours.

The PTEN (phosphatase with tensin homology) gene, which is located in chromosome 10q23.3, is mutated in approximately one-third of primary glioblastomas, but is an uncommon event in secondary glioblastomas, and may lead to a loss of the normal growth suppressive activity of this protein. In-vitro studies have shown that some other types of human malignancies with mutant PTEN are sensitive to drugs directed at the Akt pathway, although studies on glioblastomas have not been reported.

Ependymomas. Ependymomas form a clinically diverse group of gliomas that vary from aggressive intraventricular tumours of children to benign spinal cord tumours in adults. Chromosome 22q loss is common in ependymomas. A candidate glioma tumour suppressor gene on chromosome 22q was the neurofibromatosis (NF2) gene, since NF2 patients have a higher incidence of gliomas, particularly ependymomas, in addition to schwannomas and meningiomas. Analysis of the NF2 gene in ependymomas, however, has revealed only a single mutation to date, in an ependymoma that had lost the remaining wild-type allele. The paucity of NF2 mutations suggests that another, as yet unidentified, chromosome 22q gene will probably be a more integral ependymoma locus.

The p53 gene is not mutated in ependymomas or in the malignant transformation of ependymomas to anaplastic ependymoma. Transitions of ependymoma to GBM are rare, and have not been studied by molecular genetic techniques.

Stem Gliomas. Brain stem gliomas are a form of pediatric diffuse, fibrillary astrocytoma that often follows a malignant course. Brain stem GBMs share genetic features with those adult GBMs that affect younger patients: frequent p53 gene and chromosome 17p alterations without EGFR gene amplification. Since brain stem gliomas are predominantly childhood tumours, this may suggest a common oncogenic pathway for those diffuse, fibrillary astrocytic tumours that affect younger patients, regardless of their anatomic location. On the other hand, there is considerable variation in the transcription levels of particular growth factors and proto-oncogenes in different normal glial cell populations and certain astrocytes may display differential susceptibilities at different ages to the same genetic alterations.

Oligodendrogliomas. Oligodendrogliomas and oligoastrocytomas (mixed gliomas) are diffused, usually cerebral tumours that are clinically and biologically most closely related to the diffuse astrocytomas (WHO Grade II is a slow-growing oligodendroglioma and WHO Grade III is the anaplastic oligodendroglioma or oligoastrocytoma. Allelic losses in oligodendrogliomas occur preferentially on chromosomes 1p and 19q, affecting 40–80% of these tumour types. Because of the frequent loss of these loci in low-grade as well as anaplastic oligodendrogliomas, the 1p and 19q tumour suppressors are probably important early in oligodendroglial tumour genesis. Mapping of the chromosome 19q locus has demonstrated that the gene resides in the same vicinity as the astrocytoma gene. Interestingly, chromosome 1p and 19q losses are closely associated; oligodendroglial tumours with 1p loss typically also have loss of 19q, suggesting that these two putative tumour suppressor genes may be involved in biologically distinct pathways.

5.2.2. Methods used for detection of genetic mutations

Several methods have been used to detect the mutations of the genes mentioned above. Many of them are still used in a combined way to obtain an even more accurate outcome. The most significant methods for genetic tests are the following.

FISH (Fluorescence In Situ Hybridization). FISH is a laboratory technique that is used to detect genetic abnormalities at the single cell and single gene level such as numerical abnormalities (gains and losses of nucleotides), and translocations (the changing places of a gene or segment of genes on one chromosome with gene or a segment on another chromosome).

PCR (Polymerase Chain Reaction). PCR is an in vitro laboratory method that is useful for genetic testing for disease and detecting minimal residual disease, which is a small amount of disease left after treatment that may lead to recurrence and is typically not detectable with other techniques. This procedure amplifies a segment of DNA from a small sample, making it detectable. With PCR, relatively small sequences of known DNA can be replicated into millions of copies over a short period of time.

RT-PCR (Reverse Transcription-PCR). Reverse transcription (RT)-PCR is a technique that detects the degree to which genes is expressed. Complicated processes control which segment of DNA separates, gets transcribed (copied) into mRNA, and then is expressed as proteins in the cell. Not all genes are transcribed and then expressed equally. Due to many controls in the cell, some genes are over-expressed, which means they are transcribed and expressed at a higher rate than normal, while other genes are not expressed, or "turned off" so that certain functions are not manifested in the cell.

Southern Blot Analysis. Southern Blot is a hybridization-based method applied since 1975 and has been widely used in molecular biology. This method readily allows the detection of large alterations of genes such as deletions, insertions and rearrangements. Recent improvements in this technology have resulted in more rapid analysis and higher resolution of large DNA sequences.

Northern Blot Analysis. The principle of Northern Blot method is identical to that of Southern Blot, except that in this method, total RNA and mRNA are measured. Different sizes of mRNA indicate duplications, deletions and/or insertions of genes or alterations in splicing.

Protein Truncation Test. Protein Truncation Test (PPT) facilitates the deletion of mutations at the protein level rather than the DNA level. PPT consists of three main steps: (a) isolation of the RNA and amplification of the targeted sequence using RT-PCR or isolation of DNA and amplification using PCR; (b) transcription of PCR products; and (c) separation of the proteins. The shorter protein products of mutated alleles are easily distinguished from the full-length protein products of the normal alleles.

DNA Microarrays (or DNA Chips). Microarrays have advantages over other methods because, in a single analysis, it is possible to evaluate the expression of all the genes that may be involved in cancer. By graphically showing the degree to which each gene is active in the cancer, DNA microarrays can generate a "genetic signature" for a particular cancer. This possibility makes the identification of cancer subtype more precise. The ability to take a snapshot of a cancer's genetic signature may lead to a better understanding of how that cancer develops and how treatment can be individualized (Pusztai, 2003).

5.2.3. Gene therapy approaches of brain cancer

Gene therapy (Lam and Breakefield, 2001; Castro et al., 2003) refers to the introduction of genes into a person's DNA in order to treat brain tumours. Gene therapy is an emerging medical technique that involves the addition of DNA to the human genome in order to replace a defective gene or to provide a gene that the body can use to fight disease.

Several strategies as well as other novel approaches have been attempted in the treatment of malignant gliomas (Williams and Baum, 2003). They are:

- delivery of prodrug-activating genes that confer sensitivity to toxic metabolites;
- replacement of tumour suppressor genes known to be deficient in gliomas usually resulting in tumour apoptosis;
- delivery of genes resulting in suppression of angiogenesis;
- delivery of genes resulting in activation of host antitumour immune responses;
- antisense cDNA delivery to regulate negatively tumour-related protein; and
- conditionally replicating viruses that selectively infect and destroy tumour cells.

Although these approaches significantly vary in strategy, they all share a common goal: *to deliver the therapeutic gene or virus efficiently and specifically to the targeted tissue.*

5.2.4. Ex vivo versus in vivo

Gene therapy can be distinguished into two categories: ex vivo, in which cells are modified outside the body and then transplanted back, and in vivo, in which genes are changed in cells that are still in the body. The ex vivo approach was the first to be applied. In this approach, cells are removed from a patient's tumourous area and incubated with vectors (carriers) to introduce genes.

For in vivo techniques, the challenge of inserting genes is greater. Here, vectors have a more difficult task to complete. They must deliver genes to enough cells so as to have an effect. They have to remain undetected by the body's immune system and they must deliver genes into a precise spot on the genome for the body to properly produce desired proteins.

5.2.5. Vector systems

Vectors (Basillion et al., 2000; Martinez et al., 2002) are mechanisms that allow genes to be carried into the genome. Modified cells are then transplanted back into their host, where it is hoped that they will replace defective genes to correct protein problems.

Viral Vectors. Much hope has been placed on viruses to carry DNA for gene therapy. Viruses normally alter cells' DNA in order to reproduce. Common viral vectors are:

- adenovirus;
- adenoassociated virus;
- Epstein–Barr virus;
- HSV;
- papova virus;
- vaccinia virus;
- retrovirus;
- lenti virus; and
- hybrid viral vectors.

The most important viral vectors are: retroviruses and adenoviruses. retroviruses are small RNA-based viruses. They reproduce by integrating their RNA into a host's DNA. For gene therapy, scientists modify these viruses' genetic code so that none of their natural proteins are produced, meaning that they cannot replicate and damage a host. Because retroviruses target fast-growing cells, they are especially promising for possible cancer treatments. Adenoviruses are larger DNA-based viruses. They can hold more genes and are not limited to just targeting fast-dividing cells. However, their larger size makes them more difficult to manipulate.

A significant problem affecting all virus-based vectors relates to the recognition by the immune system. When familiar viruses are detected in the bloodstream, the body sends antibodies to bind to and consume them. A second problem relates to the unpredictability of where viruses will insert genes into a person's DNA. If genes are inserted in the wrong place, then they may not be expressed. Additionally, gene insertion could cause diseases, such as cancer, by adversely affecting the function of nearby genes. Thus, the insertion of genes using viral vectors can cause cells to behave irregularly and dangerously.

Non-Viral Vectors. Researchers are also examining non-viral vectors such as nanoparticles that can deliver therapeutic genes. Scientists are also considering introducing an extra chromosome into cells. Alongside existing DNA, this additional chromosome could contain therapeutic genes. Introduced into the body as a large vector, it should not be targeted by the immune system. Commonly used non-viral vectors are:

- DNA–polylysine complexes;
- liposomes;
- lipofectin;
- ligand-targeted liposomes; and
- hybrid viral and nonviral vectors.

Researchers are also examining non-viral vectors such as nanoparticles that can deliver therapeutic genes. Scientists are also considering introducing an extra chromosome into cells. Alongside existing DNA, this additional chromosome could contain therapeutic genes. Introduced into the body as a large vector, it should not be targeted by the immune system.

As mentioned above, there are several strategies used in gene therapy of brain tumours. These belong to the general principles that scientists follow and are given below:

- Immunomodulation by gene therapy;
- Apoptosis-inducing genes;
- Blocking angiogenesis; and
- Oncolytic viruses.

Therapeutic genes for brain tumour treatment based on the approaches above are summarized in Table 2.

Gene therapy cannot be considered as the “magic wand” approach in brain cancer treatment. There is a lot that has to be done yet. One of the most promising issues is not only the generation of even more accurate gene carriers, but also the invention of specific therapeutic genes for individualized treatment. These two issues become crucial due to the complexity of the brain compared to other tissues of the human body.

Several brain cancer gene expression datasets (Microarray) are already published. The most important ones are shown in Table 3.

6. CONCLUSIONS

Brain cancer is the leading cause of death from cancer in children and the second leading cause of death from cancer in general. In adults, brain cancer is proportionately less common than other cancers, yet it accounts for a disproportionate percentage of deaths from cancer. The molecular events that are crucial for normal development and function are similar between individuals. However, in brain cancer, genetic and epigenetic alterations

Table 2. Genomic based therapies and therapeutic genes

Strategy	Therapeutic genes
Immunomodulation	Cytokine genes such as *IL-2*, *Il-4*, *IL-12*, *GM-CSF*
Induction of apoptosis	*p53*, *p16*, *PTEN*, *p21*
	BAX
	hREC2
	Caspase-8
Blocking angiogenesis	Angiostatin, Endostatin
Oncolytic viruses	HSV γ34.5 minus
	RR-minus
	Ad E1B-minus

result in cascades of deregulated molecular events, which lead to genetically complex, highly individual tumours.

Primary brain tumours are among the most lethal of all cancers, largely as a result of their lack of responsiveness to current therapy. Numerous new therapies hold great promise for the treatment of patients with brain cancer, but the main challenge is to determine which treatment is most likely to benefit an individual patient. DNA-microarray-based techniques (clustering and classification), which allow simultaneous analysis of expression of thousands of genes, have already begun to uncover previously unrecognized patient subsets that differ in their survival.

The fact that DNA microarrays can be used to detect molecular subsets that differ in survival indicates that it will soon be possible to develop gene-based predictors of therapeutic response. DNA microarrays might also facilitate the functional analysis of new anti-cancer compounds and the identification of novel biomarkers and molecular-imaging probes.

The genomic revolution is transforming clinical medicine. Instead of the present model of population risk assessment and empirical treatment, we will move to one of predictive individualized care based on molecular classification and targeted therapy for brain cancer. Advanced pharmacogenetics and recent gene therapy approaches provide this option.

It is possible to imagine a day in the not-too-distant future when serum biomarkers and molecular-imaging probes that are identified by DNA microarrays will be used for screening or early detection. Tumours will undergo microarray analysis to identify pathway alterations that point to the most beneficial therapy, and response to therapy will be monitored using molecular imaging probes and/or serum biomarkers.

Although this future is not too far away, today's clinical medicine must benefit from the revolution in genomics. Traditional medical practices and state of the art biomedical approaches (DNA microarrays and nanotechnologies), offer the possibility to discover new paths in genomic-based medicine and lead to personalized healthcare.

Table 3. Published brain cancer Microarray datasets

Dataset name[1]	Description	Array type[2]	Samples[3]	Total probes[4]	Refseq genes[5]	Reference[6]
Nutt	Oligodendroglioma–glioblastoma	Affymetrix	50	12624	12000	Nutt et al. (2003)
Khatua	Astrocytoma	Affymetrix	13	12626	8257	Khatua et al. (2003)
Pomeroy	brain tumours	Affymetrix	90	7129	5418	Pomeroy et al. (2002)
Rickman	Glioma	Affymetrix	51	7069	5418	Rickman et al. (2001)
Macdonald	medulloblastoma	Affymetrix	31	2059	1309	MacDonald et al. (2001)
Ramaswamy	tumour, normal	Affymetrix	255	16063	9528	Ramaswamy et al. (2001)

[1] The brief title that is used to refer to the dataset in our data base.

[2] The array type (Affymetrix GeneChip or two-color spotted microarray).

[3] The number of samples (microarrays) in the dataset.

[4] The total number of probes on the microarray design used.

[5] The number of unique RefSeq genes represented on the array that were included for analysis. This is usually much lower than the number of probes because many probes do not refer to RefSeq genes, and a gene could be represented by more than one probe. For Affymetrix data sets, "probe" refers more precisely to "probe sets" while for spotted microarrays it refers to a spot.

[6] The reference for each dataset.

REFERENCES

Abdullah, N.D. and V.P. Mathews, 1999, Contrast issues in brain tumour imaging. Neuroimaging Clin. N. Am., 9(4), 733–749.

Aliferis, C.F., I. Tsamardinos and A. Statnikov, 2003, HITON: A novel markov blanket algorithm for optimal variable selection, AMIA Annu. Symp. Proc., Nashville, 21–25.

Alizadeh, A.A., M.B. Eisen, R.E. Davis, C. Ma, I.S. Lossos, A. Rosenwald, J.C. Boldrick, H. Sabet, T. Tran, X. Yu, J.I. Powell, L. Yang, G.E. Marti, T. Moore, J. Hudson Jr., L. Lu, D.B. Lewis, R. Tibshirani, G. Sherlock, W.C. Chan, T.C. Greiner, D.D. Weisenburger, J.O. Armitage, R. Warnke, R. Levy, W. Wilson, M.R. Grever, J.C. Byrd, D. Botstein, P.O. Brown and L.M. Staudt, 2000, Distinct types of diffuse large B-cell lymphoma identified by gene expression profiling. Nature, 403(6769), 503–511.

Alter, O., P.O. Brown and D. Botstein, 2000, Singular value decomposition for genome-wide expression data processing and modelling. Proc. Natl. Acad. Sci., 97(18), 10101–10106.

Ambroise, C. and G.J. McLachlan, 2002, Selection bias in gene extraction on the basis of microarray gene-expression data. PNAS, 99(10), 6562–6566.

Antipova, A., P. Tamayo and T. Golub, 2002, A strategy for oligonucleotide microarray probe reduction. Genome Biology, 3(12), research0073.1–0073.4.

Barkovich, A.J. 1992, Neuroimaging of pediatric brain tumours. Neurosurg. Clin., 3(4), 739–769.

Basilion, J.P., T. Ichikawa and E.A. Chiocca, 2000, Gene therapy of brain tumours: problems presented by physiological barriers. Neurosurg. Focus, 8(4), 1–7.

Bodey, B., S.E. Siegel and H.E. Kaiser, 2004, Molecular Makers of Brain Tumour Cells. Kluwer Academic Publishers, Dordrecht.

Bolstad, B.M., R.A. Irizarry, M. Astrand and T.P. Speed, 2003, A comparison of normalization methods for high density oligonucleotide array data based on variance and bias. Bioinformatics, 19(2), 185–193.

Breiman, L., J. Freidman, R. Olshen and C. Stone, 1984, Classification and Regression Trees. Wadsworth International Group, Belmont.

Carter, D.E., J.F. Robinson, E.M. Allister, M.W. Huff and R.A. Hegele, 2005, Quality assessment of microarray experiments. Clin. Biochem., 38(7), 639–642.

Castro, M.G., R. Cowen, I.K. Williamson, A. David, M.J.J. Dalmaroni, X. Yuan, A. Bigliaric, J.C. Williams, J. Hu and P. Lowenstein, 2003, Current and future strategies for the treatment of malignant brain tumours. Pharmacol. Therapeut., 98(1), 71–108.

Chuaqui, R.F., R.F. Bonner, C.J.M. Best, J.W. Gillespie, M.J. Flaig, S.M. Hewitt, J.L. Phillips, D.B. Krizman, M.A. Tangrea, M. Ahram, W.M. Linehan, V. Knezevic and M.R.E. Buck, 2002, Post-analysis follow-up and validation of microarray experiments. Nat. Genet. Supplement, 32(4) 509–514.

Cho, S.B. and H.H. Won, 2003, Machine Learning in DNA microarray analysis for cancer classification, First Asia-Pacific bioinformatics conference on Bioinformatics, Adelaide, Australia, pp. 189–198.

Davies, D.L. and D.W. Bouldin, 1979, A cluster separation measure. IEEE Trans. Pattern Anal., 1(4), 224–227.

Dayhoff, J.E. and J.M. DeLeo, 2001, Artificial neural networks: opening the black box. Cancer, 91(8) 1615–1635.

DeAngelis, L.M., 2001, Brain Tumours. N. Engl. J. Med., 344(2), 114–123.

Delbeke, D. 1999, Oncological applications of FDG PET imaging: brain tumours, colorectal cancer, lymphoma and melanomas. J. Nucl. Med., 40(4), 591–603.

Devos, A., S. van Huffel, A.W. Simonetti, M. van Der Graaf, A. Heerschap and L. Buydens, 2005, Section 8, Classification of brain tumours by pattern recognition of magnetic resonance imaging and spectroscopy data. In: A. Taktak (Ed.), A Multi-Perspective View on Outcome Prediction in Cancer. Elsevier Publishing Company.

Duda, R.O., P.E. Hart and D.G. Stork, 2001, Pattern Classification, 2nd ed. John Wiley and Sons, New York.

Dudoit, S., J. Fridlyand and T.P. Speed, 2002, Comparison of discrimination methods for the classification of tumours using gene expression data. J. Am. Stat. Assoc., 97(457), 77–87.

Dunn, J., 1974, Well separated clusters and optimal fuzzy partitions. J. Cybernetics, 4(3), 95–104.

Eisen, M., P. Spellman, P. Brown and D. Botstein, 1998, Cluster analysis and display of genome-wide expression patterns. PNAS, 95(25), 14863–14868.

Friedman, N., D. Geiger and M. Goldszmidt, 1997, Bayesian network classifiers. Mach. Learn., 29(2), 131–163.

Godard, S., G. Getz, M. Delorenzi, P. Farmer, H. Kobayashi, I. Desbaillets, M. Nozaki, A.C. Diserens, M.F. Hamou, P.Y. Dietrich, L. Regli, R.C. Janzer, P. Bucher, R. Stupp, N. de Tribolet, E. Domany and M.E. Hegi, 2003, Classification of human astrocytic gliomas on the basis of gene expression: a correlated group of genes with angiogenic activity emerges as a strong predictor of subtypes. Cancer Res., 15(63), 6613–6625.

Golub, T.R., D.K. Slonim, P. Tamayo, C. Huard, M. Gaasenbeek, J.P. Mesirov, H. Coller, M. Loh, J.R. Downing, M.A. Caligiuri, C.D. Bloomfield and E.S. Lander, 1999, Molecular classification of cancer: class discovery and class prediction by gene expression monitoring. Science, 286(5439), 531–537.

Gray, J.W. and C. Collins, 2000, Genome changes and gene expression in human solid tumours. Carcinogenesis, 21(3), 443–452.

Guyon, I., J. Weston, S. Barnhill and V. Vapnik, 1999, Gene selection for cancer classification using Support Vector Machines. Mach. Learn., 64(1), 389–422.

Hastie, T., R. Tibshirani, M.B. Eisen, A. Alizadeh, R. Levy, L. Staudt, W.C. Chan, D. Botstein and P. Brown, 2000, "Gene shaving" as a method for identifying distinct sets of genes with similar expression patterns. Genome Biol., 1(2), research 0003.1–03.21.

Herwig, R., A.J. Poustka, C. Muller, C. Bull, H. Lehrach and J. O'Brien, 1999, Large-scale clustering of cDNA-fingerprinting data. Genome Res., 9(11), 1093–10105.

Hilton, A.D. and C. Melling, 2004, Genetic markers in the assessment of intrinsic brain tumours. Current Diagnostic Pathol., 10(2), 83–92.

Hubert, L. and J. Schultz, 1976, Quadratic assignment as a general data-analysis strategy. Br. J. Mat. Stat. Psychol., 29, 190–241.

Hustinx, R. and A. Alavi, 1999, SPECT and PET imaging of brain tumours. Neuroimaging Clin. N. Am., 9(4), 751–766.

Jiang, R.C., P.Y. Pu, J. Xu, S.Z. Yu, B.H. Jiao, Z. Guo, X. Li and C.S. Kang, 2002, Preliminary analysis on the gene expression profiles of different types of gliomas with cDNA array. Ai Zheng, 21(10), 1085–1089.

Karzynski, M., A. Mateos, J. Herrero and J. Dopazo, 2003, Using a genetic aalgorithm and a perceptron for feature selection and supervised class learning in DNA microarray data. Artif. Intell. Rev., 20(1), 39–51.

Khatua, S., K.M. Peterson, K.M. Brown, C. Lawlor, M.R. Santi, B. LaFleur, D. Dressman, D.A. Stephan and T.J. MacDonald, 2003, Overexpression of the EGFR/FKBP12/HIF-2alpha pathway identified in childhood astrocytomas by angiogenesis gene profiling. Cancer Res., 15(63), 1865–1870.

Kim, S., E.R. Dougherty, L. Shmulevich, K.R. Hess, S.R. Hamilton, J.M. Trent, G.N. Fuller and W. Zhang, 2002, Identification of combination gene sets for glioma classification. Mol. Cancer Ther., 1(13), 1229–1236.

Lam, P.Y.P. and X.O. Breakefield, 2001, Potential of gene therapy for brain tumours. Hum. Mol. Gen., 10(7), 777–787.

Lee, H.K., A.K. Hsu, J. Sadjak, J. Qin and P. Pavlidis, 2004, Co expression Analysis of human genes across many microarray data sets. Genome Res., 14(6), 1085–1094.

Levin V.A., S.A. Leibel and P.H. Gutin, 2001, Neoplasms of the central nervous system. In V.T. DeVita Jr., S. Hellman and S.A. Rosenberg (Eds.), Cancer: Principles and Practice of Oncology, 6th ed. Lippincott Williams and Wilkins, Philadelphia, pp. 2100–2160.

Li, L., C. Weinberg, T. Darden and L. Pedersen, 2001, Gene selection for sample classification based on gene expression data: study of sensitivity to choice of parameters of the GA/KNN method. Bioinformatics, 17(12), 1131–1142.

MacDonald, J.T., M.K. Brown, B. Lafleur, K. Peterson, C. Lawlor, Y. Chen, J.R. Packer, P. Cogen and A.D. Stephan, 2001, Expression Profiling of medullolastoma: PDGFRA and the RAS/MARK pathway as therapeutic targets for metastatic disease. Nat. Gen., 29, 143–152.

Markert, J.M., C.M. Fuller, G.Y. Gillespie, J.K. Bubien, L.A. McLean, R.L. Hong, K. Lee, S.R. Gullans, T.B. Mapstone and D.J. Benos, 2001, Differential gene expression profiling in human brain tumours. Physiol. Genomics, 7(5), 21–33.

Martinez, A.R., I.A.M. Davila, A.H. Garcia, E.A. Gordova and H.A.B. Saldana, 2002, Gene therapy for cancer. Rev. Invest. Clin., 54(1), 56–67.

Misra, J., W. Schmitt, D. Hwang, Hsiao, L.L., S. Gullans, G. Stephanopoulos and G. Stephanopoulos, 2002, Interactive exploration of microarray gene expression patterns in a reduced dimension space. Genome Res., 12(7), 1112–1120.

Moreau, Y., F. de Smet, G. Thijs, K. Marchal and B. de Moor, 2002, Functional bioinformatics of microarray data: from expression to regulation, Proceedings of the IEEE, 90(11), 1722–1743.

Murthy, S.K., S. Kasif and S. Salzberg, 1994, A system for induction of oblique decision trees. J. Artif. Intell. Res., 2, 1–32.

Nayak, A., A.M. Ralte, M.C. Sharma, V.P. Singh, A.K. Mahapatra, V.S. Mehta, and S. Sarkar, 2004, p53 protein alterations in adult astrocytic tumours and oligodendrogliomas. Neuro. India, 52(2), 228–232.

Nutt, C., D.R. Mani, R.A. Betensky, P. Tamayo, J. Cairncross, C. Ladd, U. Pohl, C. Hartmann, M. McLaughlin, T. Batchelor, P. Black, A. Deimling, S. Pomeroy, T. Golub and D. Louis, 2003, Gene expression-based classification of malignant gliomas correlates better with survival than histological classification. Cancer Res., 63(7), 1602–1607.

Pomeroy, S.L., P. Tamayo, M. Gaasenbeek, L.M. Sturla, M. Angelo, M.E. McLaughlin, J.Y. Kim, L.C. Goumnerova, P.M. Black, C. Lau, J.C. Allen, D. Zagzag, J.M. Olson, T. Curran, C. Wetmore, J.A. Biegel, T. Poggio, S. Mukherjee, R. Rifkin, A. Califano, G. Stolovitzky, D.N. Louis, J.P. Mesirov, E.S. Lander and T.R. Golub, 2002, Prediction of central nervous system embryonal tumour outcome based on gene expression. Nature, 415(6870), 436–442.

Pusztai, L., M. Ayers, J. Stec and G. Hortobagyi, 2003, Clinical application of cDNA microarray in oncology. The Oncologist, 8(3), 252–258.

Quackenbush, J., 2002, Microarray data normalization and transformation. Nat. Genet. Supplement, 32(4), 496–501.

Quinlan, J.R., 1993, C4.5: Programs for Machine Learning. Morgan Kaufmann Publishers, San Francisco.

Ramaswamy, S. and T.R. Golub, 2002, DNA microarrays in clinical pncology. J. Clin. Oncol., 20(7), 1932–1941.

Ramaswamy, S., P. Tamayo, R. Rifkin, S. Mukherjee, C.H. Yeang, M. Angelo, C. Ladd, M. Reich, E. Latulippe, J.P. Mesirov, T. Poggio, W. Gerald, M. Loda, E.S. Lander and T. Golub, 2001, Multiclass cancer diagnosis using tumour gene expression signatures. PNAS, 98(26) 15149–15154.

Rickman, D.S., M.P. Bobek, D.E. Misek, R. Kuick, M. Blaivas, D.M. Kurnit, J. Taylor and S.M. Hanash, 2001, Distinctive molecular profiles of high-grade and low-grade gliomas based on oligonucleotide microarray analysis. Cancer Res., 61(18), 6885–6891.

Rousseeuw, P.J., 1987, Silhouettes: a graphical aid to the interpretation and validation of cluster analysis. J. Comp. App. Math., 20(1), pp. 53–65.

Sallinen, S., P.K. Sallinen, H.K. Haapasalo, H.J. Helin, P.T. Helen, P. Schrami, O. Kallioniemi and J. Kononen, 2000, Identification of differentially expressed genes in human gliomas by DNA microarray and tissue chip techniques. Cancer Res., 60(23), 6617–6622.

Shai, R., T. Shi, T.J. Kremen, S. Horvath, L.M. Liau, T.F. Cloughesy, P.S. Mischel and S.F. Nelson, 2003, Gene expression profiling identifies molecular subtypes of gliomas. Oncogene, 22(31), 4918–4923.

Shannon, W., R. Culverhouse and J. Duncan, 2003, Analyzing microarray data using cluster analysis. Pharmacogenomics, 4(1), 41–51.

Shipp, M.A., K.N. Ross, P. Tamayo, A.P. Weng, J.L. Kutok, R.C. Aguiar, M. Gaasenbeek, M. Angelo, M. Reich, G.S. Pinkus, T.S. Ray, M.A. Koval, K.W. Last, A. Norton, T.A. Lister, J. Mesirov, D.S. Neuberg, E.S. Lander, J.C. Aster and T.R. Golub, 2002, Diffuse large B-cell lymphoma outcome prediction by gene-expression profiling and supervised machine learning. Nat. Med., 8(1), 68–74.

Tamayo, P., D. Slonim, J. Mesirov, Q. Zhu, S. Kitareewan, E. Dmitrovsky, E. Lander and T. Golub, 1999, Interpreting patterns of gene expression with self-organizing maps. PNAS, 96(6), 2907–2912.

Tan, A. and D. Gilbert, 2003, Ensemble machine learning on gene expression data for cancer classification. Applied Bioinformatics, 2(3), 75–83.

Tibshirani, R., G. Walther and T. Hastie, 2001, Estimating the number of clusters in the dataset via the GAP statistic. J. Roy. Stat. Soc., 63, 411–423.

Troyanskaya, O.G., M.E. Garber, P.O. Brown, D. Botstein and R.B. Altman, 2002, Nonparametric methods for identifying differentially expressed genes in microarray data. Bioinformatics, 18(11), 1454–1461.

van den Boom, J., M. Wolter, R. Kuick, D.E. Misek, A.S. Youkilis, D.S. Wechsler, C. Sommer, G. Reifenberger and S.M. Hanash, 2003, Characterization of gene expression profiles associated with glioma progression using oligonucleotide-based microarray analysis and real-time reverse transcription-polymerase chain reaction. Am. J. Pathol., 163(3), 1033–1043.

Vapnik,V. 1998, Statistical Learning Theory. John Wiley and Sons, New York.

Viks, G.I., R. Sharan and R. Shamir, 2003, Scoring clustering solutions by their biological relevance. Bioinformatics, 19(18), 2381–2389.

Wadlow, R. and S. Ramaswamy, 2005, DNA microarrays in clinical cancer research. Cur. Mol. Med., 5(1), 111–120.

Wang, J., T. Hellem, I. Jonassen, O. Myklebost and E. Hovig, 2003, Tumour classification and marker gene prediction by feature selection and fuzzy c-means clustering using microarray data. BMC Bioinformatics, 4(60), 1–12.

Wang, Y., Y.V. Tetko, M.A. Hall, E. Frank, A. Facius, K.F.X. Mayer and H.W. Mewes, 2005, Gene selection from microarray data for cancer classification – a machine learning approach. Comput. Biol. Chem., 29(1), 37–46.

Watson, M.A., A. Perry, V. Budhjava, C. Hicks, W. Shannon and K. Rich, 2001, Gene expression profiling with oligonucleotide microarrays distinguishes World Health Organization (WHO) grade of oligodendrogliomas. Cancer Res., 61(5), 1825–1829.

Watson, M.A., D.H. Gutmann, K. Peterson, M.R. Chicoine, B.K. Kleinschmidt-DeMasters, H.G. Brown and A. Perry, 2002, Molecular characterization of human meningiomas by gene expression profiling using high-density oligonucleotide microarrays. Am. J. Pathol., 161(2), 665–672.

Williams, D.A. and C. Baum, 2003, Gene therapy – new challenges ahead. Science, 302(5644), 400–401.

Yang, Y.H. and T. Speed, 2002, Design issues for cDNA microarray experiments. Nat. Genet., 3(8), 579–588.

Yoon, K.S., M.C. Lee, S.S. Kang, J.H. Kim, S. Jung, Y.J. Kim, J.H. Lee, K.Y. Ahn, J.S. Lee and J.Y. Cheon, 2001, p53 mutation and epidermal growth factor receptor overexpression in glioblastoma. Korean Med. Sci., 16(4), 481–488.

Zhang, L., W. Zhou, V. Velculescu, S. Kern, R. Hruban, S. Hamilton, B. Vogelstein and K. Kinzler, 1997, Gene expression profiles in normal and cancer cells. Science, 276(5316), 1268–1272.

Section 5

Dissemination of Information

Chapter 14

The Web and the New Generation of Medical Information Systems

José Manuel Fonseca, André Damas Mora and Pedro Barroso

UNINOVA, Institute for the Development of New Technologies, Campus da FCT/UNL, Monte de Caparica, 2829-516 Caparica, Portugal
Email: jmf@uninova.pt
atm@uninova.pt
pnb@uninova.pt

Abstract

The advent of the Internet has allowed physicians, patients and other healthcare providers to access an unprecedented volume of information in an easy and cost-effective way. This new scenario opens up new frontiers to medical activity and changes the way physicians act with obvious repercussions on healthcare services, quality and effectiveness. However, despite the perspectives that information systems offer to healthcare professionals, their implementation is not easy. In fact, there are many difficult problems to overcome in the design of medical information systems for efficient knowledge extraction. The huge amount of information on patients accumulated in modern healthcare institutions is difficult to manage and often not as useful as it should be, because it is either inaccessible, too slow to be clinically used or too difficult to access justifying the need for more effective information management techniques and statistical analysis for knowledge discovery and extraction. The privacy of information required both for legal and ethical issues, and the quality and reliability of information are also important issues in this kind of systems. Also, in many real-world situations information is still kept on paper due to the unavailability of adequate computer support or to the traditional technophobia of many users, pushing the need for better, more appealing and user-friendly human interfaces. The interoperability of information between different healthcare institutions with different cultures and languages is another important problem that must be overcome by the use of adequate technology. New technologies such as mobile computing and wireless internet access also open up new frontiers in medical information systems by enabling the establishment of ubiquitous information networks that can be accessed virtually anywhere and anytime.

In this chapter, an overview of the state-of-the-art intelligent medical information systems are presented, the main problems in their development are identified and the currently adopted solutions are discussed. New trends in the next generation medical information systems are also pointed out.

The expected influence of the new generation intelligent medical information systems on cancer prediction, diagnosis and treatment is envisaged and related difficulties are identified.

Keywords: Internet, interoperability, medical information systems, electronic health record, web services.

Contents

© 2007 Elsevier B.V. All rights reserved

1. INTRODUCTION

The advent of Internet and its fast diffusion within the modern society, lead to a new world of opportunities that are progressively influencing the way healthcare is provided. The huge amount of scientific information currently available to everyone on the Internet, the possibility of sharing patient data and diagnostic tools, and the potential for the establishment of links both among physicians and between physicians and patients are not only creating new opportunities that can significantly improve the outcomes of cancer treatment but can also bring new problems and difficulties that must be identified and circumvented.

The Internet creates an "information highway" that can be used by different healthcare providers with different objectives. Figure 1 presents the main types of interaction that

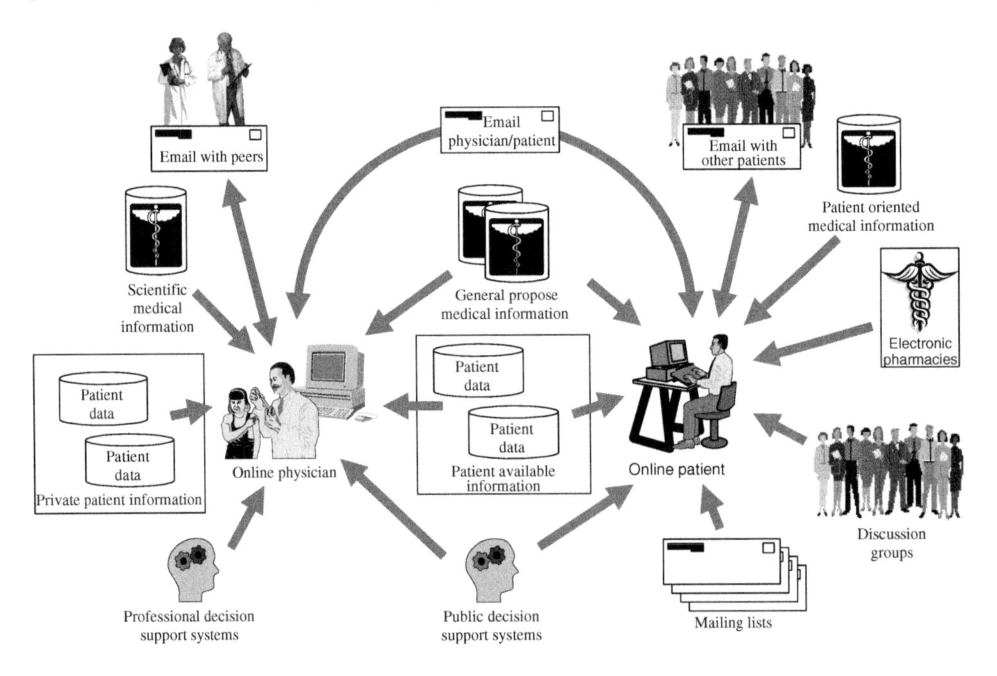

Fig. 1. Patient–physician internet-based interaction.

both physicians and patients can establish using the Internet as a communication channel. Physicians can use it to search for information about patients if this information can be made available online and adequate search tools are available. However, patient information is highly sensitive and there are a large number of technical, legal and ethical questions that must be taken into account. Physicians can also use the Internet to have access to remote diagnostic tools (ADO (2005) is an example in the cancer area) to seek help in difficult situations where support from peers is required. However, at present a great number of patients are using the Internet to search for information about their diseases, to get support from other patients with similar problems and even to communicate with their doctors or to get alternative treatment programmes. This new reality is not only opening up new possibilities for the patients suffering from cancer but is also creating new problems to patients and healthcare professionals.

In this chapter, we discuss the influence of the Internet on patient behaviour and the advantages it can present for healthcare professionals. The support technologies for efficient data sharing are discussed. We present briefly the currently developing standards for data representation essential for the achievement of true interoperability between different entities, and the most promising technologies for system integration are discussed.

2. PATIENTS ONLINE

According to Internet World Stats (IWS, 2005), 14.9% of the 6 420 102 722 world population (2005 estimation) is using the Internet at present. It means that 957 753 672 persons are now online corresponding to a growth of 165.3% in the period 2000–2005. However, penetration rate is clearly unbalanced across different continents: Africa is the continent with a lower penetration rate (2.7%), Middle East, Asia and Latin America follow next (8.2, 9.0 and 12.9%, respectively), and Europe, Oceania/Australia and North America are the continents with a higher penetration rate (37.4, 52.8 and 68.1%, respectively). However, the continents with a lower penetration rate are registering an impressive growth in user numbers with Africa growing at 428.7% during the period 2000–2005. Also, Middle East and Latin America registered an impressive growth during this period (305.4 and 291.31%, respectively). Even the continents with a high penetration rate such as North America and Oceania registered an impressive growth during the last five-year period (107.0 and 131.7%).

The numbers clearly show that the number of Internet users is already very high and is increasing significantly. However, how many of these are affected by cancer? With more than 10 million new cases every year, cancer has become one of the most devastating diseases worldwide (Stewart and Kleihues, 2003). According to the figures from the Morbidity and Mortality Weekly Report of the Centers for Disease Control and Prevention (CDCP, 2005), 9.8 million persons lived with cancer of some type in the United States during 2001 representing 3.5% of the population. Even if we reduce this number to 2% of the population due to the lower incidence of cancer in underdeveloped countries, we have approximately 128 million cancer patients.

Assuming that 14.9% of the world population is online, we can assume that about 19 million cancer patients are online worldwide. However, these figures can be influenced by many factors. The average age of cancer patients is higher than the average age of the overall population. Since Internet use is higher among the younger population, we can estimate that the number of online cancer patients might be lower. However, we can also argue that the percentage of population affected by cancer is higher in developed countries where Internet access is more common and therefore the previous number might be underestimated. In Eysenbach (2003), a study was conducted over several surveys in developed countries about the Internet usage by cancer patients. It concluded that about 39% of the cancer patients were Internet users. If we consider that a significant number of cancer patients are indirect Internet users by receiving information through relatives and friends we can estimate that the real percentage of patients relying on information from the Internet is even higher.

Of course, such a large market of very interested users (many cancer patients search the web for information about their disease and for alternative treatment plans) is attractive for business and vulnerable to false or misleading information.

The risks of misuse or misunderstanding of information downloaded from the Internet were promptly recognized by many influential institutions leading to several actions towards the warning and education of the users.

One of these efforts was conducted by the National Cancer Institute that developed a web page entitled "How to Evaluate Health Information on the Internet: Questions and Answers" (NCI, 2005), where some facts are identified to help users decide if the received information deserves credit or not. In this study, the absence of those responsible for the information, the non-identification of the sources of information, the need for the credentials of the authors and the privacy of the personal data of the users are identified as the main points to be checked by the users when visiting each website. Many other web pages dedicated to cancer also notify their visitors about the importance of information credibility.

The Internet can be used by cancer patients in at least four different ways: for communication with other patients or physicians using e-mail messages, instant messaging or voice over internet protocol (VoIP); for content retrieval by searching web pages and documents related to their disease; for community activities such as bulletin board systems, mailing lists, newsgroups, chat rooms and websites with community facilities and for e-commerce buying products and services online.

2.1. Communication with other patients and physicians

Surprisingly, it is not the huge number of web pages and the enormous quantity of information available on the Internet that a large proportion of Internet users identify as the main reason to be online (Fox and Fallows, 2003). In the USA, 93% of the web users use e-mail, 83% have searched for a product or service before buying it and 80% have searched for health information. The billions of e-mail messages exchanged every day are a testimony to the importance e-mail is assuming for the Internet users, even if a large number of the e-mail messages are currently spam many of those health related selling vitamins, penis enlargement and breast augmentation drugs, Viagra, etc.

E-mail messages are an asynchronous communication tool meaning that the message is sent and will be received by the receiver when he is available. Also, the reply can be written whenever the receiver wants, without any time limit set by the originator. Using e-mail, cancer patients can keep in touch with friends and relatives in an inexpensive way, exchange files containing health information or any other kind of information. E-mail can also be used for receiving information from special interest groups that periodically issue electronic newsletters with technical articles and replies to questions from registered users. In a recent study, cancer patients demonstrated that by joining mailing lists they were mainly looking for information about treatment, coping with side effects and treatment options (Rimer et al., 2005).

Of course, e-mail can also be used to communicate with physicians. Many patients declare that they would like to be in touch with their physicians through e-mail, according to Cyber-Dialogue (2000). About 48% of the people surveyed in 1999 wanted to communicate with their physicians through e-mail, although very few have already done so. In a survey of the American College of Physicians–American Society of Internal Medicine (Lacher et al., 2000), 82% of the physicians used computers but only 7% reported weekly use of e-mail with their patients. There are also many reasons for this: lack of time to read and answer the large number of messages they would receive if they open their e-mail to a larger community of patients, fear for the large unpaid task that would be the answering all the e-mails from their patients, the obligation of continuous monitoring of the mailbox and the problem of introducing it in their daily routine, concerns about liability, security and privacy of the messages and the preference for a face-to-face interaction with patients. Also, studies demonstrate that e-mail is used in addition to traditional services, not as a replacement, reducing the number of office visits but not the number of telephone consultations (Bergmo et al., 2005). However, e-mail is considered by some physicians as a new opportunity to get in close touch with patients, re-establishing a personal relationship that was removed by the compressed office visit that characterizes modern medicine (Morasch, 2000). Also in a study involving head and neck cancer patients, 83% of the patients declared that being able to contact care providers by electronic means had provided them an additional feeling of security (van den Brink et al., 2005). Therefore, the question does not seem to be *will they?* or *won't they?* but *when* and *how* physicians will use e-mail as a communication channel with their patients due to the advantages it can have to both.

Instant messaging is another way of contacting other people on the Internet. Being interactive and near real-time can provide cancer patients with a feeling of proximity to other patients, comparable to telephone contact. However, this is usually a time consuming communication that will be difficult to establish between patients and physicians. Nowadays, VoIP is of acceptable quality but this is mainly a replacement for the traditional phone calls with a reduced cost.

2.2. Searching information on the web

At present, the web is being widely used for health information search. In USA, 80% of the Internet users have already searched for at least one health topic (Fox and Fallows, 2003). Supposing that this picture is not very different for the rest of the world, we can have an idea about the importance of the web for the healthcare sector. On their study based on a survey of telephone interviews between 25 November and 22 December 2002, among a sample of 2038 adults aged 18 or above, Fox and Fallows (2003) concluded that the internet users search, among other things, for:

- health information at any time of the day or night;
- research diagnosis or prescriptions;
- prepare for surgery or to find the best way to recover from one;
- get tips from other caregivers and e-patients about dealing with a particular symptom;
- give and receive emotional support;
- keep family and friends informed of a loved one's condition; and
- find humour and even joy in a bad situation.

It is important to mention that although a large percentage of users have already searched the web for health information, they do it rarely. They usually do it just when they or some relative or friend have a health problem. On a typical day, 49% of the users use e-mail, 19% research a product or service and just 6% look for medical information. Also interesting is that more than half of those who recently conducted medical searches did so on-behalf of someone else. An important finding of this study is that users are increasingly going to disease-specific support sites and using e-mail to discuss health issues with more than half of the patients visiting specific diseases sites. In consequence of the higher level of information obtained, patients declared that their relationship with doctors changed (not always for better). Moreover, 70% said the web information influenced their decision about how to treat an illness or condition, 50% said the web information led them to ask a doctor new questions or get a second opinion from another doctor and 28% said the web information affected their decision about whether or not to visit a doctor (Fox and Rainie, 2000).

During July 2005, 4.5 billion information searches were done in the USA (SEW, 2005). Google has a 46.2% share with Yahoo on the second place (22.5%) and MSN the third (12.6%). Since according to Eysenbach and Köhler (2003), approximately 4.5% of all searches on the web might be health related we have a rough estimate of 200 million searches for health-related information only in July in the USA. As more than 50% of the traffic of Google is from outside the USA (Google, 2005) we can deduce that at least 400 million health-related searches are done every month worldwide. But a convenient search of the billions of pages currently available on the Internet is not an easy task. In fact, many doctors discourage patients and their support persons to search the web due to the possibility of getting erroneous or confusing information. The appeal of a "miraculous" alternative cancer treatment plan or drug available on a web page is clear when compared with a realistic treatment plan proposed by the physician. However, it can have positive economical effects for the vendor and disastrous consequences for the patient's health.

To overcome this problem, some institutions are already offering training classes to consumers and patients. One example is the Princess Margaret Hospital in Canada that developed a patient education calendar that includes a regular event on "Surfing: Finding Health Information on the Internet" for patients with cancer (UHN, 2005).

One of the main reasons for the low quality of information found on the web is the huge marketplace it is nowadays. Despite this, the number of cancer patients that buy health products or services online is unknown and it is clear that many websites visited by them are commercially motivated and information is obviously biased. Therefore, great care must be taken when considering this information. However, a considerable amount of information is provided by non-profit organizations with high scientific credibility.

Another problem that can influence the utility of information for cancer patients around the world is the predominance of the English language that is certainly an obstacle for many non-English speaking users. Finally, the lack of a common medical ontology also decreases the utility of generic World Wide Web (WWW) search engines and can also contribute to the confusion of the patient (Walczak, 2003).

Anyway, it is increasingly unlikely that health professionals will encounter patients who have not used information technology to influence their health knowledge, health behaviour, perception of symptoms and illness behaviour (Eysenbach, 2000). The twenty-first century will be the age of the net-empowered medical end user. Today's patient-driven online support networks will evolve into more robust and capable medical guidance systems that will allow end users to direct and control an ever growing portion of their own medical care (Ferguson, 2002).

2.3. Community activities

Social isolation is one of the main risk factors for cancer patients (HealthyPlace, 2005). Receiving a cancer diagnosis is often traumatic, causing emotional upset, sadness, anxiety and other negative consequences. After an initial two-week period of great abatement, patients usually start to recover to achieve normal functioning after about one month. If this does not happen, the patient must be evaluated for clinical depression (with a 25% incidence on cancer patients) (HealthyPlace, 2005). Depression can significantly affect the physical wellbeing of a cancer patient interfering with the treatment, increase the length of hospital stay, reduce the ability to care for oneself, impair the quality of life and possibly reduce the overall survival time (Straker, 1998). The psychological conditions of the patient are so important that faith and belief are identified as important factors for cancer outcome (Sherman et al., 2001).

In order to avoid depressive situations or to recover from them, it is recognized that family and friends can help significantly by encouraging the depressed person to seek or remain in treatment and fight against adversity. Participation in a support group is also considered to be of substantial importance for many patients (Rimer et al., 2005). However, the face-to-face imposed by group therapy support groups is usually difficult for patients in weak psychological (and sometimes physical) conditions. The integration of web-based discussion and support groups is much easier because no physical contact is required and the patient can participate by receiving and giving opinions and advices from the comfort of his home. In October 2005, Yahoo quoted "depression" as one of the six most popular groups on the Health session. In September 2005, in a joint effort with the American Cancer Society, Yahoo created a 30-day *Blog for Hope* event where celebrities and public figures shared insights and personal stories of how cancer has affected their lives, in an effort to connect individuals in the fight against cancer. At the same time 2755 cancer-related discussion groups were registered on Yahoo (446 groups with 100 or more members). Also, Google reports 2080 support groups on cancer and many other groups are provided by official and non-official institutions and private organizations.

Chat rooms with live interaction between the participants are also available in non-profit organizations such as BMT Support Online (BMT, 2005) or The Cancer Survivors Network (CSN, 2005) with caregivers and peer groups meeting regularly with a pre-defined schedule where patients can interact with other patients and with specialists to get advice and support. Internet-mediated support may be especially important for minorities, geographically isolated people, suffering from less common cancers, and people in rural areas because of documented disparities in their access to healthcare and health information (Rimer et al., 2005).

2.4. Buying products and services online

Internet has revolutionized the sale of medicines so that consumers can self-select and buy medicines, often delivered across national and state boundaries, without face-to-face interaction (Bessel et al., 2003). Many certified e-pharmacies are currently available on the Internet but an important number of illegal drug sellers are also operating on the web. E-pharmacies look appealing to consumers because they save trips to doctors, never have long waits in line and often offer reduced prices. Moreover, some offer private e-mail additionally to discuss medications with a druggist, tools for checking interactions with other drugs, e-mail refill reminders, and tools for tracking and viewing past orders. Some sites such as Drugstore.com (DStore, 2005) are associated with a pharmacy chain (Rite Aid (RAC, 2005) in this case) for giving customers the option of having the prescription filled at the local pharmacy where they can pick it up faster and safer.

But e-pharmacies pose many problems. In the opinion of many experts, Internet pharmacies display a disregard for the health of those buying from their websites. It is possible to buy prescription-only medicines on their sites (such as weight-loss drugs and anti-depressants) with little or no diagnosis or promise of follow-up care, making it easy for people to get their hands on powerful drugs. Usually, there is no address to write to or a phone number to complain, putting customers in limbo when they want to complain. Often there are no assurances that the doctors who prescribe the drugs are authentic or that the personal data about the patient is protected. Nor are the drugs they offer always safe or genuine. Situations where drugs are outdated, contaminated, too potent or not potent enough, improperly manufactured and handled or counterfeit are mentioned regularly in the news (FDA, 2005).

In general, to be valid, a prescription must address a legitimate medical purpose, be written by a physician or other healthcare provider authorized to prescribe medicine, and be based on a legitimate doctor–patient relationship. But some websites dispense drugs after customers simply fill out an online questionnaire or engage in some other similar cyber "consultation". This is an unacceptable situation that can create significant health problems to consumers.

Through the heavy e-mail spam that is now on the Internet, the offer of all kinds of drugs and miraculous treatments for any disease (cancer included) is such that virtually no Internet user can stay ahead of it. The main target of this commerce is people who have chronic health problems and need medications delivered regularly, and buyers who do not have medical insurance who use e-pharmacies to shop for the best deals.

Cancer patients are obviously potential clients for this kind of commerce, especially when miraculous results are promised to emotionally weakened persons. As an example, in June 2004, the US Food and Drug Administration announced the sentencing of a man who swindled cancer patients by heavily advertising and selling Laetrile, also known as vitamin B-17 or apricot pits. Although he announced it to be a dietary supplement, Laetrile is actually an unapproved drug. The highly toxic product has not shown any effect on treating cancer (FDA, 2005). Another example is the warning letter issued by FDA to the Cellular Wellness Foundation in September 2004, citing claims made on its website that the product Cellular Tea was effective in treating serious diseases such as cancer (FDA, 2005).

2.5. Accessing the Electronic Health Record (EHR) online

Since in many countries patients have the right to access their personal health record, the availability of Electronic Health Records (EHRs) to patients seems inevitable. In a recent survey (Pyper et al., 2004), 73.8% of the patients responded that they know that they have the right to see their health records but only very few (4.5%) have done so. Despite this, 79% considered it a good idea to make health records electronic and 66% believe that the advantages of electronic records outweigh the disadvantages (23.1% did not have any opinion) approximately one-half were afraid about security (50.4%). It is also important to mention that only 56.4% believed that it would be easy to understand their health records. Patients identified several benefits from accessing their own health records: better understanding of their health, easier plan of consultations, easier communication with their doctors and better decisions about their own health. The main concerns were security, cost, the need for keeping technology up to date, the distraction of addressing EHR from more important health issues, the inability in using computers and the content being frightening.

The development of adequate platforms for EHR access of patients can introduce a new dimension to the health record analysis by the patients. The support given to the patient can be greatly improved with adequate links for explanation of the scientific names and contents, with different views of information depending on the profile of the user and other support techniques that will certainly improve the usefulness and the diffusion of the health record visualization by the patients. Another important factor is the availability of decision support tools that are designed for physicians but are also made available for patients. Such decision aids can influence decisively the attitudes of the patients reinforcing the recommendations or stimulating the conflict with the doctors leading to self-medication attitudes that can negatively influence the outcome of serious diseases such as cancer (Eysenbach, 2000).

3. ELECTRONIC HEALTH RECORD

The *health record* (HR) is considered by most of the people to be the history of the care they received from various clinicians. However, this same expression may be applied in different ways depending on the healthcare practitioners providing the care.

3.1. Healthcare records history

In earlier times, paper-based techniques for recording and keeping medical information were well accepted by caregivers and their patients. During that time, most people had a single physician (a General Practitioner or family doctor) over many years and much of their medical history resided in physician's memory or was kept in physician's own healthcare record. There was no integration of the data collected by various clinicians that had contact with the patient. Therefore, a patient was most likely to have many different HRs.

The traditional paper-based HR had served as a starting point for the conception of all current versions of Electronic Health Record (EHR). Because currently the medical practice is more complex and sophisticated involving many healthcare providers, greater mobility of citizens, complex medical examinations and others, an adequate patient information system is required.

The paper-based HR has become an obsolete way of medical care delivery. Some examples of its importance are the number of evitable medical errors that produced patient death (according to Kohn et al. (2000) more people die from medical mistakes each year than from highway accidents, breast cancer, or AIDS), the need for laboratorial analysis just because earlier tests were not available (Tierney et al., 1987), prescription errors which are potentially life threatening (Barker et al., 2002), increase in health insurance costs (Balabanova, 2004) and others. Therefore, a redefinition of current health records is an urgent need.

3.2. Today's health record

The lack of access to up-to-date information, the limited time for research and the poor information organization, are some examples of knowledge dissemination barriers clinicians face everyday. Significant progress on healthcare quality would be achieved if new information could be quickly and efficiently delivered to all clinical working places, such as hospitals, clinics and doctors' offices.

An EHR is a computer-based health record that embraces all information, clinical and administrative, including practitioners of all specialities involved in a patient healthcare over his lifetime from prenatal to post-mortem.

To have an idea about the change of paper-based to computer-based health record, Geiger et al. (1995) from Toronto University made a guideline to develop a strategic plan to implement an EHR. The report mentioned that of the 143 in-patients records, 18 654 physical pages were found using 165 different forms. The average for each patient was 130–569 pages, containing 26 different forms. The duplication of data fields within actual charts followed a pattern similar to the duplication found on the forms. The duplication magnitude seen, leaves little doubt that significant amount of time could be saved with appropriate modification of health-care delivery processes. This study demonstrated that hospital charts contained many copies of the same information, such as medication lists, allergies, etc. Due to manual replication of data fields, there is no mechanism to ensure that each copy within a chart actually contains the same information.

The benefits of adopting EHRs are obvious. Using HER systems, healthcare entities can enhance patient care, reduce medical errors and minimise paper-handling costs. However, the development of HER systems without any kind of standards lead to heterogeneous systems unable to share information between them.

To achieve a truly interoperable scenario, there is a special need for standards that include system interoperability, ontologies and architecture. Based on a largely diffused HER, retrieval systems, using concepts and modifiers entered directly by clinicians or automatically by EHR systems, can display relevant information and provide links to support evidence and analysis.

3.3. Future of health records

Without a unifying standard, it requires an enormous effort to get contents, resources, methods and interfaces accessible worldwide. To amalgamate work, the definition of standards is essential. Information science must define standards of how to structure contents to get optimal performances in information retrieval, how to develop powerful search interfaces for professional users, how to integrate information from various sources into one reliable view and how to select the best resource to answer a particular question. In recent years, multidisciplinary medical informatics is focusing on important areas such as information, decision and computer science, biomedicine and psychology. Technology is the keyword for delivering up-to-date, well-structured, high-quality contents to clinicians' desktops. World Wide Web (WWW) has also enabled high-speed networks, standard protocols and cross-platform applications as important requirements for efficient EHR.

Each jurisdiction in Europe is moving from a fragmented situation to a comprehensive and cooperative deployment of e-health solutions based on interoperability standards. In the beginning of the 1990s, Europe decided that several subjects that required standards for health informatics would best be resolved on a European scale rather than at the national level (CEN, 2005). This position evolved in the creation of ISO-TC215 and the emergence of HL7 as an international standard. European Standard Development (CEN) has moved to a position of sharing and cooperation in the international community.

The grand vision for a future EHR is converging to EHR systems that are based on standard protocols for enabling the system's interoperability. The standards organizations involved in defining these healthcare-specific standards are mainly:

- ISO/TC 215 – health informatics;
- CEN/TC251 – European standard development;
- HL7 – clinical messaging standards (CDA and RIM based);
- *open*EHR – reference model and archetype approach;
- IEEE – medical device standards;
- DICOM – imaging standard.

3.4. Standard health records

The first question to be answered is "why the use of standards in healthcare?" The primary reason for the adoption of standards is the huge amount of data that is to be shared, and the different types and forms of this data. It is in fact important, even for economical reasons, to have both data and knowledge shared to achieve a successful and coordinated evolution in healthcare quality. According to the IEEE Standard Computer Dictionary (1990) interoperability is the "*ability of two or more systems or components to exchange information and to use the information that has been exchanged*". Only the adoption of data representation and communication standards can guarantee true interoperability between different medical entities.

Communication standards are increasingly important in healthcare systems. Without standards, there is the necessity of using two different interfaces for connecting each pair of healthcare systems, making information exchange between heterogeneous systems too expensive or even impossible. Solutions to this problem are being developed by several research groups (Standards Developing Organizations (SDOs) that are studying optimal ways to standardize these interoperability issues: International Standards Organization (ISO), Committee European Normalization (CEN) and Health Level 7 (HL7) are the most relevant. In the following sections, the main contributions for the establishment of standards for medical data representation are presented.

3.4.1. ISO/TC 215

The view of ISO/TC 215 Ad Hoc Group on Standards Requirements for the Electronic Health Record, is that EHR standards should be limited to the structure and function of the data and systems that process it (i.e. EHR systems) (Schloeffel and Jeselon, 2002). Using this view, EHR standards can be organized into several different groups within health informatics: the core EHR standards, standards for EHR-related services, EHR standards for specific purposes and finally EHR meta-standards.

The first group, *Core EHR standards*, includes standards for the structure and content of EHRs and the functionality and interoperability of EHR systems. The *EHR-related services* include the non-basic functionalities such as patient and clinician identification. *EHR standards for specific purposes* enclose standards for EHR systems related to specific technologies or standards for the record in particular, health sectors or concern groups. These last standards are so particular, that are avoidable whenever possible, since there is a high risk of incompatibility with basic EHR standards. Finally, *EHR meta-standards* contain a group of high-level standards.

Although ISO/TC 215 is already seven-year old, it is still considered a newcomer to health informatics standards. It is the most influential international standards body for EHR and other informatics standards. It was created with the following objective: "*Standardization in the field of information for health, and Health Information and Communications Technology (ICT) to achieve compatibility and interoperability between independent systems. Also, to ensure compatibility of data for comparative statistical purposes (e.g. classifications), and to reduce duplication of effort and redundancies*". Access control standardization would be an important feature of the standard, but it is very difficult and challenging because of the variety of current access control policies and procedures in different countries, jurisdictions and institutions. Despite these problems, the propagation of information technology in healthcare cannot achieve its full potential without interoperability, and that is why it is an urgent need for healthcare systems. An important help for this problem comes from the new technologies developed around the World Wide Web (WWW) bringing an entirely new environment for electronic data exchange.

Within the TC 215 working group, there are some developed standards that were produced from scratch such as ISO/TS 18308 "Requirements for an EHR Reference Architecture", but many others use existing standards from either national or international standards organizations as a basis for an ISO standard. Some of the organisations are Institute of Electrical and Electronics Engineers (IEEE), European Committee for Standardization (CEN), Health Level 7 (HL7) and Digital Imaging and Communication in Medicine (DICOM).

In addition to the EHR definition, scope and context technical report, there are a number of EHR standards, technical specifications and technical reports currently under development within TC 215. Some of them are:

- Architectural Requirements for EHR Systems – core EHR standard in early stage development as a de novo ISO standard.
- Identification of Subjects of Care – EHR-related service standard which is being developed based on the Australian Health Client Identification standard.
- Patient Health card Data: Limited Clinical Data – specific technology standard which is one of the eight health card standards, which are being adapted by ISO from their CEN equivalents.
- Framework for Emergency Data Sets – this is an EHR meta-standard being developed de novo within TC 215.

3.4.2. CEN/TC 251

If ISO is the most internationally known standard organisation, then CEN is the most-watched European standards organisation whose authority exceeds the national standards organisations of its 28 member countries – EU plus Norway, Switzerland and Iceland (CEN, 2005).

The scope of CEN/TC 251 is to create "*Standardization in the field of Health Information and Communications Technology (ICT) to achieve compatibility and interoperability between independent systems and to enable modularity. This includes requirements on health information structure to support clinical and administrative procedures, technical methods to support interoperable systems as well as requirements regarding safety, security and quality*".

The work is fragmented in four workgroups:

WGI – *information models* – whose scope is the development of European standards to facilitate communication between independent information systems within and between organisations, for health-related purposes;

WGII – *terminology and knowledge representation* – the objectives of this working group are the semantic organization of information and knowledge so as to have practical use in the domains of health informatics and telematics and the provision of information and criteria to support harmonisation. This encompasses clinical, managerial and operational aspects of the medical record and enabling access to other knowledge;

WGIII – *security, safety and quality* – it provides a legal structure to ensure that information systems used in healthcare have appropriate levels of quality, safety and security;

WGIV – *technology for interoperability* – the aim of this workgroup is to develop and promote standards that enable the interoperability of devices and information systems in health informatics.

CEN has two main taskforces developing EHR standards. The first is CEN13606 "*Electronic Health Record Communication*" which was originally published in 1999. According to Schloeffel (2004), it is still the only comprehensive EHR interoperability standard in the world. In 2001, a decision was taken by CEN to update 13606 and to adopt the *openEHR* archetype methodology. This revision would be done by CEN workgroups and also by members of *openEHR* foundation. CEN13606 should be a standard consisting of the Reference Model, Archetype Interchange Specification, Reference Archetypes and Term Lists, Security Features and Exchange Models. CEN has also predicted that the introduction of 13606 into ISO/TC 215 as the basis for the international EHR interoperability standard and this should be achieved by 2006.

Other CEN EHR standard in development for European norm is CEN12967 "*Health Informatics Service Architecture*" (HISA) which is a major revision of "Health Information Systems Architecture" published in 1998. HISA is a high-level service-based architecture, which is compatible with CEN 13606 and similar lower level standards such as HL7 CDA. The HISA standard will provide a reference model for healthcare information technology (IT) services, facilitating the creation and acquisition of interoperable systems. There are several other working standards within this organization related with health informatics such as: patient health card data, blood transfusion related messages, messages for maintenance of supporting information in healthcare systems, messages for the exchange of healthcare administrative information, messages for maintenance of supporting information in healthcare systems, international transfer of personal health data covered by the EU data protection directive – high-level security policy, etc.

3.4.3. HL7

Health Level Seven (HL7) is the most important US health informatics standard organization. In the last four years, its membership has tripled to over 1600 health industry members including most of the major healthcare information systems consultants and vendors and 90% of the healthcare system vendors. The HL7 standard, supported by most information system vendors, is at present being used in the majority of large US hospitals and in many other countries (HL7, 2005). In the beginning it was concerned only with messaging standards, but in the recent years it also became involved in standardization of decision support tools, terminology and ontology.

HL7 is an ANSI-accredited not-for-profit voluntary organization, whose mission is to provide standards inside healthcare organizations for the exchange, integration, sharing and retrieval of electronic health information; support clinical practice; and support the management, delivery and evaluation of health services. This standard makes possible the transfer of laboratory results, pharmacy data and other information between heterogeneous computer systems.

HL7 standards domain is within clinical and administrative data, while other standard developing organizations are involved in other areas like medical devices, imaging, pharmacy, etc. As a not-for-profit organization, its members (providers, vendors, payers, consultants, government groups and others) develop the standards. A frequent misunderstanding about HL7 is that it produces and develops software. The most widely used HL7 standard is a messaging standard that enables heterogeneous healthcare applications to exchange clinical and administrative data (HL7, 2005).

The name "Health Level Seven" is related with the *application level* of Open System Interconnection (OSI), the highest level of the ISO communications model. The OSI model is a layered model that explains how information travels from two different applications running on two different networked computers. Fundamentally, the OSI model regulates the steps to transfer data over a transmission channel between two network devices. The seventh layer or the application layer provides network services to the software (end users). It should be remembered that normal computer applications are not on this layer, but programs such as browsers, file transfer protocol (FTP) clients, and mail clients are.

There are several SDO efforts currently underway to develop standards to healthcare domain, but HL7 has a particular speciality, it is focused on the interface requirements of the entire health-care organization, instead of being focused on the requirements of a particular department. Being stakeholder oriented, the definition of standard within HL7 is fast because its members develop, analyse and ballot the ongoing standards.

The HL7 functional model consists of a set of functions and their associated functional descriptors. These functions are divided into three main sections: direct care, supportive and information infrastructure (see Fig. 2).

HL7 defines the Clinical Document Architecture (CDA), as a document markup standard that specifies the structure and semantics of a clinical document, such as a billing summary or progress medical note, for the purpose of exchange. A CDA document is an object-oriented document that can include text, images, sounds and other multimedia content. Although it is not strictly an EHR standard it forms an important sub-component of an EHR which has already been integrated with the equivalent structures in CEN 13606 and *open*EHR. CDA is encoded as Extensible Markup Language (XML) documents based on the HL7 Reference Information Model (RIM) attached with terminology.

Section	Code	Function
Direct Care - Electronic health record system (EHR-s) functions for providing direct health care to, or direct self-care for, one or more persons	DC 1.0	Care Management
	DC 2.0	Clinical Decision Support
	DC 3.0	Operations Management and Communication
Supportive - EHR-s functions that most frequently use existing EHR data to support the management of Health care services and organizations	S 1.0	Clinical Support
	S 2.0	Measurement, Analysis, Research, Reporting
	S 3.0	Administrative and Financial
Information Infrastructure - Critical backbone elements of Security, Privacy, Interoperability, Registry and Vocabulary	I 1.0	EHR Security
	I 2.0	EHR Information and Records Management
	I 3.0	Unique identity, registry and directory services
	I 4.0	Support for Health Informatics & Terminology Standards
	I 5.0	Interoperability
	I 6.0	Manage business rules
	I 7.0	Workflow

Fig. 2. HL7 functional model.

CDA release 1.0 became an ANSI-approved HL7 Standard in 2000, representing the first specification derived from the HL7 RIM. The major difference between the CDA R1 and the new R2 (released in 2005) is that CDA R2 model is richly expressive, enabling the formal representation of clinical statements (observations, medication administrations and adverse events) such that they can be interpreted and acted upon by a computer (Dolin et al., 2006).

HL7 messages were developed for several years using a bottom–up approach to reach each individual problem. Thus, such an ad hoc methodology created the HL7's success due to its flexibility. It contains many optional data elements and data segments, making it adaptable to almost any application. While providing great flexibility in its version 2, the different options available made the design of reliable conformance tests of any vendor's implementation quite difficult, and also forced implementers to use more time analyzing and planning their interfaces to guarantee that both parties were using the same optional features. To overcome this, the HL7 version 3 was released in 2005 using a well-defined methodology based on a reference information model mainly because objectivity is mandatory for reliable conformance tests. With fewer options vendors would have their conformance certification, because the primary goal of HL7 was to offer a standard that is objective and testable. This very limited-options version was reached by the use of message building techniques, adding more trigger events and limiting message formats. This new version for creating messages uses a development of object-oriented methodology and a Reference Information Model. RIM is an essential part of the new version, because it provides a clear illustration of the semantic and lexical connections that exist between the diverse information carried in the HL7 message fields.

3.4.4. DICOM

The committee responsible for maintaining international standards for communication of biomedical diagnostic and therapeutic information in disciplines that use digital images and associated data is the Digital Imaging and Communications in Medicine (DICOM) Standards Committee. Like HL7, DICOM has the same way of developing and improving a cooperative standard, getting together the stakeholders of its research topic.

The aim of DICOM is to achieve compatibility and to improve workflow efficiency between imaging systems and other information systems in healthcare environments worldwide. Currently, almost all diagnostic medical imaging vendors had integrated the standard into their product design and most are actively participating in the enhancement of the standard (DICOM, 2005). Every member can propose enhancements for the standard, and these proposals are considered for inclusion in future editions of the standard.

DICOM is used or will soon be used by virtually every medical professional who makes use of images within the healthcare industry. These include cardiology, dentistry, endoscopy, mammography, ophthalmology, orthopaedics, pathology, paediatrics, radiation therapy, radiology, surgery, etc. This imaging standard obviously also deals with the integration of information produced by various specialty applications in the patient's EHR. It defines the network and media interchange services allowing storage and access to these DICOM objects for EHR systems.

4. DISTRIBUTED ELECTRONIC HEALTHCARE RECORDS

The increase of medical information in digital format along with the definition of standards for electronic healthcare records and the wide availability of the internet are some of the factors that are enabling and motivating the adoption of a worldwide view of EHRs of patients. The possibility of gathering all patient clinical records is opening up new frontiers in healthcare delivery.

A wider access to EHRs will provide doctors with a complete view of clinical history of the patients, increasing not only their efficiency but also preventing clinical errors. Because at present there is no efficient communication between medical entities, significant quantities of patient clinical information must be transmitted by the patient to the doctor every time he is seen by a different doctor. Suppose for example a patient were unconscious, the information which could be critical is not transmitted resulting in unpredictable consequences.

The benefits of accessing distributed EHRs are not only on direct healthcare delivery. It can have a significant importance for scientific advances, by providing the research community with increasingly diverse clinical data. This gives the possibility of analyzing the patient from birth to death and find correlations between different types of clinical information. This can be especially interesting for identifying symptoms, lifestyle, clinical history and other factors that can be used for cancer prediction.

This worldwide view of EHR of patients brings up several ethical considerations that must be carefully evaluated when designing distributed medical information systems. Information security, authentication of users and information access rules are probably the most important ones that can dictate the success or failure of a high-technology system.

4.1. Distributed EHRs requirements

The creation of a system that can gather medical information will require medical entities to be interconnected and to speak with each other in an automatic manner. The first requirement is becoming a reality. However, it can be useless if each medical entity speaks in a different language. As it was seen earlier in this chapter, HL7 (HL7, 2005), CEN/TC 251 (2005), ISO/TC 215 (2005) and others are standards for information interchange that can be used to communicate between these entities. This is one of the most important requirements for any distributed EHR system.

For establishing communication between medical entities, both a common language and a common communication protocol for exchanging this information are needed (see Fig. 3). Medical entities which are involved in the system should provide a set of functionalities (searching patient information, selling clinical information, managing appointments, sharing or renting computer-aided diagnosis tools and others) for external entities to use in a standard way.

The architecture for a widely distributed EHR system will inevitably be composed of a network of medical entities having an external interface composed of a software application that processes external requests. This distributed architecture is mainly due to the sensitive nature of clinical information. The centralization of the information on a single

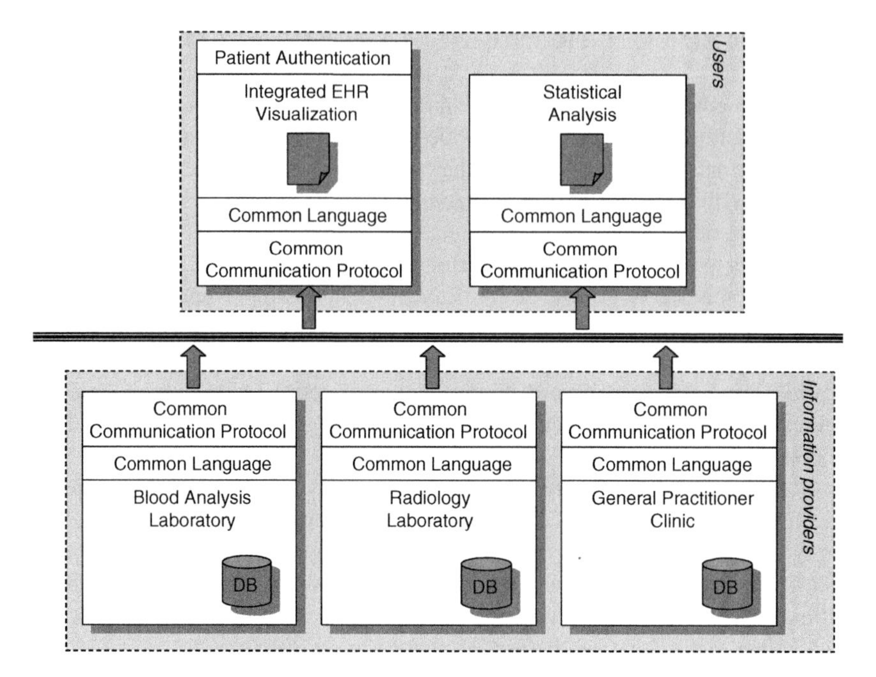

Fig. 3. General distributed EHR architecture.

system would certainly create important difficulties in the ownership and security of data. Keeping information distributed but accessible when required will guarantee that information is accessed only in specific cases where it is really necessary.

Information security is another important requirement for these systems. Medical information is valuable and if stolen, in most of the cases, it can no longer be retrieved. For example, suppose it is found, by analyzing some patient clinical information, that his/her probability of having cancer in the future is very high. Insurance companies and employers will certainly not want to maintain or will renegotiate their contracts with the patient, only based on cancer probabilities.

4.2. Development technologies

The interoperability technologies used in these initiatives vary from database sharing (Willard et al., 1994) to more sophisticated messaging systems, such as Multi-Agent Medical Information System (MAMIS) (Fonseca et al., 2005) or Integrated Electronic Health Record (I-EHR) (FORTH-ICS, 2005). Database sharing has several limitations since every medical entity involved must have the same database architecture, that is very difficult to implement, or it publicizes its architecture for others to interpret and use, putting a big interoperability effort on the external users. The more accepted solution has been to create software programs that can be automatically invoked to interact with EHRs data and return the results. This solution can also offer more sophisticated functionalities and not only to give access to the raw data. For example, in a cardiology laboratory these functionalities can be used to automatically analyse ECG data and report only the pathologies encountered.

For developing software to automatically process requests, intelligent Multi-Agent Systems (MASs) and Remote Procedure Calls (RPCs) technologies are the most efficient and commonly used. Both have been designed for creating distributed systems and are already being used in many commercial applications.

Many definitions for intelligent MASs can be found in literature, but one of the most widely accepted was proposed by Wooldridge and Jennings (1995). According to these authors, agents are software applications that have autonomy to take decisions without external intervention, social capabilities to communicate with other agents, reactivity to process requests and initiative to undertake autonomous actions. Besides the concept of initiative, that is optional, these are the main requirements for an application to interoperate in a medical network. Although organizations like Foundation for Intelligent Physical Agents (FIPA) (FIPA, 2005) tried to standardize agents message format, the communication is made using messages that are still dependent on the MAS platform being used. For developing agents several MAS platforms are now-a-days available, such as JADE (2005), JACK (2005) and Sun's Java Dynamic Management Kit (Java DMK, 2005).

RPC technology is also being used for developing distributed systems, it is not as ambitious as MAS in terms of local intelligence and autonomy, but is less complex, more efficient and has the support from big software companies such as Microsoft, IBM, SUN and others. This support is probably one of its major advantages since a common communication platform is needed for the success of distributed EHR systems. In spite of this support for developing a common RPC platform, several RPC technologies have been developed over the last years, such as, the Common Object Request Broker Architecture (CORBA, 2004), Java Remote Method Invocation (RMI) (Java RMI, 2003), Distributed Component Object Model (DCOM) (Microsoft, 2005a), Extensible Markup Language RPCs (XML-RPCs) and Web Services (W3C, 2005).

Basically, RPC technology is composed of applications with public methods that can be remotely evoked by other applications. Methods interface (inputs and outputs) is known a priori by the developers or in some RPCs there are interface description languages and interface description servers for a wider reusability. The communication platform is also an important interoperability issue which differs between RPCs. CORBA uses Internet Inter-ORB Protocol (IIOP) a standard communication protocol from Object Management Group (OMG) that runs over TCP/IP. Java RMI is a language-dependent RPC that uses direct sockets connection for communicating between applications. DCOM developed by Microsoft is more devoted to MS-Windows platforms and uses TCP/IP protocol for communication, therefore, relies on dynamically assigned ports.

Web Services technology appeared in the year 2000, joining the efforts of big software companies like IBM, Microsoft, Sun and others. The goal was to create a new RPC technology based on the most widely deployed, supported and understood web technologies for communication and interface description that could make interoperable applications developed in different languages. Web Services explored the increasing standardization of Extensible Markup Language (XML) in several domains. HL7 version 3.0 is already based on XML technology, and uses the widely adopted Hypertext Transfer Protocol (HTTP) as a communication standard. Since HTTP is a core protocol of the web, most organizations have already a network infrastructure that supports HTTP and people who understand how to manage it, turning it a de facto standard. Along with an XML services description language (WSDL) and a unified services publishing and discovery mechanism (UDDI) it created a powerful tool to develop distributed systems over the web.

The question that is being raised now is what technology to use in the development of a distributed EHR system that will be in use in the next decade (AMHA, 2005; CFH, 2005). This question is particularly important since diversity of local EHR systems will always happen and systems interoperability will be required. Both technologies (MAS and RPCs) have their own advantages and disadvantages. MAS paradigm has more local intelligence and autonomy, although it lacks standardization. RPCs with the introduction of Web Services brought an easy way to provide systems interoperability and their disadvantages are only on communication efficiency due to XML language overheads (Laurent et al., 2001). Proof of its importance lies in the updating of most development languages to support it and the adoption of the Web Services technology on the most recent MAS platforms (Moreau, 2002). Also, the promising GRID computing (GLOBUS, 2005), that takes unused resources from many computers in a network to solve problems too complex for one single machine, is considering converting its middleware services to Web Services (Hagel and Brown, 2002).

The aim of this chapter is to give an overview of the possible technologies to develop distributed EHR systems and to detail the one that is becoming more promising to do so, i.e. the Web Services. This opinion is supported by the involvement of W3 Consortium in defining and recommending the use of XML standards in medical domains (W3C, 2003), Microsoft by releasing its Collaborative Health Tools (Microsoft, 2005b) based on HL7 and Web Services and the involvement of other standards organizations. There are also several pilot projects being developed all over the world using these technologies (Clair, 2003; Bicer et al., 2005), however these have, at the moment, only a local or regional scope.

4.3. Inside Web Services

Web Services were conceived to allow loosely coupled applications, i.e. services that can exist independent of each other within an application. This allows applications to be developed using service-oriented architecture, code reutilization, and easier system maintenance and updating. A Web Service that gathers EHRs of the patients will involve - issuing requests to other Web Services to find clinical information about the patient, requesting special data analysis, finding recommended prescriptions, etc., leading to an "n-tier" application.

The success of Web Services over other technologies such as the very promising CORBA, DCOM or RMI came from its easy integration, simplicity and by the adoption of de facto standards like XML and HTTP. Web Services are language independent and therefore they can be used in different interfaces, such as web pages, graphical interfaces, PDAs and others, covering almost every entity involved.

When using Web Services technology the architecture proposed in Fig. 3 is extended as shown in Fig. 4, including services discovery (UDDI), services description (WSDL),

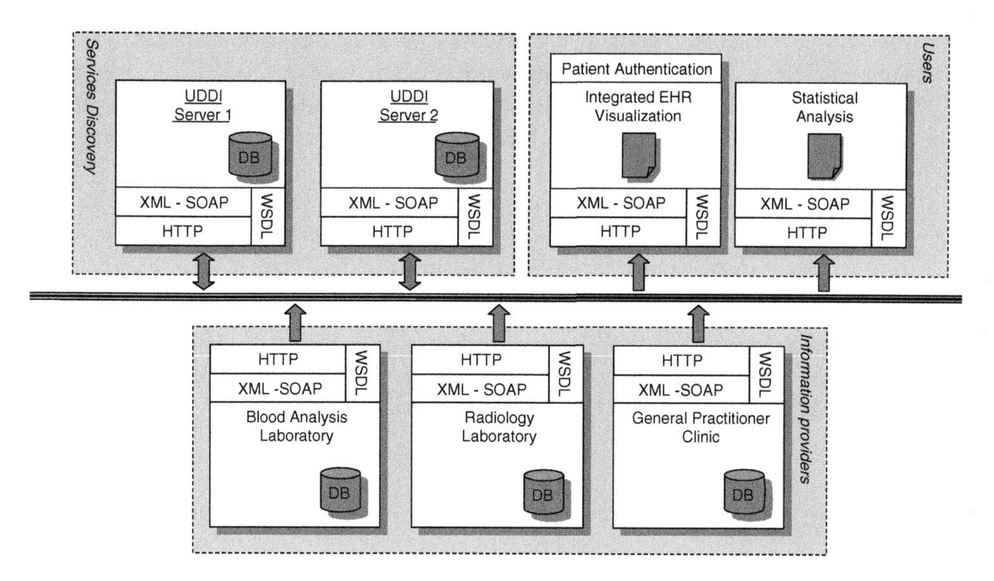

Fig. 4. Web Services-based distributed EHR system architecture.

a common language (XML-SOAP) and a standard communication protocol (HTTP). These modules are described below.

4.3.1. SOAP (Simple Object Access Protocol)

SOAP is a lightweight extensible communication protocol designed for use over the internet. It defines rules for creating RPC messages to be sent to remote servers in an XML and HTTP standard-based form. Although HTTP is the standard defined in SOAP specification, it can be used in other communication protocols such as MSMQ, MQ Series, SMTP or TCP. The advantage of using HTTP is that it uses a simple low-cost web server, is easy to maintain and SOAP messages can go across firewalls. Security is not currently addressed in SOAP standard. It assumes that security is a transport issue and is silent on security issues.

SOAP messages are composed of three major components:

- SOAP envelope – defines the overall framework for expressing the message content, the recipients and whether these are optional or mandatory.
- SOAP encoding rule – defines the rules for describing data in an XML format.
- SOAP RPC representation – a convention for representing RPC requests and responses.

4.3.2. WSDL (Web Service Description Language)

WSDL is an optional component used to describe Web Services in a standard XML language. It is used to promote systems interoperability by describing services operational information.

This way, service consumers (developers) can easily integrate the service into their system, increasing reusability of services and reducing developing time.

WSDL file describes the SOAP messages and how the messages are exchanged to talk with the service. It describes also the service location and the communication protocol used by the service.

4.3.3. UDDI (Universal Description, Discovery and Integration)

UDDI is a platform-independent way to advertise and subscribe Web Services. These are servers that contain WSDL description of Web Services, which are available for consumers to use. The service providers, in order to take better return for their services, publicize them in a UDDI which means they are publicizing them all over the web. Users that are searching for Web Services consult UDDI servers in real time and negotiate the use of such services.

5. CONCLUSIONS

Internet and information technologies are definitely installed in the health sector, offering numerous advantages but bringing with it also significant problems. This information highway cannot be ignored by healthcare professionals and healthcare institutions. The access to complete electronic health records (EHRs) of patients is currently quite difficult, but it will be certainly possible in the near future. The availability of online decision support tools is already a reality that is being continuously enhanced. Patients are already using the information available on the Internet to know more about their diseases and make their own decisions, changing their behaviour and modifying their relationship with physicians. However, there is still a long way to go until we have a stable and really widespread use.

The adoption of standards for data and knowledge representation and communication between healthcare entities, the definition and acceptance of ethical protocols to regulate the access to information on patients both by physicians and patients, and the development of secure communication protocols acceptable for the transference of health data are some of the main technical barriers that must be overcome to achieve a truly ubiquitous network of medical information. Patients must be educated in order to find the most accurate information and certification mechanisms have to be created in order to guarantee the quality of the information and services found on the Internet.

Despite the numerous difficulties in the achievement of a ubiquitous medical network of information using the Internet, benefiting both physicians and patients, we can say that it is a certain possibility and the attempts to ignore it can only represent a loss of time.

REFERENCES

ADO, 2005, Adjuvent Online [online]. Available from: http://www.adjuvantonline.com/

AMHA, 2005, Road map for Healthconnect, Australian Minister for Health and Ageing, Australia.

Balabanova, D., 2004, Funding health care: Options for Europe. European Observatory on health care systems series. Eur. J. Public Health, 14, 108.

Barker, K.N., E.A. Flynn, G.A. Pepper, D.W. Bates and R.L. Mikeal, 2002, Medication errors observed in 36 health care facilities. Arch. Internal Med., 162, 1897–1903.
Bergmo, T.S., P.E. Kummervold, D. Gammon and L.B. Dahl, 2005, Electronic patient-provider communication: Will it offset office visits and telephone consultations in primary care? Int. J. Med. Inform., 74, 705–710.
Bessel, T.L., J.N. Anderson, C.A. Silagy, L.N. Sansom and J. E. Hiller, 2003, Surfing, self-medication and safety: buying non-prescription and complementary medicines via the internet. Qual. Saf. Health Care, 12, 88–92.
Bicer, V., O. Kilic, A. Dogac and G. Laleci, 2005, Archetype-based Semantic Interoperability of Web Service Messages in the Healthcare Domain. IJSWIS, 1, 1–22.
BMT, 2005, Bone Marrow Transplant Support Online [online]. Available from: http://www.bmtsupport.org/
CDCP, 2005, Centers for Disease Control and Prevention [online]. Available from: http://www.cdc.gov/
CEN, 2005, Committee European Normalization (CEN) [online]. Available from: http://www.centc251.org
CFH, 2005, Linking Health Care Information – Proposed Methods for Improving Care and Protecting Privacy. Report from Connecting for Health, Markle Foundation. [online]. Available from: www.connectingforhealth.org/
Clair, D.S., 2003, Healthcare's Last Mile: Linking Disparate Information Systems. Health Management Technology, Nelson Publishing, Nokomis, USA, Feb. 2003.
CORBA, 2004, OMG CORBA®/IIOP® Specifications [online]. Available from: http://www.omg.org/
CSN, 2005, Cancer Survivors Network [online]. Available from: http://www.acscsn.org
Cyber-Dialogue, 2000, Ethics Survey of Consumer Attitudes about Health Web Sites, 2nd ed. California Health Care Foundation and Internet Healthcare Coalition.
DICOM, 2005, Digital Imaging and Communications in Medicine (DICOM) [online]. Available from: http://medical.nema.org
Dolin, R., L. Alschuler, S. Boyer, C. Beebe, F. Behlen, P. Biron and A. Shabo, 2006, HL7 Clinical Document Architecture, Release 2. J. Am. Med. Inform. Assoc. (JAMIA), 13(1):30–39.
DStore, 2005, Drugstore.com [online]. Available from: http://www.drugstore.com
Eysenbach, G., 2000, Recent advances – Consumer health informatics. Br. Med. J., 320, 1713–1716.
Eysenbach, G., 2003, The impact of the Internet on cancer outcomes. CA Cancer J. Clin., 53, 356–371.
Eysenbach, G. and C. Köhler, 2003, What is the prevalence of health-related searches on the world wide web? Qualitative and quantitative analysis of search engine queries on the internet, Proc AMIA 2003 Annual Fall Symposium, Washington DC, 225–229.
FDA, 2005, US Food and Drug Administration [online]. Available from: http://www.fda.gov/
Ferguson, T., 2002, From patients to end users – Quality of online patient networks needs more attention than quality of online health information. Br. Med. J., 324, 555–556.
FIPA, 2005, FIPA – IEEE Foundation for Intelligent Physical Agents [online]. Available from: www.fipa.org.
Fonseca, J.M., A.D. Mora and A.C. Marques, 2005, MAMIS – A Multi-Agent Medical Information System, Proc Biomed–2005, Innsbruck, Austria.
FORTH-ICS, 2005, Integrated Electronic Health Record [online]. Available from: http://www.ics.forth.gr/eHealth/technology.html
Fox, S. and D. Fallows, 2003, Internet Health Resources: Health Searches and Email have Become More Commonplace, but there is Room for Improvement in Searches and Overall Internet Access [online]. Available from: http://www.pewinternet.org [29 October 2005].
Fox, S. and L. Rainie, 2000, The Online Health Care Revolution: How the Web Helps Americans Take Better Care of Themselves [online]. Available from: www.pewinternet.org [29 October 2005].
Geiger, G., K. Merrilees, R. Walo, D. Gordon and H. Kunov, 1995, An analysis of the paper-based health record: information content and its implications for electronic patient records, Proc 8th World Congress on Medical Informatics (MEDINFO 95), Vancouver, July 23–27.
GLOBUS, 2005, Towards Open Grid Services Architecture [online]. Available from: http://www.globus.org/ogsa/
Google, 2005, Google: Corporate Information [online]. Available from: http://www.google.com/corporate/facts.html
Hagel, J. and J.S. Brown, 2002, Service Grids: The Missing Link in Web Services, Release 1.0, December.
HealthyPlace, 2005, HealthyPlace [online]. Available from: http://www.healthyplace.com/
HL7, 2005, HL7 – Health Level Seven [online]. Available from: http://www.hl7.org/
IEEE, 1990, IEEE Standard Computer Dictionary: A Compilation of IEEE Standard Computer Glossaries, IEEE, New York, USA.
ISO, 2005, International Organization for Standardization (ISO) [online]. Available from: http://www.iso.org
IWS, 2005, Internet World Stats [online]. Available from: http://www.internetworldstats.com/stats.htm

JACK, 2005, JACK Development Environment (JDE) [online]. Available from: http://www.agent-software.com
JADE, 2005, Java Agent DEvelopment Framework [online]. Available from: http://jade.tilab.com/
Java DMK, 2005, Java Dynamic Management Kit [online]. Available from: http://java.sun.com/products/jdmk/
Java RMI, 2003, Java Remote Method Invocation (Java RMI) [online]. Available from: http://java.sun.com/products/jdk/rmi/
Kohn, L.T., J.M. Corrigan and M.S. Donaldson (Eds.), 2000, To Err Is Human: Building a Safer Health System. National Academy Press, Washington, DC, USA.
Lacher, A., E. Nelson, W. Bylsma and R. Spena, 2000, Computer use and needs of internists: A survey of members of the American College of Physicians – American Society of Internal Medicine. Proc AMIA Symp. 53–456.
Laurent, S.S., J. Johnston and E. Dumbill (Eds.), 2001, Programming Web Services with XML-RPC: Chapter 8 – XML-RPC and the Web Services Landscape, O'Reilly & Associates, Sebastopol USA.
Microsoft, 2005a, COM: Component Object Model Technologies [online]. Available from: http://www.microsoft.com/com/
Microsoft, 2005b, Infrastructure Integration Solutions for Healthcare Providers [online]. Available from: www.microsoft.com/industry/healthcare/
Morasch, L.J. 2000, Making the most of Physician-Patient email, Hippocrates, 14(11), 33–39.
Moreau, L., 2002, Agents for the Grid: A Comparison with Web Services, Proc 2nd IEEE/ACM International Symposium on Cluster Computing and the Grid (CCGRID.02), Berlin, Germany, 21–24 May 2002.
NCI, 2005, National Cancer Institute [online]. Available from: http://www.cancer.gov/cancertopics/factsheet/Information/internet
Pyper, C., J. Amery, M. Watson and C. Crook, 2004, Access to electronic health records in primary care – a survey of patients' views. Medical Science Monitor, 10(11), 17–22.
RAC, 2005, Rite Aid Corporation [online]. Available from: http://www.riteaid.com/
Rimer, B.K., E.J. Lyons, K.M. Ribisl, J.M. Bowling, C.E. Golin, M.J. Forlenza and A. Meier, 2005, How new subscribers use cancer-related online mailing lists. J. Med. Internet Res., 7(3), e32.
Schloeffel, P., 2004. Current EHR developments: an Australian and international perspective, Proc Health Informatics New Zealand Conference (HINZ2004), Wellington, New Zealand.
Schloeffel, P. and P. Jeselon, 2002, Final Report: Standards Requirements for the Electronic Health Record & Discharge/Referral Plans. ISO/TC 215 EHR Ad Hoc Group.
SEW, 2005, Search Engine Watch [online]. Available from: http://searchenginewatch.com
Sherman, A.C., S. Simonton, D.C. Adams, U. Latif, T.G. Plante, S.K. Burns and T. Poling, 2001, Measuring religious faith in cancer patients: Reliability and construct validity of the Santa Clara Strength of Religious Faith Questionnaire. Psychooncology, 10, 436–443.
Stewart, B.W. and P. Kleihues, 2003, World Cancer Report. World Health Organization, Geneva.
Straker, N., 1998, Psychodynamic Psychotherapy for Cancer Patients. J. Psychother. Pract. Res., 7, 1–9.
Tierney, W.M., C.J. Mcdonald, D.K. Martin, S.L. Hui and M.P. Rogers, 1987, Computerized Display of Past Test-Results - Effect on Outpatient Testing. Ann. Intern. Med., 107, 569–574.
UHN, 2005, University Health Network [online]. Available from: http://www.uhn.ca/pmh/
van den Brink, J.L., P.W. Moorman, M.F. de Boer, J.F.A. Pruyn, C.D.A. Verwoerd and J.H. van Bemmel, 2005, Involving the patient: A prospective study on use, appreciation and effectiveness of an information system in head and neck cancer care. Inter. J. Med. Inform., 74, 839–849.
W3C, 2003, W3C and the Medical Sector [online]. Available from: http://www.w3c.rl.ac.uk/QH/WP5/handouts/health_w3c.html
W3C, 2005, W3C Web Services Activity [online]. Available from: http://www.w3.org/2002/ws/Activity.html
Walczak, S., 2003, A multiagent architecture for developing medical information retrieval agents. J. Med. Syst., 27, 479–498.
Willard, K.E., J.H. Hallgren and D.P. Connelly, 1994, W3 based medical information systems vs custom client server applications, Proc 2nd International WWW Conferencex '94: Mosaic and the Web, Geneva, Switzerland, May 25–27.
Wooldridge, M. and N.R. Jennings, 1995, Intelligent Agents – Theory and Practice. Knowl Eng Rev, 10, 115–152.

Chapter 15

Geoconda: A Web Environment for Multi-Centre Research

Christian Setzkorn, Azzam F. Taktak and Bertil Damato

Royal Liverpool University Hospital, UK
Email: C.Setzkorn@csc.liv.ac.uk

Abstract

The collection of data for the validation and generation of hypotheses is a fundamental scientific endeavour. To achieve a low margin of error, it is necessary to obtain sufficient numbers of samples. However, this is often difficult, especially if the process being observed is very rare and/or if the collection of data is expensive. This is, for example, the case for uveal melanomas, which have an occurrence rate of six per million per year. Research into uveal melanoma has motivated the Geoconda system. Geoconda is an abbreviation for General Ocular Oncology Database. It uses a dynamic website and a database to facilitate international collaborations via the Internet and helps, apart from other things, to accumulate sufficient numbers of samples.

To collect data from several different centres around the world requires the standardization of variables. This is achieved using an interactive multi-stage process. The same process is also used for other tasks within the Geoconda system. For example, it is used for the standardization of terminologies, which is of great importance for the success of international collaborations where people from different backgrounds and countries work together. The Geoconda system also contains a mailing list and a discussion forum, which simplify the communication between the members.

Geoconda has sixty members from twelve countries at the moment. The system is currently used for several international collaborations between sixteen different countries.

The collaborations evaluate, for example, different approaches for survival analysis and classification in a double-blind manner. Another collaboration compares the performance of several international centres.

Acknowledgements

Geoconda is funded by a grant from the European Network of Excellence Biopattern, which was awarded in January 2004 (Grant Number: FP6-2002-IST-1 N 508803). Matching funds were provided by the Eye Tumour Research Fund of the Royal Liverpool University Hospital.

Contents

Outcome Prediction in Cancer
Edited by A.F.G. Taktak and A.C. Fisher
© 2007 Elsevier B.V. All rights reserved

1. INTRODUCTION

The collection of data for the validation and generation of hypotheses is a fundamental scientific endeavour. To achieve a low margin of error, it is necessary to obtain sufficient numbers of samples. However, this is often difficult, especially if the process being observed is very rare and/or if the collection of data is expensive. This is, for example, the case for uveal melanomas, which have an occurrence rate of six per million per year (Damato, 2005) and arise from melanocytes in the uvea. The uvea consists of the choroid, ciliary body, and iris. The choroid is a cup-shaped layer of tissue lying between the sclera and the retina, which it nourishes.

The ciliary body is a ring-shaped muscular tissue located at the rim of the choroid and encircling the lens, which it stretches to adjust the focal length of the eye. The ciliary body is lined by a secretory epithelium that pumps water into the eyeball, so that its spherical shape is maintained. The iris is a muscular sphincter, which adjusts to the size of the pupil thereby controlling the amount of light entering the eye and improving visual acuity. Patients with uveal melanoma usually have symptoms, such as blurred vision, flashing lights, and visual field loss.

Without treatment, many eyes become blind, painful and cosmetically unsightly. For many years, the standard form of treatment was enucleation (i.e. removal of the eye). This has been superseded by a variety of methods aimed at conserving the eye with as much vision as possible.

These consist of various types of radiotherapy, laser treatment and local resection. The chances of preserving vision and the eye are related to factors such as tumour size and location as well as secondary effects of the tumour on the eye and unrelated concomitant ocular disease.

Approximately 50% of all patients with uveal melanoma ultimately die of this disease, nearly always as a result of haematogenous spread of tumour (i.e. through the blood circulation) to the liver. The probability of metastatic disease is related to tumour size and extent at the time of treatment, various microscopic features such as cell type, and cytogenetic abnormalities, particularly those affecting chromosomes 3 and 8. Metastatic disease rarely responds to treatment and is usually fatal in a few months. The need for multicentre research into uveal melanoma has motivated the Geoconda system described in this chapter. It has to be noted that the principles described here could also be applied in other research areas. Geoconda is an abbreviation for **Ge**neral **Oc**ular **On**cology **Da**tabase. It uses several web pages and a database to facilitate international collaborations via the Internet and helps, apart from other things, to accumulate sufficient numbers of samples from several different centres around the world. Such collaborations require the standardization of variables. This is achieved using an interactive multi-stage process that is described in Section 2. This interactive multi-stage process is also used for other tasks within the Geoconda system. For example, it used for the standardization of terminologies.

Standardization is of great importance for the success of international collaborations where people from different backgrounds work together. Other objectives of Geoconda are to:

- develop and maintain rules for collaboration;
- understand essential jargon from different research areas;
- become acquainted with collaborators;
- host discussions; and
- collaborate in the preparation of protocols, consent forms and other documents.

This chapter is organized as follows. Section 2 briefly describes the technologies that were used to implement the Geoconda system. Section 3 provides an exhaustive description of the Geoconda system. This section is followed by the discussions, summary and conclusions. The chapter concludes in Section 6, which provides avenues for future research.

2. MATERIAL AND METHODS

The Geoconda system utilizes several web pages and a relational database. The websites are described in greater detail in Section 3. The system has been implemented using the ASP.NET technology version 1.1, the C-sharp programming language and the development environment Visual Studio.NET 2003. These technologies are property of the company Microsoft. ASP.NET is an abbreviation for Active Server Pages.NET. The interested reader is referred to Homer et al. (2004) for more details about the ASP.NET technology. The relational database was implemented using the database system MySQL version 4.0.20a-nt.

To gain more freedom in developing the Geoconda system it was decided to host the website and the database using a professional Internet service provider (the website of the ISP can be accessed at http://www.titanhosts.net.) rather than the computing service provided by the British National Health Service. The latter has many restrictive measures, which are necessary but hinder the development of systems like Geoconda.

As mentioned in Section 1, the collection of data requires the standardization of variables, which is necessary because different centres might, for example, take measurements using different scales. It is therefore important to arrive an agreement about the variables to be measured before the data are collected. This is achieved using the aforementioned interactive multi-stage process, which is also used to come to an agreement about other items such as glossary items, which are used to standardize terminologies. The Geoconda system allows members to propose different items. Currently, there are seven items, which are listed as follows:

- FAQs;
- positions;
- variables;
- glossaries;
- projects;
- links; and
- online papers.

The interactive multi-stage process works as follows. After an item has been proposed (using a particular web form) it has the status "open" and is stored in the database. The item is then visible to other members of Geoconda who can add comments to it. If a comment is added, an email is sent to the member who proposed the item. The member can then edit the item, allowing him/her to refine it by incorporating comments added by other members. A committee of experts" reviews open items on a regular basis. The Chairman of Geoconda can invite the experts who are requested to add reviews to items. After the review process, the Chairman decides whether the status of the item is changed from "open" to "accepted" or "rejected". This implements a somewhat democratic system to reach agreements within an international multi-user environment such as Geoconda. Section 3.1 provides more details about the aforementioned items.

3. DESCRIPTION OF THE GEOCONDA WEBSITE

The main web page of the Geoconda system can be accessed at *www.geoconda.com*. A screen shot of this page is shown in Fig. 1. The entry page summarizes aims and key principles of the Geoconda system and acknowledges sources of funding. It has to be noted,

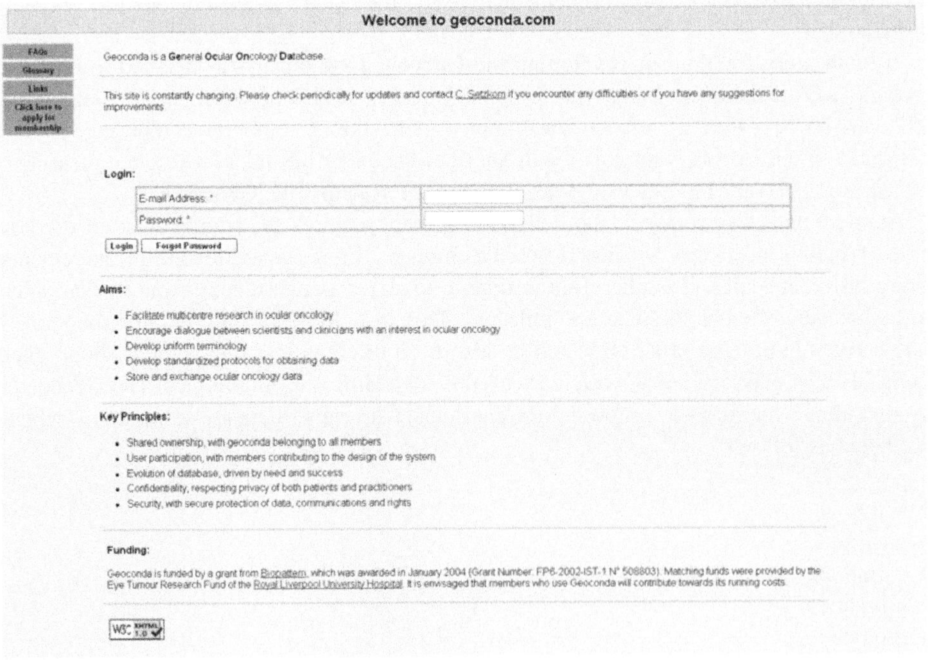

Fig. 1. The main/entry page.

that only a restricted number of web pages and functionalities can be accessed from the main page without login. These pages include the *FAQs*, *glossaries*, *links* and the *discussion forum*.

The Geoconda system contains many more pages. Their content is dynamic as the members always then change it. To access these pages, accepted members have to login using their email address and a password. Members who forget their passwords can request a randomly generated password by clicking on the button "Forgot Password". The password is sent to the provided email address, which is double-checked against the database. Members can then change their password after accessing their personal details.

People interested in becoming members of Geoconda can apply for membership. Potential members are usually invited by already existing members, for example, at international conferences. However, people interested in contributing to uveal melanoma research are also encouraged to join. Clicking on the button: "Click here to apply for membership" starts the application process. A form has to be completed, which contains the details summarized in Table 1. The details are temporarily stored in a database and reviewed by a committee of existing members who decide whether or not the member is accepted. Only applicants who have the potential to contribute to the Geoconda system are likely to be accepted.

Table 1. Details of the membership application form

Field	Description
First name	First name of the applicant.
Surname	Surname of the applicant.
Email	Email address of the applicant.
Password	Password chosen by the applicant. It has to be noted that the password is encrypted before it is stored in the database. This ensures further security.
Retype Password	Repeated password. The password has to be exactly the same as the one provided above.
Image	This field allows the user to upload a picture of himself/herself.
Title(s)	Titles of the applicant (e.g. Prof., Dr. etc.).
Qualifications	A list of recent qualifications of the applicant.
Positions	This field contains professional positions of the applicant.
Contributions	A list of potential contributions of the applicant to the Geoconda project.
Date of Birth	Birth date of the applicant.
Gender	Gender of the applicant.
Address Line 1	First line of the address.
Address Line 2	Second line of the address.
Address Line 3	Third line of the address.
Street	Street of the address.
City	City of the address.
Postcode	Postcode of the address.

Table 1. cont'd

Field	Description
Country	Country of residence of the applicant. The country has to be selected from a dropdown list.
Phone Number	Phone number of the applicant.
Fax Number	Fax number of the applicant.
Further Details (Research Interests etc.)	This field allows the member to provide further information about himself/herself.
Proposer First Name	First name of the person who encouraged the applicant to apply for membership.
Proposer Surname	Surname of the person who encouraged the applicant to apply for membership.

Figure 2 shows the Geoconda main page, which can only be accessed by accepted members. Several other sections/pages can be reached from here by clicking on one of the buttons shown in the navigation panel on the left-hand side.

There are currently thirteen sections, which are listed as follows:

- officers;
- FAQs
- positions;
- members;

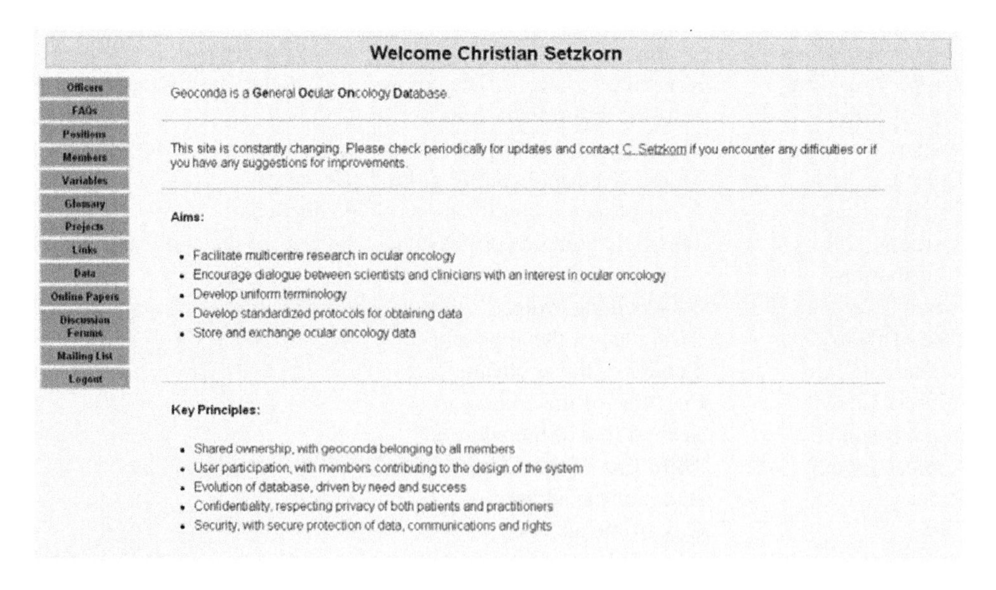

Fig. 2. The main page of the Geoconda website.

- variables;
- glossary;
- projects;
- links;
- data;
- online papers;
- discussion forum;
- mailing list; and
- logout.

The "officers" section contains a list of accepted members who were assigned to a particular position. The reader is referred to Section 3.1 for further details about these positions. A part of the officers section is depicted in Fig. 3.

Further details about an officer and the corresponding position can be obtained by clicking on the name or the position respectively. The member section can be reached by clicking on the button "Members". Additional details about a particular member can be obtained by clicking on his/her name. Members can change their details by clicking on their name and then on the button "Edit". It has to be noted that the "Edit" button is only visible for the member himself/herself because the Geoconda system knows the identity of the member who has logged in. The details of a particular member are shown in Fig. 4.

When a member clicks on the button "Edit", his/her details can be edited as shown in Fig. 5. Changes can be stored by clicking on the button "Update". The changes are not stored if the member clicks on the button "Cancel".

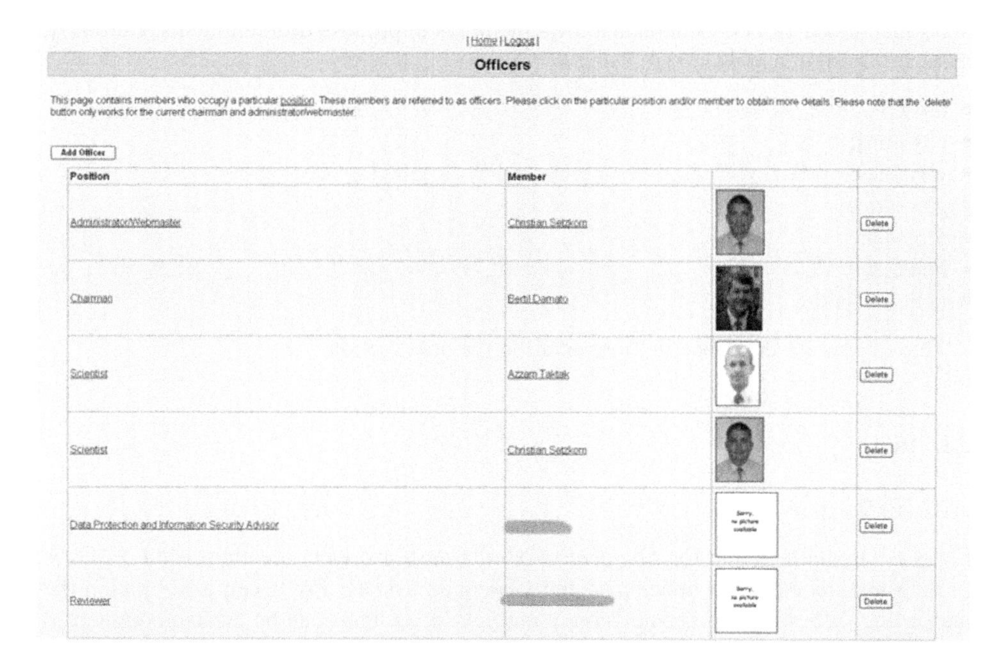

Fig. 3. List of current officers. The names of Geoconda members who are not authors of this chapter are hidden for privacy reasons.

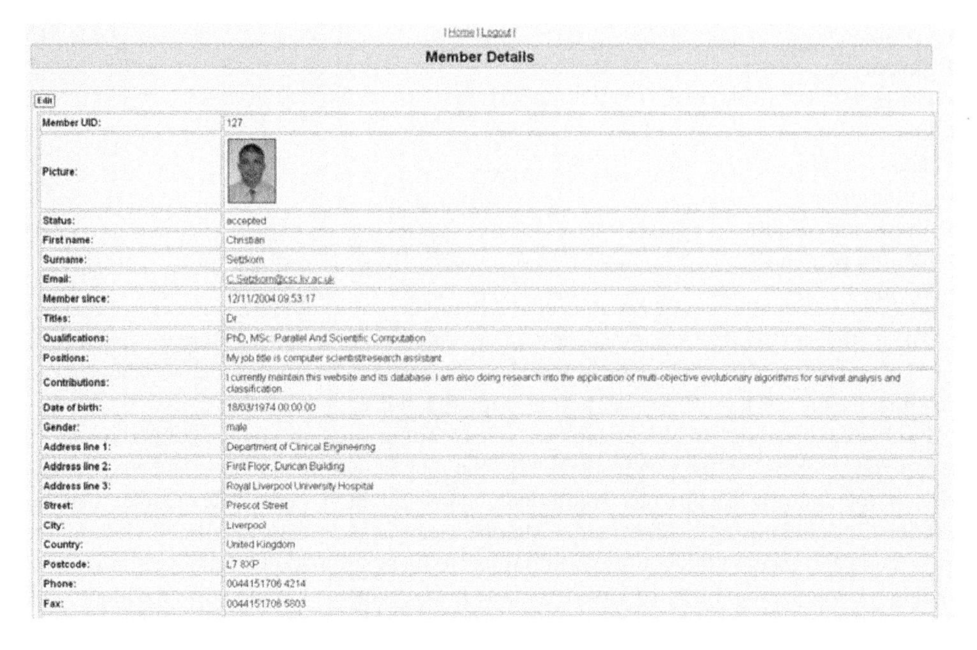

Fig. 4. Details of a particular member.

As mentioned earlier, Geoconda allows members to propose different items. Currently, there are seven items, which are listed as follows:

- FAQs;
- positions;
- variables;
- glossaries;
- projects;
- links; and
- online papers.

These items are described in more detail in the next section.

3.1. Items

3.1.1 FAQs

FAQs is an abbreviation for *Frequently Asked Questions*. One intention of the FAQs is to help new members to understand the Geoconda system. FAQs can also contain the underlying rules of the Geoconda community. As FAQ items can be created/commented by all members, the creation of these rules is therefore democratic (see Section 2). FAQ items contain the information summarized in Table 2.

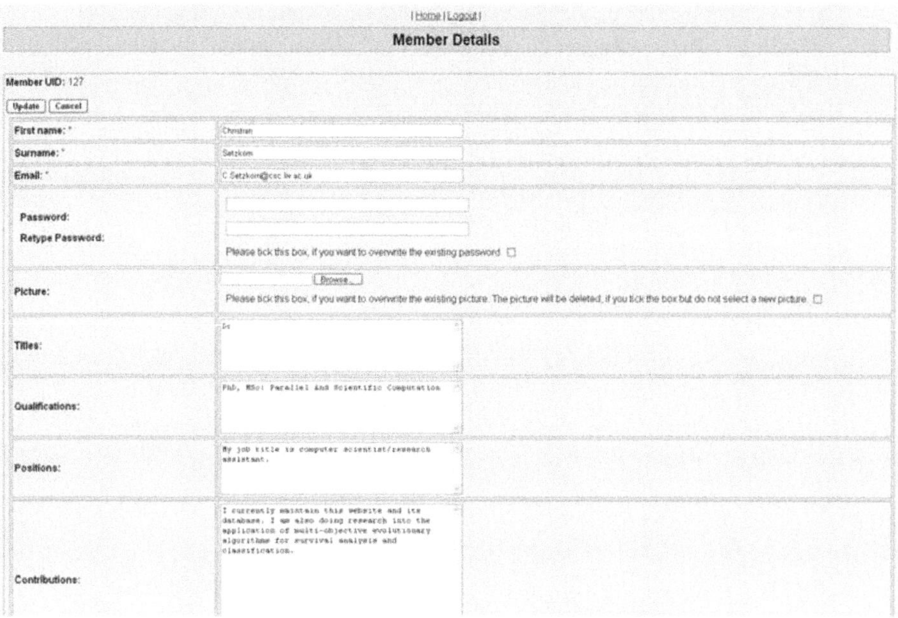

Fig. 5. Member details in the edit mode.

Figure 6 depicts the FAQ proposal form. The member has to provide the information in the mandatory fields. The item is added to the database (and consequentially the website) after pressing the "Submit" button.

Members can assign a FAQ item to one of the headings in the dropdown list. The headings help to categorize FAQ items. New headings can be added to the dropdown list by completing the field "Heading" and pressing the button "Add New Heading". It has to be noted that a new heading is only added if it does not already exist in the database/dropdown list.

FAQ items that currently exist for the heading/category "Links" are shown in Fig. 7. The member can press the button "More Details" to obtain further information about a particular FAQ item. Members can also obtain more details about the member who proposed an item by clicking on his/her name.

Table 2. The fields of a FAQ item

Field	Description
Question	Question of the FAQ item.
Answer	Answer to the question of the FAQ item.
Heading	FAQs can be categorized using headings that correspond to categories. An already existing heading can be chosen from a dropdown list. Members can modify this dropdown list and add new headings.

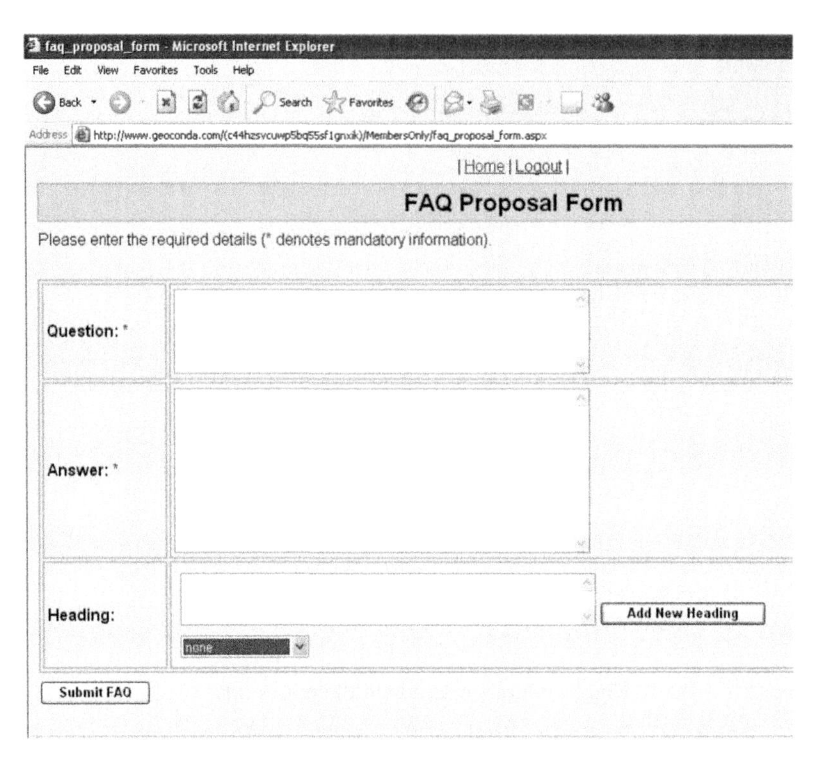

Fig. 6. The FAQ item proposal form.

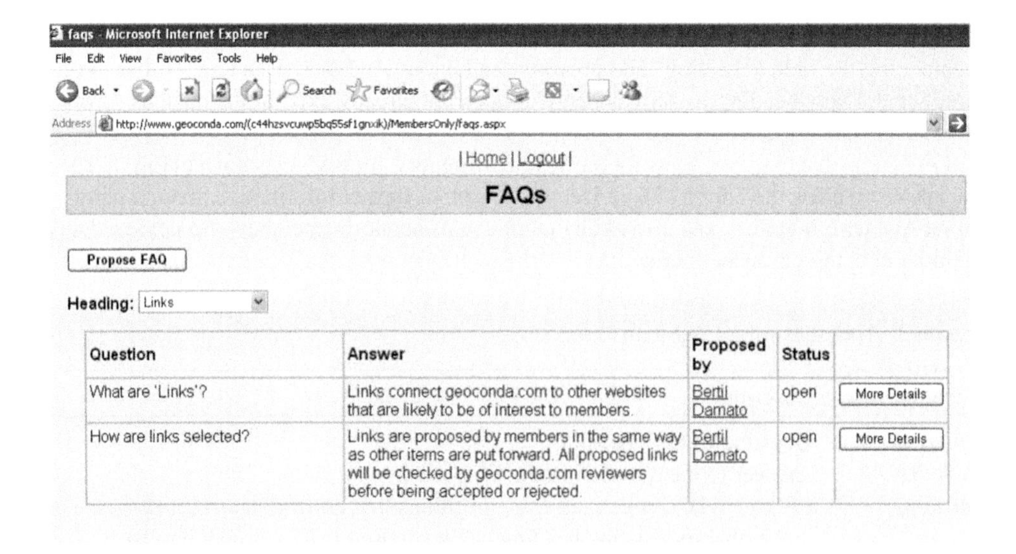

Fig. 7. FAQs for the heading/category “Links”.

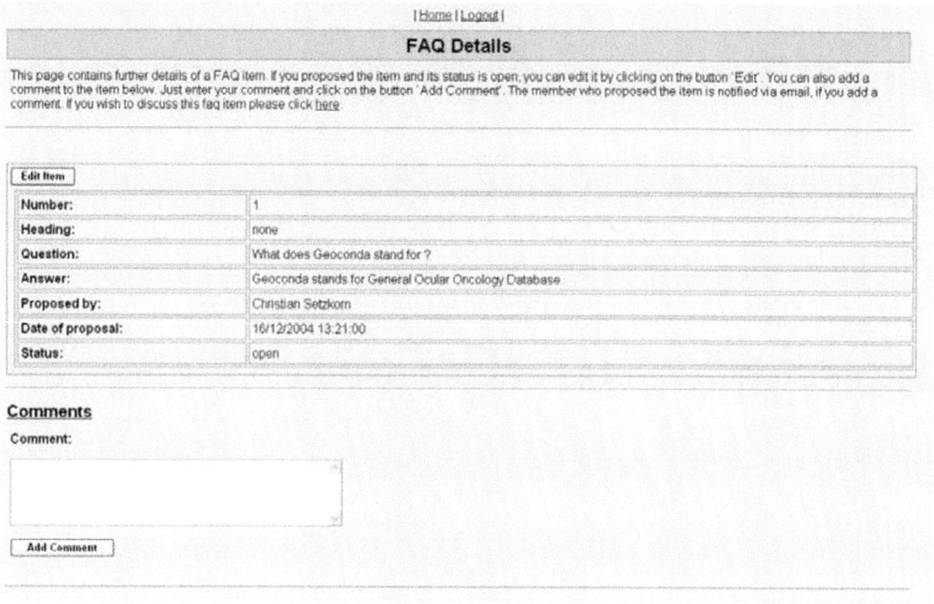

| Home | Logout |

FAQ Details

This page contains further details of a FAQ item. If you proposed the item and its status is open, you can edit it by clicking on the button 'Edit'. You can also add a comment to the item below. Just enter your comment and click on the button 'Add Comment'. The member who proposed the item is notified via email, if you add a comment. If you wish to discuss this faq item please click here.

Edit Item

Number:	1
Heading:	none
Question:	What does Geoconda stand for ?
Answer:	Geoconda stands for General Ocular Oncology Database
Proposed by:	Christian Setzkorn
Date of proposal:	16/12/2004 13:21:00
Status:	open

Comments

Comment:

Add Comment

Fig. 8. Details of a FAQ item.

Figure 8 shows the details of a particular FAQ item. It has to be noted that the button "Edit" is only visible for members who proposed the item and as long as its status is "open". Members are encouraged to add comments to items by completing the textbox "Comment" and pressing the button "Add Comment". This principle is followed for all other items within the Geoconda system. It helps members who proposed items to refine them and to make them more likely to be accepted by the committee of reviewers (see Section 2).

Figure 9 depicts the form, which allows the member who proposed the item to edit it. Changes are stored by pressing the button "Update". They are ignored, if the button "Cancel" is pressed. The field "Number" allows members to change the order of FAQ items within a category (items are ordered according to this number).

3.1.2. Positions

As in other organizations, the smooth functioning of the Geoconda community requires the existence of official positions that can be occupied by members of the Geoconda community. However, because the Geoconda system is a distributed rather than centralized organization, the positions have to be created dynamically by the Geoconda community. Hence, similar to other items, members can propose "position" items. These items are put forward in the same manner as FAQ items. They can have the status: "open", "accepted", and "rejected" and are subject to a review process (see Section 2). The fields of a position item are summarized in Table 3.

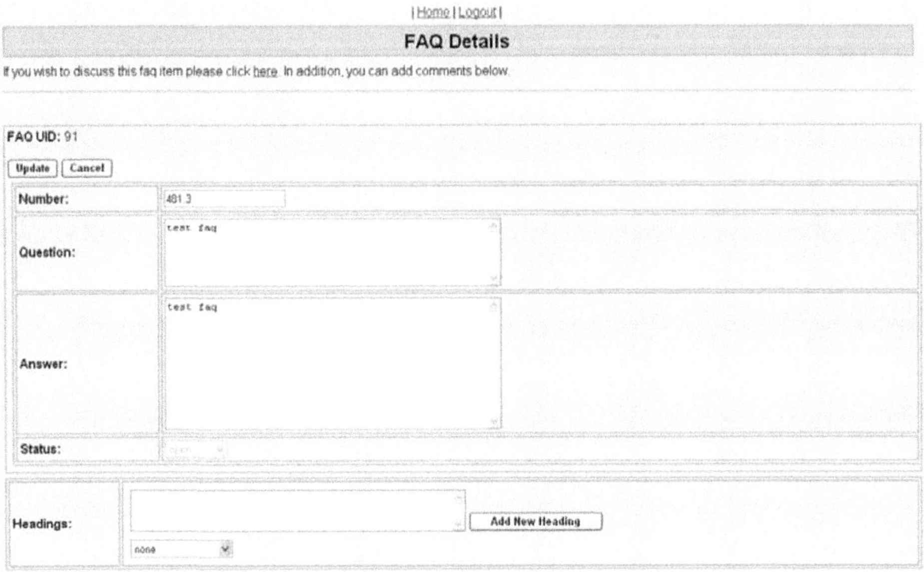

| Home | Logout |

FAQ Details

If you wish to discuss this faq item please click here. In addition, you can add comments below.

FAQ UID: 91

Update Cancel

Number: 481.3

Question: test faq

Answer: test faq

Status:

Headings: Add New Heading

none

Fig. 9. An FAQ item in the edit mode.

The member who proposed a position can edit the item, as long as its status is "open". Other members can also add comments to an item. This allows a somewhat democratic creation of positions within the Geoconda environment/organization (see also Section 2). Positions can be assigned to members by members with special rights as shown in Fig. 10.

A member is chosen from the top drop down list and a position from the bottom drop down list. The assignment is finalized by pressing the button "Add Officer" (members who occupy a position are referred to as officers).

3.1.3. Variables

As mentioned earlier, one of the main objectives of Geoconda is to allow the collection of data from several international institutions via the Internet. To facilitate this, the data

Table 3. Details of the position item

Field	Description
Position name	Name of the position.
Description	Further details about the position that could, for example, describe the duties of the member who occupies the position.
Max number members	Maximum number of members who could be assigned to this position. If the field is left empty, an unlimited number of could be assigned to the position.

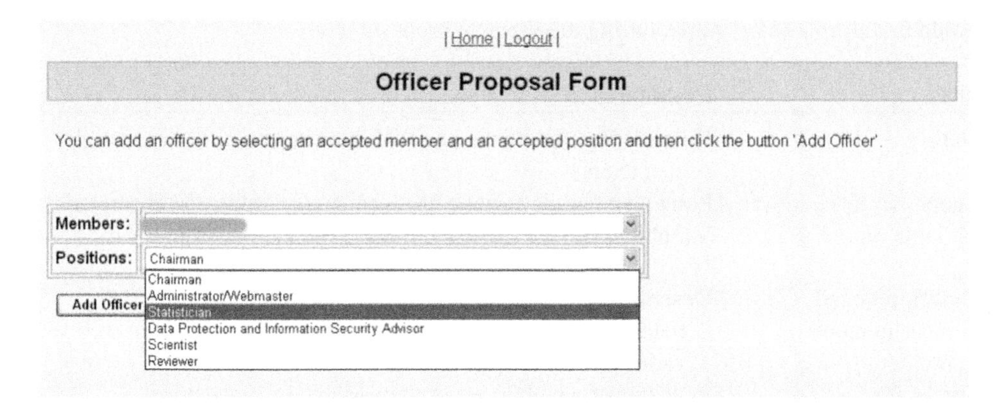

Fig. 10. Assigning a position to a member. The names of Geoconda members who are not authors of this chapter are hidden for privacy reasons.

collection process has to be standardized. This is necessary, for example, because different institutions might measure particular features using different scales. The standardization is achieved by variable items, which are proposed by members similar to other items. A member has to choose between six alternative variable types, which are summarized in Table 4.

Apart from specifying a variable type, the member must also provide the information summarized in Table 5. It has to be noted that some of the fields are only available for

Table 4. Possible variable types

Variable Type	Description
Nominal	This variable type can be used to model variables with a finite number of two or more unordered values. Hair colour is an example of a nominal variable. It could have the values: blonde, brown, brunette and red.
Ordinal	This variable type can be used to model variables with a finite number of two or more ordered values. The Likert scale is an example of an ordinal variable. It has the values: strongly disagree, disagree, neutral, agree and strongly agree. Please note that no distance is defined between the values of an ordinal variable.
Real	This variable type can be used to model variables with an (infinite) number of ordered values such as age, weight and blood pressure.
String	This variable type can be used to model variables, which correspond to strings such as general comments and postcodes.
Date	This variable type can be used to model variables, which correspond to dates such as the birth date of a patient.
File	This variable type enables members to add files, such as pictures and other arbitrary documents to a sample.

Table 5. Information required during the variable proposal

Field	Description
Name	Unique identifier of the variable that can contain at most eight characters.
Label	Long name of the variable that can contain up to 255 characters.
Variable type	Variable type (see Table 4). It has to be chosen from a dropdown list.
Description and measurement protocol	Description of how the variable is obtained/measured. This field might also contain further information about the variable.
Optional	Indicator of whether or not the variable is mandatory. A dropdown list provides a choice between "yes" and "no".
Unit	This information is only required for the variable type "real". It indicates the measurement unit of the variable.
Minimum number of decimal points	This information is only required for the variable type "real". It determines the precision of the measurement (minimum number of decimal points).
Minimum value	This information is only required for the variable type "real". It determines the smallest possible value.
Maximum value	This information is only required for the variable type "real". It determines the largest possible value.
Category values/category labels	This information is only required for the variable types "nominal" and "ordinal". It can be used to model concepts such as gender. Here the category value "1" might, for example, correspond to the category label "male" (see also table 6). It has to be noted that at least two category values/category labels have to be provided.

particular variable types. For example, it would not make sense to define a minimum value or measurement unit for a nominal variable.

If the variable type is "nominal" or "ordinal", the member has to propose at least two pairs of category values/category labels. A category value is a number, whereas the category label describes the "meaning" of this number in the form of a string. This allows the member to model concepts, such as gender shown in Table 6.

Table 6. Possible implementation of the nominal variable gender

Category Value	Category Label
0	Female
1	Male

| Home | Logout |

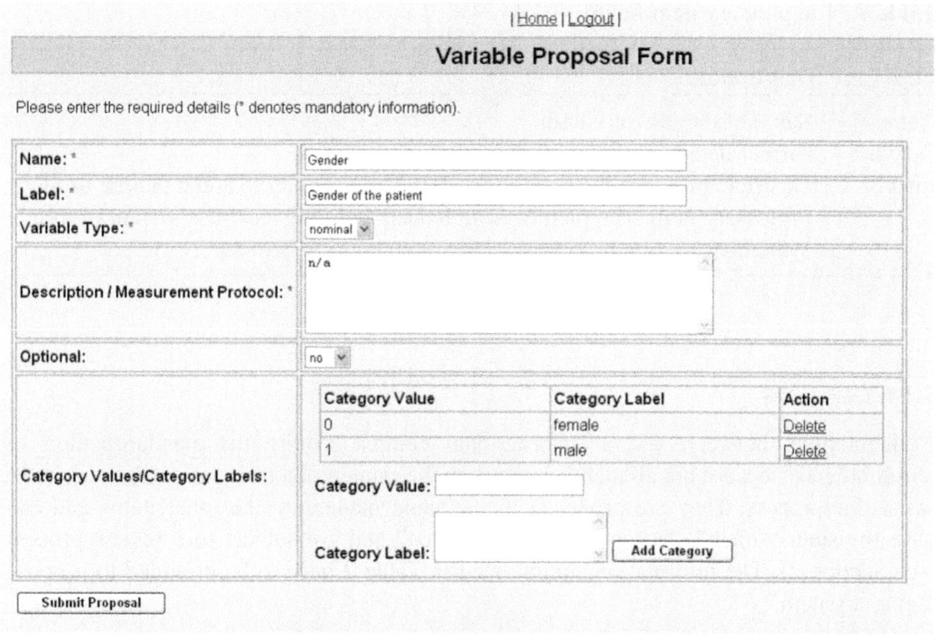

Variable Proposal Form

Please enter the required details (* denotes mandatory information).

Name: *	Gender
Label: *	Gender of the patient
Variable Type: *	nominal
Description / Measurement Protocol: *	n/a
Optional:	no
Category Values/Category Labels:	

Category Value	Category Label	Action
0	female	Delete
1	male	Delete

Category Value:

Category Label: Add Category

Submit Proposal

Fig. 11. Proposal form with the details of the gender variable.

The proposal of the nominal variable gender is illustrated using Fig. 11. The form already contains the category values/labels described in Table 6. They were added by completing the fields "Category Value"/ "Category Label" and then clicking on the button "Add Category". Categories can be removed by clicking on the hyperlink "Delete" beside them. The fields "Category Value"/"Category Label" are filled with the details of the category being deleted. This allows the member to edit the category and possibly add it again. It has to be noted that category values/labels are only accepted if they are unique.

The proposal of a variable takes place in the same manner as for other items. The item is submitted by clicking on the button "Submit Proposal". It can have the status: "open", "accepted", and "rejected" and undergoes a review process. Other members can also add comments. Members who proposed a variable item can edit it, as long as its status is "open". This allows members to refine the item and to incorporate the comments of other members. Hence, it increases the chance that the review committee will accept the variable and that the variable is actually used in multi-centre studies (see also Section 2).

All proposed variable items are listed in the variable section of Geoconda. It is possible to view the variables in chronological or alphabetical order. Furthermore, for practical reasons it is possible to restrict the number of shown variables according to their usage (i.e. the number of times the variable is used in a project) and their status.

Table 7. The glossary item fields

Field	Description
Name	Name of the glossary item.
Details	Further details of the glossary item.
Image	This field provides the member with the opportunity to add a picture to the glossary item. The picture is uploaded from the local file system of the member using a browsing facility (see button "Browse").

3.1.4. Glossaries

Collaborations between several international centres require the standardization of terminologies, because not all members work in the same problem domain. Glossary items assist this process. They are proposed in the same manner as the other items and can have the status "open", "accepted", and "rejected" and are subject to a review process (see Section 2). The information summarized in Table 7 have to be provided to propose a glossary item.

Members who propose glossary items can edit them as long as their status is "open". This allows members to incorporate comments from others, making the acceptance of the glossary item by the committee of reviewers more likely (see also Section 2).

3.1.5. Projects

To encourage international collaborations, members can propose project items. It has to be noted, however, that projects require the existence of accepted variables (each project must contain at least one accepted variable). Variables are assigned to a project during the proposal process. Members can also be assigned to a project. They are referred to as participants and can share project specific data with the member who proposed the project (after the project has been accepted). It has to be noted that each participant has the right to delete/edit his/her own data. Data can be shared as described in Section 3.2. A member who would like to propose a project has to provide the information summarized in Table 8.

Similar to other items, project items have the status "open" after their proposal and other members can add comments to them. Project items also undergo a review process after which their status is either changed to "accepted" or "rejected" (see Section 2). It has to be noted that the member who proposed a project can add new participants to the project, even if the project is already accepted. This makes the member who proposed the project more flexible to create additional collaborations to share data.

Members who propose project items can also transfer the "authorship" of the project to other members. Whoever owns the authorship can change the content of the project details as long as its status is "open". It has to be noted that the member with the authorship can pass it on to other members. However, the member who proposed the project can always recover the authorship by assigning it to himself/herself.

Table 8. Details of a project item

Field	Description
Short title	Unique short name for the project.
Full title	Title of the project that would appear in the published article.
Public	This field indicates whether or not the project is public. A dropdown list offers a choice between "yes" and "no". If "no" is chosen; only the member who proposed the project, the participants, and the current author can view the project details. If "yes" is chosen, everyone can view the project details.
Aims	Aims of the study as they would appear in the published article.
Background	Background information that would form the basis of any grant or ethical committee applications, patient information sheets, and the introduction of any published articles.
Patients	Inclusion/exclusion criteria for patients considered for enrolment in the study.
Material	Descriptions of any materials, such as pharmaceutical or other agents, which will be used in the project.
Methods	Description of the methods such as the examination and treatment techniques, statistical methods and follow-up protocols.
Main results	Main results of the study.
Discussion	Brief summary of the most important findings; the main strengths and weaknesses of the study, comparisons with other studies; scope for further work; clinical implications; and the conclusions.
Comments	Any comments relevant to the project, such as pending issues relevant for the successful completion of the project.
Ethical required, committee	Statement as to whether or not ethical committee approval is together with information on where specimen application forms, consent forms, patient information sheets can be obtained.
References	This field contains literature references relevant to the study.
Co-workers	Information about people who are involved in the design of the study, analysis of the results and/or writing of the manuscript.
Participants	The member who proposes a project can assign other members (participants) to the project. The participants can share the data submitted to the project. Each participant has the right to delete/edit his/her own data.
Variables	The member who proposes a project must assign at least one accepted variable to the project. Samples for this project will consist of these variables.

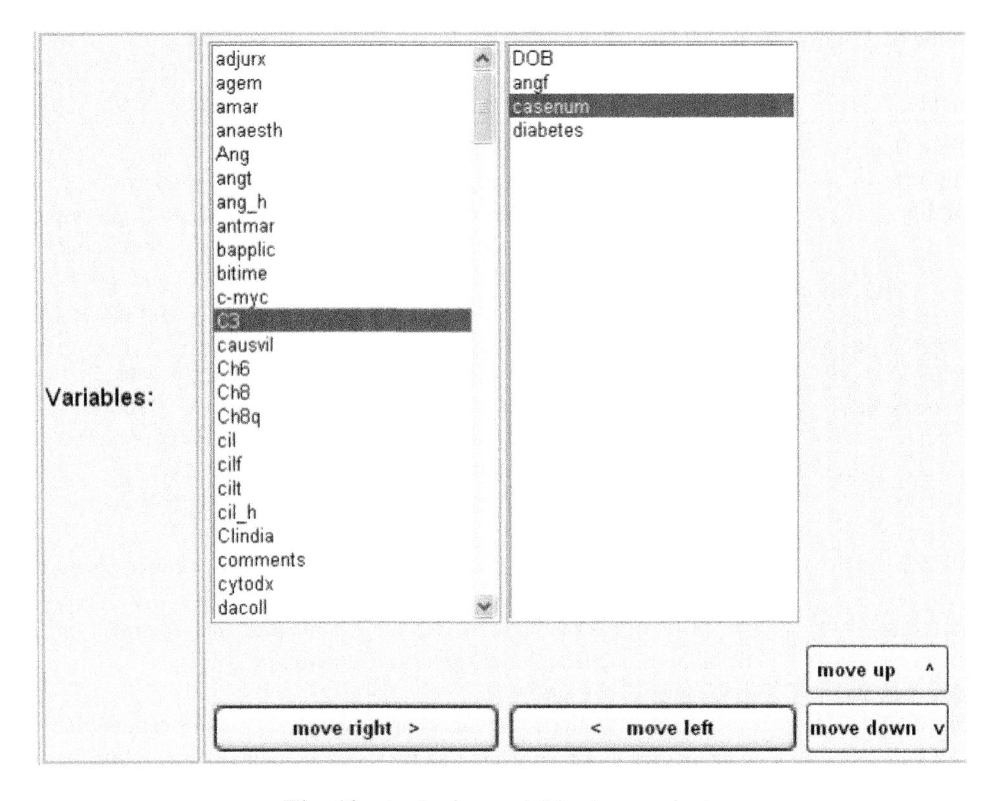

Fig. 12. Assigning variables to a project.

Variables can be assigned to a project as illustrated in Fig. 12. The left list shows all variables that were not assigned to the project in alphabetical order. A selected variable can be assigned to the project by pressing the button "move right". Variables appear in the right list in the order they have been assigned to the project. The order of the variables can be changed by selecting a variable and pressing the button "move up" and "move down". The proposed order is used to dynamically generate the online forms for the collection of data for this project. To impose a particular order of the variables can be beneficial, for example, in a clinical environment where the data are collected according to a semantic rather than an alphabetical order.

Accepted members can be assigned to the project as described for the variables. These members are referred to as participants.

3.1.6. Links

Link items enable members to make other members aware of other relevant and interesting web pages. They are proposed in a similar manner as other items. The member has to provide the information summarized in Table 9.

Table 9. Details of a link item

Field	Description
Name	Short name for the link that can contain at most 45 characters.
Link	Link to the actual website, which is also often referred to as URI (Uniform Resource Identifiers) or URL (Uniform Resource Locator).
Description	Short description of the referred web page.

Similar to all the other items, a link has the status “open” after its proposal. It also undergoes a review process, which is described in Section 2. Other members can also add comments to link items.

3.2. Data

To share and accumulate large amounts of data is the main objectives of the Geoconda system. Data consist of samples, which consist of values of variables that were assigned to a particular project. To ensure the smooth functioning of multi-centre data submission, particular rules for the submission of data were agreed on by the developers of the Geoconda system. For example, data can only be submitted to accepted projects. Furthermore, only the member who proposed a project and the participants of the project can submit/retrieve data to/from a project. Data can be submitted from files (located on the computer of the particular member) or manually via dynamically created forms (the forms contain entries for the variables that were assigned to the project). There are additional rules for the submission of data from files. Before these rules are detailed, the concept of the Local Unique Identifier (LUID) has to be introduced.

LUIDs are strings that are necessary to allow members to identify their samples after they were submitted to a particular project. As the name suggests, each LUID string has to be unique for all the samples a particular member submits to a project. The database itself assigns a Global Unique Identifier (GUID) to each sample. Both the LUID and the GUID allow the merging of data from different research centres/members without losing the information about the origin of a sample. Please note, however, that other members do not know the LUIDs of samples from other members to maintain confidentiality. The following list summarizes the rules for the submission of data from files.

- Datasets can only be submitted from files if the associated project does not contain variables of type “file”. If the project contains variables of type “file”, samples can only be submitted manually.
- Dataset columns can be delimitated by the characters “—”, “,”, or “;”. The particular delimiter is chosen from a dropdown list.
- The first row of a dataset file can only contain variable names associated with the project. The order of the variable names is not relevant and the number of variable names must not be complete. Missing variable values are left blank and can be edited later.

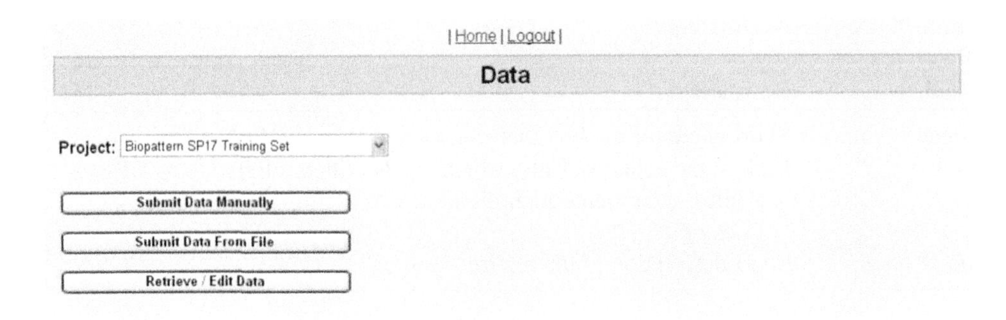

Fig. 13. First page of the data section.

- The first row of the dataset file must contain a LUID column. If it does not contain a LUID column, the dataset file is rejected.
- Each LUID variable value in the LUID column must be unique. Otherwise, the dataset is rejected.
- If a member resubmits samples from a file (samples with the same LUID value in the database) the original samples in the database are automatically overwritten without warning.
- Files can only contain variable names that are associated with the project. The dataset file is rejected if it contains unknown variable names.

Members can submit data to a project by clicking on the button "Data" shown in Fig. 2.

Figure 13 shows the first page of the data section. The dropdown box lists all the projects the member proposed or participates in (the Geoconda system knows the identity of the member after his/her login). Figure 13 also contains three buttons. The first two buttons allow you to submit data manually or from a file respectively. The third button allows the member to retrieve or edit data. It has to be noted that the button "Submit Data From File" only appears for projects that do not contain variables of type "file".

The retrieved data for the "test project" are shown in Fig. 14 and Fig. 15. They were obtained by clicking on the button "Retrieve/Edit Data". The member can either view his/her own data (see Fig. 14) or all project data which were submitted by all the participants of the project (see Fig. 15).

Members who proposed the project or its participants can also edit and delete their own samples and submit additional samples either manually or from a file. The member can retrieve the visible data by pressing the button "Send Visible Data As Email". Internally a comma delimited file containing the depicted data is assembled and send via email as attachment to the participant.

The manual submission of data is illustrated in Fig. 16. All variables associated with the project are shown in the order defined during the project proposal, apart from the LUID variable which is always at the top of the list. The chosen project contains variables of type file, which means that the members can upload files from their local file system. Files can be of any kind but their size is, for practical reasons, restricted to one mega byte. It is

| Home | Logout |
Data Retrieval For Project: test_project
Delete All Your Data
Submit Data From File
Submit Data Manually
Send Visible Data As Email
All Project Data Your Project Data
Database ID (GUID)
Your ID (LUID)
Gender
Edit
Delete
9514
x##91
1
Edit
Delete
9515
2
0

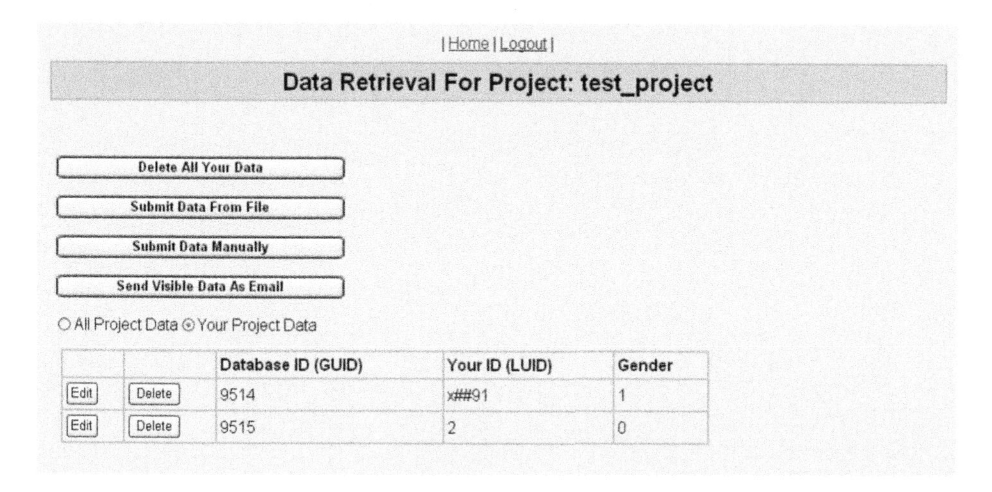

Fig. 14. Retrieved data for the "test project". This view only shows samples that were submitted by the member who is logged in.

important to note that the Geoconda system stores the file under a unique name and the original name is stored in the database.

Figure 17 illustrates the retrieval of data for a project that contains variables of type "file". Participants of a project can retrieve data by clicking on the button "Send Visible Data As Email". However, these data do not contain the files that were submitted to the project. To obtain the actual files, participants have to click on each file name individually.

| Home | Logout |
Data Retrieval For Project: test_project
Delete All Your Data
Submit Data From File
Submit Data Manually
Send Visible Data As Email
All Project Data Your Project Data
Database ID (GUID)
Submission Date
Last Update Date
Gender
9514
17/05/2005 10:25:03
17/05/2005 10:25:03
1
9515
17/05/2005 10:25:10
17/05/2005 10:25:10
0
9516
17/05/2005 10:27:20
17/05/2005 10:27:20
0
9517
17/05/2005 10:27:27
17/05/2005 10:27:27
1
9518
17/05/2005 10:27:46
17/05/2005 10:27:46
1

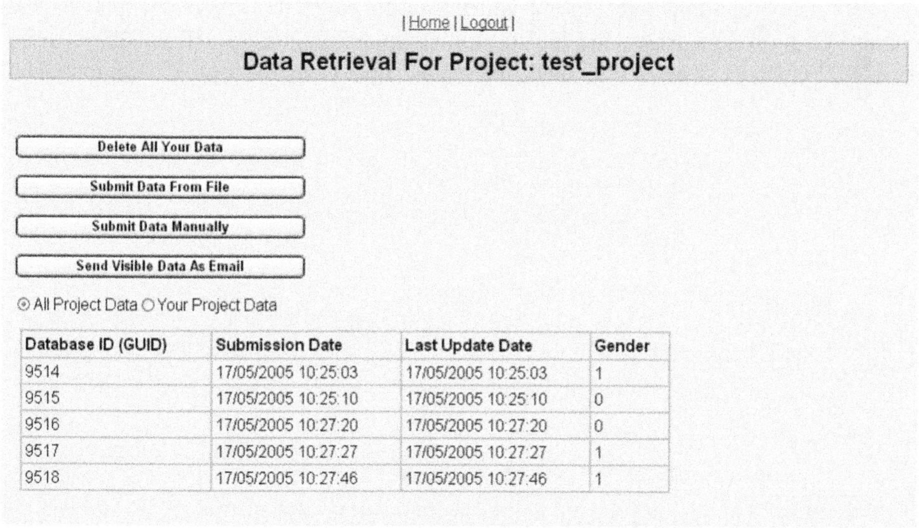

Fig. 15. Data for the "test project". The data consist of all samples that were submitted by all members who participate in the chosen project.

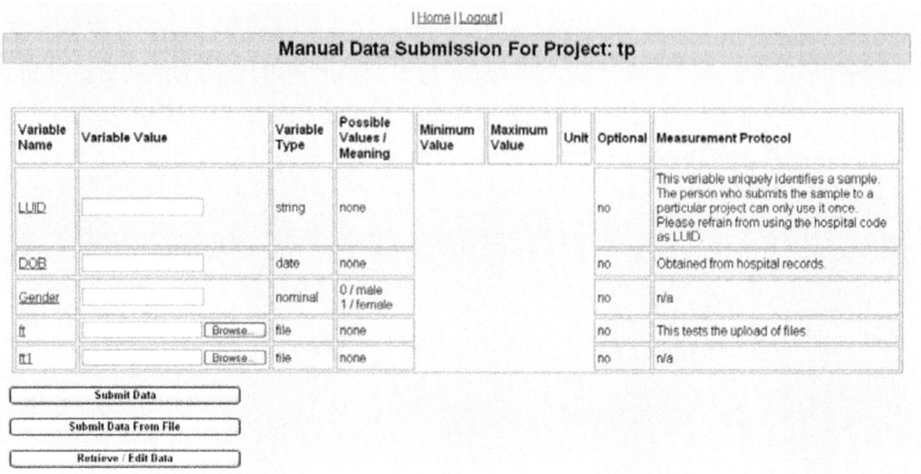

| Home | Logout |

Manual Data Submission For Project: tp

Variable Name	Variable Value	Variable Type	Possible Values / Meaning	Minimum Value	Maximum Value	Unit	Optional	Measurement Protocol
LUID		string	none				no	This variable uniquely identifies a sample. The person who submits the sample to a particular project can only use it once. Please refrain from using the hospital code as LUID.
DOB		date	none				no	Obtained from hospital records.
Gender		nominal	0 / male 1 / female				no	n/a
ft	Browse...	file	none				no	This tests the upload of files.
ft1	Browse...	file	none				no	n/a

Submit Data

Submit Data From File

Retrieve / Edit Data

Fig. 16. Manual submission of data to a chosen project that contains variables of type file.

The file name is shown as a hyperlink. An email is sent to the participant containing the file as attachment.

3.3. Online papers

Members can propose online papers, which can be edited by several people via the Internet. To propose a paper, the information summarized in Table 10 will have to be provided. Figure 18 shows a fraction of the online paper proposal form. Co-authors, who

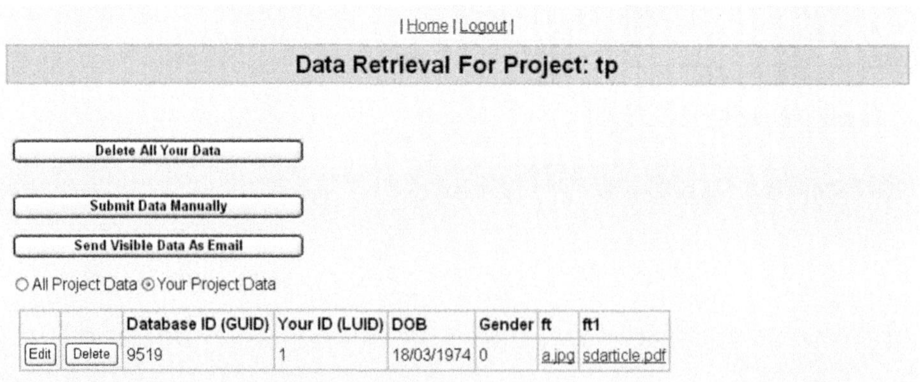

| Home | Logout |

Data Retrieval For Project: tp

Delete All Your Data

Submit Data Manually

Send Visible Data As Email

○ All Project Data ⊙ Your Project Data

		Database ID (GUID)	Your ID (LUID)	DOB	Gender	ft	ft1
Edit	Delete	9519	1	18/03/1974	0	a.jpg	sdarticle.pdf

Fig. 17. Data retrieval for a project that contains variables of type file.

Table 10. The online paper item fields

Field	Description
Title	The title of the online paper.
Public	This field indicates whether the paper is public (value "yes") or not (value "no"). If the paper is not public, only the member who proposed the paper and the co-authors can access its content. Otherwise, every member can view the content of the paper.
Abstract	The abstract of the paper.
Co-authors	A list of co-authors who can edit the paper together with the member who proposed the paper.

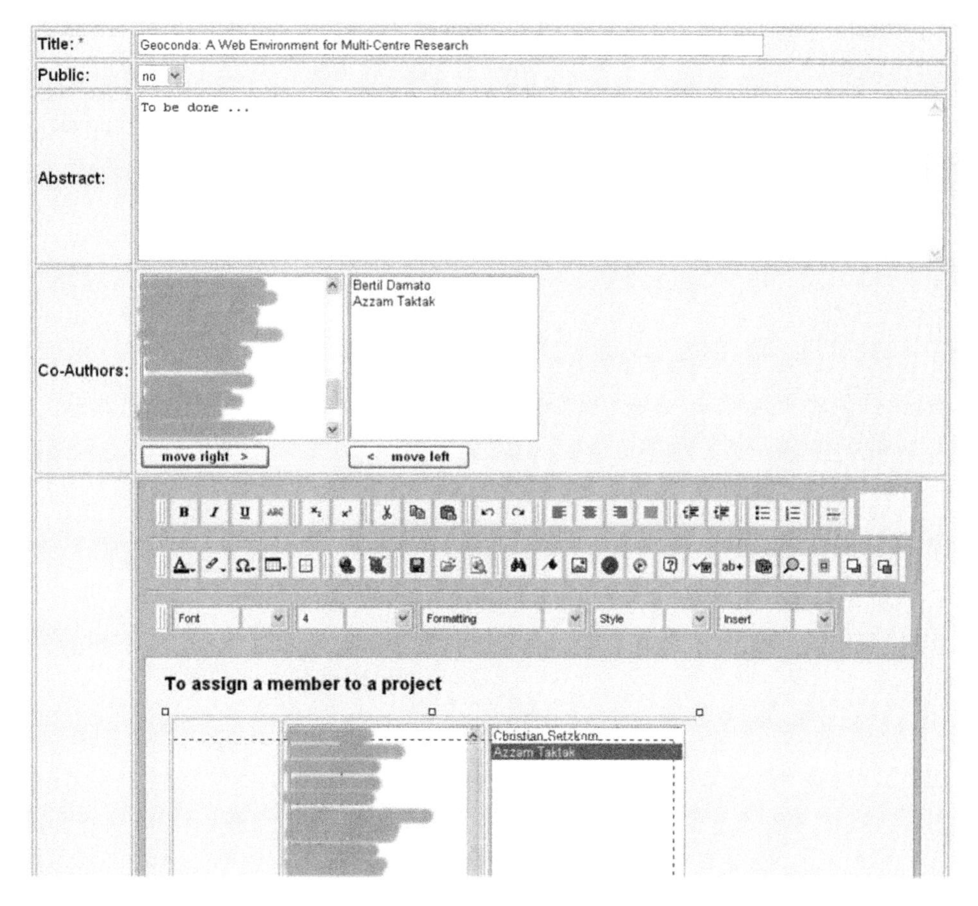

Fig. 18. Proposal of an online paper. The names of Geoconda members who are not authors of this chapter are hidden for privacy reasons.

can edit the paper later together with the member who proposed the paper, can be assigned to the paper by selecting a member from the list on the left-hand side and clicking the button "move right".

The content of the paper can be edited similar to a standard text editor. This enables one to, for example, format the text and create tables. In fact, the editor allows one to insert pictures and even animations.

It has to be noted that the online paper facility can cope with multi-user updates. This is important, as many people could try to change the same paper at the same time.

3.4. Discussion forums

The Geoconda system also contains several discussion forums, which were implemented using an existing tool called phpBB (which can be downloaded free from http://www.phpbb.com/.). The discussion forums allow members to exchange information on particular subjects in a very interactive manner. There are currently five forums as shown in Fig. 19.

Some of these forums are moderated and require members to register. This means that not everyone can submit/retrieve entries to/from a discussion forum. This ensures privacy, because confidential forums could be accessed from the Internet.

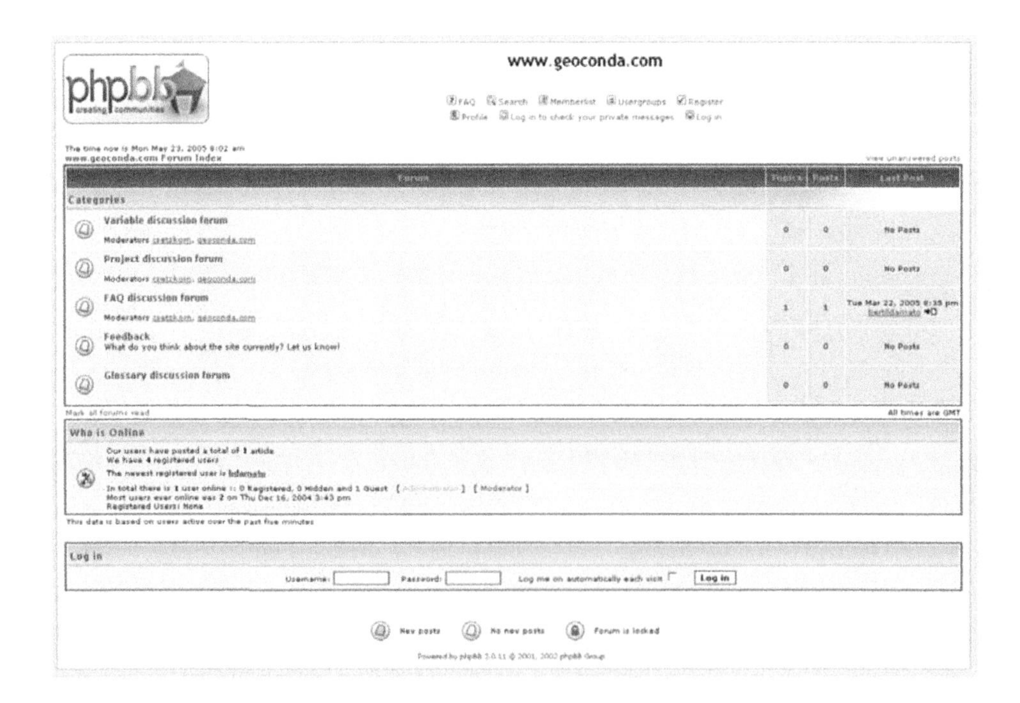

Fig. 19. The current discussion forums.

3.5. Mailing list

The Geoconda system also hosts a mailing list. The mailing list simplifies the communication between the members. In addition, it will help to broadcast news. It has to be noted that the mailing list is moderated. This means that not everyone can post messages, which decreases the likelihood of Spam e-mails.

4. DISCUSSION

Several requirements have to be fulfilled for successful multi-centre research. For example, all members must be able to communicate with each other in a free and convenient manner. All data must be collected and stored in a standardized manner. The data must be stored securely, respecting the confidentiality of both patients and project participants. There must be full compliance with all relevant regulations pertaining to matters such as data protection, human rights, and publication rights. The website we have created facilitates this.

An environment is provided for clinicians and scientists from different disciplines to communicate with each other, by means of e-mail (lists), comments, and discussion forums. Special measures were taken to enable each individual to obtain information on members, positions, regulations, variables, projects etc. quickly and conveniently.

The website is designed to be very dynamic to be responsive to the needs of the members. To enable continuous and efficient evolution, a variety of forms allow the proposal of new items, their discussion, amendment, and review by experts. Such transparency provides all members with a sense of ownership and collective responsibility.

Patient confidentiality is guaranteed by disallowing storage of hospital number, surnames, addresses, telephone number or any other personal details that would allow an individual to be identified. Practitioner/centre confidentiality is respected allowing project participants to identify only their own patients.

It is recognized that teams of researchers will wish to protect their intellectual property. Each project can therefore be classified as non-public, so that all details are only available to participants of that project. The chairperson and other officials do not have access to details regarding private studies.

Responsibility for compliance with national laws, local hospital regulations, and ethical committee requirements lies entirely with the member who proposed a project. The committee is unable to police all projects, particularly those that do not have public access. Consideration is being given to appointing a compliance officer, who would have access to all projects, public or private, to ensure that standards are maintained. It is also the responsibility of each project leader to organize validation and verification of data, selection of appropriate statistical methods, and prevention of fraud and plagiarism.

Using ASP.NET form authentication ensures the security of the Geoconda system. Each member has to use a password to log into the system. The passwords are stored in encrypted form in the database to ensure further security. The Internet service provider generates backups every day.

5. SUMMARY AND CONCLUSIONS

This chapter has introduced the Geoconda system, which uses a website and a relational database to facilitate international research collaborations. Table 11 provides some statistics of the website, which is online since December of 2004.

The Geoconda system is currently used for several international collaborations between four different countries: Greece, Italy, Netherlands and the United Kingdom. These projects evaluate different approaches for survival analysis and classification in a double-blind manner. Survival analysis is used to estimate the probability of survival following treatment of uveal melanoma. Estimating the probability of survival in cancer has a number of benefits. It allows clinicians to review their practice and advise their patients on the best course of treatment. It also allows patients to plan their lives and provide future care for their dependents.

There are numerous algorithms for estimating the probability of survival including the Kaplan–Meier non-parametric model, the proportional hazard model by Cox and Artificial Neural Networks (Kleinbaum, 1996; Taktak et al., 2003; Setzkorn et al., 2005). Although some researchers have conducted direct comparison between different models, as far as we are aware, none have conducted multi-centre studies on a common dataset.

6. FUTURE WORK

To provide the user with more flexibility and expressiveness in adding content to the Geoconda system, standard text boxes are currently replaced with so-called WYSIWYG entry fields (WYSIWYG stands for: "what you see is what you get"). Standard text boxes only allow users to submit fields that contain text. This is not very useful, if one would

Table 11. Current statistics of Geoconda

Item	Number of items	Number of accepted items	Further details
Officers	10	n/a	n/a
Positions	7	0	n/a
FAQs	52	0	n/a
Members	46	46	Members are from 13 different countries.
Variables	252	185	n/a
Glossary	70	6	n/a
Projects	19	10	n/a
Links	10	0	n/a
Samples	5863	n/a	n/a
Online Papers	1	0	n/a

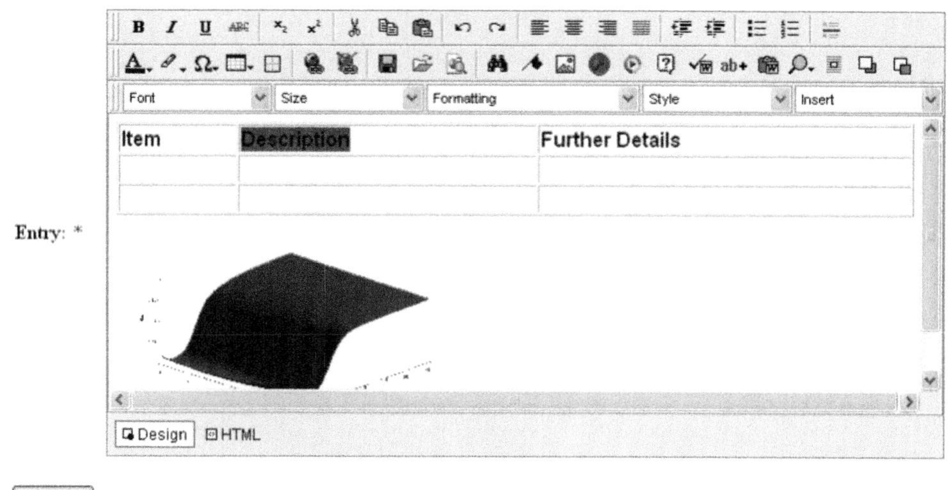

Fig. 20. A WYSIWYG (what you see is what you get) entry field.

like to submit more complex information (e.g. tables, pictures, animations). A WYSIWYG entry field is shown in Fig. 20. It contains several buttons, which allows the user to add, for example, tables and pictures. It also enables one to format the text similar to other well-known editors.

A WYSIWYG entry field is currently only used for the item "Online Papers" described in Section 3.1. However, it could also be very useful for items such as "glossaries", which could contain pictures and tables or variable definitions.

REFERENCES

Damato, B., 2005, Current management of uveal melanoma. Eur. J. Cancer Suppl., 3(3), 433–435.

Homer, A., D. Sussman, R. Howard, B. Francis, K. Watson and R. Anderson, 2004, Professional ASP.Net 1.1. Hungry Minds Inc., US.

Kleinbaum, D., 1996, Survival analysis: A self-learning text. Springer.

Setzkorn, C., A. Taktak and B. Damato, 2005, Survival analysis using a multi-objective evolutionary algorithm. In: Proceedings of the Second International Conference on Computational Intelligence in Medicine and Healthcare – CIMED 2005. pp. 224–230.

Taktak, A., A. Fisher and B. Damato, 2003, Modelling survival after treatment of intraocular melanoma using artificial neural networks and bayes theorem. Phys. Med. Biol., 49 (1), 87–98.

Chapter 16

The Development and Execution of Medical Prediction Models

Michael W. Kattan[1], Mithat Gönen[2] and Peter T. Scardino[3]

[1]*Department of Quantitative Health Sciences, The Cleveland Clinic Foundation, Cleveland, OH, USA*
Email: kattanm@ccf.org
[2]*Departments of Biostatistics and Epidemiology and*
Email: gonenm@msku.org
[3]*Urology, Memorial Sloan-Kettering Cancer Center, New York, NY, USA*
Email: scardinp@msku.org

Abstract

Multivariable regression models are firmly established as the standard method in medical literature for obtaining adjusted estimates and adjusted tests of association. Prediction of individual patient outcome is a different area than testing for associations.

The purpose of this chapter is to present the strategy, developed by others, which we use for building and implementing several regression-based prediction models. One of our software products is the most common prognostic tools in cancer for the personal digital assistant, according to a survey by the American Society of Clinical Oncology. One of the specific messages we will convey here is that building prediction models require a different strategy even though the statistical models are the same.

We will emphasize achieving high predictive accuracy as the goal rather than building a model with statistically significant factors. We will also review the importance of model validation and calibration as indispensable steps before finalizing a predictive model. Finally, we will focus on simple and effective communication of the results. The particular tool that we use for this purpose is the nomogram. This graphical depiction of a multivariable model has been used for a long time, but not as widely as one might expect given its advantages.

Finally, we will describe the software implementation for personal digital assistants and our web-based experience in distribution.

Keywords: Nomogram, prediction, software.

Contents

Outcome Prediction in Cancer
Edited by A.F.G. Taktak and A.C. Fisher
© 2007 Elsevier B.V. All rights reserved

1. INTRODUCTION

Many consider multivariable regression models to be the standard method in the medical literature to adjust for influential variables when computing estimates and testing associations. In fact, most retrospective analyses use a multivariable regression model following model selection. The statistically significant factors (e.g. $p < 0.05$) are usually called "independent" risk factors (Tseng, 2004).

An important goal in medical research is to determine the risk factors that have a substantial influence on patient outcome. These risk factors usually clarify the biology of the disease, trigger further research, and determine prognosis. They generally comprise a discrete risk score (e.g. the number of risk factors), resulting in rather crude predictions for the individual patient. Alternatively, the goal of a prediction model is to provide accurate patient-level predictions. A prediction model predicts far more accurately than does a list of independent prognostic factors (Spiegelhalter, 1986).

While we will tend to use these terms interchangeably, some authors make a distinction among risk, prediction and prognosis. Risk is often used to describe the calculation of a patient's probability of developing a condition, such as a particular form of cancer. Prognosis usually means the probability that a patient will do well assuming no treatment is administered. Prediction is sometimes reserved for the calculation of an outcome probability assuming a specific form of treatment is applied (e.g. surgery). However, because the modeling concepts are generally the same, we will use these terms interchangeably.

Predicting an individual patient outcome is different from testing for associations (Korn and Simon, 1990). For example, a statistically significant factor can be of limited use for predicting outcome (Healy, 1990). Kattan et al. (2003c) reported that the percent of biopsy cores that were positive, despite being statistically significant, had essentially no effect on the area under the receiver operating characteristic curve for the prediction of prostate cancer recurrence. The reason for this is that significance tests are sensitive to the sample size and the effect size, whereas prediction is a function of only the effect size. Statisticians have known this for quite some time and have developed several excellent prediction models (D'Agostino et al., 2001). In general, however, the medical literature has made little attempt to distinguish prediction from association. For example, when a test of association is significant, it is common to conclude that the significant variable is a "predictor" of outcome despite the fact that the factor is merely associated with the outcome.

Most adjusted tests of association utilize regression modeling. A predictive model is multidimensional also because patient outcome is complex and depends on multiple factors. As an alternative to regression, other methodologies exist for building prediction models such as tree-based methods, neural networks, and support vector machines. However, none of these methods is considered to be uniformly more accurate than other. In fact, regression models often predict at least as accurately. Schwarzer et al. (2000) and Sargent (2001) have carefully compared regression and machine learning methods and concluded that when fair comparisons were made, regression models performed just as well. We have found this also (Kattan, 2003a), and therefore limit our discussion to regression models only.

Prediction models are clearly needed for patient counseling, medical decision-making, and medical research in general. They provide the most accurate predictions and outperform clinical judgment (Ross et al., 2002), risk groups (Kattan, 2003b), or chance (See Fig. 1).

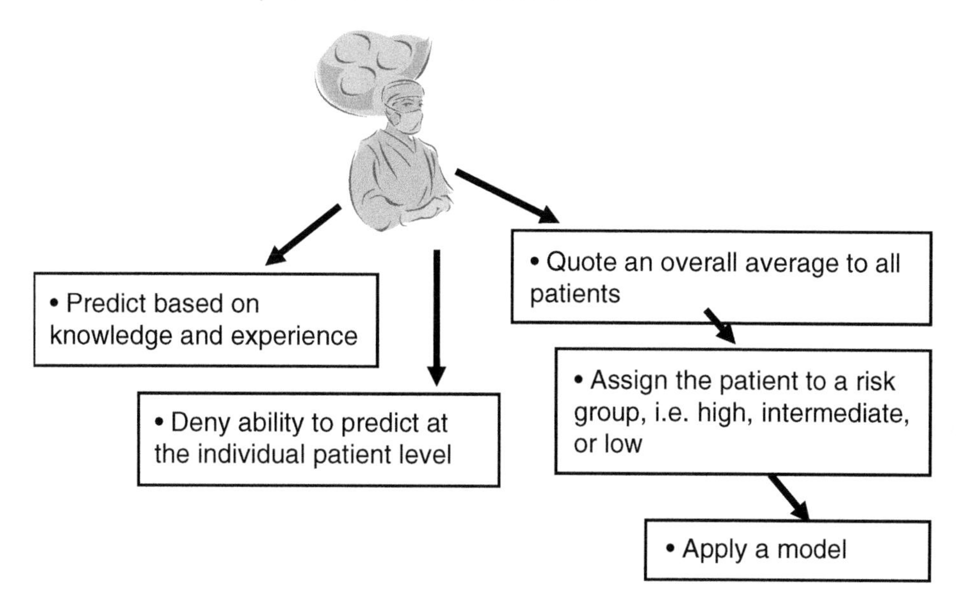

Fig. 1. Options for the patient who desires a prediction of outcome.

The purpose of this chapter is to present the strategy that we use for building and implementing regression-based prediction software. Using a survey by the American Society of Clinical Oncology survey, we have developed the most commonly used prognostic tool in cancer for the personal digital assistant (Blumberg, 2004). On the surface, constructing a regression model for testing associations may not differ from building a regression model for making predictions. However, the latter requires a different strategy. The goal here is high predictive accuracy, and not simply building a model with statistically significant factors. Illustrating and applying the model graphically is greatly facilitated by the use of a nomogram (Harrell, 2001). However, software implementation on personal digital assistants and the World Wide Web is preferable.

1.1. An example

For example, imagine that a clinician wants to predict the probability that a patient with soft tissue sarcoma will die of this (Kattan et al., 2003a). If likely, a novel therapy may be useful. Soft tissue sarcoma is rare. Only 8000 cases and 4000 deaths annually are due to this disease. About half of the patients who receive surgery alone relapse within a decade, and many who do will die of their disease. From July 1982 to May 2000, 2327 adult patients underwent surgery for primary soft tissue sarcoma at the Memorial Sloan-Kettering Cancer Center.

As of February 18, 2001, 355 of these patients had relapsed locally. These patients are typically very concerned about their risks of dying of sarcoma. In this setting, proportional hazards regression would be the default method for developing a prediction model.

2. METHODOLOGY

2.1. Variable selection

The decision regarding which variables to include in the prediction model should be based on the judgment of the physician and/or analyses of completely separate datasets (Harrell et al., 1996). The physician should rely on his or her knowledge base, training, and patient experience to form a mental model of variables believed to be predictive. In particular, decisions should not be made based on significance testing in the dataset to be modeled. No univariable screening or stepwise variable selection should be performed (Altman and Royston, 2000). Rather, the clinician should be asked to provide a list of variables he or she thinks, theoretically, should be prognostic and are commonly measured. Next, the clinician should be asked for a direction of effect. "Should the patient have a better or worse prognosis as some variable increases?" If the clinician cannot answer this question, this variable should be omitted because of insufficient evidence for a theoretical relationship between the variable and the outcome of interest. Univariable screening or selection of variables as further reduction of this list produces a prediction model that, on average, will be less accurate (Spiegelhalter, 1986). In particular, the coefficients of this smaller model would have large bias in absolute value. As long as the variables are routinely measured, they are retained. Thus, the p values of the predictors are irrelevant (Sterne, 2002). Maximally selected statistics do not follow the standard normal asymptotic theory, and therefore, a model based on univariate screening or stepwise selection and subsequently analysed using standard asymptotics will be biased (Miller and Siegmund, 1982).

2.2. Model fitting

Missing values often need imputation. However, if a variable is very widely missing, it should be omitted because it is not routinely available. Otherwise, multiple imputation methods should be used, whereby missing values are predicted based on the levels of other predictor variables using regression models. All imputation of predictor variable values is thus done without regard to the outcome. Then, the full model is fit to this imputed dataset, using restricted cubic splines (Ambler et al., 2002) with ordinal or higher level variables that have a sufficient number of unique levels. The splines often improve the predictive ability of the model by relaxing linearity assumptions. They are especially useful for uncovering non-monotone relationships that would be poorly modeled by linear forms. For example, both low and high levels of hemoglobin portends a high likelihood of post-operative complications in patients undergoing major liver surgery (Jarnagin et al., 2002). Occasionally, rare levels of categorical variables need to be combined with other levels, as theoretically appropriate. If the clinicians feel that such combinations would produce inconsistent groups, those patients should be excluded. The presumed benefit of simplicity, often cited as a reason for model reduction, largely disappears while assuming that the prediction model will be distributed in software.

2.3. Model assessment

Models should be assessed and compared for their discrimination and calibration (Harrell et al., 1996). Importantly, discrimination can be quantified on an interpretable scale (Begg et al., 2000), making it valuable for comparing new versus previous prediction models (Kattan et al., 2003c), classic staging systems (Kattan et al., 2003b), and human judgment (Ross et al., 2002), and judging whether improvement in prediction is really being made.

While it is important to compute discrimination, such as using the concordance index, such a measure is of limited use in isolation. To compute the concordance index, one first obtains predictions for each individual patient. Then, all possible pairs of patients are formed. However, analysis is restricted to those pairs of patients where the patient with the shorter follow-up time experiences the event of interest (i.e. fails). The concordance index is the proportion of pairs of patients where the prediction model predicts a worse outcome for the patient, who fails first. It is context dependent as to whether a model is useful, and the concordance index alone cannot provide all the necessary information for this evaluation. Some rules of thumb exist, such as a certain minimum concordance index, or area under the receiver operating characteristic curve, is necessary before the model may be used in clinical practice or for medical decision-making. However, it is very difficult to justify a cutoff. Misclassification costs need to be considered to make this decision, and those are difficult to specify. Furthermore, specification of a minimum cutoff tends to imply that the current approach for prediction, whatever that is, exceeds this cutoff. For example, if a prediction model is developed that has a concordance index of 0.58, some would say that is insufficient for clinical use, and that this model should be discarded. Presently, however, it could be that human judgment is responsible for the prediction, and that may be no better than chance. In this example, discarding the "insufficient" prediction model results in inferior prediction by human judgment. Therefore, the most useful place for calculating the discrimination of a model is for comparison with other models. One could compute predicted probabilities from both a prediction model and a staging system for each patient. The concordance indices for these rival models could be computed and compared in the same set of patients. To be fair, if the set of patients is not a true validation set, the predicted probabilities from the prediction model should be computed on a left-out basis (e.g. jackknife or cross-validated). Assuming misclassification costs are equal, one should prefer the prediction method with the higher discrimination, all else being equal, regardless of the actual value. Figure 2 displays the concordance indices of various models we have developed and offer in software.

The fundamental weakness of discrimination is that it does not reflect absolute predictive accuracy, but only ranking. Calibration, on the other hand, helps to illustrate graphically the predicted versus observed accuracy of the prediction model and complements

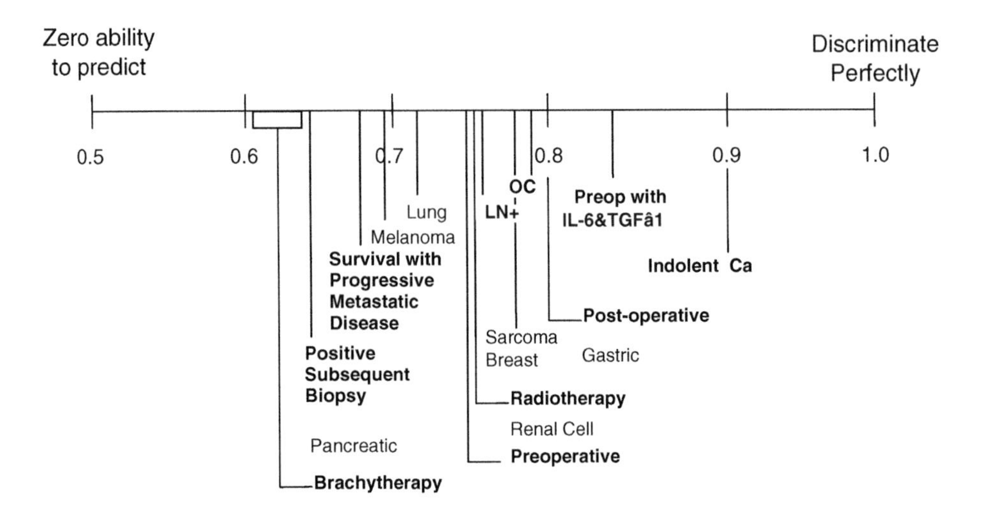

Fig. 2. Levels of discrimination for some prediction tools. Models in bold are prostate cancer related.

discrimination (Harrell, 2001). This determination is more critical than discrimination but not easily quantified. Instead, the calibration plot provides a visual interpretation of the model's performance, but does not lend itself to a hard and fast decision rule. There are two obvious exceptions. First, if calibration were really poor, one might dismiss the prediction model entirely, despite whether it had acceptable discrimination. The formation of such a decision rule, however, is difficult, because the calibration assessment is visual. Second, in the presence of acceptable discrimination, the calibration plot can help to adjust the predictions from the model when calibration is in error. In other words, the calibration plot may reveal that some or all of the predictions could be helped by adjusting them, as we have done with one of our models (Koh et al., 2003). This is especially attractive when using software, as the tedious calibration adjustment can be performed automatically by the software.

Both discrimination and calibration need to be carried out in an overfit-corrected fashion (van Houwelingen and le Cessie, 1990). If a validation dataset is not available, some sort of cross-validation or bootstrapping method is necessary. Bootstrapping offers the advantage (Altman and Royston, 2000) of validating the actual prediction model, rather than a prediction model development process. With the bootstrapping approach (Harrell, 2001), one first calculates the apparent concordance index of the full model using the entire dataset. This value will be optimistic. A sample of the same size is drawn with replacement. A model is fit to this new sample, and the concordance index is measured. The original dataset is also used to measure the concordance index of this new model. Optimism is defined as the difference between these last two concordance indices. After repeating this process 200 times, the mean optimism is subtracted from the original value, to obtain a bootstrap-corrected concordance index.

2.4. Model validation

It is easy to declare that external validation is the gold standard of prediction model. Similarly, it is easy to say that a prediction model should not be used until it has been externally validated. However, such a view essentially places very high costs on the use of a bad prediction model, and very low value on the benefits of using a truly better prediction model. At the expense of this strategy is the potential to benefit patients immediately, if indeed the prediction model works better. It can be an ethical challenge to choose between the older, more trusted prediction model and the newer one that appears to predict better, yet has not been as extensively validated. Furthermore, one could argue that a single validation dataset does not comprise validation, in that a future validation dataset may provide findings, which contradict that of the first validation dataset. In this sense, true validation can never be achieved, only disproven. In some cases, we have chosen to provide software prediction models when validation datasets were not available. In the case of soft tissue sarcoma (Kattan et al., 2002), validation datasets were requested, but not supplied, and because this is a very rare form of cancer, we felt release of the prediction model would do more good than harm. Recently, a validation dataset was provided, and our concordance index and calibration appeared to be similar to that reported from bootstrapping (Eilber et al., 2004). In another example, a gastric cancer model (Kattan et al., 2003b) had no validation dataset, yet in our data, it appeared to predict better than did the present method in place, a staging system. We chose to release the prediction model despite lacking a validation dataset. Recently, validation data were made available, and although the discrimination index of our model shrank a little on the validation dataset, it remained superior to that of the staging system (Peeters et al., 2005). Thus, in these instances we were potentially not premature in the release of the software. In each of the examples above, the development datasets were quite large, each comprising more than thousand patients. Certainly, one would tend to be more cautious with models developed from smaller datasets.

Therefore, rigorous same-sample validation is required before the release of a prediction model for public use, but external validation is not necessary but it should still be performed. Ultimately, users vote with their feet, and more extensive validation raises the comfort level that a clinician has with a predictive model. Thus, our philosophy is that the fundamental requirement prior to the use of a prediction model is rigorous, same-set comparisons of discrimination against the existing prediction tool. A new prediction model should have a greater concordance index. Beyond this, clinicians have to decide for themselves how compelling the evidence is in favor of the new prediction tool.

To assess the accuracy of our sarcoma prediction model, we generated predicted probabilities for each case by leaving it out of the dataset, refitting the model on the $N-1$ patients, and predicting the probability of failure for the left-out case. This is comparable to the asymptotic jackknife given the size of the sarcoma dataset. Quartiles were then formed from the predicted probability of failure for each year. Subjects within each quartile were used to compute the marginal cumulative incidence of failure by that year and the mean predicted conditional probability of failure by that year (Kalbfleisch and Prentice, 1980). The concordance index, based on these jackknifed predicted probabilities, was 0.73. The calibration plot was generated to compare the mean predicted conditional probabilities to the non-model-based marginal cumulative incidence probability within each quartile and

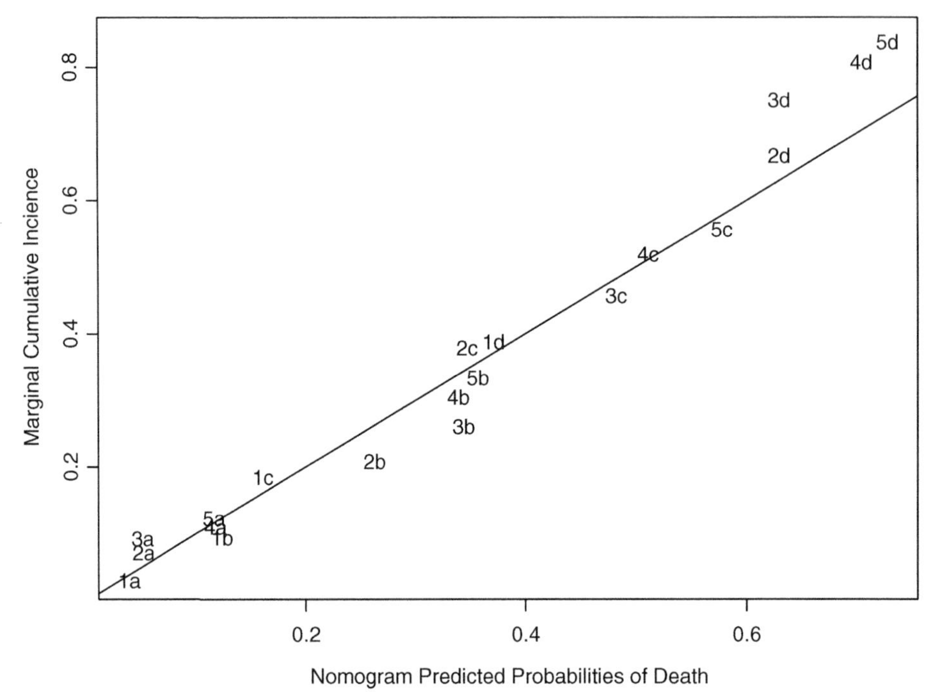

(*X* axis is mean predicted probabilities of the conditional cumulative incidence model. *Y* axis is the marginal cumulative incidence probability for the respective cohort. Plotting symbol is year of prediction (numeric) combined with quartile (a letter). For example, point "2c" is the 3rd quartile of the 2-year nomogram predictions. Solid line represents equality between predicted (conditional cumulative incidence from nomogram) and observed marginal cumulative incidence. Reprinted with permission from Kattan et al. (2003a)).

Fig. 3. Calibration plot.

shown in Fig. 3. A perfectly accurate nomogram prediction model would result in a plot where the marginal/conditional probability pairs would fall along the 45° line through the origin.

3. NOMOGRAM

Implementation is a key obstacle in using statistical prediction models at the bedside. It is impractical to obtain a patient's predicted probability by having a clinician execute a statistical package routine. An attractive, paper-based implementation method is the nomogram. This is a graphical device which implements a regression model in a friendly manner, enabling the user to relate the subject-specific covariates to the probability of an event. The first nomogram has been attributed to Professor Maurice d'Ocagne in 1989 (Banks, 1985). However, among the first medical applications was an acute myocardial infarction nomogram by Lubsen et al. (1978). Nomograms are particularly attractive when models contain continuous predictors. Most alternatives to the nomogram, such as tables, require categorization of continuous variables, and as such, serve to estimate the continuous functions, rather than graphically illustrate them. This reduces predictive accuracy.

The nomogram for computing the probability that an individual patient will die from sarcoma is shown in Fig. 4. The mechanics of this tool are as follows. The user determines the patient-specific index. This is accomplished by calculating how many points the patient receives for values of each of his prognostic factors, and summing these to arrive at his total points. The total points can then be used to determine the patient's probability of death from sarcoma.

4. SOFTWARE

For paper-based implementation of a prediction model, the nomogram has clear advantages. It provides an intuitive display of the model, nicely illustrating the effects of the predictors. Its graphical nature appears to preserve accuracy, relative to simpler to use point-based tables. Nonetheless, drawing lines is the trade-off, relative to tables. If paper-based

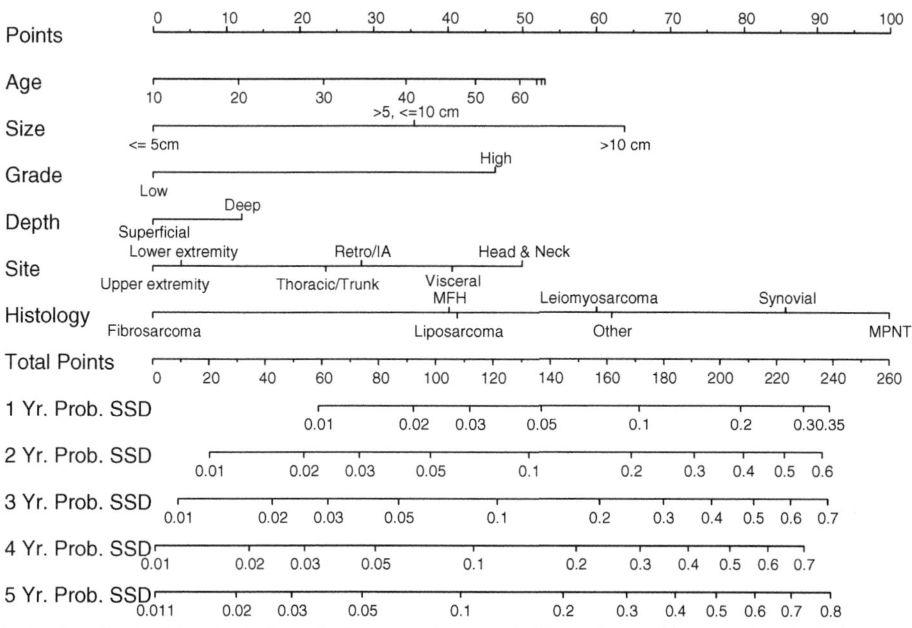

Instructions for physician: locate the patient's age on the age axis. Draw a line straight upwards to the **Points** axis to determine how many points towards sarcoma-specific death the patient receives for his age. Repeat this process for the other axes, each time drawing a line straight upward to the **Points** axis. Sum the points achieved for each predictor and locate this sum on the **Total Points** axis. Draw a line straight down to find the patient's probability of dying from sarcoma each year within 5 years.
Instruction to Patient: "If we had 100 patients exactly like you, we would expect <predicted percentage from nomogram> to die of sarcoma within *X* years."
(Abbreviations: MFH – malignant fibrous histiocytoma, MPNT – malignant peripheral-nerve tumour, SSD – sarcoma-specific death. Age is age at time of primary surgery. Size refers to primary tumour. Note that comorbidities should be taken into account.)

Fig. 4. Nomogram for probability of death from sarcoma following local recurrence in the presence of competing risks. Reprinted with permission from Kattan et al. (2003a).

implementation is not a requirement, software is clearly a preferred method. One can easily code the regression model in software for handheld or desktop computers, as we have done with nearly all our prediction tools (freely downloadable from www.nomograms.org, see Fig. 5).

We have tried many platforms for model implementation. Initially, the desktop software versions were created in Microsoft Access, and the handheld versions in Codewarrior for the Palm operating system and Embedded Visual C++ for Pocket PC versions. The desktop applications were later rewritten using Macromedia Flash. This was done for cosmetic reasons and to allow the nomograms to be directly integrated into a website for online use, in addition to remaining downloadable. Also, the Macromedia implementation only required that the user had the free, small, Flash plug-in for his or her web browser, rather than having the full commercial Microsoft Access software package. Visual Basic (VB) later replaced C/C++ as the language for model implementation on the handheld units. The AppForge MobileVB product was chosen because its implementation of VB for handhelds allowed the same code for both Palm OS and Pocket PC devices. This, combined with the much greater simplicity of the VB language compared to C/C++, meant that development time required for the handheld applications was greatly reduced. With AppForge, however, the user is required to install a free AppForge Booster run-time programme. This is problematic for some older Palm devices (OS 1-4.x) because the Booster can take up a large portion of memory (about 1 MB). Furthermore, the AppForge Mobile VB applications run much slower than the previous C/C++ versions. This has led us to consider some alternatives. First, we examined the very inexpensive PDAToolbox development platform, but found that it did not allow any programming and was totally form based, which greatly limited the features we could include. Next, we examined NSBasic, which is also a very inexpensive and simpler implementation of VB but lacked many of AppForge's advanced programming features, actually making it substantially harder and more complex to programme. Furthermore, different codes would be required for the Palm OS and Pocket PC versions.

To date, over 15 000 downloads of our software have been registered, and the prostate cancer tool was named in an ASCO survey as the most frequently mentioned handheld prognostic tool (Blumberg, 2004). Table 1 presents download statistics by model and by platform.

It is widely accepted that regression models provide more accurate predictions than discrete risk scores and tabular point systems. The latter methods seem to have prevailed based on their simplicity in use. However, our efforts to make prediction models available on PDAs and desktop computers have made them as accessible as any other prediction model. The popularity of these tools attests to their usefulness for the clinicians and the patients.

Prediction models will prove to be even more useful as targeted patient management philosophies gain ground. In colorectal cancer, for example, the number of therapeutic options increased exponentially over the past few years with no one option dominating the other in terms of efficacy. Therefore, the search for identifying patients who are more likely to respond to a given therapy (or similarly who are likely to fail a given therapy) is becoming widely important. Similarly, as genomic data becomes widely available, it is likely to contribute substantially to patient selection (Stephenson and Kattan, 2004). However, evidence would suggest we are not quite there yet. From Stephenson et al. (2005), we developed prediction models from gene expression data and compared their

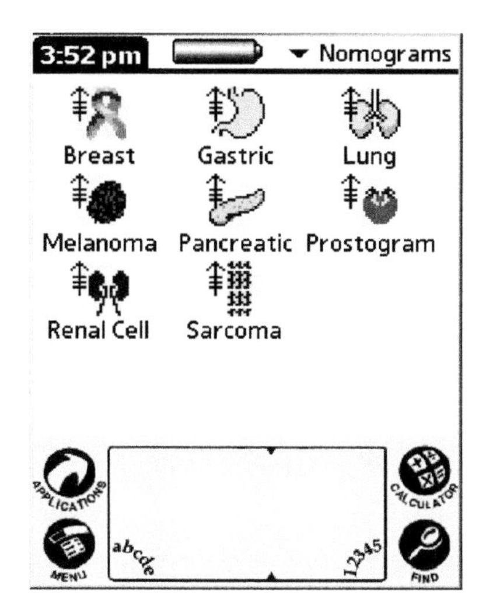

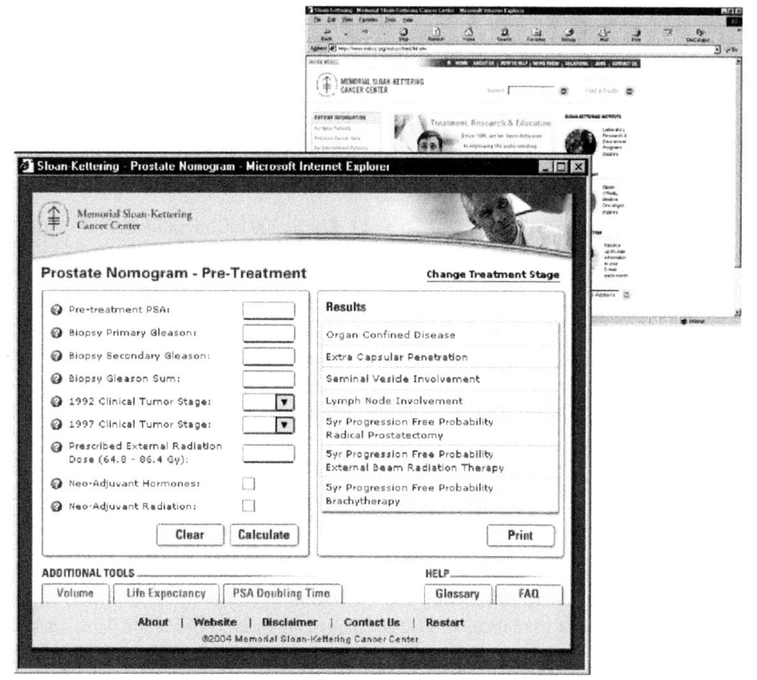

Fig. 5. Screenshots of software available from www.nomograms.org.

performance to that of an established nomogram. on data with the nomogram proved even better than either alone. The challenge with data like this is the difficulty in accommodating the complexity of the gene expression data. We chose to build stepwise models, which is clearly suboptimal. Other approaches may be performed more accurately. One can envision that prediction models have a central role to play in these efforts.

Table 1. Downloads by platform and type of cancer

	N	%
By platform:		
Palm	6780	44
Pocket PC	1744	11
Desktop	6984	45
By cancer:		
Breast	1053	7
Gastric	610	4
Lung	1142	7
Prostate	7168	46
Renal cell	3179	20
Sarcoma	2356	15

REFERENCES

Altman, D.G. and P. Royston, 2000, What do we mean by validating a prognostic model? Stat. Med., 19, 453–473.

Ambler, G., A.R. Brady and P. Royston, 2002, Simplifying a prognostic model: a simulation study based on clinical data. Stat. Med., 21, 3803–3822.

Banks, J., 1985, Nomograms. Wiley, New York.

Begg, C.B., L.D. Cramer, E.S. Venkatraman and J. Rosai, 2000, Comparing tumor staging and grading systems: a case study and a review of the issues, using thymoma as a model. Stat. Med., 19, 1997–2014.

Blumberg, J.W., 2004, PDA applications for physicians. ASCO Technology News, 4–6.

D'Agostino, R.B., S. Grundy Sr., L.M. Sullivan and P. Wilson, 2001, Validation of the Framingham coronary heart disease prediction scores: results of a multiple ethnic groups investigation. JAMA, 286, 180–187.

Eilber, F., M. Brennan, F. Eilber, W. Dry, S. Singer and M. Kattan, 2004, Validation of the postoperative nomogram for 12-year sarcoma-specific mortality. Cancer, 101, 2270–2275.

Harrell Jr., F.E., 2001, Regression Modeling Strategies with Applications to Linear Models, Logistic Regression, and Survival Analysis. Springer-Verlag, New York.

Harrell Jr., F.E., K.L. Lee and D.B. Mark, 1996, Multivariable prognostic models: issues in developing models, evaluating assumptions and adequacy, and measuring and reducing errors. Stat. Med., 15, 361–387.

Healy, M.J.R., 1990, Measuring importance. Stat. Med., 9, 633–637.

Jarnagin, W.R., M. Gonen, Y. Fong, R.P. Dematteo, L. Ben-Porat, S. Little, C. Corvera, S. Weber and L.H. Blumgart, 2002, Improvement in perioperative outcome after hepatic resection: analysis of 1,803 consecutive cases over the past decade. Ann. Surg., 236, 397–406.

Kalbfleisch, J.D. and R.L. Prentice, 1980, The Statistical Analysis of Failure Time Data. John Wiley and Sons, New York.

Kattan, M.W., 2003a, Comparison of Cox regression with other methods for determining prediction models and nomograms. J. Urol., 170, S6–S10.

Kattan, M.W., 2003b, Nomograms are superior to staging and risk grouping systems for identifying high-risk patients: preoperative application in prostate cancer. Curr. Opin. Urol., 13, 111–116.

Kattan, M.W., D.H.Y. Leung and M.F. Brennan, 2002, A postoperative nomogram for 12-year sarcoma-specific death. J. Clin. Oncol., 20, 791–796.

Kattan, M.W., G. Heller and M.F. Brennan, 2003a, A competing-risks nomogram for sarcoma-specific death following local recurrence. Stat. Med., 22, 3515–3525.

Kattan, M.W., M.S. Karpeh, M. Mazumdar and M.F. Brennan, 2003b, Postoperative nomogram for disease-specific survival after an R0 resection for gastric carcinoma. J. Clin. Oncol., 21, 3647–3650.

Kattan, M.W., S. Shariat, B. Andrews, K. Zhu, E. Canto, K. Matsumoto, M. Muramoto, P. Scardino, M. Ohori, T.M. Wheeler and K.M. Slawin, 2003c, The addition of interleukin-6 soluble receptor and transforming growth factor $beta_1$ improves a preoperative nomogram for predicting biochemical progression in patients with clinically localized prostate cancer. J. Clin. Oncol., 21, 3573–3579.

Koh, H., M.W. Kattan, P.T. Scardino, K. Suyama, N. Maru, K.M. Slawin, T.M. Wheeler and M. Ohori, 2003, A nomogram to predict seminal vesicle invasion by the extent and location of cancer in systematic biopsy results. J. Urol., 170, 1203–1208.

Korn, E.L. and R. Simon, 1990, Measures of explained variation for survival data. Stat. Med., 9, 487–503.

Lubsen, J., J. Pool and E. van Der Does, 1978, A practical device for the application of a diagnostic or prognostic function. Methods Inf. Med., 17, 127–129.

Miller, R. and D. Siegmund, 1982, Maximally selected Chi square statistics. Biometrics, 38, 1011–1016.

Peeters, K., M. Kattan, H. Hartgrink, E. Kranebard, M. Karpeh, M. Brennan and C. van de Velde, 2005, International validation of nomogram for predicting disease-specific survival following a RO resection for gastric cancer. Cancer, in press.

Ross, P.L., C. Gerigk, M. Gonen, O. Yossepowitch, I. Cagiannos, P.C. Sogani, P. Scardino and M.W. Kattan, 2002, Comparisons of nomograms and urologists' predictions in prostate cancer. Semin. Urol. Oncol., 20, 82–88.

Sargent, D.J., 2001, Comparison of artificial neural networks with other statistical approaches: results from medical data sets. Cancer, 91, 1636–1642.

Schwarzer, G., W. Vach and M. Schumacher, 2000, On the misuses of artificial neural networks for prognostic and diagnostic classification in oncology. Stat. Med., 19, 541–561.

Spiegelhalter, D.J., 1986, Probabilistic prediction in patient management and clinical trials. Stat. Med., 5, 421–433.

Stephenson, A.J. and M.W. Kattan, 2004, Stratification of risk for disease progression following initial therapy for prostate cancer: nomograms do it better. New Urology: Prostate Cancer, 1, 1–9.

Stephenson, A., A. Smith, M. Kattan, J. Satagopan, V. Reuter, P. Scardino and W. Gerald, 2005, Integration of gene expression profiling and clinical variables to predict prostate carcinoma recurrence after radical prostatectomy. Cancer, 104, 290–298.

Sterne, J.A., 2002, Teaching hypothesis tests – time for significant change? Stat. Med., 21, 985–994.

Tseng, C.H., 2004, Lipoprotein (a) is an independent risk factor for peripheral arterial disease in Chinese type 2 diabetic patients in Taiwan. Diabetes Care, 27, 517–521.

van Houwelingen, J.C. and S. Le Cessie, 1990, Predictive value of statistical models. Stat. Med., 9, 1303–1325.

Subject Index

Printed and bound by CPI Group (UK) Ltd, Croydon, CR0 4YY
08/05/2025
01865009-0002